Medical Immunology

Medical Immunology

Malcolm S. Thaler, M.D.
Duke University School of Medicine
Durham, North Carolina

Richard D. Klausner, M.D.
Duke University School of Medicine
Durham, North Carolina

Harvey Jay Cohen, M.D.
Chief, Medical Service
Veterans Administration Hospital;
Associate Professor of Medicine
Duke University School of Medicine
Durham, North Carolina

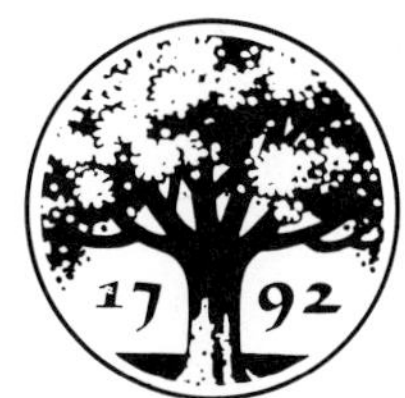

J. B. Lippincott Company
Philadelphia Toronto

ISBN 0-397-52081-6
Library of Congress Catalog Card Number 77-3656

Library of Congress Cataloging in Publication Data

Thaler, Malcolm S
Medical Immunology.

Includes bibliographical references and index.
1. Immunology. 2. Immunopathology.
I. Klausner, Richard D., joint author. II. Cohen,
Harvey Jay, joint author. III. Title.
QR181.T45 616.07'9 77-3656
ISBN 0-397-52081-6

Printed in the United States of America

1 3 5 6 4 2

Preface

Our experience with a short course in immunology for first-year medical students offered at the Duke University Medical Center left us with a sense of dismay at the complexities of the cellular and molecular events that together comprise the immune response and, at the same time, conveyed an appreciation for the vast implications that this relatively young science has for the practice of clinical medicine. These feelings, at first only somewhat discomforting, gradually crystallized into a desire to understand as fully as possible this rapidly expanding field that seemed to offer unique insights into many disease processes that previously had remained enigmas. This book is the result of our inquiries.

We have attempted to write the very book that we would have liked to have had available when we were first exposed to immunology in all its many forms and faces. To this end we have tried to remain faithful to certain principles that we believe are necessary for a clear, simple, yet comprehensive approach to the subject: We have tried to expand as completely as possible upon the basic scientific aspects of immunology while emphasizing the relevance of this material to clinical medicine. We have emphasized experimental studies in humans wherever possible, and, when animal models have been relied upon, have tried to make clear which systems are under discussion. The introductory chapter was designed with the hope of providing an overview of the cellular and molecular events of the immune system and their functions, in order to provide a framework for the more detailed discussion to follow.

Finally, we have tried to avoid creating a catalog of all phenomena and diagnoses and instead have tried to focus on the application of immune principles in those situations where their importance and behavior has been most carefully studied.

We hope that we have succeeded in some measure in these attempts and that this text will arouse the curiosity of those who will themselves some day become a part of this rapidly expanding field as physicians or researchers as well as those who wish simply to share in one of the great adventures of human thought.

MALCOLM S. THALER
RICHARD D. KLAUSNER
HARVEY JAY COHEN

Acknowledgments

We wish to thank the many people who contributed so much to the writing of this book. In particular, we want to thank several persons whose input and support were of crucial importance to us. We would like to express our appreciation to Dr. Wendell Rosse, whose knowledge and insight into clinical immunology we tapped often and whose flexibility provided the institutional space within which this project took place; Dr. Nelson Levy, who truly made this book a reality through his generous teaching, continuous criticism, support, and friendship; and Dr. Ralph Snyderman, who not only provided a knowledge and perspective of immunology but whose creative and challenging questions both puzzled and excited us and led us continually to reexamine our work.

Several people were invaluable readers of the rough and developing manuscript. These included Drs. Doug Kelling, James Niedel, Roger Kurlander, Marty Arthur, and Nels Anderson. Many people provided criticism and guidance in their fields of expertise, including Drs. Rebecca Buckley, Jerry Logue, Ed Holmes, and John Hamilton.

We would like to give special mention to the extraordinary work done by our illustrator, Linda Kohl. Her tremendous ability to make graphic and visual images of even our most vague and convoluted ideas resulted in the excellent illustrations for this book. Our thanks also to Mr. Paul Greenwood for his help in photomicrography.

Finally, we would like to acknowledge those people without whose influence this book would probably not have been written: Philip Zaeder, who has taught that communication is a difficult struggle between language and ideas, tempered by the patience of silence; Shalom Baranes, whose gentle creative expectations actually provided the stimulus for the writing of this book; Glen Schneider, who showed us again and again that a humoral response can mean much more than the production of antibodies; David Margulies, whose affirmation of the individual spirit in each of us gave us the courage to attempt a task that often seemed beyond our reach; and Drs. Ludwig Eichna, Eugene Stead, and R. Wayne Rundles, who helped mold the sense of scientific inquiry modified by a touch of healthy skepticism which provided the background and milieu for the completion of this task.

It goes without saying that this endeavor could not have even been initiated, much less completed, without our families' support, tolerance, love, and good humor.

M.S.T.
R.D.K.
H.J.C.

Foreword

Immunology is clearly a burgeoning, active science. Great increases in our understanding of the workings of the body's defense mechanisms over the past 20 years and our beginning understanding of the malfunction of this system in clinical situations during the same period of time has been truly amazing and almost unparalled in any other area of biological sciences, with the possible exception of molecular genetics. This increased information has encompassed a spectrum from very highly sophisticated, quantitative science, such as the elucidation of the structure of immunoglobulins, to the more phenomenologically interpretable but nonetheless vitally important observations concerning the cellular biology of the immune response.

In parallel with this great increase in basic knowledge concerning the immune system, there has been an increasing awareness of its clinical importance. Formerly, immunology was taught largely in terms of infectious disease and response to infectious disease. More and more, it has become clear that the abnormalities of the immune system account for a number of diseases and that only by a thorough understanding of the immune system and of the body's responses within that system can the causes and effects of many common diseases be understood. This has led to an emphasis on clinical immunology both at the medical school and at the postgraduate level. More and more, freestanding divisions of Clinical Immunology or "hyphenated services," such as Rheumatology-Immunology, have been formed, and the role of immunology has begun to assume a central role in the teaching for medical students.

One manifestation of this greatly increased knowledge in immunology has been a proliferation of journals and books documenting these advances. This has been true in basic as well as in clinical immunology. The number of journals dealing primarily with immunological subjects has more than doubled every 5 years, and the number of books on immunological subjects is now legion. Given this proliferation of immunological writing, one may legitimately ask, Why is another book necessary? That question must be asked by the authors before undertaking the writing of a new book on immunology, by the publishers before publishing it, by the reader before reading it. If good reasons don't exist, then the project should be stopped at any point along the way.

The authors of the present book perceived a gap in the spectrum of immunological writing. They felt that there was not a recent, readable, up-to-date, short textbook for the medical student and the clinically oriented physician which described the latest knowledge from the basic sciences as applied to the clinical sciences. In many medical schools, including Duke University, courses in clinical immunology are now being taught; in general, the textbooks for such courses either arise from the notes of the teachers or are abstracted from some of the currently available great compendia of immunological knowledge. The current book tries to make available to the medical student a simply written text from which he can extract both the basic science and clinical information needed to interpret the manifestations of immunologically related disease.

This has necessitated an extensive literature review, particularly of the most recent literature. The sources of the information are carefully documented by the authors. Thus, the book is also a valuable reservoir of references for the student of immunology who wishes to look further into specific questions using original texts.

Immunological writing has two problems to overcome. On the one hand, there is a tendency to overemphasize the theoretical and imaginative aspects of immunology. While these theories may be based on some facts and interpretations of them, they frequently are not firmly rooted in the factual world. Although this system has been quite successful at times in moving immunological knowledge forward, it is difficult for the uninitiated and sometimes even the initiated to distinguish fact from fancy.

On the other hand, immunological writing can be so very rooted in factual detail as to become obscure in meaning. Although the professional immunologist requires detail in order to ascertain whether the conclusions are correct, the nonprofessional immunologist sometimes can be bogged down in trying to elicit from such writing the information that he needs.

In writing a concise text of immunology, it has been necessary for the authors to steer a course between this Scylla and Charybdis, on the one hand writing carefully so that the reader can see the broad outlines, but understand what is known and what is imaginative and, on the other hand, extracting what is necessary from masses of detail. In general, they have succeeded admirably, and if one does take exception on occasion to the course that they have steered, one must only read the sources from which they have synthesized the text to understand how helpful they have been.

Part of the problem of the current state of immunological writing is a generalized problem affecting all scientific writing. It appears to be increasingly difficult for the scientist to write a simple declarative sentence devoid of decorations and usages which tend to obfuscate rather than elucidate. Although there may be exceptions in the present text, it has been written with intelligence and the ability to write in simple English about a complex subject.

These have been the objectives of the authors. It remains for the scientific community and for the readership to evaluate how well they have achieved these objectives. If, as I believe, they have achieved them, they have filled an important gap in immunological writing.

WENDELL F. ROSSE, M.D.
Professor of Medicine and
Associate Professor of Immunology
Duke University School of Medicine

Foreword

The study of immunology began with the demonstration of acquired immunity of infection, almost 100 years ago. Substances in serum, later identified as immunoglobulins, of an animal injected with a foreign agent such as a bacterium had many properties. They could, for example, inhibit bacterial growth, agglutinate bacteria, or precipitate or neutralize their toxic products, and when transferred to a new host they could passively transfer immunity. Thus the early studies of Pasteur, of Koch, of Bordet, of Ehrlich and of many others established the existence of humoral immunity and its interrelationship with the complex set of serum proteins collectively known as complement. Pursuing the properties of the immunoglobulins, Landsteiner demonstrated the exquisite specificity of individual antibodies.

The antibody response was easy to detect, so progress was spectacular. Moreover, antibodies could be used to give quantitative measurements. They could, if directed against red blood cells, distinguish between species or even between different members of the same species. From the microbial studies came the many successful vaccination programs that have saved millions of lives and contributed to the very existence of industrial civilizations. From the quantitative determinations developed the science of immunochemistry; the procedures of immunochemistry have now pervaded every biologic science. From the studies of red cell agglutination by Landsteiner came the fundamentals of blood transfusion and of the rapidly expanding subspecialties of immunohematology and immunogenetics.

Yet while still in the halcyon days when every experiment, no matter how trivial, could yield an exciting result, immunology became deeply divided by the finding of Mechnikoff that mononuclear cells could carry out many of the same tasks of protection against infection that had been ascribed to the humoral system. Popularized by George Bernard Shaw in the *Doctor's Dilemma,* the study of cellular immunity began. Unlike the early explosive growth of knowledge of humoral immunity, progress in cellular immunology was at first very slow because techniques *in vitro* were not available. It is now appreciated that the reaction *in vivo* is almost invariably a compound of humoral and cellular responses. Many cell types, some collaborating with each other and some inhibiting, are drawn into the response. Cellular immune responses presently occupy center stage. The molecular pathways, the differentiation steps, the products released by the responding cell, and the nature of the cell-surface interactions are all still the subjects of extensive investigation and vigorous controversy. Much of the impetus to further study comes from these uncertainties.

Not surprisingly, immunology is not easy to comprehend because it has so many ramifications. Like a smoothly running machine, in the healthy individual it tends to go unnoticed. As soon as parts of it fail, or even get out of phase, the malfunction soon becomes manifest as a disease or as a group of diseases. Thus, for the student or practitioner of medicine a thorough grasp of immunology is a necessity. Autoaggression follows a break in the usual protective curtain of self-tolerance; atopies such as allergic rhinitis or hay fever reflect the predominance of one class immunoglobulin, IgE. Many rheumatoid diseases, and a variety of gastroenterologic upsets have strong immunologic overtones. Immunologic deficiencies allow skin and respiratory infections to become rampant. These are but few of the many well established relationships to medicine. Less well explored are the effects of declining immune function with age on the diseases of old age, while interrelationship between cancer and immunity has been highly controversial for over 50 years.

Available information about immunity and the exploitation of immunological reagents is of immediate value in the diagnosis and in the evaluation of the prognosis of a wide range of diseases. Much more is to be expected as we continued to probe the full dimensions of immune responsiveness. The reader of this volume (which explains basic mechanisms and then their implications in clinical medicine, often within the same chapter) will gain a good insight into this fascinating system. The inquiring few may be stimulated to follow the footsteps of Landsteiner and the other great minds of the past century who have spent their lives in the frustrating, but rewarding, elucidation of that which we call the immune response.

D. BERNARD AMOS, M.D.
Chief, Division of Immunology;
James B. Duke Professor of Immunology and Experimental Surgery
Duke University School of Medicine

Contents

Medical Immunology

1 The Foundations of the Immune Response

The fundamental role of the immune system is the preservation of the body's integrity against invasion by microorganisms and chemical agents. Molecules that are viewed as foreign by the host are called *antigens*. The presence of any antigen may pose a threat to the homeostasis of the body, and it is the immune system that is responsible for defending against such insults. Its importance in this regard is most dramatically illustrated in individuals born without an intact immune system. Although there are many ways such immunologic deficiencies can manifest themselves, each has serious consequences for the individual, sometimes culminating in death from unchallenged and overwhelming infection. The immune system has developed many means for preventing such catastrophes. These include the removal of antigen from the body, the neutralization of infectious organisms and biologically active molecules, and the lysis of foreign cells. In this chapter we will attempt to give an overview of the role of the immune system in host defense, emphasizing the organ systems where the immune response occurs and the cells and molecular species that are the actual generators of the response.

ANATOMY OF THE IMMUNE SYSTEM

THE CELLULAR UNITS

The Lymphocyte

Lymphocytes are generally small cells, about 8 to 10μ in diameter, that are almost entirely filled with nucleus (Fig. 1-1). They are mobile and circulate throughout the body, an important characteristic for cells involved in defense of the whole host against infection wherever it may occur. Lymphocytes can be found in almost every body tissue.

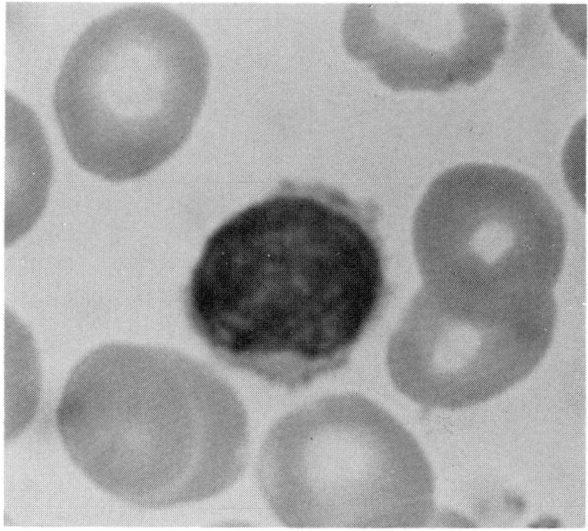

Fig. 1-1. A lymphocyte in the peripheral blood.

The lymphocyte is not the most aggressive cell in the body (neutrophils, for example, are more efficient at disposing of antigens) but it is thus far the only cell shown to be intrinsically capable of *specifically* recognizing an antigen as foreign—as something not intrinsic to the host—and initiating mechanisms to get rid of the invader. Just as importantly, the lymphocyte can recognize a component of the host tissue as "self" and direct the vast resources of the immune system to remain still and unreactive. This ability to distinguish self from nonself, the foreign and potentially harmful from the body's own tissue components, is an essential feature of the lymphocyte. It is the starting point for all immune reactivity.

The recognition of antigen by the lymphocyte triggers a series of events that leads to the destruction and/or removal of the antigen. Initially the lymphocyte undergoes some striking morphologic alterations. Its size increases dramatically, a direct reflection of an increase in the cytoplasmic mass. The new cell is called an *immunoblast* (Fig. 1-2). This activated lymphocyte can carry out many immunologic effector functions, but further differentiation is required in order to achieve a maximum and fully mature response. The various immunologic effector functions have been classified into two broad categories:

1. *Humoral immunity* refers to the production of *antibodies*, glycoprotein molecules capable of binding the stimulating antigen.

2. *Cell-mediated immunity* refers to a wide range of functions carried out directly by cells or products of those cells other than antibody molecules.

Humoral Immunity. Some lymphocytes progress beyond the immunoblast

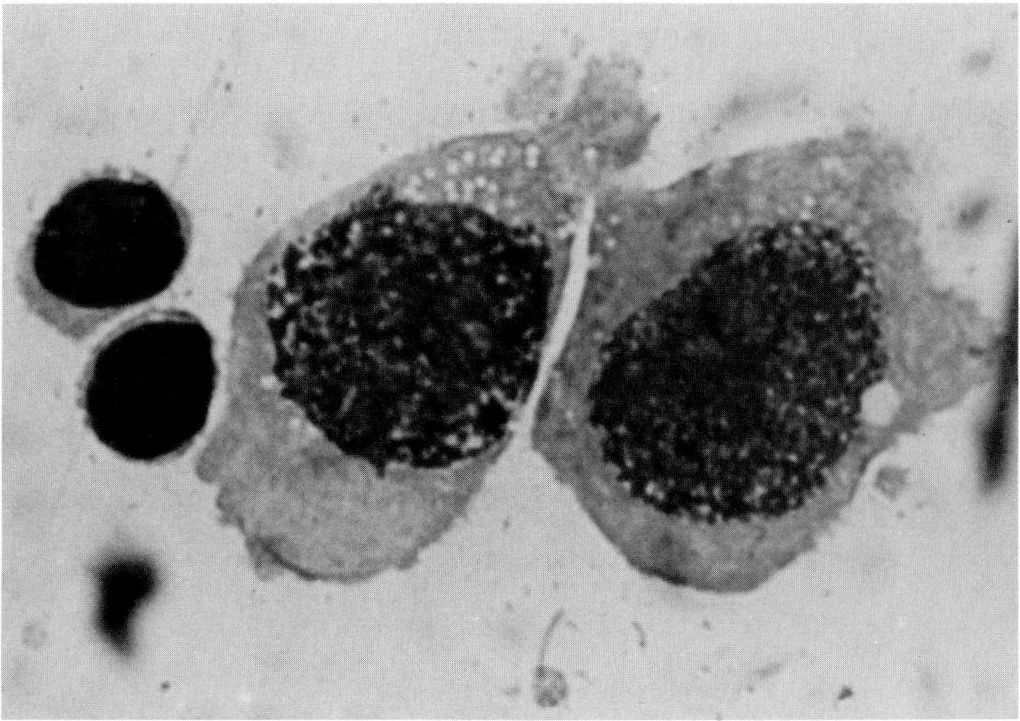

Fig. 1-2. The two large cells on the right are immunoblasts resulting from antigenic stimulation of lymphocytes in vitro. Two normal small lymphocytes are seen on the left.

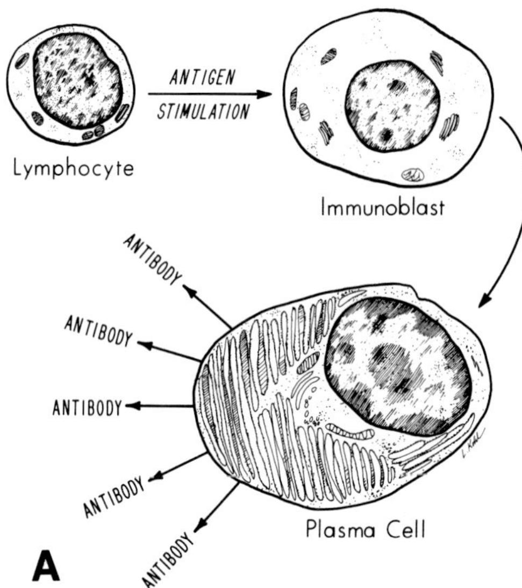

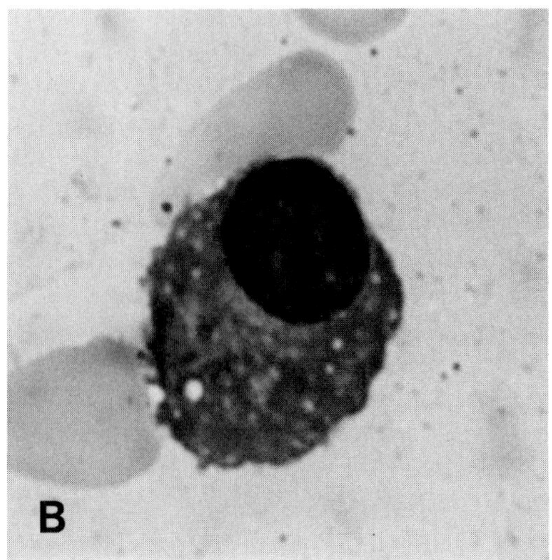

Fig. 1-3. (*A*) The differentiation of a lymphocyte into a plasma cell following antigenic stimulation. (*B*) Light micrograph of a plasma cell.

stage and differentiate into *plasma cells* (Fig. 1-3). The plasma cell is a medium-sized cell with a low nucleus-to-cytoplasm ratio. Its cytoplasm is stuffed with endoplasmic reticulum, indicative of active protein synthesis. The product of the plasma cell's synthetic machinery is the antibody molecule, and the plasma cell is largely responsible for humoral immunity. Antibody (or immunoglobulin)* is secreted by the plasma cell into the surrounding milieu where it may bind the inciting antigen.

All antibodies share certain structural features. The basic unit of which all antibodies are composed is a symmetrical structure of four polypeptides, two light chains and two heavy chains defined by molecular weight, that are linked to each other by several disulfide bridges (Fig. 1-4). There are five classes of immunoglobulin, each displaying its own particular variations on this underlying architectural theme. The five classes are called IgG, IgM, IgA, IgE and IgD. In the next chapter we shall explore in detail the structure of the immunoglobulin molecule.

The immunoglobulin is a *bifunctional* molecule, a characteristic that can be demonstrated by splitting the molecule with the enzymes pepsin and papain (Fig. 1-5). One fragment retains the antigen-binding properties of the molecule, and is referred to as the $F(ab)_2$ portion. The second, or Fc portion possesses a variety of biological functions, including the ability to activate proteins that are instrumental in initiating an inflammatory response, and the ability to adhere to the surfaces of several cell types, including neutrophils, macrophages and a subpopulation of lymphocytes.

The body has the ability to produce many unique antibody molecules, each capable of binding only certain antigens. Although it is not known precisely how many different antibodies can be produced, most estimates are on the order of 10^5 to 10^6 distinct molecules. These estimates are based upon our current under-

*The term *antibody* is usually used when a target antigen has been identified. Otherwise, the term *immunoglobulin* is used to denote molecules which presumably have the capacity to bind a particular antigen, but for which the target antigen has not yet been identified.

THE ANTIBODY MOLECULE

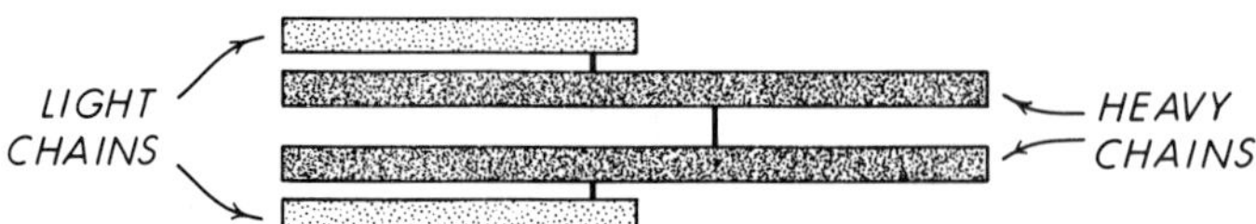

Fig. 1-4. The basic structural design of an antibody molecule. Each light chain is linked to a heavy chain by a disulfide bridge. The heavy chains are similarly joined by a variable number of disulfide linkages.

standing of the nature and extent of antibody specificity.

Specificity has long been known to be a basic property of the immune system. From the very first use of Jenner's vaccine for smallpox it became apparent that immunity to one disease, such as smallpox, did not confer protection against other diseases, such as measles or chickenpox. With the discovery of the immunoglobulin molecule and the demonstration of its antigen-binding properties, a molecular basis for this specificity was established. It was first assumed that each antibody could bind one and only one antigen. Although antibody molecules *are* remarkably specific in their ability to bind selectively only certain antigenic structures, such a simple interpretation of antibody specificity is no longer considered to be valid. Instead, we now view each antibody as having a unique *spectrum* of binding affinities. Any single antibody will bind any antigen whose structure allows it to fit into the antigen-binding region of that antibody. Some structures fit better than others. Thus, antibody A may bind antigen A very well (high affinity), structurally related antigen B fairly well (moderate affinity), and structurally unrelated antigen C poorly, if at all (low affinity; Fig. 1-6). Thus, when we talk about antibody specificity, we are really referring to a range of binding affinities* that is

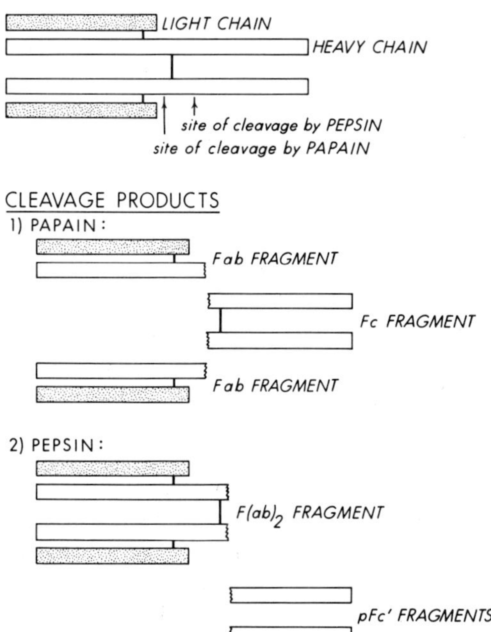

Fig. 1-5. Papain cleaves the immunoglobulin molecule on the proximal (amino terminus) side of the inter-heavy-chain linkages, yielding three cleavage products: two identical Fab fragments and the Fc fragment. Pepsin splits the molecule on the distal (carboxy terminus) side of the inter-heavy-chain linkages, so that the Fab fragments remain joined to form a single $F(ab)_2$ fragment. The Fc fragment does not remain intact.

***Affinity* can be defined as the strength of binding of a single antibody combining site to a target antigen. However, antibodies have more than one antigen-binding site. Thus, affinity must be distinguished from *avidity*, which is the strength of binding of an entire antibody molecule to an antigen. Avidity is the sum of the affinities of each antibody combining site with each bound part of the antigen. This sum is generally greater than the sum of the individual affinities considered separately.

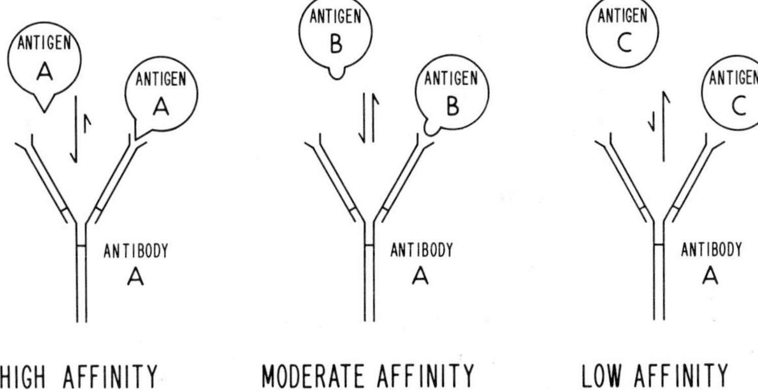

Fig. 1-6. A given antibody molecule can bind a spectrum of related antigens. The strength of binding to any particular antigen (affinity) depends upon how well the antigen's structure fits into the antigen-binding site of the antibody.

uniquely defined for each individual molecule.

One of the basic concepts of immunology, the *clonal selection theory*, states that each antibody-producing cell (or clone of identical cells) is committed to making one particular antibody of a unique specificity (Fig. 1-7). When antigen A is injected into a host, all the cells capable of producing antibody against antigen A are stimulated. Some of these antibodies bind with high affinity to the antigen, others with moderate or low affinity. Antigen B elicits the response of a different population of cells. How much overlap there is between the populations of cells activated against antigen A and antigen B depends upon how structurally similar the antigens are. The amount of overlap is a measure of the *crossreactivity* between antigens A and B. Crossreactivity is one way of assessing the similarity of two antigens. A large degree of crossreactivity indicates that antigens A and B

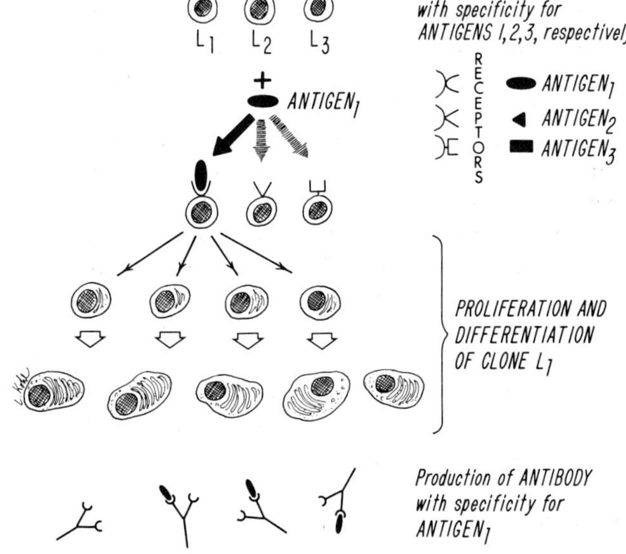

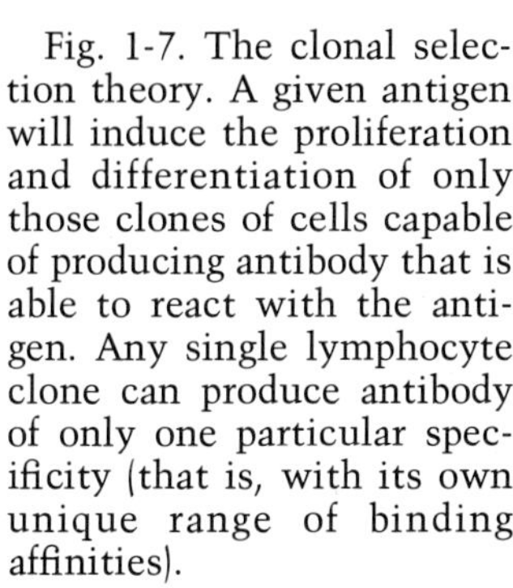

Fig. 1-7. The clonal selection theory. A given antigen will induce the proliferation and differentiation of only those clones of cells capable of producing antibody that is able to react with the antigen. Any single lymphocyte clone can produce antibody of only one particular specificity (that is, with its own unique range of binding affinities).

are structurally alike, since many of the antibodies directed against one will also bind the other, although with a different binding affinity. A small degree of cross-reactivity is an indication of structural incongruity.

Thus, each antibody is specific in that it binds one particular antigenic structure most effectively, but that same antibody can also bind other similar structures, although not as intensely. The specificity of each antibody resides in the amino acid sequence of its polypeptide chain which determines the three-dimensional structure of the antibody and therefore the conformation of its antigen-binding region. Each antibody has a unique specificity because it has a unique amino acid sequence.

The antibody molecule is effective in several ways in combating antigenic invasion. When antibody complexes with antigen it greatly facilitates the phagocytosis and clearance of that antigen. This process is called *opsonization*. Antibody can also coat the surfaces of viruses, bacteria and chemical agents such as enzymes and structurally interfere with their normal functions, thereby effectively neutralizing these agents. There are other ways in which antibody contributes to the elimination of antigen, and we shall explore these later.

Cell-Mediated Immunity. Antibody production is by no means the only mechanism by which lymphocytes oppose an antigenic challenge. Some cells do not differentiate into antibody-secreting plasma cells but instead acquire the ability to partake in what is termed *cell-mediated immunity*. These cells participate directly in the destruction of antigen. When the foreign substance is a cell, lymphocytes are activated which specifically bind that cell and, by mechanisms not yet completely understood, are able to destroy it. Rejections of skin grafts and kidney transplants are examples of cell-mediated immune destruction.

Activated lymphocytes are also able to produce a variety of soluble effector substances that are active in the immune response (Fig. 1-8). These are called *lymphokines*, and include: (1) *interferon*, which blocks the reproduction of viruses; (2) *cytotoxic factors*, which kill foreign cells; (3) *cell growth inhibitors*, which prevent cellular proliferation; (4) *factors that activate lymphocytes; (5) factors chemotactic* for (that is, they attract) macrophages, monocytes and granulocytes; and (6) *macrophage inhibition factor (MIF)*, which has profound effects on macrophage activity.

The Macrophage

It is the lymphocyte's task to specifically recognize antigen and set into motion the complex machinery of the immune system. There is another cell that appears to act nonspecifically but whose importance in an immune response is perhaps just as great. This is the macrophage (Fig. 1-9). The macrophage is derived from the circulating blood monocyte. The monocyte remains in the circulation for, at most, several days, and its fate appears to be unidirectional egress into the tissues, where it becomes the highly active macrophage. The monocyte is capable of many immunologically related functions which are further enhanced by its transformation within the body tissues to the macrophage form.

The macrophage, once considered to be only a peripheral component of the immune system, is now emerging as a central cell in the immune response. It is capable of at least three immune-related activities. First, the macrophage is a potent phagocyte and thus plays a crucial role in the clearance and degradation of foreign substances within the body. Like the lymphocyte, the macrophage must undergo a process of activation in order to become maximally efficient. One of the ways in which this can occur is through the release of stimulatory soluble sub-

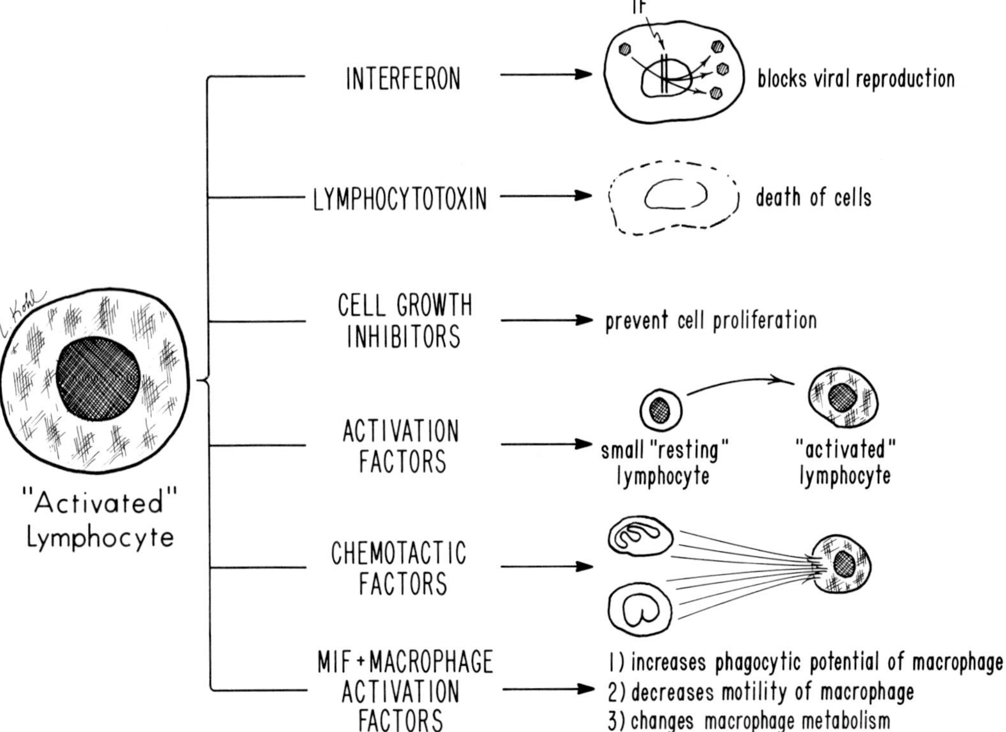

Fig. 1-8. Lymphokines are soluble substances produced by activated lymphocytes.

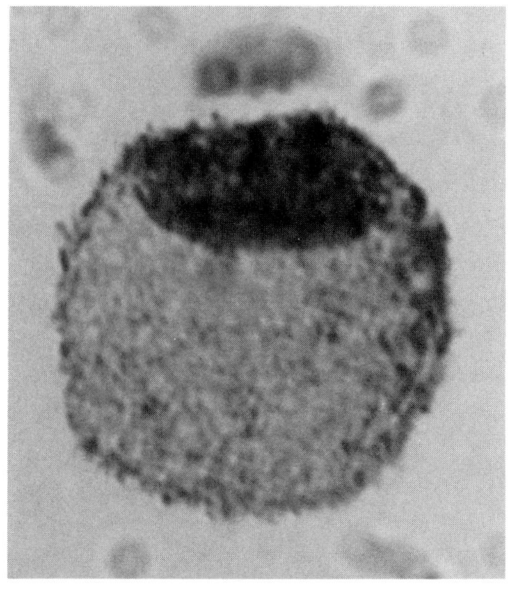

Fig. 1-9. Light microscopic view of a macrophage.

stances by antigen-activated lymphocytes. This phenomenon links macrophage phagocytosis directly to the lymphocytic immune response.

The second macrophage function is its capacity for *chemotaxis*, the directed migration of a cell along an increasing concentration gradient of a soluble substance. The macrophage can be actively summoned to the site of an immune reaction by factors released during the course of an immune response.

Third, the macrophage can express antigen on its surface. Antigen presented in this manner is *immunogenic* (that is, it is capable of eliciting an immune response), and lymphocytes that interact with macrophage-bound antigen become immunologically activated. Antigen that escapes this macrophage "processing" will stimulate only a weak immune response or may fail to evoke any response at all. It is this aspect of macrophage activity that has been most instrumental in conferring upon this cell a new importance as a critical component of the immune response.

Perhaps the major immunologic distinction between the macrophage and the lymphocyte concerns antigenic specificity. Whereas each clone of lymphocytes displays a particular antigenic specificity, no such clonal distinction is known for the macrophage. The macrophage appears to be nonspecific in that any macrophage deals with a given antigen in much the same way as with any other antigen. There is also no evidence that the macrophage is capable of making the distinction between components of self and nonself. Nevertheless, it seems likely that certain controls exist over macrophage activity that limit its response against self-components; clearly, the macrophage does not recklessly devour its host. Whether such controls are extrinsic or intrinsic to the macrophage is unknown.

The importance of the macrophage in host defense is emphasized by the observation that this phagocytic cell is the first cell devoted primarily to defense against microbial invasion to appear phylogenetically. The macrophage is associated ontologically with the gut, suggesting that the development of an immune system derived from the necessity for host protection against pathogens in the gastrointestinal tract. It is interesting in this regard that the major organs associated with lymphocyte maturation are also gut-associated.

The Inflammatory Cells

Although the lymphocyte and macrophage are the most prominent cellular elements of the immune system, the immune system also has wide-ranging interactions with other cellular systems in the body. A complete understanding of immunologic mechanisms requires a knowledge of these other cell lines as well. Most important is the inflammatory system, whose principal cells are the granulocytes. The immune and inflammatory systems interact via a considerable variety of soluble substances, including immunoglobulin molecules and lymphokines.

Neutrophils are the predominant circulating white cells and primary phagocytes of the body. There are two major ways in which these cells are allied to the immune system. First, they are capable of *chemotaxis*. Among the lymphokines released by activated lymphocytes is one called *neutrophil chemotactic factor* (NCF) which guides neutrophils to the site of an immune response.

The second immunologically related function of neutrophils is called *immune adherence* (Fig. 1-10). Antibody binds antigen via the $F(ab)_2$ end of the antibody molecule, leaving the Fc portion free. Neutrophils possess a surface receptor for the Fc portion and will bind the antibody, thereby forming a neutrophil-antibody-antigen complex. This binding greatly enhances the phagocytosis of the antigen.

Phagocytosis by the neutrophil is a remarkably efficient process. Foreign substances, such as bacteria, are engulfed by the cell in membrane-bound vacuoles. Enzyme-containing lysosomes fuse with these vacuoles to form phagolysosomes. The release of the destructive potential of these enzymes into the vacuole leads to the death of the bacteria (or degradation of the antigen, Fig. 1-11). There are several congenital disorders of neutrophil function in which the normal processes of intracellular digestion are defective. One such disorder is chronic granulomatous disease (see Chap. 11). Children afflicted with this disease die very young of overwhelming bacterial infections, dramatically illustrating the necessity for healthy neutrophils in the defense of the body.

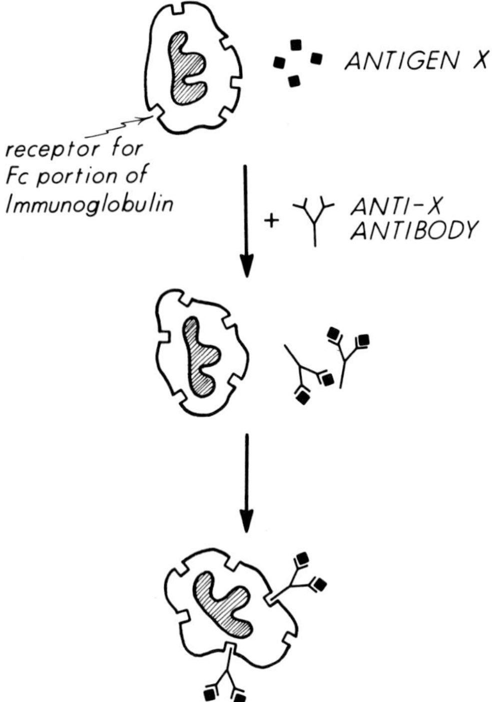

Fig. 1-10. Immune adherence. Neutrophils and other cell types (see Chap. 3) can bind antigen-antibody complexes by the Fc end of the antibody molecule. Following attachment, phagocytosis of the complex may ensue.

Basophils and Mast Cells. The basophil possesses receptors specific for the Fc portion of IgE molecules and binds them to its surface. When two of these surface-bound IgE molecules are bridged by the binding of antigen (Fig. 1-12), the basophil becomes activated and releases a variety of substances which have powerful effects on the body's vasculature and pulmonary system. These include the inflammatory substances *histamine, slow-reacting substance of anaphylaxis* (SRS-A), and *eosinophil chemotactic factor of anaphylaxis* (ECF-A). In sufficiently high concentrations these substances can induce the clinical state of anaphylaxis, typified by profound shock associated with increased vascular permeability, contraction of smooth muscle, and an influx of inflammatory cells.

The circulating basophil represents only a very small proportion of the body's total population of inflammatory cells. Another cell, present in much greater numbers, is also capable of performing all of the activities attributable to basophils. This is the *mast cell*, a noncirculating cell

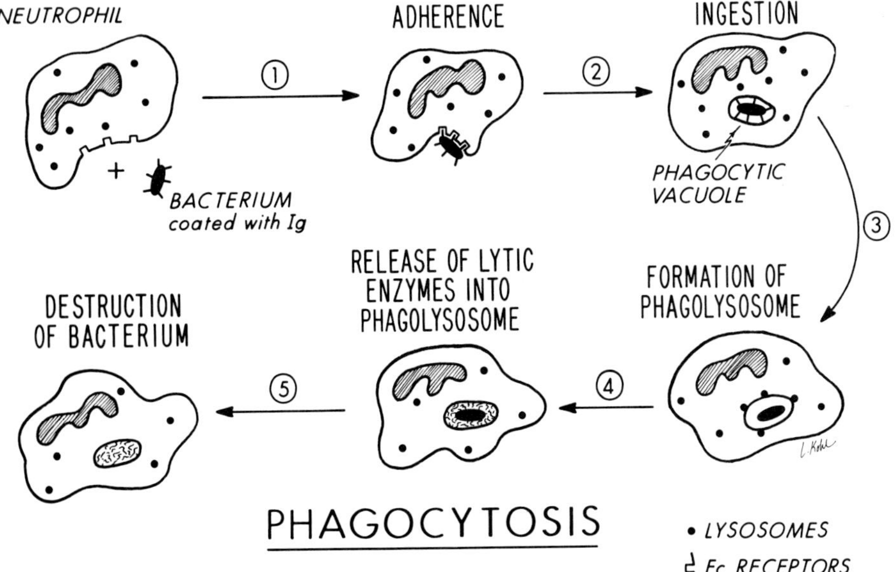

Fig. 1-11. The events leading to the phagocytosis and intracellular destruction of an antibody-coated bacterium.

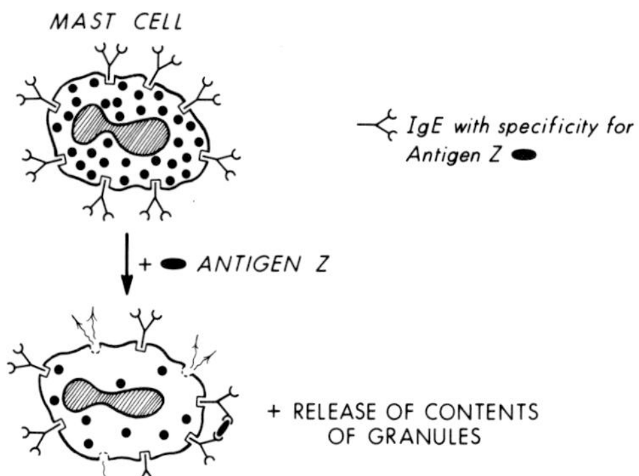

Fig. 1-12. Degranulation of a mast cell following the bridging of two surface-bound IgE molecules by antigen.

found solely in the body tissues. Although on superficial examination it closely resembles the basophil, finer analysis reveals morphologic features distinct from those of the basophil. Its cell membrane is less regular, its nucleus rounder, and, instead of containing a few large granules, the mast cell contains many smaller ones. Like the basophil, the mast cell binds IgE and releases a similar array of chemical mediators when antigen bridges two IgE molecules. These observations have led to a long and yet unresolved debate as to whether or not the basophil and mast cell are simply the blood-borne and tissue-borne states of the same cell. That this may not be so has been suggested by recent data. Careful morphologic studies have demonstrated that even when basophils enter the body tissues they maintain their morphologic distinction from the mast-cell population. In addition, basophilic leukemia rarely affects the mast-cell population, and the mast-cell proliferation of urticaria pigmentosa (a rare disease characterized by an infiltration of mast cells in the skin) is rarely accompanied by blood basophilia.

Eosinophils. Eosinophils are closely allied to the events of immune reactivity and are often found at the site of an immune response. Eosinophilia is associated with many states of heightened immune reactivity such as allergies, drug reactions and hypersensitivity states. In many of these situations, the presence of eosinophils may be the result of the release of ECF-A by activated basophils. The eosinophil is a powerful phagocyte with a marked predilection for antigen-antibody complexes.

Summary

The lymphocyte and the macrophage are the two cell types most directly involved in immune activities. The lymphocyte is capable of recognizing an antigen as foreign and responding in either of two general ways: some lymphocytes differentiate into plasma cells and are responsible for humoral immunity, that is, the elaboration of antibody molecules that can specifically bind antigen. It is believed that any single lymphocyte or clone of lymphocytes produces one particular antibody of unique specificity. Other lymphocytes differentiate into cells which carry out cell-mediated immunity, the direct destruction of antigens by the cells themselves. The macrophage appears to be much less specific in its actions—there is no apparent clonal restriction—but is nevertheless critical in host defense both as a phagocyte and through its ability to present antigen in immunogenic form to the lymphocyte population. The complex interactions between macrophages and lymphocytes will be discussed in later chapters. Other cell lines, notably those of the inflammatory system, interact extensively with the immune system via soluble substances such as lymphokines and immunoglobulins.

SOLUBLE SUBSTANCES OF THE IMMUNE SYSTEM

Soluble substances are a basic part of the immune system; antibodies and lymphokines are just two examples.

There is a third group of substances, complement, that is also crucial in the defense of the body.[1] Its importance in the immune system is such that a relatively detailed discussion is warranted here. (The complement pathways are discussed more fully in Appendix A.)

Complement

Complement is a series of proteins, named in the order of their discovery, many of which circulate in inactive forms in the extracellular fluid. The activation of complement resembles the activation of the coagulation pathway in that it involves a sequence of steps, each one generating a new active component that in turn activates the next complement component.

There are two major pathways of complement activation, the *classical pathway* and the *properdin pathway.* As shown in Figure 1-13, these two pathways join at the level of the C3 component, and a single sequence of reactions finishes out the complement cascade. At each step in the complement sequence molecules are activated which have important and potent biological activities (list p. 15).

The classical pathway is more intimately tied to the immune response, because it is initiated by the binding of antigen to antibody (Figure 1-14). The C1 component binds to the Fc portion of the antibody molecule and gets the classical pathway under way. The binding of C1 to antigen-antibody complexes may also increase the strength of the antigen-antibody interaction and may influence the rapidity with which the complex is cleared from the body.

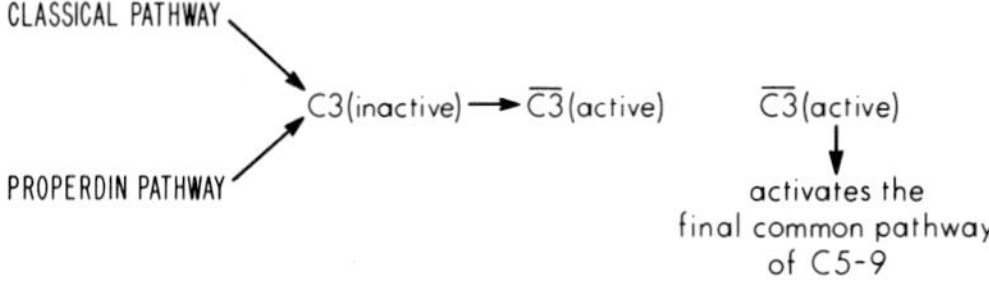

Fig. 1-13. The two major pathways of complement activation, the classical and properdin pathways, converge at the level of C3. Activated C3 then initiates the remainder of the complement cascade.

$+ C1 \longrightarrow \overline{C1} + C4 \text{ and } C2 \longrightarrow \overline{C142}$

$C\overline{142} + C3 \longrightarrow C\overline{1423b} + C\overline{3a}$

$C\overline{1423b} + C5 \longrightarrow C\overline{5b} + C\overline{5a}$

$C\overline{5b} + C6 \text{ and } C7 \longrightarrow C\overline{5b67}$

$C\overline{5b67} + C8 \text{ and } C9 \longrightarrow C\overline{5b6789}$

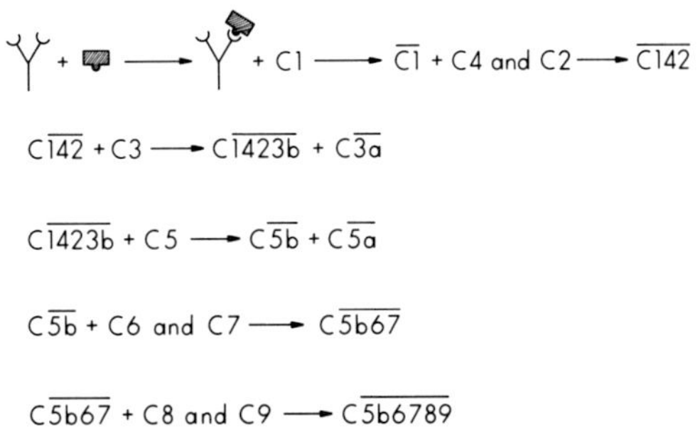

Fig. 1-14. The classical complement pathway is initiated by the binding of antigen by antibody. Each activated complement component then acts upon the next substrate in line to generate the entire complement cascade.

With the activation of C4 by C1, a basic property of several of the complement components first becomes evident: the activated component, in this case C4, binds to the surface of the target antigen to which the antibody has been bound. The coating of antigens with C4 may contribute to their neutralization.

The C$\overline{142}$ complex activates C3. (A bar placed over the complement numbers signifies that those components are in an activated form.) C3a is split off and has powerful biological potential as an *anaphylatoxin.*[2] This means that it is capable of causing the degranulation of mast cells with the release of their intracellular store of vasoactive amines. C3b, like C4, can bind to the surface of the target antigen. The antigen is therefore coated with both C4 and C3b. The coating of antigen by these complement components can lead to *immune adherence.*[3] Phagocytic cells, such as neutrophils and macrophages, possess surface receptors for complement components (see Chap. 3), including receptors specific for C3b and for C4. Any antigen which has these complement components adhering to its surface can be readily bound to the phagocytes via these receptors. Many lymphocytes also have receptors for C3b and C4 as well as for C3d (a breakdown product of C3b), but their biological function has not been established.

C5 is activated next. C5a is released and, like C3a, is an anaphylatoxin. C5a (and possibly C3a) is also chemotactic for neutrophils.[4] This latter function may be important in coordinating the immune reaction against an antigen with the nonspecific inflammatory response. C5b adheres to the antigen surface.

The late components of complement are responsible for the most widely known property of complement, cell lysis.[5] The stable trimolecular complex $\overline{C5b67}$ can attach to cell surfaces and, with the addition of C8, produce a "hole" in the cell membrane, leading to cell death (Fig. 1-15). C9 may not be needed for cell lysis but accelerates the process. This cytolytic mechanism may be important in the destruction of foreign cells, including bacteria and tissue transplants. Complement-mediated cell lysis may also be significant in autoimmune disease where the host's own tissues are susceptible to immunologic attack.

Little is known about the biological activities of the individual components of the properdin pathway. The properdin pathway can be activated by endotoxin, bacterial cell wall polysaccharides, and probably all classes of immunoglobulin.[6] The key to the importance of the

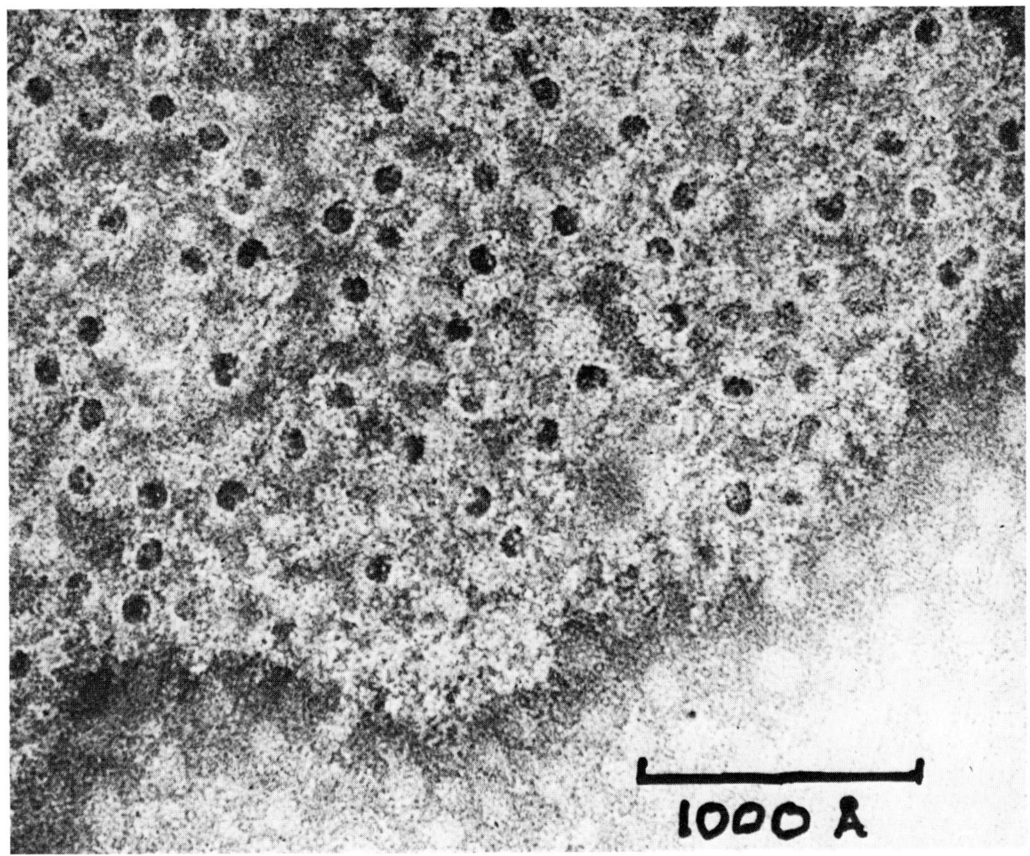

Fig. 15-1. Membrane lesions produced by the action of complement on the red blood cell surface. (Courtesy of Dr. W. F. Rosse)

Functions of Various Complement Components

C1	Initiates the classical complement pathway May increase the affinity of some antibodies Promotes aggregation of antigen-antibody complexes
Properdin pathway	May be activated directly by antigen, without requiring the production of antibody
$C\overline{14}$	May contribute to viral neutralization
C2	Cleavage product may have kininlike activity
C4b	Immune adherence
C3a	Anaphylatoxin May be chemotactic
C3b	Immune adherence
C5a	Anaphylatoxin Powerful chemotactic agent
$C\overline{5b67}$	May be chemotactic Initiates reactive lysis
C8, 9	Induces cell lysis

properdin pathway is that it can be activated directly by antigens (such as endotoxins) without requiring the presence of antigen-specific antibody. Thus, the properdin pathway defines a first line of defense and can activate the complement cascade without waiting for an immune response to evolve. This may be especially important during a host's first exposure to an antigen when antibody may take from one to three weeks to appear in substantial amounts (see below).

The importance of complement in the normal defense and homeostasis of the body is most evident in the many pathologic conditions, including a high susceptibility to infections, that may be seen with certain congenital complement deficiencies. The congenital absence of specific complement components has been documented in many individuals (the consequences of such deficiencies are discussed in Chap. 10).

It is evident that the complement pathway generates an impressive array of bioactive factors. Many of these can also be potentially harmful to the host, including the lytic complexes and the anaphylatoxins. The body must therefore control this system very carefully. It is likely that the complement system is constantly being activated in the body in response to a continual low-grade antigenic invasion, primarily from the gut, and this may explain why the turnover rate of these proteins is so rapid. The complement system therefore demands a dynamic interplay of stimulatory and inhibitory mechanisms that strike a balance between continual defense of the body and potential self-destruction. Several complement inhibitors have now been identified, and include the C1 esterase inhibitor, the C3 inactivator (which splits C3b to C3c and C3d), and the C6 inhibitor. There is also an inhibitor of the C3a and C5a anaphylatoxins. Absence of these inhibitory molecules destroys this balance and can result in serious pathology. For example, the absence of C1 esterase inhibitor is the cause of hereditary angioneurotic edema, and a lack of C3 inhibitor leads to recurrent infections (see Chap. 10).

Other Humoral Systems

The processes of immunologic reactivity and inflammation are closely linked. We have seen much evidence of this already in the elaboration of lymphokines by lymphocytes and in the activation of complement. Communication between these two systems relies heavily on humoral factors. There are actually six such humoral systems which interact to produce an optimal immunologic and inflammatory response. These are the (1) immunoglobulin; (2) lymphokine, (3) complement, (4) coagulation, (5) fibrinolytic, and (6) kinin systems. Some of these interactions are diagrammed in (Figure 1-16). The picture is confusing and complex, and that is probably its most accurate feature. Even so, much has been

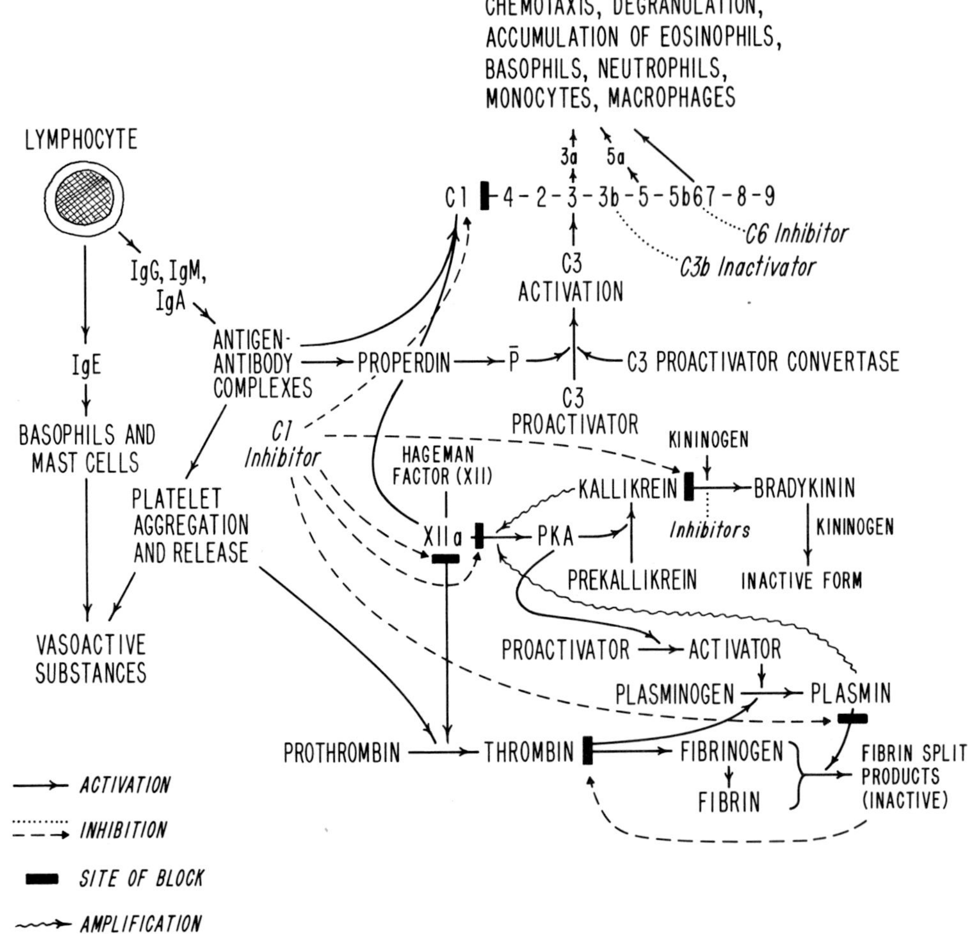

Fig. 1-16. A simplified version of the interactions among the six major humoral systems involved in immunologic and inflammatory reactions.

omitted, such as the influence of hormones and prostaglandins, in order to keep the scheme readable.

Each of the various systems plays a unique role in the overall host response. There are three key substances whose actions affect several systems:

Antigen-antibody complexes may activate complement via either the classical or properdin pathway. They can also lead to the release reaction of basophils. Their effect on platelets may feed into the coagulation pathway by inducing the release of platelet procoagulant activity.

Hageman factor in its activated form can initiate the coagulation sequence as well as the powerful kinin system. Activated Hageman factor can also activate the C1 esterase, perhaps via several intermediary steps, in the absence of antigen-antibody complexes.

C1 esterase inhibitor has an inhibiting and thus a regulatory effect on many of these interlocking systems. It can block the complement pathway, the coagulation pathway, the kinin system and the fibrinolytic system.

The lesson of this complex scheme is that the effects of the interaction of antigen with antibody may include the activation and modulation of many disparate systems.

Summary

Communication among the different cellular elements that contribute to the defense of the host is affected by a variety of soluble substances, notably antibody, lymphokines and complement. Complement is a series of protein molecules that is activated in a progressive cascade. There are two pathways for complement activation, the classical and properdin pathways. The former is initiated by the binding of antigen to antibody, the latter may be directly activated by antigen alone. The complement system is under the regulation of several inhibitory molecules and interacts extensively with other soluble systems of the body.

THE ORGANS OF THE IMMUNE SYSTEM

Several organs and tissues have been grouped under the heading "immune system" out of regard for their concentrated efforts on behalf of host defense.[7] This is purely a functional definition. Anatomically, the immune system is actually a part of the larger reticuloendothelial system (RES). The RES comprises a set of organs characterized by a unique architectural theme. The basic structure consists of a complex meshwork of reticular fibers, collagenous proteins embedded in a mucopolysaccharide matrix. Fixed phagocytic cells which inhabit the mesh complete the pattern. The reticuloendothelial design can be found throughout the body in the bone narrow, liver, lung, thymus, spleen and lymph nodes.

The Central Organs

The bone marrow appears to be the source of stem cells for all the cellular elements of the blood.[8] Lymphocytes comprise up to 20 per cent of all the nucleated cells in the marrow. Plasma cells are commonly found only in low numbers (up to 3 to 5% of the marrow cells), and their presence in sheets or nodules of cells is usually associated with certain pathologic conditions.

There is some evidence that a single pluripotential stem cell serves as the precursor of the lymphocyte, granulocyte, erythrocyte and megakaryocyte populations. The various cell lines separate from each other early in their development. In animal systems, stem cells can repopulate the entire lymphocyte pool of a host who has been deprived of his lymphocytes by x-irradiation.[9]

T and B Lymphocytes. There are two pathways along which precursor lymphocytes may further differentiate (Fig. 1-17). Some cells migrate to the thymus where they are induced to differentiate into a subpopulation of mature lymphocytes known appropriately as *T (thymic) lymphocytes*. These are the lymphocytes responsible for cell-mediated immunity. A second population of cells avoids thymic processing. In the chicken, these lymphocytes migrate to a hind gut organ called the bursa of Fabricius where they mature into *B (bursal) lymphocytes*. These cells are responsible for the production of immunoglobulin. No bursal equivalent has yet been found in humans.[10]

Under the light microscope T and B lymphocytes appear identical. They can be distinguished by their electrophoretic properties and their location in lymph nodes (see below). There are also several functional tests which can be used to distinguish them, the most obvious being the production of antibody as a measure of B-cell function and cell-mediated cytotoxicity for T-cell function. B and T cells also differ in the various receptor molecules present on their surface (see Chap. 3). Additionally, some people have felt that they could be distinguished by their appearance under the scanning electron microscope.[11] Thus, B cells have been described as appearing "hairy," possessing a remarkably villous surface, and T cells as appearing "bald," with a rela-

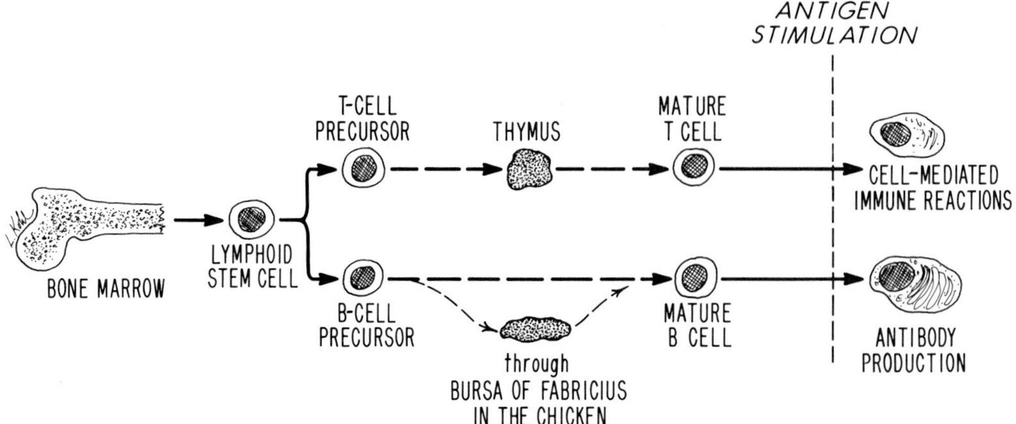

Fig. 1-17. The origin of T and B lymphocytes. Both cell types are derived from a marrow stem cell. T-cell precursors mature within the thymus into T cells capable of carrying out cell-mediated immune reactions. B-cell precursors may either mature directly into fully competent B cells or, as in the chicken, require processing in a second organ in order to achieve full immunologic competence.

tively smooth surface. Recent evidence, however, indicates that these distinctions are probably only experimental artifacts, and that microscopically these two cells are most likely indistinguishable.[12]

Over the past decade, the distinction between T and B lymphocytes and between cell-mediated and humoral immunity in general has been at the center of our growing understanding of the immune system. More recently, investigators have begun to uncover a complex array of interactions between these two aspects of immune reactivity that is blurring these once sharp distinctions. The discovery of additional subpopulations of lymphocytes has further muddied this once clear dichotomy. These new intricacies will be amplified in the next several chapters. However, we must emphasize that the concept of distinct subpopulations of lymphocytes, each with different developmental and functional characteristics, remains essential to our current conception of the immune system. At present, the T-cell/B-cell distinction is the best studied and most carefully defined in cellular immunology.

The Thymus. Many people have come to view the thymus as the master organ of the immune system.[13] The thymus is not only responsible for the maturation and development of T lymphocytes but may also be important in the overall control and maintenance of the immune system. This latter role has been established by the discovery of several "thymic hormones" which have been found to have profound effects on the immune system (see Chap. 5).[14]

The thymus consists of a reticular network stuffed with lymphocytes. It is one of the most active sites of lymphocyte proliferation. Precursor cells migrate from the bone marrow to the thymus where they mature into T lymphocytes. This maturation process involves many divisional steps, and only the emergent progeny are capable of carrying out T-cell-related functions. Only 5 per cent of the cells produced in the thymus actually leave the organ; the remainder survive only a few days and die within the thymus. These dead cells are probably rapidly phagocytosed, as there is no histologic evidence of massive cell death.

What is the meaning behind this massive and seemingly wasteful proliferation? Two explanations have been offered. The first claims that it represents the elimination of lymphocyte clones reactive against self-antigens that are present in the thymus. Such lymphocyte clones have been called forbidden clones since ordinarily they would not survive in the host. The second suggests that the proliferative process enables somatic mutation to occur, thus generating the diverse specificities needed by the immune system to recognize the thousands of different antigens that might be encountered. Most cells, therefore, die, since the vast majority of mutations are lethal. It is interesting in this latter regard to consider the recent discovery of an enzyme normally present in large amounts only in the human thymus. Terminal deoxyribonucleotidal transferase (TDT) is a DNA polymerase with the unique feature of not requiring template nucleotides to be active. It has been suggested that TDT may act as a generator of somatic mutation.[15]

The activity of the thymus appears to be under the control of an intrinsic biological clock.[16] The thymus reaches peak activity in childhood, and it attains its largest size at puberty. The size of the thymus is an important clinical parameter. Often it can be measured by a routine chest roentgenogram, whereas at other times special techniques are required. A smaller-than-normal thymus can be found in a number of situations. These include congenital thymic hypoplasia, hypercorticalism (as in Cushing's disease, malnutrition, and any condition of stress), pregnancy and lactation, drug therapy with steroids and neoplastic agents, and x-irradiation. Large thymuses are found most commonly in hyperthyroidism, especially thyrotoxicosis, but also in Addison's disease, anencephaly, acromegaly, myasthenia gravis, and various neoplasms, especially thymoma and metastatic lymphoma.

There have been several reports that soluble substances derived from the thymus can replace the intact thymus in inducing T-cell development. There is no longer any question that thymic factors (thymic hormones) exist which have powerful effects on lymphocytes, but many investigators still feel, and recent evidence supports the contention, that at least one step in T-cell maturation requires the passage of the cell through an intact thymus.[17]

Early in life the thymus is critical for T-cell maturation. Thus thymectomy in neonatal animals induces a state of severe immunodeficiency. No T-cell function is evident in these animals. They develop a wasting syndrome of poor growth, diarrhea and early death attributable to massive infection by organisms that are not usually pathogenic. Interestingly, B-cell function is also compromised in these thymic-deficient animals. We will explore the meaning of this finding shortly.

In the adult the thymus may serve mainly as a regulator of the immune system via the secretion of thymic hormones. Thymectomy in adult animals has less severe consequences, presumably because the long-lived recirculating T cells are relatively independent of thymic control. In humans, many adult thymectomies have been performed primarily for the treatment of myasthenia gravis and thymoma. The effect on immunologic function is still being evaluated.

The Peripheral Organs

The peripheral lymphoreticular system consists of the spleen, lymph nodes, and a network of channels for the flow of lymph, the lymphatics.[18]

The Lymph Node. It is in the lymph node particularly that the body tries to localize an immune response against an offending antigen. The structural organization of a lymph node is depicted below (Fig. 1-18). The interior of the lymph node is laced by a fine reticular matrix.

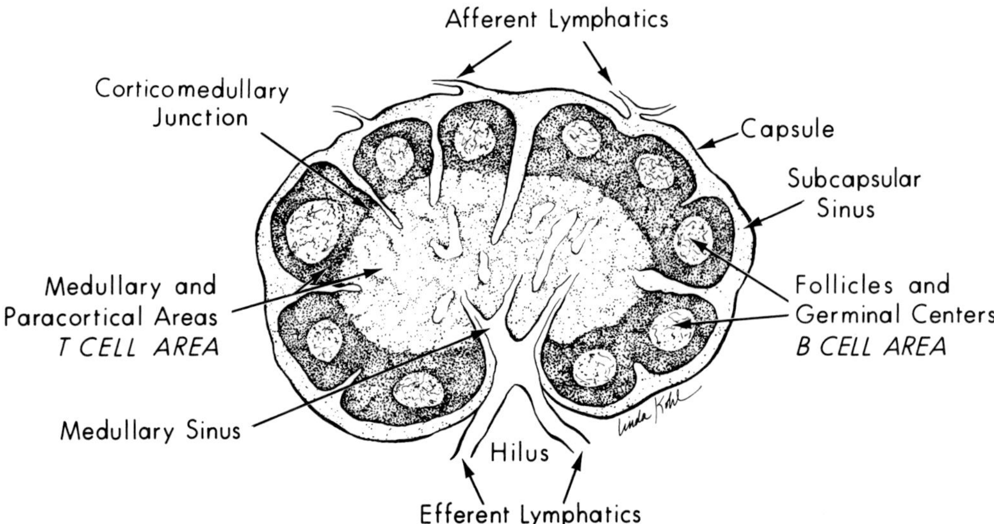

Fig. 1-18. The internal structure of a lymph node. The follicles are heavily populated with B cells; the medullary and paracortical areas contain a high percentage of T cells.

Sprawled out along these fibers are reticular cells possessing long, dendritic extensions. This reticular system serves as an efficient filter of the lymph that continually passes through the node. If a large dose of antigen is placed in a lymphatic entering a node, over 99 per cent of the antigen will be trapped within the lymph node.[19]

The reticular matrix also provides an effective scaffolding for the localization and organization of immunocompetent cells, including lymphocytes and macrophages. Most of the lymph node consists of a diffuse, poorly organized arrangement of lymphocytes. However, in the cortex dense spherical clusters of lymphocytes called *follicles* can be found. The follicles are comprised primarily of B cells, whereas T cells occupy the diffusely patterned areas of the medulla and paracortical region.[20]

The spleen also displays diffusely packed T-cell areas and follicles composed primarily of B cells. Its relationship to the circulatory system is analogous to the lymph node's association with the lymphatics. The spleen serves as a major filter for blood-borne antigens.

Circulation of Lymphocytes. Lymphocytes are constantly passing out of the central organs of the immune system into the peripheral system. Within the periphery, many lymphocytes take part in a complex circulatory pattern.[13,14] Figure 1-19 illustrates the path by which lymphocytes recirculate between the blood and the lymph. It takes about 24 to 48 hours to complete one cycle.[21] The recirculating pool is composed primarily of long-lived cells (both B and T cells), with a lifetime of longer than 20 years. Ten to 40 per cent of the white cells in the blood are lymphocytes, and of these about 80 per cent are T cells. The percentage of T cells is even greater in the thoracic duct. When the lymphocytes enter the lymph nodes they rapidly migrate to their specific areas of residence.[22] What guides this homing process is unknown. The lymphocytes remain in these locations for varying lengths of time and then rejoin the circulating pool.

PHYSIOLOGY OF THE IMMUNE SYSTEM

In this section we will outline the events that unfold when the body is ex-

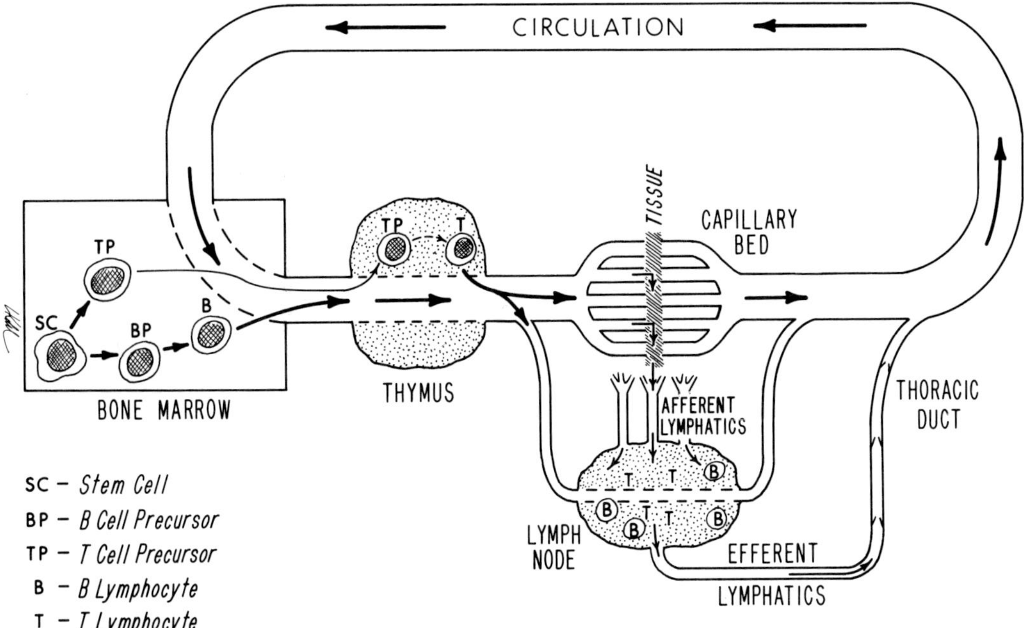

Fig. 1-19. The circulation of lymphocytes. Once released from the central organs, lymphocytes move back and forth between the blood and the lymph. B cells and T cells home to their particular areas within a lymph node and are then released again into the circulation. Not all lymphocytes appear to recirculate. Primarily the long-lived cells, most of which are T cells, participate in this continual pattern of movement.

posed to antigen. The setting for these responses is the lymphoreticular system described above. The physiology and dynamics of the immune response will be explored in much greater detail in the succeeding chapters.

THE FATE OF ANTIGEN WITHIN THE BODY

It is within the lymph node that the most dynamic events of an immune response take place. When antigen enters the body through a break in the skin, for example, it is carried within minutes by the lymphatic flow to the subcortical and medullary areas of the regional lymph nodes (Fig. 1-20). The macrophages and reticular cells are the first to engage the antigen. They can either phagocytose and degrade the antigen or else hold it on their surface where contact with lymphocytes stimulates a specific immune response against the antigen.[23]

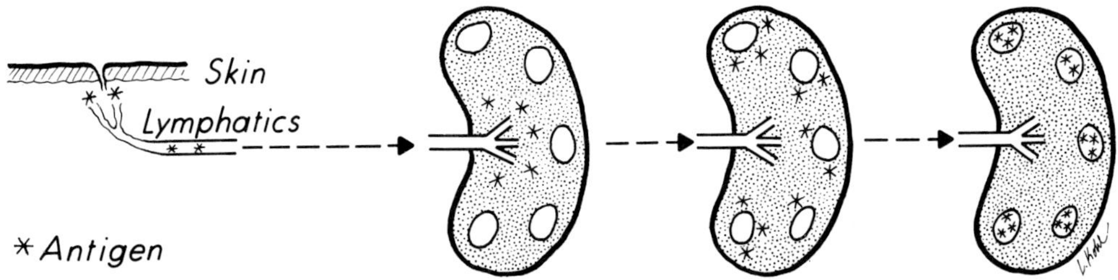

Fig. 1-20. Antigen entrapment in a lymph node following entry through the skin.

Within one day after it has entered the body, much of the antigen will be found in the cortical areas, for the first time encountering the cortical follicles. At first it forms a halo around the cortical nodule, but later antigen can be observed to have penetrated within the follicle itself.[24]

Antigen which escapes entrapment by the lymph node enters the circulation where it is filtered by the spleen, liver, lung and kidney. Of these, the spleen is the most important, and events analogous to those in the lymph node take place.[25]

THE IMMUNE RESPONSE

Having described the movement of antigen and lymphocytes within the lymphorecticular system, we must investigate the actual response of the immunocompetent cells to the presence of antigen. There is a wide spectrum of immune reactivity; the precise pattern of reaction differs for different antigens. In general, it has been convenient to consider three basic types of immune responses to antigen: those that are primarily humoral, those that primarily involve cell-mediated immunity, and combined responses.

The Humoral Response

Certain antigens elicit a response typified by the production and secretion of antibody. Like all antigens, these rapidly concentrate in the local lymph node after administration. It is not until one to six days later, however, that the first cytologic changes occur within the node.[26,27] The small lymphocyte undergoes transformation first into an immunoblast, and several days later immature plasma cells can be seen. These cells arise primarily in the center of the cortical follicles and because of their low nuclear/cytoplasmic ratio the central area of the follicle becomes lighter in color than the rest of the follicle. These central regions are termed *germinal centers*.

With the appearance of plasma cells we can begin to detect antibody secretion within the lymph node. This antibody has the ability to bind the inciting antigen. One to two weeks after antigen injection, specific antibody can be detected in the blood. The number of plasma cells continues to increase and peaks in three to five weeks. Circulating antibody titers also achieve a maximum at this time. The number of plasma cells then begins to decline, and the level of antibody falls. The active phase of the humoral immune response is over.[27]

The type of response we have just described is called a humoral response because the immune system has responded to the presence of antigen by directing the synthesis of a soluble protein, antibody, against the antigen. This took place in the center of the cortical follicle, a B-cell area, and hence what we have just described is a typical B-cell response to antigen. It is the role of the B cells to specifically interact with antigen and then undergo a sequence of developmental changes giving rise to the plasma cell. The result of B-cell stimulation is thus the secretion of antibody directed against the offending antigen.

Within the first four days of germinal-center activity, many new cells are produced.[28] All of the activity that occurs in the follicle leaves its mark on that structure. The germinal center remains visible within the follicle. It is now called a *secondary nodule* and is composed of many "sensitized" cells. This means that these cells will respond rapidly and forcefully to any subsequent exposure to the original antigen. They have been *primed* by that antigen and are prepared to respond even more vigorously to a second exposure.

The Cellular Response

Certain antigens elicit a markedly different kind of immune response. These provoke two phases of response, one in the regional lymph node and the other at the site of antigen entrance into the body. Within the lymph node, there is mitotic activity in the paracortical and medullary areas, regions of T-cell concentration. These lymphocytes divide and differentiate, becoming immunoblasts. The cells enlarge and their cytoplasm becomes packed with ribosomes. However, there is no evidence of antibody synthesis and the cortical nodules remain quiet and undisturbed.

Similar events unfold at the site of antigen administration, and there is a marked infiltration of blast cells, lymphocytes and macrophages. Thus, unlike the humoral response where the cells remain in the node and exert systemic effects by the secretion of antibody molecules, here the cells themselves migrate to wherever antigen might be. Not surprisingly, this is termed *cell-mediated immunity* and it is attributable to the T-cell population. The activated T cells participate directly in the destruction of the inciting antigen against which they are specifically sensitized. Such T cells are referred to as *T killer cells*.

The Combined Response

The separation of the immune response into a B-cell-mediated humoral immunity and a T-cell-mediated cellular immunity is somewhat misleading. Most antigens do *not* elicit *pure* B- or *pure* T-cell responses as we have so far described; rather *both* types of responses are evoked. This is the case with a commonly employed experimental antigen, the sheep erythrocyte (SRBC). Injection of this antigen leads to blast-cell activity in the T-cell paracortical areas by two days. Several days later follicular activity is noted, germinal centers are formed, and antibody is produced. Thus, the pattern of lymph node reaction is actually a combination of the two patterns described above, and both effector limbs of the immune system, humoral and cellular, are activated to counteract the potential threat of this and *most* other antigens.

The Systemic Response to Antigen

Despite the best efforts of the host to localize an immune response within the local lymph nodes, this is not always possible. If the antigen is introduced via a systemic route (for example, in a blood transfusion), if the antigen is an extremely aggressive pathogen, or if the dose of antigen is too large to be contained by the local lymph nodes, antigen may then enter the circulation and spread throughout the body. When this occurs, the task of removing the antigen falls on those tissues of the RES associated with the circulatory system. These include the spleen, liver and lung. Their structure allows them to function as both filter and phagocyte for circulating antigens.

The ability of the RES to clear an antigen from the circulation is a function of several factors. Of great importance are the physical properties of the antigen. Large, particulate or colloidal molecules are readily cleared: the liver can remove 80 to 90 per cent of such antigens in a single passage. Small, soluble particles are much less easily removed. The presence of antibody directed against the antigen enhances clearance. The removal of antigen-antibody complexes from the circulation can be of great significance, since free complexes can play a nefarious role in the pathogenesis of several diseases, including serum sickness and several types of glomerulonephritis. A third factor is the ability of some antigens to nonspecifically stimulate RES activity. Prominent among these are bacterial cell wall components such as lipopolysaccharides (LPS).

A large challenge of antigen can induce proliferation of the RES and hypertrophy of the involved organ. It has been suggested that an excessively large dose of antigen can exhaust the RES, leaving the host vulnerable to secondary infection.

Among the organs of the RES, the liver probably serves as the major filter for antigen. The spleen, however, is constructed much like the lymph node, and events closely analogous to the events of an immune response within a lymph node can occur there. The spleen can therefore mount a specific immune response and rapidly release antibody and sensitized cells directly into the circulation.

The Effect of Antigen on the Circulation of Lymphocytes

Not only can lymphocytes that are specifically reactive against the inciting antigen proliferate within the lymph nodes and spleen, but the large population of recirculating cells can be mobilized to the site of reactivity.

The introduction of antigen disrupts the normal pattern of lymphocyte circulation. There is a rapid disappearance of cells capable of reacting to the antigen from the recirculating pool.[29] They are specifically sequestered in the lymph nodes draining the site of antigen invasion. At this time, a second administration of antigen at a site distal to the original one will evoke a very poor response in the local lymph nodes. This may be because all the antigen-specific cells have been summoned to the site of the initial attack and it may take a while to reapportion these cells between the two locales.

Also serving to localize the antigen-specific lymphocytes in the lymph nodes is the nonspecific influx of granulocytes into the involved nodes. These cells plug up the lymphatics and prevent lymphocyte egress. Not all of the factors leading to the dramatic decline in the rate of lymphocyte egress from a lymph node have been defined.[30,31]

It appears that the antigen itself does not necessarily have to be carried to a lymph node in order to incite a reaction there. It is clear that such antigen localization does occur, but recent evidence suggests that circulating lymphocytes can contact an antigen, become sensitized to it, and then migrate to the nearest lymph node carrying a stimulatory message to the resident lymphocytes. This process has been demonstrated only for the T-cell population and is called "recruitment." The recruiting T cell does not carry antigen back to the node. The only requirement for this activity described thus far is that the T cell needs a surface-expressed protein of an, as yet, unspecified nature in order to recruit effector cells.[32] Recruitment may be one way by which host sensitization and eventual rejection of a renal transplant takes place. The release of donor-tissue antigens directly into the blood is probably important as well (see Chap. 9).

Interdependence of Humoral and Cellular Responses

Thus far we have presented a very simple picture of an immune system neatly divided into two parts, a cellular limb and a humoral limb. Work of the past decade, however, has forced a revision of this uncomplicated view. Essential to attaining a new sophistication in our understanding of the immune response has been the observation that the ability to mount a humoral response to most antigens requires the concomitant activity of T cells. Such T-cell activity is called *T helper activity*, and the cells involved are called *T helper cells* (Fig. 1-21).[33] Antigens that demand T-cell cooperation in eliciting a B-cell humoral response are called *T-cell-dependent antigens*. There are some exceptions, and antigens which seem to require only B-cell activity in order to induce a humoral response are called *T-cell-independent antigens*. T helper cells do not make antibody. Rather their role is to interact with the B-cell population so that the latter can mount an effective humoral response. How this is accomplished will be discussed in Chapter 5.

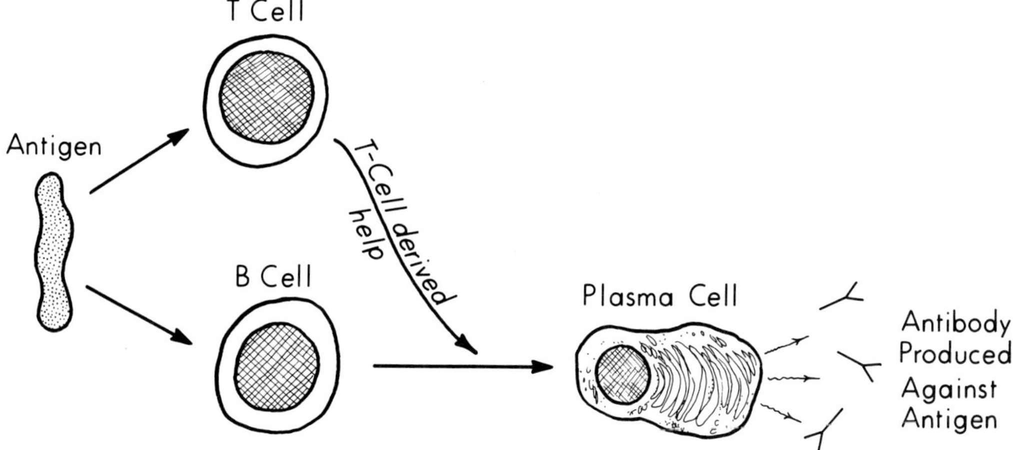

Fig. 1-21. T helper cells are required for the production of a B-cell-mediated humoral response to many antigens.

The existence of T helper cells explains the observation we alluded to earlier, namely, that neonatal thymectomy not only compromises T-cell function but also significantly reduces the B-cell humoral response against most antigens.[34] Thymectomy removes T cells involved in both effector and helper functions.

Are these T helper cells a distinct subpopulation from the T killer cells, or can one cell subserve both functions? The answer to this is not clear at present, but most evidence indicates that two separate T-cell subpopulations are involved (see Chap. 5).

The Secondary Response and Immunologic Memory

Up to this point we have investigated the immune response to antigens that the immune system has never seen before. The responses we have described are therefore called *primary* and differ significantly from the body's response to a second exposure to an antigen. A *secondary* response is more rapid and of greater intensity than a primary response. This observation illustrates another basic characteristic of the immune system—*memory*. Secondary responses are called *anamnestic* because the immune system"remembers" having encountered the antigen before. The first encounter has primed the host so that upon subsequent exposure the immune system is effectively alerted and prepared to deliver a devastating blow against the antigen.[35]

Immunologic memory is a characteristic of both B and T cells. The responsibility for anamnestic responses is felt to reside in specialized B and T lymphocytes called memory cells, generated during initial exposure to antigen.

The secondary response in the lymph nodes and the spleen appears much like the primary response, but events happen more quickly and the degree of cellular activity is greater.[36] Antigen penetrates rapidly into the cortical follicles where it is rapidly bound to the surface of reticulum cells and macrophages. This rapid immune adherence of the secondary response is due to the presence of antibody molecules that can bind to the surface of these cells and hence are termed *cytophilic*. These cytophilic antibodies exist as the result of the previous primary response. Upon second introduction of antigen into the lymph node, the antigen can combine with these antibody molecules and the resulting complexes rapidly bind to the dendritic reticulum cells of the follicles via receptors for the Fc portion of antibody present on those cells. In this way the antigen is efficiently localized within the follicles during the secondary response.[37] This localization is in contrast to the primary response where the antigen is found throughout the medullary sinuses as well as in the cortical follicles. During a secondary immune response the germinal centers proliferate rapidly and often so extensively that they spill over into the medullary areas. Cellular activity is also pronounced in the T-cell regions. In Chapter 6 we shall examine the cellular basis of immunologic memory.

LYMPHADENOPATHY AND SPLENOMEGALY

We have just described a great deal of cellular activity that occurs in the lymph node during an immune response. The lymph nodes in which these reactions occur often enlarge. The clinical finding of enlarged lymph nodes is almost always an important one. An understanding of the structure and function of lymph nodes provides a way to approach the problem of lymph node enlargement. If the lymphadenopathy is localized, the clue to the anatomical source is obtained by a knowledge of the area drained by each set of lymph nodes.

There are two major aspects of lymph node enlargement. First, the nodes are filters. This is part of the reason for lymph node enlargement in metastatic disease. Tumor cells are picked up by lymphatics and filtered out by the appropriate nodes. Second, the nodes are also the sites of normal immune lymphocytic proliferation. Therefore, enlargement is seen (1) in infections, due to viruses, parasites, bacteria and fungi, (2) in immune-associated states such as the rheumatic diseases, sarcoidosis, autoimmune hemolytic anemia and drug-sensitivity reactions, and (3) in the case of intrinsic neoplasms such as lymphomas and Hodgkin's disease.

Localized lymphadenopathy in cancer can be viewed from two perspectives. Viewing the nodes as a filter, it is an indication of tumor extension. However, upon node biopsy such enlarged nodes often show immunologic activation. There is evidence that in some of these cases these nodes are the site of lymphocyte proliferation directed against tumor antigens. In this situation the enlarged nodes may be better left alone than removed.

Often no clear-cut cause is found in people with lymph node enlargement—whether local or generalized—and with vague constitutional symptoms. Biopsy of these lymph nodes reveals "atypical hyperplasia."[38] This diagnosis is nonspecific and usually refers to an increase in the number and immaturity of cells as well as the presence of follicles with active germinal centers. Many patients so afflicted may eventually develop serious and often fatal diseases.

Splenomegaly can be understood in the same way as lymph node enlargement but is more often associated with systemic diseases such as bacterial endocarditis, malaria and other generalized parasitic infections, rheumatic diseases, lymphomas, and disseminated cancer.

SUMMARY

The organs of the immune system can be conveniently divided into two groups. The central organs (the bone marrow and thymus) provide the cell precursors for the immunocompetent cells. Some lymphocytes emerge from the bone marrow and are processed in the thymus. These become T cells and are responsible for cell-mediated immunity. A second population of cells avoids thymic processing. These are the B cells and can transform into antibody-secreting plasma cells. Most of the action of host defense occurs in the peripheral lymphoreticular system. The lymph nodes serve as the primary site of local defense against antigen, the spleen as the principal systemic defense.

The primary cells of the immune system are the macrophage and the lymphocyte. The macrophage acts as a nonspecific phagocyte and also can present antigen in immunogenic form to the lymphocyte. The lymphocyte specifically recognizes antigen and initiates and carries out numerous processes aimed at its destruction or removal. Toward this end certain lymphocytes (B cells) differentiate into plasma cells and secrete antibody molecules capable of specifically binding the antigen. Other cells (T cells) partake in what is termed cell-mediated immunity and can directly destroy foreign substances by mechanisms that are only now being elucidated. The activation of T helper cells is also required for the generation of a maximal B-cell antibody response to most antigens. Both B and T cells secrete lymphokines with various biological activities, including the ability to attract inflammatory cells to the site of immunologic reactivity. The other major link of the immune system with the inflammatory system is the complement system. All of these elements of the host defense are involved to some degree in the response against most (but not all) antigens.

Second exposure to an antigen elicits a more rapid and powerful response than does initial exposure and is due to the generation of memory cells during the primary response. Both B and T populations can be primed by an antigen and will respond vigorously to a second challenge with that same antigen.

REFERENCES

1. Frank, M. M., and Atkinson, J. P.: Complement in clinical medicine. D. M., January, 1975.
2. Dias da Silva, W., and Lepow, I. H.: Complement as a mediator of inflammation. J. Exp. Med., *125*:921, 1967.
3. Henson, P. M.: The adherence of leukocytes and platelets induced by fixed IgG antibody or complement. Immunology, *16*:107, 1969.
4. Ward, P. A., and Hill, J. H.: Biological role of complement products. J. Immunol., *108*:1137, 1972.
5. Müller-Eberhard, H. J.: Complement. Ann. Rev. Biochem., *38*:389, 1969.
6. Osler, A. G., and Sandberg, A. L.: Alternate complement pathways. Prog. Allergy, *17*:51, 1973.
7. Weiss, L.: The Cells and Tissues of the Immune System, Englewood Cliffs, N.J., Prentice-Hall, 1972.
8. Till, J. E., McCulloch, E. A., Phillips, R. A., and Siminovitch, L.: Analysis of Differentiating clones derived from marrow. Cold Spring Harbor Symp. Quant. Biol., *32*:461, 1967.
9. Miklem, H. S., Ford, C. E., Evans, E. P., and Gray, J.: Interrelationship of myeloid and lymphoid cells. Proc. R. Soc. Lond.[Biol.], *165*:78, 1966.
10. Claman, H. N., and Chaperon, E. A.: Immunologic complementation between thymus and bone marrow cells. Transplant. Rev., *1*:92, 1969.
11. Polliak, A., *et al.*: Identification of human B and T lymphocytes by scanning electron microscopy. J. Exp. Med., *138*:607, 1973.
12. Alexander, E., Sanders, S., and Braylan, R.: Purported difference between human T- and B-cell surface morphology is an artefact. Nature, *261*:239, 1976.
13. Good, R. A., and Gabrielson, A. E. (eds.): The Thymus in Immunobiology: Structure Functions and Role in Disease. New York, Harper and Row, 1964.
14. Levey, R. H., Trainin, N., and Law, L. W.: Evidence for function of thymic tissue in diffusion chambers implanted in neonatally thymectomized mice. J. Natl. Cancer Inst., *31*:199, 1963.
15. Gallo, R. C.: Terminal transferase and leukemia. N. Engl. J. Med., *292*:804, 1975.
16. Goldstein, G., and Mackay, I. R.: The Human Thymus. London, William Heinemann Medical Books, 1969.
17. Stuttman, O., Yunis, E. J., and Good, R. A.: Studies on thymus function. J. Exp. Med., *132*:583, 1970.
18. Yoffey, J., and Courtice, F.: Lymphatics, Lymph and Lymphoid Tissue. Cambridge, Mass., Harvard University Press, 1956.
19. Drinken, C., Field, M. E., and Ward, H. K.: The filtering capacity of lymph nodes. J. Exp. Med., *59*:393, 1934.
20. Parrott, D. M. V., deSousa, M. A. B., and East, J.: Thymic-dependent areas in the lymphoid organs of neonatally thymectomized mice. J. Exp. Med., *123*:191, 1966.
21. Sprent, J.: Migration of T and B lymphocytes in the mouse. Cell. Immunol., *7*:40, 1973.
22. Howard, J. C.: The life span and recirculation of marrow-derived small lymphocytes from the rat thoracic duct., J. Exp. Med., *135*:185, 1972.
23. Nossal, G. J. V., Abbot, A., Mitchell, J., and

Lummus, Z.: Antigens in immunity. J. Exp. Med., *127*:277, 1968.
24. Nossal, G. J. V., Austin, C. M., Pye, J., and Mitchell, J.: Antigens in immunity. Aust. J. Exp. Biol. Med. Sci., *42*:311, 1964.
25. ——: Antigens in immunity. Int. Arch. Allergy Appl. Immunol., *29*:368, 1966.
26. Langevoort, H. L.: The histophysiology of the antibody response. Lab. Invest., *12*:106, 1963.
27. Avrameas, S., and Leduc, L. E.: Detection of simultaneous antibody synthesis in plasma cells and specialized lymphocytes in rabbit lymph nodes. J. Exp. Med., *131*:1137, 1970.
28. Makinodan, T., Sado, T., Groves, D. L., and Price, G.: Growth patterns of antibody-forming cell populations. Curr. Top. Microbiol. Immunol., *49*:80, 1969.
29. Sprent, J., and Miller, J. F. A. P.: Effect of recent antigen priming on adoptive immune responses. J. Exp. Med., *138*:143, 1973.
30. McConnell, I., Lachmann, P. J., and Hobart, M. J.: Restoration of specific immunological virginity. Nature, *250*:113, 1974.
31. Ford, W. L.: Lymphocyte migration and immune responses. Prog. Allergy, *19*:1, 1975.
32. Livnat, S., and Cohen, I. R.: Recruitment of effector lymphocytes by initiator lymphocytes. Eur. J. Immunol., *5*:357, 1975.
33. Miller, J. F. A. P., and Mitchell, G. F.: Cell to cell interaction in the immune response. J. Exp. Med., *128*:801, 1968.
34. Miller, J. F. A. P.: Effect of neonatal thymectomy on the immunological responsiveness of the mouse. Proc. R. Soc. Lond. [Biol.], *156*:415, 1962.
35. Celada, F.: The cellular basis of immunologic memory. Prog. Allergy, *15*:223, 1971.
36. Hanna, M. G., and Szakel, A.: Localization of ^{125}I-labelled antigen in germinal centers of mouse spleen. J. Immunol., *101*:949, 1968.
37. Lang, P. G., and Ada, G. L.: Antigen in tissues. Immunology, *13*:523, 1967.
38. Moore, R. D., Weisberger, A. J., and Bowerfind, E. J.: An evaluation of lymphadenopathy in systemic disease. Arch. Intern. Med., *99*:751, 1957.

2 Antigens and Antibodies

ANTIGENS AND ANTIGENIC DETERMINANTS

Antigens are molecules which can be bound by antibody. However, the antigen-binding site of an antibody is much smaller than typical antigens such as viral subunits, enzymes and bacterial cell wall glycoproteins, and therefore only a small part of any antigen can be bound by any single antibody (Fig. 2-1). The actual part of an antigen that fits within the antibody combining site is called an *antigenic determinant.*

The maximum size of a determinant is limited by the size of the antigen-binding region of the antibody. The ability to bind antigen resides in the $F(ab)_2$ portion of the antibody molecule. Within this region an IgG molecule contains two identical cup-like structures where antigen can be bound, each with a volume of about 3000 cubic Å. These antigen-binding regions can accomodate structures no larger than five to seven amino acids of a protein or five to seven glucose residues of a polysaccharide.[1,1a] These measurements therefore represent the maximum size of an antigenic determinant.

Antigens are not bound covalently within the antibody combining regions, but are bound by weak forces such as hydrogen and hydrophobic bonds, Van der Waals forces, and perhaps ionic forces. Each antigen-binding region is specific in that it is able to bind certain structures with high affinity, others with lower affinities, and still others not at all (see Fig. 1-6).[2] For example, antibody capable of binding aminobenzene in the meta configuration will not bind para-aminobenzene nearly as well. Similarly, antibody which binds an intact protein may fail to bind the same protein when it is denatured.[3] The measurement of the similarity of two antigens is expressed in the concept of *crossreactivity*: an antibody that binds a given antigen will also bind antigens with similar conformations. Thus, a certain percentage of antibody molecules directed against one antigen may also react with another antigen depending upon the extent of crossreactivity between them. Specificity is retained in the strength of binding, for each antibody is uniquely suited to bind one particular molecular structure best. Those molecules which are not of the specific target conformation will be only weakly bound if, in fact, they can be bound at all.

Most antigens have several antigenic determinants. The humoral response to any antigen is the sum of the responses to each individual determinant. On the basis of size alone, one would expect polypeptides with 100 amino acid residues to

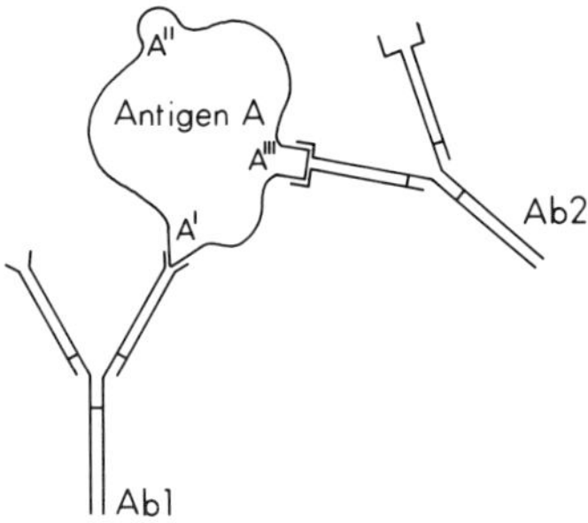

Ab1 is specific for determinant A′ of Antigen A

Ab2 is specific for determinant A‴ of Antigen A

Fig. 2-1. The part of an antigen bound by an antibody is called an antigenic determinant. Most antigens possess many determinants which are bound by different antibody molecules.

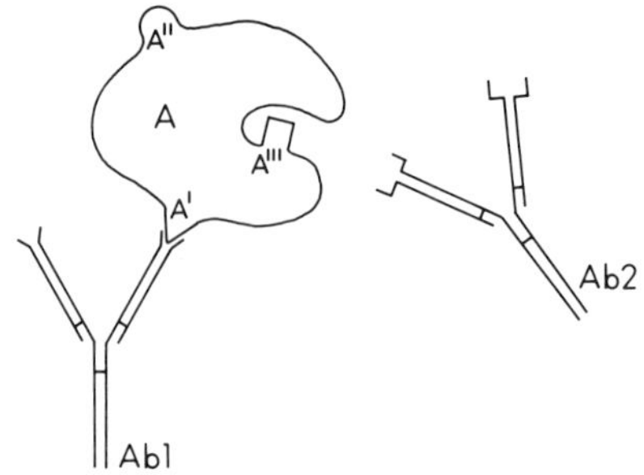

Ab2 does not have access to "hidden" determinant A‴

Fig. 2-2. Only determinants expressed on the surface of an antigen can be bound by antibody. Thus the antigen above has, effectively, only two determinants.

contain approximately 14 to 20 nonoverlapping determinants. However, a typical globular 100-residue protein may contain only a very few determinants. Why is this? When a protein is in its natural state it is folded upon itself with much of its structure totally hidden from the outside. Only the surface of the protein is available for interacting with antibody (Fig. 2-2). The conformation of a protein determines not only which potential determinants are exposed to the surface but, further, which determinants are accessible to enter the antigen-binding site.[4]

IMMUNOGENS

We must distinguish the concept of antigen from that of immunogen. In order for a molecule to be considered an antigen, it need be capable only of being bound by an antibody molecule. Whether or not a molecule can induce an *active* immune response such as we described in Chapter 1 is of no consequence as far as its definition as an antigen is concerned. *Immunogens* are those antigens that are capable of eliciting an active immune response.

What qualities must an antigen possess in order to be an immunogen, and how are the characteristics of an immunogen related to the type of immune response that is evoked? The immunogenicity of a molecule is dependent upon several general molecular characteristics:

Size. There is a correlation between the size of a molecule and its ability to elicit an antibody response. Many small molecules can be bound by preformed antibody but cannot by themselves stimulate an immune response. These molecules are called *haptens*. Haptens are nothing more than antigenic determinants. If a hapten is coupled to a larger molecule, called the *carrier*, it becomes immunogenic and can stimulate an immune response. Thus, antigenic determinants by themselves are not immunogenic, and must be part of a larger molecule in order to evoke immune reactivity.

Careful studies have been done to determine the minimal size requirement for immunogenicity. For peptides, it seems that a minimum of seven amino acids is required.[5] There is an interesting distinction between cell-mediated and humoral immunity with regard to the size of an immunogen. The smaller the antigen the more likely it is to induce cell-mediated immunity without any antibody formation.[6]

Foreignness. There is a relationship between a substance's immunogenicity and its foreignness.[7] For example, within a given species, the more a protein varies in its amino acid sequence from the homologous protein in the host, the more potent an immunogen it will be. However, this must not be taken as a hard and fast rule. As we shall see, there are several human disease states associated with the production of antibodies against the host's own tissues (autoantibodies). In these situations, autologous proteins and polynucleotides are able to act as immunogens.

Conformation and Charge. Most any molecule of any conformation can be immunogenic provided it meets the requirements for size and foreignness discussed above. There is no evidence that an antigen needs to be electrically charged to be immunogenic. Not surprisingly, the charge of an immunogen bears an inverse relationship to the net charge of the antibodies produced in response to it.[8]

Solubility. The physical state of a molecule also contributes to its immunogenicity. The more insoluble a molecule is, the more immunogenic it is.[9] Therefore, intermolecular cross-linking, heat aggregation and attachment to insoluble carriers all increase immunogenicity.

Other Factors. Since the measure of immunogenicity is the elicitation of an immune response, factors other than those intrinsic to the immunogen may modify the host's response and enhance the molecule's apparent immunogenicity. *Adjuvants* are experimental agents that can be administered along with an antigen and which may cause any of three effects:[9a] (1) they can enhance the immune response to an immunogen; (2) they can confer immunogenicity on substances incapable of inducing an immune response by themselves; and (3) they can alter the nature of the response to a given immunogen. Some adjuvants commonly employed in experimental work include water-in-oil emulsions (incomplete Freund's adjuvant), endotoxin, aluminum hydroxide ($AlOH_3$), and live or killed microorganisms such as mycobacteria, *Bordetella pertussis* or *Corynebacterium parvum*. Complete Freund's adjuvant is a water-in-oil emulsion with killed mycobacteria in the oil phase. BCG is a live, attenuated strain of *Mycobacterium bovis*. Some of these, notably BCG and *C. parvum*, have found their way into clinical practice in attempts to boost a patient's faltering immune system. There is as yet no clear understanding of how these adjuvants work. It has been suggested that they may nonspecifically stimulate immunoreactive cells, increase macrophage activity, or alter the traffic of recirculating lymphocytes through the lymph nodes. As with many situations in which several possible mechanisms have been proposed, the true explanation may rest with some combination of all.

The intrinsic ability of the host to respond to an antigen will also partly determine an antigen's immunogenicity. Perhaps most important in this regard are the recently discovered *immune response* (Ir) *genes*. The ability to mount both humoral and cellular responses against a given antigen is inherited as an autosomal dominant trait. Every individual has many Ir genes controlling immune reactivity against many antigens. Ir genes have been demonstrated in several animal species, but there is as yet little evidence of their presence in man (see Chap. 9).

Thus far we have described those characteristics of a molecule that determine its immunogenicity. However, immunogens do not all behave alike. Some elicit predominantly humoral responses, whereas others induce primarily cellular responses. Many immunogens provoke powerful humoral and cellular responses. Can we define the characteristics of an immunogen that determine the type of response that it will induce?

There are certain types of antigens that will elicit almost exclusively humoral responses.[10] In addition, some molecules not only selectively provoke humoral immunity but can do so without stimulating T-cell helper activity. These antigens can evoke an antibody response even in individuals lacking T cells. Such antigens are called *T-cell-independent antigens*.[11] They share two general characteristics: they are multivalent repeating molecules with identical antigenic determinants expressed many times on their surfaces, and they are poorly degraded by the body and therefore persist in the host for a long time. Polysaccharides and lipopolysaccharides comprise most of these molecules.

Other antigens can selectively stimulate a T-cell response. There are no well-defined structural requirements for such molecules. T cells appear to be more sensitive to antigenic stimulation than B cells, and hence low doses of some antigens as well as antigens of poor immunogenicity may preferentially stimulate a cellular response.[3,12]

Some antigens appear to demonstrate an inverse relationship between their ability to evoke a powerful T-cell response and the ability to stimulate a strong humoral response.[13] For example, polymerized bacterial flagellin (POL) is an excellent B-cell immunogen and can evoke a strong antibody response. If this molecule is chemically modified by the successive addition of acetoacetyl groups it loses the capacity to induce a humoral response and begins to stimulate a stronger and stronger T-cell response. Just how generalizable this inverse cellular/humoral relationship may be is not known.

THE HAPTEN-CARRIER PHENOMENON

We have defined haptens as small molecules capable of binding preexisting antibody but which by themselves are incapable of inducing an immune response. Only when they are bound to larger molecules, carriers, can they become immunogenic. This observation has been designated the *hapten-carrier phenomenon*.[11] An understanding of the hapten-carrier phenomenon allows us further to define immunogenicity; in particular, it provides the first step toward the understanding of immunologic memory and the role of the T helper cell in the humoral response.

The hapten most often utilized in studies of the hapten-carrier phenomenon is the 2,4-dinitrophenyl (DNP) radical. By itself this small molecule cannot elicit an immune response. If, however, it is conjugated to a carrier, an excellent antibody response against DNP can be observed. Thus, when DNP is conjugated to ovalbumin (OVA), a typical primary response occurs. Subsequent challenge with DNP-OVA evokes a powerful secondary (anamnestic) response. If a different carrier is used for the second challenge (for example, DNP conjugated to bovine gammaglobulin—BGG), a secondary anti-DNP response is *not* observed. One can then measure only a primary response to DNP (Fig. 2-3).[14]

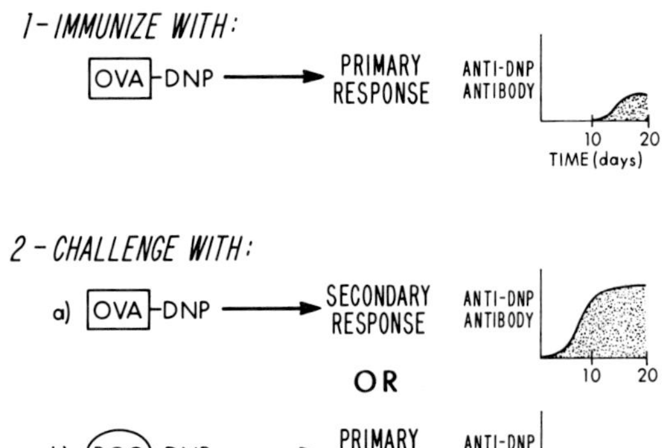

Fig. 2-3. The hapten-carrier phenomenon. Following immunization with the hapten DNP coupled to the carrier OVA, only rechallenge with DNP on that same carrier will elicit a secondary (anamnestic) response.

The hapten-carrier phenomenon is one of the fundamental observations of modern immunology. It becomes clear from the discussion above that the carrier does not serve merely to add bulk to the hapten but is intimately associated with the regulation of the humoral response to the hapten. In this first example we saw the importance of the carrier in immunologic memory. Thus, only rechallenge with carrier to which the animal had been previously sensitized could evoke a secondary antihapten response. We can extend this observation even further. If an animal is immunized with just the carrier OVA and then rechallenged with the complex DNP-OVA, a secondary anti-DNP response is seen. Thus immunologic memory is determined to a large extent by the carrier moiety (Fig. 2-4).[15]

Many experiments have shown that the T cell is responsible for the recognition of carrier and the B cell for the recognition of hapten.[16] Thus, when we speak of the role of the carrier in regulating an antibody response to a hapten, we are really referring to the ability of T helper cells to recognize carrier and then modify the B-cell antihapten response. This is the basis of the T helper activity described in Chapter 1. In essence, any antigen can be considered as a complex of haptens and carriers. We can look at a simple example, that of glucagon. Bovine glucagon elicits a marked humoral response in guinea pigs. It can be split into two fragments by trypsin. One fragment is capable of inducing T-cell blastogenesis and the other is very efficient at binding antiglucagon antibody and has no effect on T-cell function. Thus, one end of glucagon acts as the carrier and the other as the hapten.[17]

Not all antigens are so simple. A red blood cell bears many antigenic determinants, each of which can be considered a hapten. In this sense, hapten becomes a functional definition: a hapten is the determinant against which we are measuring antibody production. Consider two distinct antigenic determinants on the red-cell surface, X and Y. When we measure the production of anti-X antibody, determinant X is the hapten. If we measure the production of anti-Y, Y is the hapten. Since different B cells are involved in the recognition of determinants X and Y, the response to X and Y may differ markedly. Both these responses, as well as the responses against other red-cell determinants, will ordinarily occur at the same time, and thus many different lymphocyte populations are active in the response to any complex antigen.

How can we understand the way in which T and B cells interact to produce

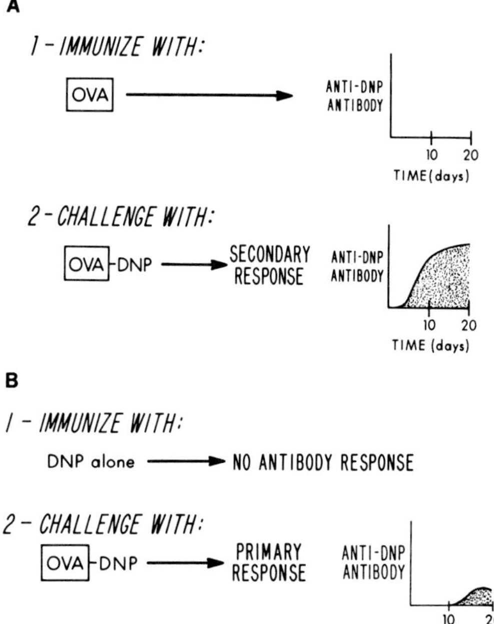

Fig. 2-4. (*A*) Following exposure to the carrier OVA, immunization with DNP-OVA elicits a secondary anti-DNP response. This result indicates that immunologic memory may be determined largely by the carrier moiety in some situations. (*B*) Immunization with DNP followed by challenge with DNP-OVA does not elicit a secondary anti-DNP response, further emphasizing the importance of the carrier in immunologic memory. However, hapten memory has been demonstrated to exist in other situations (see Chap. 6).

the hapten-carrier phenomenon? It is believed that T cells must first recognize the carrier and then communicate this fact to the hapten-specific B cells (Fig. 2-5). It is important to emphasize that such a communication *must* occur, since no one cell recognizes both hapten and carrier. Thus, the interpolation of "spacer" molecules between the hapten and the carrier does not affect the ability to mount a secondary antihapten response.[18] Further, if an animal has been primed to both DNP-OVA and to the carrier BGG, subsequent challenge with DNP-BGG elicits a secondary anti-DNP response. No cell has previously "seen" the DNP-BGG conjugate, yet we observe a secondary response. Thus, T cells which have seen the carrier BGG alone and B cells which have seen the hapten DNP, but never attached to BGG, can interact to produce a secondary response. Clearly, carrier and hapten are functionally distinct entities. The ways in which B cells and T cells communicate are discussed in Chapter 5.

SUMMARY

Antigens are molecules that can be bound by antibody. The structural parts of an antigen that actually fit into the antigen-binding site are referred to as antigenic determinants. Most antigens express several determinants on their surface.

Immunogens are antigens that can elicit an active immune response. Immunogenicity is determined by several

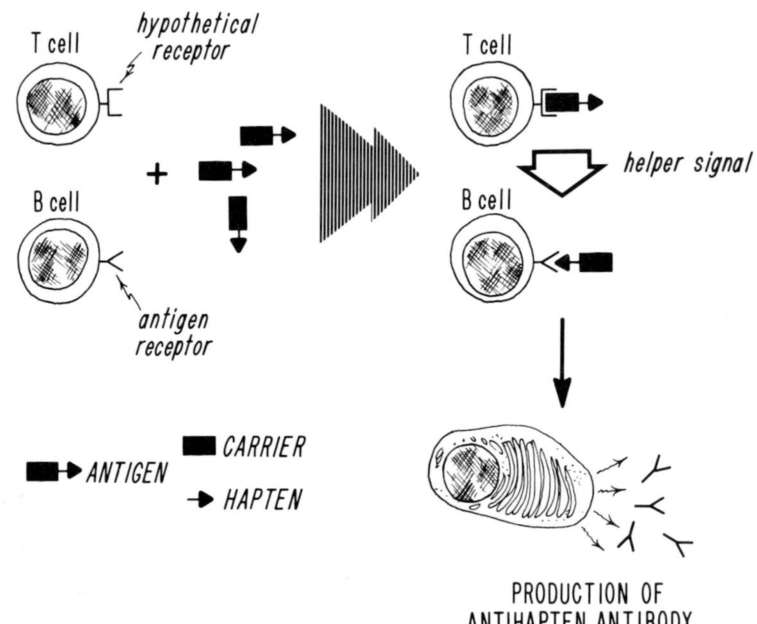

Fig. 2-5. Cooperation between T and B cells in the hapten-carrier phenomenon. The T cell recognizes carrier and is induced to deliver a helper signal to the hapten-binding B cell. The end result is the differentiation of the B cell into a plasma cell capable of producing antibody against the hapten.

factors, including the size, foreignness, conformation, charge and solubility of the molecule, as well as by other factors such as the presence of adjuvants and the immunologic status of the host.

Haptens are antigenic determinants, and as such are unable to elicit an immune response by themselves. However, when a hapten is coupled to a carrier molecule, an antihapten response can ensue. Only by rechallenging with that hapten on the same carrier can a secondary (anamnestic) antihapten response be elicited. Thus, the carrier moiety provides more than mere bulk to the hapten, and is itself an important determinant of immunologic memory and therefore of the type of response that is observed. T helper cells recognize the carrier moiety and B cells recognize the hapten. Communication between these two cell types is necessary for an effective humoral response against most antigens. Only a small subclass of molecules termed T-cell-independent antigens can elicit a significant humoral response without T-helper-cell activity.

For the remainder of this chapter we shall be focusing on the immunoglobulin molecule. The elucidation of the structure of this molecule has been one of the signal triumphs of modern science. Virtually our entire understanding of immune recognition stems from our knowledge of the interaction of antibody and antigen. For this reason an appreciation of the structure and function of the immunoglobulin molecule is essential to achieving an understanding of the workings of the immune system.

THE IMMUNOGLOBULIN MOLECULE

Basic Structural Considerations

Pictured in Figure 2-6, in highly schematic form, is an immunoglobulin molecule. The basic unit of every immunoglobulin is a symmetrical four-polypeptide chain structure composed of two types of polypeptide chains, distinguishable on the basis of their molecular weights, and referred to as heavy (H) and light (L) chains.[19] In addition, a varying amount of carbohydrate is bound to the protein skeleton, primarily to the heavy chains.

The structural formula for any immunoglobulin can be represented as $(HL)_{2n}$ where $(HL)_2$ represents the basic four-polypeptide unit and where $n = 1, 2, 3, 4$ or 5. Thus, the smallest immunoglobulin contains two light and two heavy chains (1 basic unit; for example, IgG) and the largest, ten light and ten heavy chains (5 basic units; for example, IgM).

The heavy chains have been divided into five classes (γ, μ, α, ϵ, δ) based upon their serologic characteristics.[20] By this we mean the following: human immunoglobulins, like most human proteins, behave as antigens and elicit an immune response when they are injected into a foreign host such as a rabbit. The rabbit's immune system responds against determinants on the surface of the immunoglobulin molecules which it views as foreign, and produces anti-immunoglobulin antibody. This resultant rabbit antibody (antisera) has been used to define five serologically distinct classes of

THE ANTIBODY MOLECULE

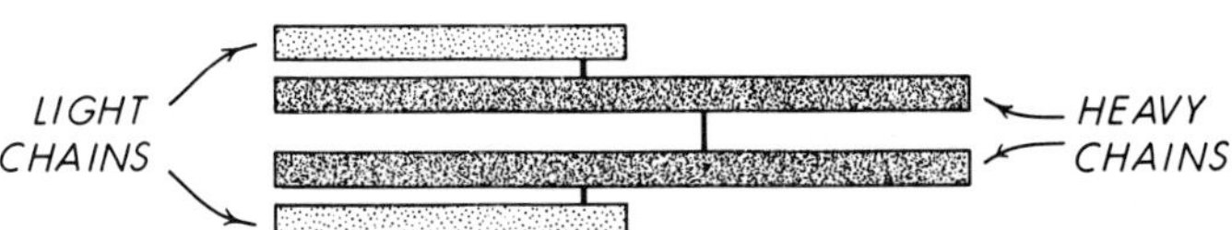

Fig. 2-6. The basic structure of the immunoglobulin molecule.

immunoglobulin heavy chains. All heavy chains of a given class share certain antigenic determinants, called class-specific antigenic determinants, and react with identical antisera.

Any one immunoglobulin possesses heavy chains of only a single class; one never finds a molecule containing, for example, one γ and one α chain. Those immunoglobulins containing two γ heavy chains are called IgG, those containing μ heavy chains are called IgM, and those possessing α, ϵ and δ heavy chains are called, respectively, IgA, IgE and IgD. The γ and α heavy chains have been further subdivided into the serologically definable subclasses IgG_1, IgG_2, IgG_3, and IgG_4, and IgA_1 and IgA_2. μ Sublcasses have been proposed but at present have not been well defined.[20] All of the heavy chains in a given molecule are identical.

There are only two types of serologically defined light chains, κ and λ, each of which can associate with any class of heavy chain. Like the heavy chains, all of the light chains present in a given immunoglobulin molecule are of one kind; they are never mixed within a molecule. Thus, for example, an IgG molecule is composed of two heavy and two light chains (n=1) and can have the structural formula $(\gamma\kappa)_2$ or $(\gamma\lambda)_2$, but never $\gamma_2\kappa\lambda$ (Fig. 2-7). κ Chains are present in about two thirds of human immunoglobulin molecules, λ chains in about one third. The light chains contained in any single molecule are identical to each other.

The light chains are bound to the heavy chains by disulfide bridges (thus far, only one genetic variant of the IgA_2 subclass has been found to lack such linkages)[21] and, probably more importantly, by hydrogen and hydrophobic bonds. The heavy chains are also bound to each other by disulfide linkages. Different classes and subclasses of immunoglobulin have different numbers of interchain disulfide bonds. Intrachain disulfide bridges are also present at regular intervals on all light and heavy chains, each enclosing 60 to 70 amino acids. Schematic diagrams of the classes and subclasses of immunoglobulin are shown in Figure 2-8.

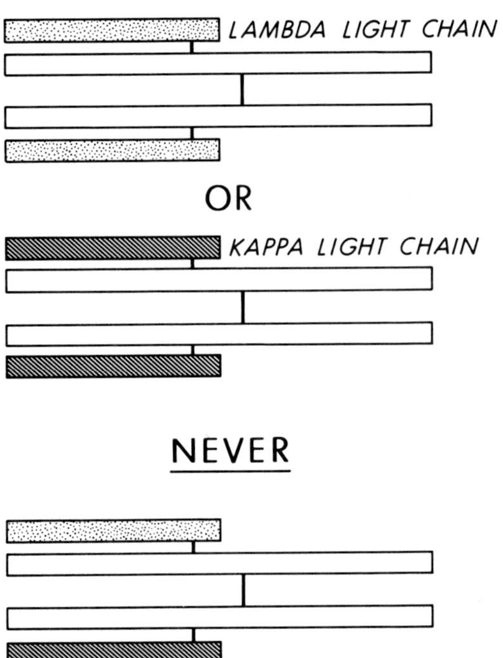

Fig. 2-7. Any single immunoglobulin molecule possesses only one type of light chain.

The Subunit Structure of the Immunoglobulin Molecule

Despite their substantial difference in size, the light and heavy chains exhibit a remarkable structural similarity. Each polypeptide chain is built up out of small subunit structures, regions of approximately 110 amino acids centered around an intrachain disulfide bridge (Fig. 2-9).[22] Light chains are composed of two such regions, heavy chains of four or more. These repeating subunits are called *homology domains* because of their great structural similarity to one another, and are believed to have derived from the duplication and subsequent mutation of a single gene coding for a peptide of about 110 amino acids.[23]

There are two types of homology do-

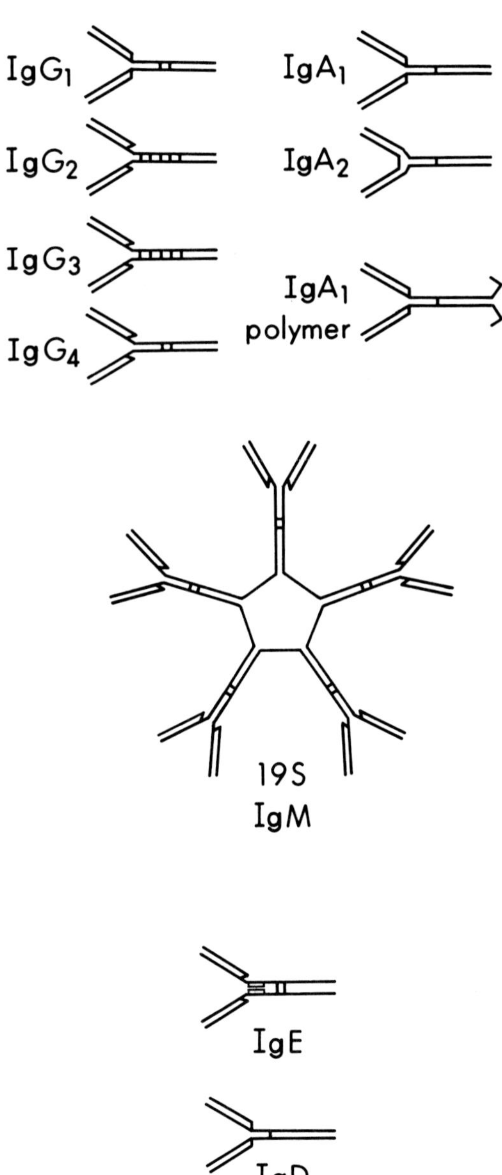

Fig. 2-8. The structures of the various immunoglobulin classes and subclasses.

mains, referred to as *variable* and *constant* regions.

Variable Regions. The homology domain found at the amino terminal end of each polypeptide chain is called the variable (V) region. Within this domain there is a marked variability in the amino acid residues present at a number of positions. The variability is so great that the variable regions of an immunoglobulin produced by any given clone of cells are different from those of all other immunoglobulin molecules. Certain amino acid positions are especially highly variable and have been designated *hypervariable loci*. The relationship between amino acid variability and position can be plotted on a graph as shown in Figure 2-10.[24] This graph reveals that the hypervariable loci are grouped into several hypervariable subregions. Light-chain variable regions have three such hypervariable subregions and heavy-chain variable regions have four. The positions between the hypervariable subregions are called *framework residues* and are relatively constant among all polypeptides.

All of this variability in the placement of amino acids is not without its purpose. The variable regions are responsible for the antigenic specificity of the immunoglobulin molecule. When the intact molecule is assembled, the variable domains of the light and heavy chains overlap at the amino terminus of the molecule, forming cuplike regions where antigen can be bound (Fig. 2-11). The antigen-binding site is approximately the size of a hexapeptide or hexasaccharide.[1,1a,25] Each antigen-binding region is composed of the variable regions of one light and one heavy chain. An IgG molecule thus has two *identical* antigen-binding sites. The amino acids which define the internal geometry of the binding region and thus determine the antigenic specificity of the molecule are, not surprisingly, the hypervariable loci. Their variability permits the construction of many diverse antigen-binding sites, each with its own unique antigenic specificity.

Confirmation that the hypervariable subregions define the antigen-binding site has been derived from affinity-labelling studies (see Fig. 2-12).[26] This technique utilizes small haptens to which a reactive group, such as a diazo group or a photoac-

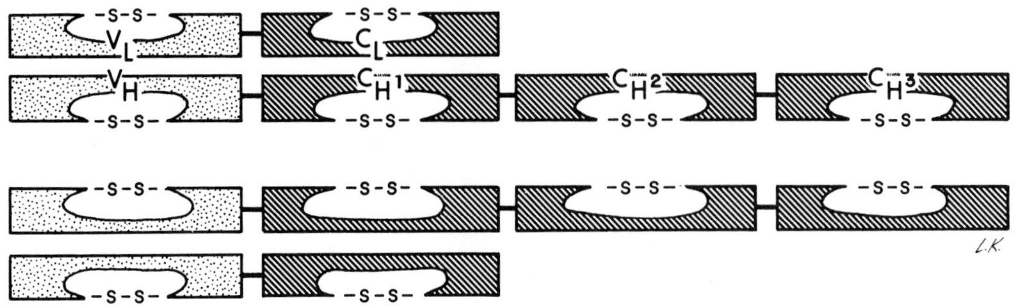

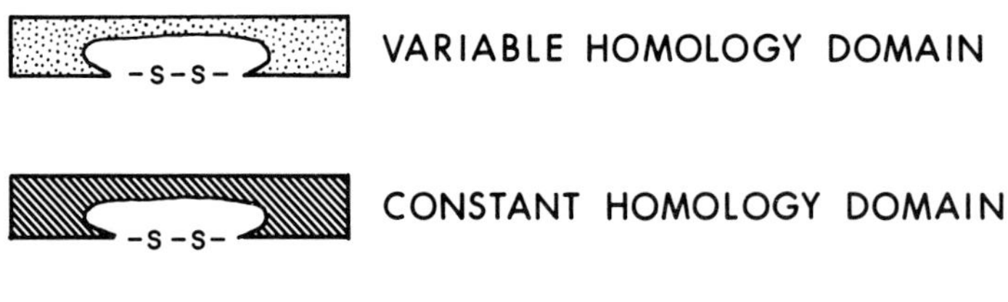

V_L VARIABLE REGION OF THE LIGHT CHAIN

C_L CONSTANT REGION OF THE LIGHT CHAIN

V_H VARIABLE REGION OF THE HEAVY CHAIN

$C_H{}^{1,2,3}$ CONSTANT REGIONS OF THE HEAVY CHAIN

Fig. 2-9. Each polypeptide chain of an immunoglobulin molecule consists of a linked repetition of several homology domains, regions of about 110 amino acids centered around an intrachain disulfide bridge and bearing a remarkable structural resemblance to each other.

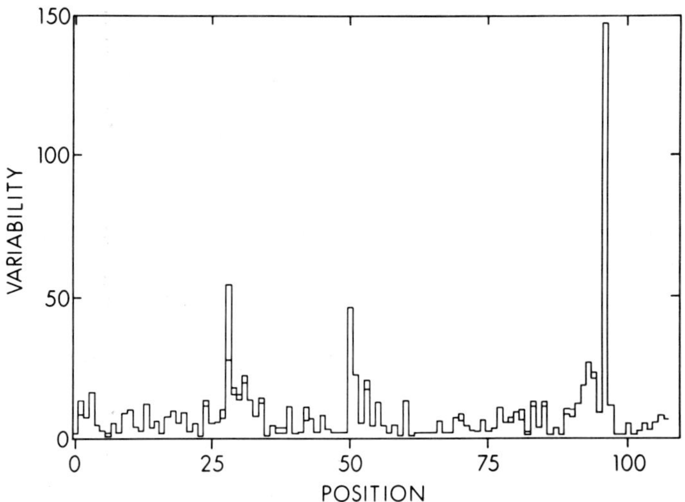

Fig. 2-10. A graph of the amino acid variability plotted for each amino acid position of immunoglobulin light chains. Note the grouping of the hypervariable loci into hypervariable subregions. (Adapted from Wu, T. T., and Kabat, E. A.: An analysis of the sequences of variable regions of Bence-Jones proteins and myeloma light chains and their implications for antibody complementarity. J. Exp. Med., *132*:211, 1970.)

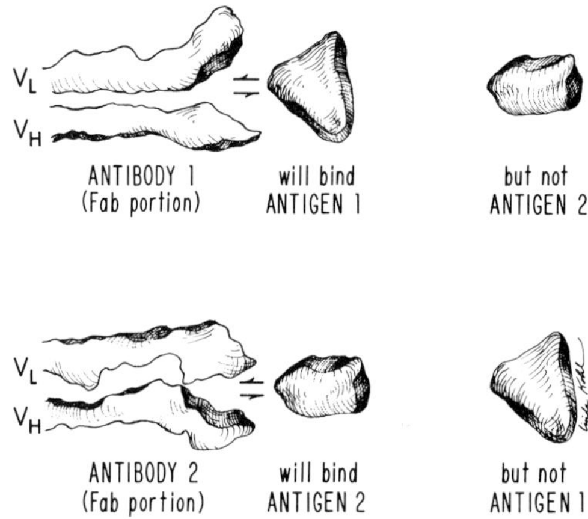

Fig. 2-11. The antigen-binding region of an antibody molecule can bind certain antigens well, others poorly if at all.

tivated aromatic azide, is attached. When the hapten is bound by antibody, the reactive group is transferred and binds covalently at or near the antibody combining site. The antibody is then hydrolyzed and the resultant peptides are analyzed to see where labelling has occurred. With recent refinement of the technique, affinity labelling appears to be restricted to the hypervariable subregions.

Since the antigen-binding site of every immunoglobulin molecule is structurally unique, each immunoglobulin should itself have unique antigenic determinants within its structure that it does not share with other immunoglobulin molecules. Antibody directed against these unique determinants of an individual immunoglobulin molecule is referred to as *anti-idiotype antiserum,* and the unique determinant(s) is called the *idiotype* of the particular immunoglobulin (Fig. 2-13).[27] Ideally, an idiotype should be the serologic expression of the antibody combining site of a unique immunoglobulin molecule. Although it is presently impossible to prove that a given anti-idiotype antiserum is in fact directed against a unique antigen-binding site, idiotype remains at present the best serologic approximation of the structure responsible for antigen recognition.

Constant Regions. The second type of homology domain does not display the conspicuous amino acid variability of the variable regions, and is called the constant domain. Light chains have only one constant region and heavy chains have several, the precise number depending upon the class of the molecule. Aside from a limited number of amino acid irregularities at some positions (substitutions, deletions, additions), the constant regions are basically *equivalent within a given class.* Comparison of the constant regions between *different classes* of immunoglobulin reveals a greater variation in the precise number of amino acids present, the sequence of amino acids and the amount of bound carbohydrate. The constant regions are not involved in antigen recognition, and a large degree of amino acid variability is not required. Nevertheless, as we shall see, the constant regions do more than simply supply a structural backbone for the antigen-binding portion of the molecule.

The constant domains, and the Fc portion in particular (recall that the Fc portion consists of all the constant regions except CH_1 and the constant domains of the light chains), convey biological activ-

Fig. 2-12. Affinity labelling. A hapten is labelled with a reactive group which can be transferred to the antibody molecule where the hapten is bound. Affinity labelling is limited to the hypervariable subregions of the antibody.

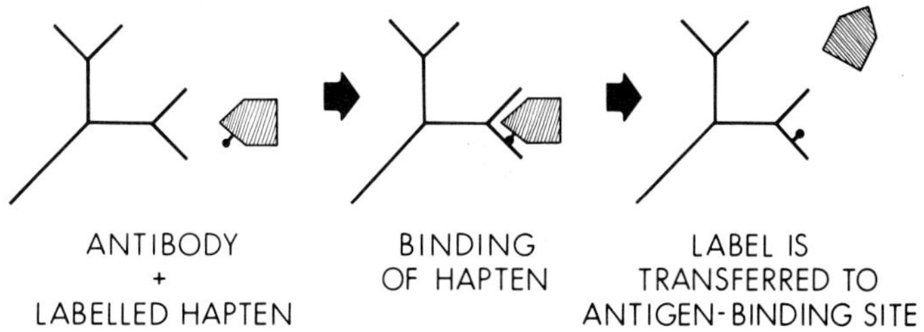

ANTIBODY + LABELLED HAPTEN

BINDING OF HAPTEN

LABEL IS TRANSFERRED TO ANTIGEN-BINDING SITE

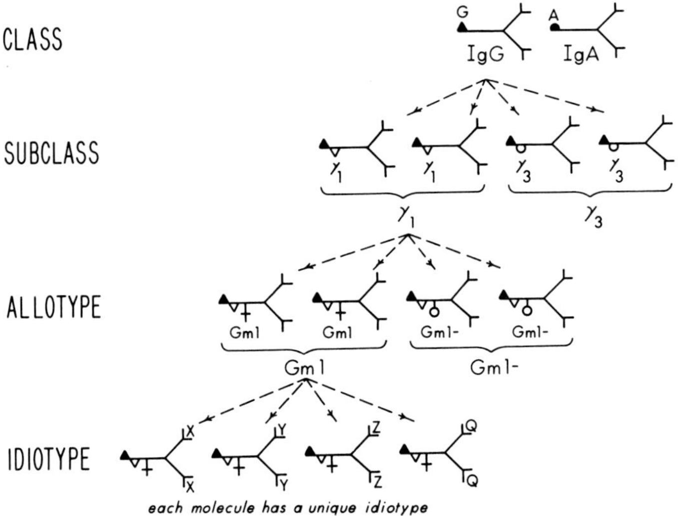

Fig. 2-13. The relationship between immunoglobulin class, subclass, allotype and idiotype is depicted in highly schematic form. These illustrations are designed to simplify these often difficult concepts and should not be taken literally. Fuller descriptions appear in the text. All molecules of the same class share some antigenic identity. Immunoglobulin molecules within a given class can be further broken down into serologically defined subclasses, for example, γ_1 and γ_3. Allelic forms associated with specific amino acid substitutions have been identified at certain loci within the genetic region coding for immunoglobulin polypeptides. The antigenic determinants associated with these genetically determined substitutions are called allotypes. Thus, as shown above, a γ_1 molecule can express either the Gm1 or the Gm1− allotype. Finally, the antigen-binding region of each individual antibody molecule should itself be antigenically unique, distinguishable from all other antibody molecules. The best serologic expression of the antigen-binding region is called the idiotype.

ity to the antibody molecule. Complement fixation, transplacental transfer, skin fixation, binding to macrophages and granulocytes, and mast-cell histamine release are all functions of the Fc portion of the immunoglobulin molecule. Each class and subclass of immunoglobulin differs in its ability to carry out these functions (Table 2-1).[20] Some of these activities have been further localized to specific parts of the Fc regions; for example, the second constant region of the heavy chain (CH_2) appears to be responsible for binding and activating complement.[28]

The rate of synthesis and catabolism of

Table 2-1. Characteristics of Immunoglobulin Molecules Determined by the Nature of Their Fc Regions

Immunoglobulin Function	*IgG*	*IgM*	*IgA*	*IgE*	*IgD*
Complement activation	$IgG_{1,3}$ + IgG_2 ±, IgG_4 −	+	Properdin pathway only	Properdin pathway only	Properdin pathway only
Cross placenta	$IgG_{1,3,4}$ + IgG_2 ±	—	—	—	—
Cytophilic to macrophages	$IgG_{1,3}$ + $IgG_{2,4}$ −	—	—	—	—
Fix to mast cells	—	—	—	+	—

an immunoglobulin molecule is determined by the Fc portion. The rate of clearance and hence the efficiency with which antigen-antibody complexes are removed from the body is largely determined by the biological properties of the antibody in the complex, and thus the Fc portion is a critical determinant of the rate of antigen removal.

Many of the functions of the Fc portion are only activated when the Fab portion of the antibody binds antigen. One of the more perplexing questions of immunology is how the binding of antigen by the Fab portion activates functions attributable to the distal end of the molecule. Investigators have sought to observe conformational changes in the Fc region associated with antigen binding (Fig. 2-14(1)), but such alterations have been difficult to detect.[29] Nevertheless, some recent studies have begun to produce data suggestive of a measurable degree of intramolecular mobility, and many investigators are convinced that interactions between the Fab and Fc portions of the antibody molecule will eventually be demonstrated.

An alternative hypothesis to explain the antigen-binding dependency of several Fc functions is that, rather than inducing an intramolecular conformational shift, the binding of antigen effects the aggregation of several antibodies, and thus brings into close approximation two or more Fc portions. It is postulated that Fc aggregation effectively creates an intermolecular active site and thereby generates the potential to carry out Fc-related functions (Fig. 2-14 (2)). Several Fc functions could theoretically be explained on this basis, notably mast-cell activation, the binding of cytophilic antibody to macrophages and granulocytes and complement fixation. Thus, the cross-linking of two or several IgE molecules on a mast cell is known to lead to mast-cell release. Similarly, antigen-aggregated cytophilic antibody binds more strongly to inflammatory cells than do single immunoglobulin molecules. Finally, several IgG molecules must bind to an antigen in order to activate complement, whereas only one IgM molecule—which is essentially an aggregate of five basic immunoglobulin units—is often sufficient. This last observation is especially intriguing in light of the recent visualization of the C1q molecule (the first component of the classical pathway that interacts with the Fc portion of antibody) by electron microscopy (Fig. 2-15).[30] It is readily apparent

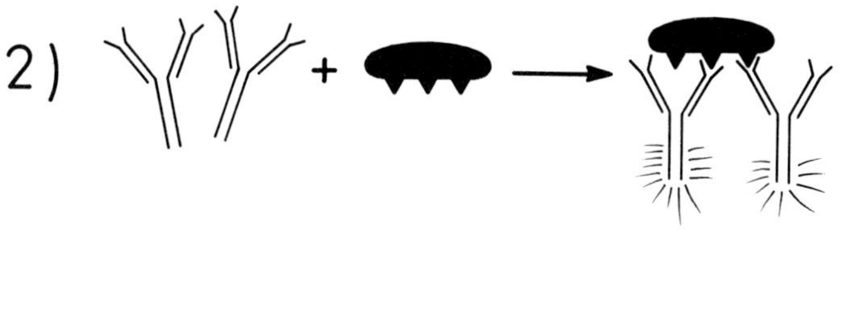

Fig. 2-14. Two theories of how antigen binding by the $F(ab)_2$ portion of an antibody molecule activates the biological potential of the Fc portion. (*1*) Antigen binding induces a conformational change in the Fc portion. (*2*) The aggregation of two or more antibody molecules brings their Fc portions into close proximity. It has been postulated that the drawing together of two or more Fc regions is responsible for inducing Fc-mediated immunologic function, perhaps via molecules which can sense such an aggregation phenomenon.

1)

2)

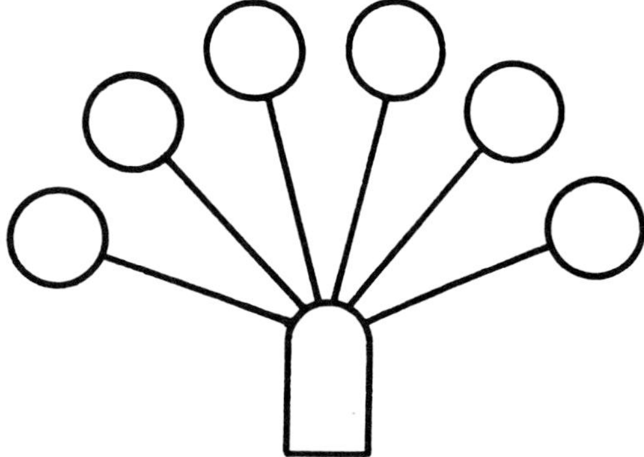

Fig. 2-15. Schematic rendering of the C1q molecule.

dimensional structure almost completely independent of the rest of the molecule. The three-dimensional structure of a variable and a constant region linked together as one continuous polypeptide chain is shown in Fig. 2-16.[31] Within each domain the chain weaves alternately back and forth to form two opposing planes, with four polypeptide segments forming one plane (white arrows) and three forming the other (black arrows). At the amino terminus of the molecule, the four-chain planes form the outer surface of the variable regions. The three-chain planes of one light-chain variable domain and one heavy-chain variable domain face each other to form a cavity about 10 Å deep and 15 Å across where antigen is bound. The amino acids lining the cavity belong to the hypervariable subregions.

that the structure of C1q with its six terminal projections emerging from a central subunit, is remarkably suited to recognize an aggregation phenomenon. Of course, this interpretation is only conjecture at present, and additional data will be needed before firm conclusions can be drawn.

The Three-Dimensional Structure of Variable and Constant Regions. Each constant and variable domain has a three-

Other Structural Features of the Immunoglobulin Molecule. There are two regions of the immunoglobulin molecule that do not conveniently fit into the pattern of repeating homology domains. In the region of the inter-heavy-chain bridg-

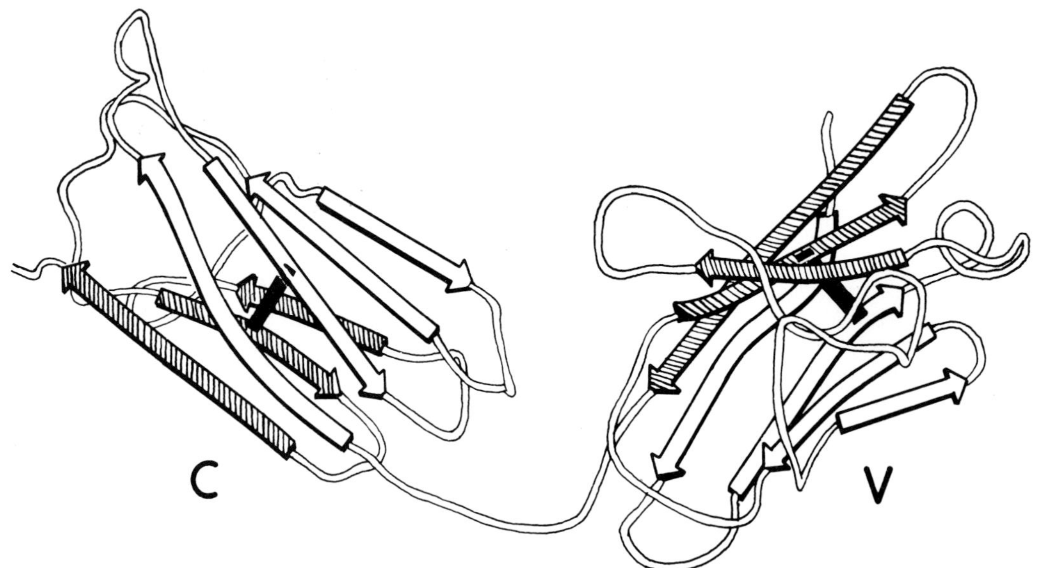

Fig. 2-16. Three-dimensional structure of a variable and a constant region of an immunoglobulin molecule. Note the structural independence of each homology unit. (Adapted from Schiffer, M., *et al.*: Structure of a λ-type Bence-Jones protein at 3.5-Å resolution. Biochem., *12*:4620, 1973.)

ing, there are a number of proline residues. This part of the molecule is called the *hinge region*, for here the molecule might be free to rotate upon binding antigen (Fig. 2-17). The prolines may serve to stabilize this region, since rotation of peptide bonds next to a proline residue is difficult.

Just distal to each variable region (in both light and heavy chains) there is a stretch of amino acids containing several glycine residues. Because of their small size glycine residues offer little structural restriction to molecular movement, and therefore this segment might allow movement of the combining sites to permit the closest fit between antibody and antigen.

Molecules that Are Incorporated into the Immunoglobulin Structure

Pentameric IgM and polymeric IgA include another molecule within their structures. This is a small polypeptide called *J chain* (Fig. 2-18).[32] It is made by the same plasma cell that produces the immunoglobulin molecule to which it is bound and is probably added on just before the immunoglobulin is released from the cell. It is linked to the Fc portion of the immunoglobulin by disulfide linkages. J chain may be necessary for the polymerization of IgA and IgM.

IgA, when present in the secretory fluids (secretory IgA), contains still another small polypeptide moiety in its structure. *Secretory component*[33] (or transport piece) is made by epithelial cells and represents an addition to the IgA molecule subsequent to its release from the plasma cell (Fig. 2-19). Its function is not understood, but it has been suggested that it may aid in the uptake of free IgA by the epithelial cells for eventual excretion into the gastrointestinal and respiratory tracts, and may also protect against proteolysis in the gut.

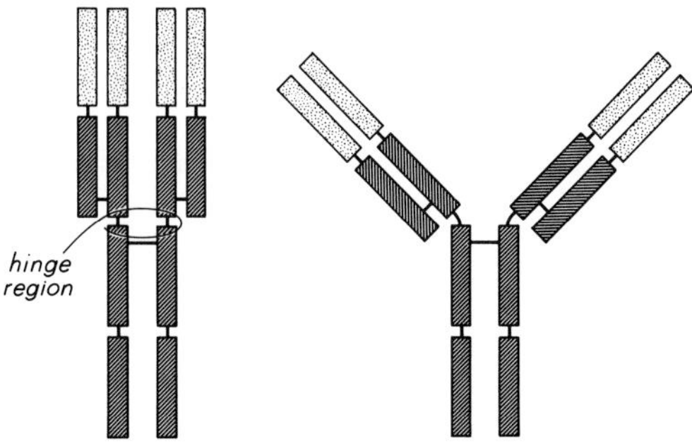

Fig. 2-17. The hinge region, where the arms of an antibody molecule may be free to rotate upon binding antigen.

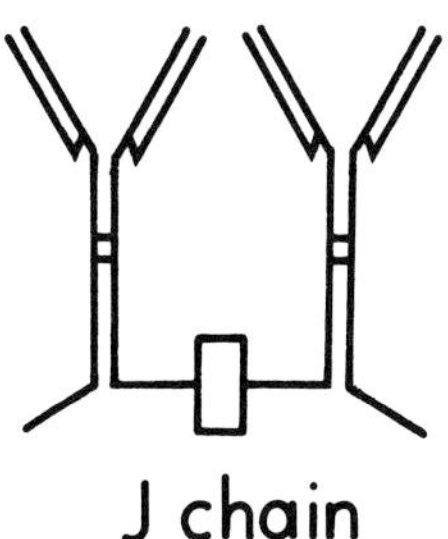

Fig. 2-18. J chain appears to be required for the polymerization of IgA and IgM.

Immunoglobulin Carbohydrate

All classes of heavy chains contain at least one oligosaccharide moiety. The carbohydrate is bound to an asparagine that is part of an Asn-X-Ser/Thr sequence (where X is any amino acid), with the exception of the carbohydrate located at the hinge region of IgA_1 which is bound to a serine. In IgG, carbohydrate is attached within the CH_2 domain. IgM, IgA, IgE and IgD have carbohydrate attached within several constant regions and the hinge region.[1a]

GENETIC MARKERS ON HEAVY AND LIGHT CHAINS

Various genetic markers have been identified within the constant regions of both light and heavy chains.[34] These markers are detected serologically as inheritable antigenic determinants present within the immunoglobulin structure, and are due to specific amino acid substitutions in the polypeptide chains.

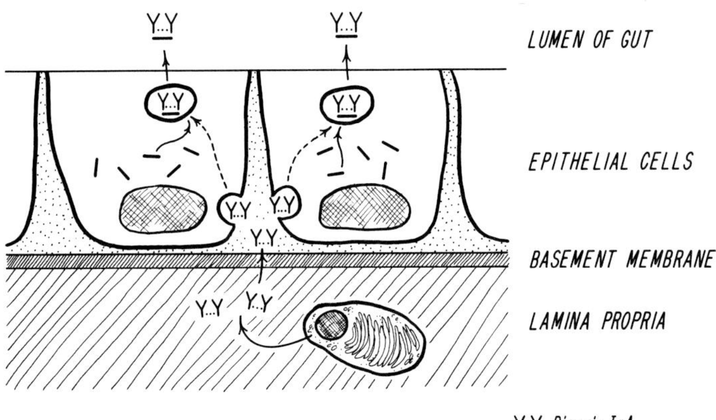

Fig. 2-19. Dimeric IgA, secreted by plasma cells in the lamina propria, binds secretory component which is produced by the epithelial cells of the gastrointestinal tract. The resultant secretory IgA is then released into the lumen of the gut.

Light Chains[35]

The κ-chain constant region shows remarkable conservation of primary structure and the only variability that has been detected serologically and associated with specific amino acid substitutions is the Inv allotypic marker. An *allotypic marker,* or allotype, is an antigenic specificity representing one of any possible number of allelic markers present on a significant percentage of immunoglobulin molecules (Fig. 2-13). When human immunoglobulin is injected into a rabbit, thus itself acting as an antigen, all immunoglobulin molecules of the same allotype will react with the resulting rabbit antiserum. An allotype is therefore nothing more than an antigenic specificity traceable to the particular product or products of a genetic allele. The Inv allotypic markers reflect amino acid substitutions at positions 191 and 153 of the κ chain. A person can inherit only one Inv marker from each parent, and hence they are true alleles.

The constant region of the λ chain demonstrates greater variability than the constant regions of the κ chains. Several variations in amino acid sequence have been defined for the λ chain, but these are not true allotypic markers. One example is the Oz variant. This is associated with the presence of lysine (Oz+) or arginine (Oz−) at position 193. All individuals, however, express both Oz+ and Oz− variants. Therefore, they are not alleles but probably represent a duplicated gene locus with subsequent mutation affecting amino acid expression at the mutated locus. All antigenic specificities of type, subtype, and also class and subclass are called *isotypic markers.* A more detailed discussion of the λ-chain isotypes and the κ-chain allotypes can be found in Appendix B.

Heavy Chains[26,34]

Many allotypic markers have been described for the alpha and gamma classes of heavy chains. In the human they are all located within the constant regions. The markers are called Am for the alpha chains and Gm for the gamma chains and, like the light-chain allotypes, are defined by reactivity with particular antisera. Most of the Gm markers are found in only one of the four IgG subclasses. No Gm markers have been found for IgG_4.

Although a large number of allotypic markers representing products of a genetic allele have been described, in only a few cases have allotypic markers representing products of two allelic forms of the same locus been defined (see Table 2-2). The term *homoallele* has been used to describe two alternate DNA sequences at the same genetic locus. Homoalleles are thus mutually exclusive. An example of two homoalleles that code for different allotypes are the Gm 4 and Gm 17 markers. Gm 4 is present on IgG_1 molecules and represents an arginine at position 217; Gm 17 represents a lysine at the same position. An individual may inherit both the Gm 4 and Gm 17 alleles, one from each of his parents, but any single antibody-producing cell will make antibody with only one of the markers. This principle is called *allelic exclusion* (Fig. 2-20). A heterozygous individual will thus have a population of cells making antibody with each phenotype but no single cell will make antibody of more than one phenotype.

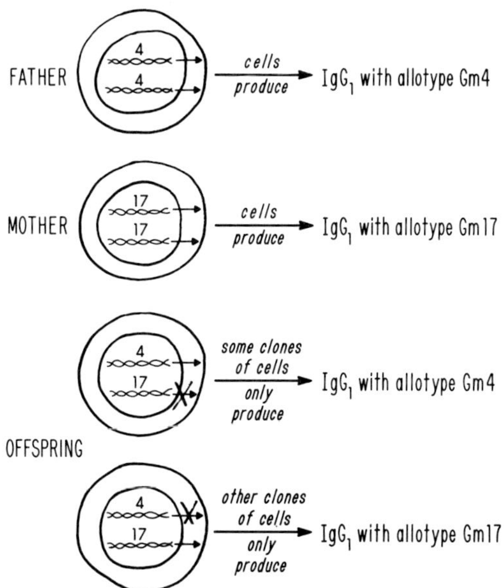

Fig. 2-20. Allelic exclusion. Although a lymphocyte may possess the genetic information to produce immunoglobulin of two different allotypes (a different allotype inherited from each parent), any single cell will synthesize immunoglobulin of only one allotype.

THE FIVE CLASSES OF IMMUNOGLOBULIN

IgM and IgG

Those functions generally attributed to the humoral immune response are due primarily to the activity of these two immunoglobulin classes (see Chap. 6). While IgA, IgE and perhaps IgD have specific and localized actions, IgM and IgG are present in high concentrations throughout most of the body and comprise a major part of the systemic humoral reaction to an antigenic challenge.

IgM usually exists as a multivalent molecule with ten potential antigen-binding sites; thus, it is effectively five antibody units bound together by J chain. This provides IgM with a great avidity for binding antigen. However, only five combining sites appear to bind antigen strongly, perhaps as a result of steric interference by adjacent binding sites. IgM has a molecular weight of about 900,000 and a sedimentation coefficient (reflecting molecular size) of 19S. It is the major immunoglobulin of the early part of the primary humoral response. Some antibodies directed against the blood group antigens and the natural antibodies to many bacteria and other microorganisms are most often of the IgM class. IgM is not cytophilic but it can fix complement.

Table 2-2. The Gm Allotypic Markers

IgG_1	1, 1−, 2, 3, 4, 7, 17, 18, 19, 20
IgG_2	23
IgG_3	3, 6, 10, 11, 12, 13, 14, 15, 16, 21
IgG_4	None

	Homoalleles	*Amino Acid Substitutions*	*Position*
IgG_1	1	Asp Glu Leu	356, 358
	−1	Glu Glu Met	
IgG_1	4	Arg	214
	17	Lys	
IgG_3	5	Phe	436
	21	Tyr	

Table 2-3. Molecular Properties of the Immunoglobulin Classes

	IgG	*IgM*	*IgA*	*IgE*	*IgD*
Heavy-chain class	γ	μ	α	ϵ	δ
Heavy chain (mol. wt.)	50,000	70,000	55,000	65,000	65,000
Intact molecule (mol. wt.)	150,000	900,000	$(160,000)_n$	180,000	180,000
Sedimentation coefficient	7S	19S	7S, 9S, 11S	8S	7S
Carbohydrate	3%	12%	7.5%	12%	12%
Serum conc. (mg./ml.)	8–16	0.6–2	1.5–4	Trace	Trace

IgG is the major immunoglobulin of the secondary humoral response. Its great versatility in providing for host defense stems from its ability to diffuse into almost any of the body tissues and to interact there with antigen. It consists of two heavy and two light chains with very little carbohydrate. IgG has a molecular weight of about 150,000 and a sedimentation coefficient of 7S. About 80 per cent of serum immunoglobulin is IgG. The ability of IgG to perform various biological functions differs according to subclass. IgG_1 and IgG_3 can cross the placenta, fix complement, and will bind to macrophages. IgG_4 will cross the placenta as well, but does not contribute significantly to complement fixation and macrophage binding. IgG_2 does not readily cross the placenta, nor will it strongly fix complement or bind to macrophages.

IgA

IgA is the major immunoglobulin of the secretory immune system. Although it is found in low concentration in the blood and in the body's internal secretions, IgA is the dominant immunoglobulin in the external secretions, which include the lacrimal secretions, nasal secretions, tracheobronchial secretions, intestinal secretions, saliva and bile.[33,36] In humans, serum IgA exists primarily as a 7S monomer, although polymeric forms may also be seen. Serum IgA is rapidly catabolized and has a half-life of only five to six days. The IgA of external secretions, the so-called secretory IgA, exists predominantly as a dimer joined by the J chain and linked to a glycoprotein called secretory component. This 11S dimer is made by plasma cells in the lamina propria throughout the body, and is excreted into the lumina of the gastrointestinal tract and tracheobronchial tree. The IgA molecule binds secretory component as it crosses the epithelial barrier.

IgA plays a key role in providing initial protection against external pathogens and perhaps in regulating the distribution of the normal flora. Precisely how IgA functions as an antipathogen is unknown. Although IgA does not fix complement by the classical pathway, there is evidence that IgA-antigen aggregates may activate complement by the properdin pathway. IgA has been demonstrated to aggregate certain bacteria and to prevent the attachment of bacteria to the gastrointestinal mucosa.[37,38] Its ability to neutralize viruses is also well established.

One out of every 300 to 700 people has a deficiency of IgA. In such people, one can often measure an increased concentration of IgM at the mucosal surfaces which may compensate for the lowered IgA, and many of these individuals remain asymptomatic. Not uncommonly, however, patients with IgA deficiency will have problems with respiratory or gastrointestinal infections (see Chap. 10). The IgA system is late to mature, and during the immediate neonatal period IgA-secreting plasma cells are difficult to demonstrate. It is of interest in this regard that young children are generally more susceptible to respiratory and gastrointestinal infections than are older children and adults.

IgE

IgE,[39-41] also called reaginic antibody or homocytotropic antibody, has a molecular weight of about 190,000. It has a short serum half-life and is present in very low serum concentrations. Higher serum levels can often be found in atopic (allergy-prone) individuals. IgE is cytophilic and binds avidly to mast cells and basophils. The number of bound IgE molecules is several times higher in atopic persons than in normal individuals. Plasma cells producing IgE may be found throughout the body but are located primarily in the gastrointestinal submucosa and in the respiratory tract.

IgE is the antibody responsible for *immediate hypersensitivity* (see Chap. 6). The bridging of two cell surface-bound IgE molecules by divalent antigen in the presence of calcium serves as the signal to trigger mast cell and basophil release of their contents; these include histamine, slow-reacting substance of anaphylaxis, and eosinophil chemotactic factor of anaphylaxis. These substances are responsible for the signs and symptoms of allergy and anaphylaxis.

The physiologic role of IgE is not known. There is limited data to suggest that it may play a role in host defense against parasites. It has been observed that the shedding of parasites from the guts of rodents reaches a maximum at the same time that IgE titers peak.

IgD

IgD was discovered in 1965 when it was recognized that the serum monoclonal spike of a patient with multiple myeloma constituted an entirely new class of antibody.[42] The serum concentration of IgD is very low. However, within this low range there is considerable variation, with concentrations ranging from 4 to 400 ng./ml. (Only IgG_4 shows a similar variability.) Although it is present in very low concentrations in neonatal serum, a high percentage of neonatal lymphocytes display positive surface staining for IgD.[43]

Like IgE, IgD is very unstable. It is extremely susceptible to proteolysis, especially by plasmin, and has a short half-life *in vivo*. Sufficient IgD has been obtained from the few patients with IgD multiple myeloma to allow a determination of its molecular weight, between 170,000 to 200,000. IgD is composed of two heavy and two light chains and has a high carbohydrate content.[44]

Recently, IgD has been found to be capable of antibody activity such as complement fixation,[45] but most likely its physiologic role is not as free antibody. Recent reports suggest that IgD is present on the surfaces of most adult B lymphocytes, a finding that has been interpreted by some to indicate that IgD may act primarily as a cell-surface receptor (see Chap. 3).

ANTIBODY DIVERSITY

It was originally estimated that the human immune system can produce about one million unique antibody molecules. With refinement of the concept of crossreactivity and the observation that a single antibody can bind several related molecular structures, albeit with varying affinities, this figure may represent an overestimation of the immune system's potential. However, even with this qualification, we are clearly dealing with a vast number of unique protein molecules. Much attention has therefore been focused upon the genetic basis for this enormous molecular diversity.[34]

All theories offering explanations of antibody genetics make several simplifying assumptions that are based upon structural considerations of the antibody molecule. Since an antibody is composed of two identical light chains and two identical heavy chains which, without compelling evidence to the contrary, can be assumed to combine at random, we need to account for only 1,000 light chains and 1,000 heavy chains in order to achieve the maximum figure of 1,000,000 unique antibody molecules (1,000 × 1,000). Secondly, since each polypeptide chain is divided into variable and constant regions, it is further assumed that each polypeptide chain is coded for by one variable (V) gene and one constant (C) gene. The several constant regions of heavy chains are so nearly identical that one can reasonably assume limited gene duplication of a single C gene as a mechanism for heavy-chain production.

There are three major hypotheses that attempt to explain the genetics of antibody production:

The first theory proposes that each cell contains the genetic material required to code for all 1,000,000 antibodies, that is, 1,000 light and 1,000 heavy chains (Fig. 2-21). Each V gene is visualized to be adjacent to a C gene; the resultant mRNA thus contains the information necessary to create an intact protein chain. This is a simple Mendelian genetic model, the validity of which depends upon the presence of as many V and C genes per cell as there are possible antibody molecules. However, several lines of evidence indicate that at most several C genes are present in a cell, and hence this model is no longer favored.[46]

The finding that there are only several C genes is neither surprising nor particularly disconcerting since antibody diversity rests in the variable regions of the light and heavy chains. The second model therefore argues that each cell possesses the genetic material for all possible antibodies, but goes further in stating that C genes are represented only a few times on the genome. A process of *translocation* at the level of DNA is required to place a C gene adjacent to a V gene in order to allow production of a single mRNA strand coding for a complete chain.[22] As depicted below (Fig. 2-22) translocation is a process that joins two distant DNA regions to each other. Subsequently, a single RNA polymerase can read them without interruption in one pass, producing an mRNA molecule with all the information necessary to create a complete polypeptide chain.

The third model deviates even more significantly from standard Mendelian genetics (Fig. 2-23). As in the second model, the genome is depicted as carrying only several C genes. However, it is further hypothesized that V genes are also present only a few times on the genome. Diversity results from *somatic mutation* of these V genes during cell division. The major impetus behind this idea is twofold: (1) to maximally conserve genetic material by limiting the amount of DNA devoted to antibody synthesis, and (2) to account for the homology among variable regions. According to this model, the DNA coding for antibody synthesis must undergo random mutation in the

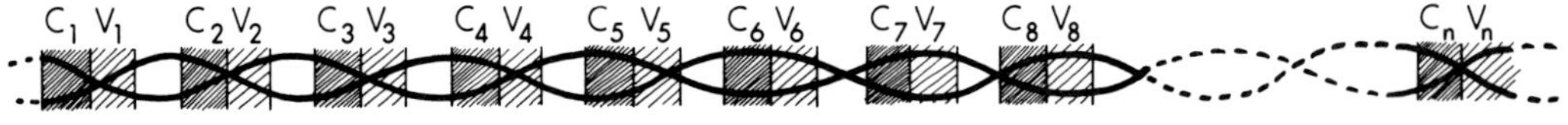

C_x V_x

each region codes for a unique light chain L_x

a similar scheme would account for heavy-chain diversity

Fig. 2-21. The first theory of antibody diversity. Each lymphocyte possesses the genetic information to code for every possible antibody molecule. Every V and C region is coded for separately on the genome such that the V and C genes necessary to construct an intact polypeptide are adjacent to each other. Thus, for light-chain synthesis, there are as many C genes as V genes.

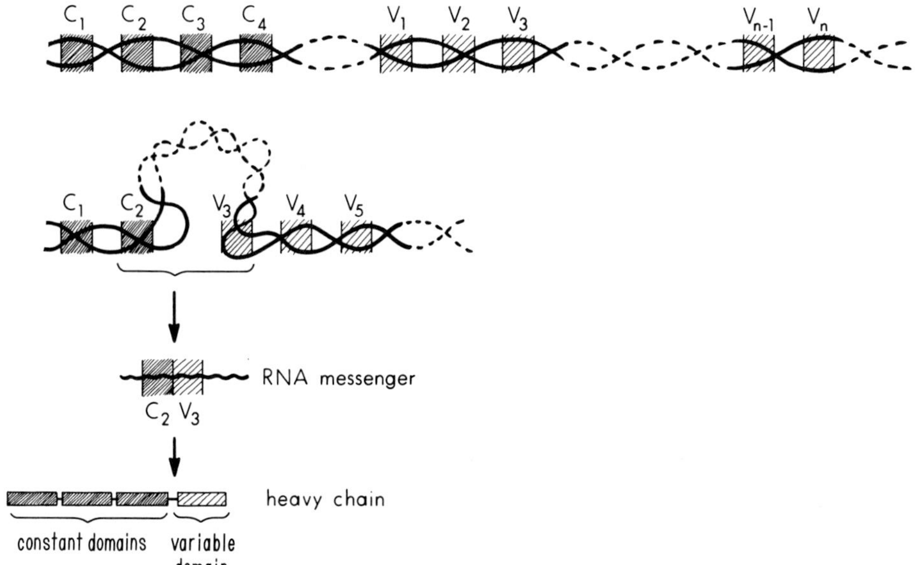

Fig. 2-22. The second theory of antibody diversity. Each lymphocyte possesses the genetic material to make all possible antibody molecules. However, the C genes are present only a few times on the genome, and a process of translocation is required to bring the V and C genes together to code for an intact polypeptide.

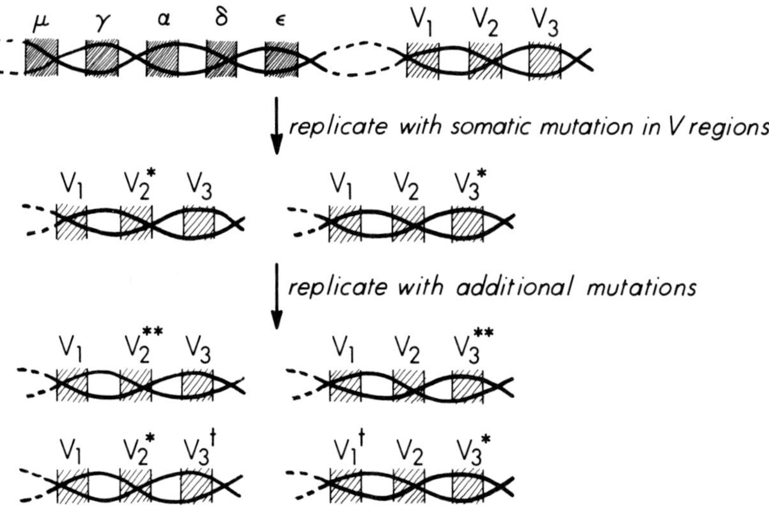

Fig. 2-23. The third theory of antibody diversity. Each cell does *not* possess the genetic information for all possible antibodies. Instead, a process of somatic mutation leads to a diverse set of V genes dispersed among the lymphocyte population. A given mutated V gene may therefore be present in only a very few lymphocytes.

process of cell division. Genetic regions coding for the hypervariable subregions are considered to be hypermutable. Somatic mutation could occur either during development of the organism or during the stimulation to cell division evoked by an antigenic challenge. Recent evidence indicates that in the fetal mouse 4 days before birth a range of antigen-binding specificities is present similar to that found in the adult animal.[47] This finding strongly suggests that antibody diversity, whatever the mechanism, arises during ontogeny.

It is not yet possible to finally discriminate between the latter two hypotheses. The somatic mutation theory stands in opposition to some firmly established genetic principles. DNA, as a relatively immutable carrier of heredity, has been undeniably successful in accounting for the genetic basis of many biochemical systems. Nevertheless, molecular hybridization studies in the mouse indicate that the number of V genes may be limited to only a very few per genome, suggesting a potentially important role for somatic mutation in generating antibody diversity.[48,49]

REFERENCES

1. de Weck, A. L.: Low molecular weight antigens. *In* Sela, M.: The Antigens. Pt. II, p. 141. New York, Academic Press, 1974.

1a. Kabat, E. A.: Structural Concepts in Immunology and Immunochemistry. Ed. 2. New York, Holt, Rinehart and Winston, 1976.

2. Eisen, H. N., and Siskind, G. W.: Variations in affinities of antibody during the immune response. Biochemistry, *3*:996, 1964.

3. Thomsen, K., Harris, M., Benjamini, F., Mitchell, G., and Noble, M.: Cellular and humoral immunity: a distinction in antigenic recognition. Nature (New Biol.), *238*:20, 1972.

4. Lindsley, H., Mannick, M., Bornstein, P.: The distribution of antigenic determinants in rat skin collagen. J. Exp. Med., *133*:1309, 1971.

5. Schlossman, S. F., and Levine, H.: Immunochemical studies on delayed and arthus-type hypersensitivity reactions. J. Immunol. *98*:211, 1966.

6. Schlossman, S. F., Yaron, A., Ben-Efraim, S., and Sober, H. A.: Immunogenicity of a series of α-DNP-L-Lysines. Biochemistry, *4*:1638, 1965.

7. Crumpton, M. J.: Protein antigens: the molecular bases of antigenicity and immunogenicity. *In* Sela, M.: The Antigens. Pt. II, p. 1. New York, Academic Press, 1974.

8. Mozes, E., and Sela, M.: Distribution of antibody activities after simultaneous immunization with two antigens. Biochem. Biophys. Acta., *130*:254, 1966.

9. Anderer, A. A., and Schlumberger, H. D.: Antigenic properties of protein cross-linked by multidiazonium compounds. Immunochemistry, *6*:1, 1969.

9a. Myrvik, Q. N.: Adjuvants. Ann. N.Y. Acad. Sci., *221*:324, 1974.

10. Borek, F.: Delayed-type hypersensitivity to synthetic antigens. Curr. Top. Microbiol. Immunol., *43*:126, 1968.

11. Bullock, W., and Möller, E.: The continuing carrier problem. Transplant. Rev., *18*:3, 1974.

12. Gell, P. G. H., and Benacerraf, B.: Studies on hypersensitivity. Immunology, *2*:64, 1959.

13. Parish, C. R.: The relationship between humoral and cell-mediated immunity. Transp. Rev., *13*:35, 1972.

14. Rajewsky, K., Schirrmacher, V., Nase, S., and Jerne, N. K.: The requirement of more than one antigenic determinant for immunogenicity. J. Exp. Med., *129*:1131, 1969.

15. Katz, D. H., Paul, W. E., Goidl, E. A., and Benacerraf, B.: Carrier function in anti-hapten immune responses. J. Exp. Med., *132*:261, 1970.

16. Mitchison, N. A.: The carrier effect in the second response to hapten-protein conjugates. Eur. J. Immunol., *1*:18, 1971.

17. Senyk, G., Williams, E. B., Nitecki, D. E., and Goodman, J. W.: The functional dissection of an antigen molecule. J. Exp. Med., *133*:1294, 1971.

18. Mitchison, N. A.: Antigenic recognition responsible for the induction in vitro of the secondary response. Cold Spring Harbor Symp. Quant. Biol., *32*:431, 1967.

19. Fleischman, J. B., Porter, R. R., and Press, E. M.: The arrangement of the peptide chains in gammaglobulin. Biochem J., *88*:220, 1963.

20. Spiegelberg, H. L.: Biological activities of immunoglobulins of different classes and subclasses. Adv. Immunol., *19*:259, 1974.

21. Jerry, L. M., and Kunkel, H. G.: Special characteristics of the IgA_2 subclass. Adv. Exp. Med. Biol., *45*:151, 1974.

22. Edelman, G. M.: Antibody structure and molecular immunology. Science, *180*:830, 1973.

23. Edelman, G. M., *et al.*: The covalent structure of an entire immunoglobulin molecule. Proc. Natl. Acad. Sci. U.S.A. *63*:78, 1969.

24. Wu, T. T., and Kabat, E. A.: An analysis of the sequence of the variable regions of Bence-Jones proteins and myeloma light chains and their implications for antibody complementarity. J. Exp. Med., *132*:211, 1970.

25. Porter, R. R.: Structural studies of immunoglobulins. Science, *180*:713, 1973.

26. Porter, R. R., Defense and Recognition. P. 159. Baltimore, University Park Press, 1973.

27. Natvig, J. B., and Kunkel, H. G.: Human immunoglobulins: classes, subclasses, genetic variants, and idiotypes. Adv. Immunol., *16*:1, 1973.
28. Kehoe, J. M., and Fougerau, M.: Immunoglobulin peptide with complement fixing activity. Nature, *224*:1212, 1969.
29. Metzger, H.: Effect of antigen binding on the properties of antibody. Adv. Immunol., *18*:169, 1974.
30. Knobel, H. R., Villiger, W., and Isliker, H.: Chemical analysis and electron microscopy studies of human C1q prepared by different methods. Eur. J. Immunol., *5*:78, 1975.
31. Schiffer, M., Girling, R. L., Ely, E. R., and Edmundson, A. B.: Structure of a λ-type Bence-Jones protein at 3.5-Å resolution. Biochemistry, *12*:4620, 1973.
32. Inman, F. P., and Mestecky, J.: The J chain of polymeric immunoglobulins. Cont. Top. Mol. Immunol., *3*:111, 1974.
33. Tomasi, T. B., and Grey, H. M.: Structure and function of immunoglobulin A. Prog. Allergy, *16*:81, 1972.
34. Fudenberg, H. H., Pink, J. R. L., Stites, D. P., and Wang, A. C.: Basic Immunogenetics. Oxford, Oxford University Press, 1972.
35. Solomon, A.: Bence-Jones proteins and light chains of immunoglobulins. N. Engl. J. Med., *294*:17, 1976.
36. Lanim, M. E.: Cellular aspects of immunoglobulin A. Adv. Immunol., *22*:223, 1976.
37. Williams, R. C., and Gibbons, R. J.: Inhibition of bacterial adherence by secretory immunoglobulin A: a mechanism of antigen disposal. Science, *177*:697, 1972.
38. Gibbons, R. J.: Bacterial adherence to mucosal surfaces and its inhibition by secretory antibodies. Adv. Exp. Med. Biol., *45*:315, 1974.
39. Ishizaka, K., and Dayton, D. H.: The biological role of the immunoglobulin E system. Washington, D.C., U.S. Dept. H.E.W., 1972.
40. Stanforth, D. R.: Immediate Hypersensitivity. Amsterdam, North-Holland Publ. Co., 1973.
41. Johansson, S. G. O., Bennich, H. H., and Berg, T.: The clinical significance of IgE. Prog. Clin. Immunol., *1*:157, 1972.
42. Rowe, D. S., and Fahey, J. L.: A new class of human immunoglobulin. J. Exp. Med., *121*:171, 1965.
43. Rowe, D. S., Hug, K., Faulk, W. P., and McCormick, J. N.: IgD on the surface of peripheral blood lymphocytes of the human newborn. Nature [New Biol.], *242*:155, 1973.
44. Spiegelberg, H. L., Prahl, J. W., and Grey, H. M.: Structural studies of human γD myeloma protein. Biochemistry, *9*:2115, 1970.
45. Konno, T., Hirai, H., and Inai, S.: Studies in IgD. Immunochemistry, *12*:773, 1975.
46. Leder, P., *et al.* The organization and diversity of immunoglobulin genes. Proc. Natl. Acad. Sci., U.S.A., *71*:5109, 1974.
47. D'Eustachio, P., and Edelman, G. M.: Frequency and avidity of specific antigen-binding cells in developing mice. J. Exp. Med., *142*:1078, 1975.
48. Rabbitts, T. H., and Milstein, C.: Mouse immunoglobulin genes. Eur. J. Biochem., *52*:125, 1975.
49. Tonegawa, S.: Reiteration frequency of immunoglobulin light chain genes: further evidence for somatic generation of antibody diversity. Proc. Nat. Acad. Sci. U.S.A., *73*:203, 1976.

3 The Lymphocyte Surface

The first step in the initiation of an immune response is the recognition of antigen by the immune system. The ability to recognize antigen resides in receptor molecules expressed on the surface of lymphocytes. These receptors sample the environment around them and, when appropriately stimulated, activate the complex machinery of the immune response. The lymphocyte receptors for antigen have two basic characteristics: (1) they are capable of selectively binding specific antigenic determinants, and (2) they are able to signal the interior of the cell that antigen binding has occurred so that a proper response can be effected. The second aspect—the way in which antigen recognition leads to immune activation—will be discussed in Chapter 4. In this chapter we shall look at the nature of the lymphocyte receptors and the process of antigen recognition, and also examine other immunologic activities that can be attributed to lymphocyte surface structures.

SURFACE RECEPTORS FOR ANTIGEN

We have already described a molecule capable of interacting specifically with antigen: the antibody molecule. The antibody, therefore, seems a likely candidate for the role of cell-surface antigen receptor, and early investigations were directed at detecting immunoglobulin on the surface of lymphocytes. These studies were successful, and the presence of membrane immunoglobulin on a large percentage of lymphocytes is now well established. Nevertheless, as we shall see below, the precise characteristics of these immunoglobulin molecules are still in doubt.

Lymphocytes with Membrane-Bound Immunoglobulin

Many experimenters have employed fluorescein-labelled antiserum directed against immunoglobulin and looked for staining of lymphocyte surfaces (Fig. 3-1).[1] When such studies were done on normal adult human cells it was found that 10 to 20 per cent of peripheral blood lymphocytes were positive for immunoglobulin (Ig+).[2] Only a small percentage of thoracic duct cells, almost no thymic lymphocytes, 25 to 50 per cent of tonsillar tissue cells, and 25 to 45 per cent of spleen cells were Ig+ (Table 3-1). Immunoglobulin could be identified by using fluorescent antisera directed against Fc fragments, Fab fragments, or κ and λ light chains. Only the carboxy terminal end of the Fc portion was found to be inaccessible to the fluorescent antisera, suggesting that it is this portion of

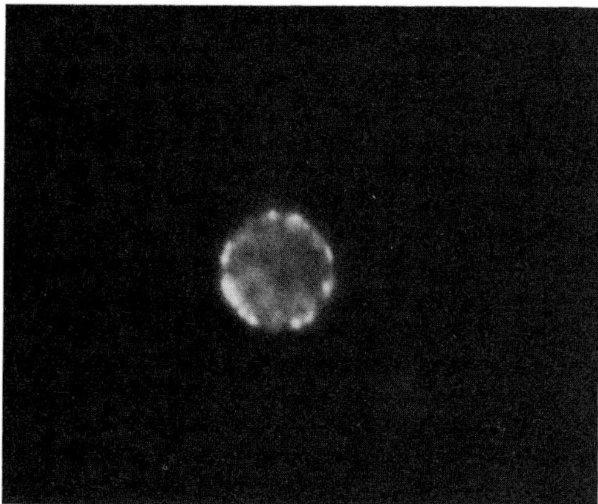

Fig. 3-1. An immunoglobulin-bearing lymphocyte stained with fluorescent antisera directed against the immunoglobulin molecules on the cell surface.

the molecule that is attached to and hidden in the membrane (Fig. 3-2).[3]

Only B lymphocytes appear to express easily detectable surface immunoglobulin.[4] Evidence supporting this conclusion derives from several sources:

Patients who have infantile X-linked hypogammaglobulinemia have virtually no lymphocytes that bear surface immunoglobulin. These patients lack any detectable B-cell function. On the other hand, patients with deficiencies in T-cell function, such as congenital thymic hypoplasia, have either a normal or greater than normal proportion of Ig+ cells in their blood.

More straightforward evidence arises out of correlations between surface characteristics and lymphocyte functions. Ig+ cells can be removed from a mixed population of lymphocytes by passing them through an anti-immunoglobulin column (that is, an affinity column containing antibody directed against antigenic determinants on immunoglobulin molecules). The remaining cells, virtually none of which are Ig+, cannot secrete antibody in short-term cultures. Thus, B-cell function disappears along with the Ig+ cells. *In vitro* tests of T-cell function remain unaltered.

Table 3-1. Percentages of Ig+ Lymphocytes

Human Cells	*Ig+ (%)*
Peripheral blood lymphocytes	10–20
Thoracic duct cells	<10
Thymic lymphocytes	~0
Tonsillar tissue cells	25–50
Spleen cells	25–45

From these results, investigators have concluded that only B cells carry easily detectable surface immunoglobulin, whereas T cells do not. This does not mean that T cells do not express immunoglobulin on their surfaces, but that if they do, it is not readily detected by standard techniques. We will consider the reasons for this qualification later.

The surface immunoglobulin on B cells is the antigen receptor for those cells.[5] In addition, most studies have further shown that all of the immunoglobulin molecules present on the surface of any single cell or clone of related cells share the same antigenic specificity.[6] This principle is called *clonal restriction.* Clonal restriction applies not only to antigenic specificity but also to idiotype[7] and light-chain type (κ or λ). In each of these aspects the immunoglobulin molecules on a single clone of cells are identical.

Still unresolved is the question of whether clonal restriction applies as well to immunoglobulin allotype (allelic exclusion). Some animal studies have shown that more than one allotype may be expressed on the surface of a single B cell,[8] whereas studies with human B cells have thus far supported the notion that each clone of cells expresses only a single immunoglobulin allotype on its surface.[9]

Another point of contention is whether clonal restriction applies to the class and subclass of surface immunoglobulin. Early studies utilizing class-specific fluorescent antisera supported the clonal restriction of immunoglobulin classes and subclasses. Accordingly, any single clone of B cells appeared to express either IgM or IgG or IgA but never more than one class of immunoglobulin on its sur-

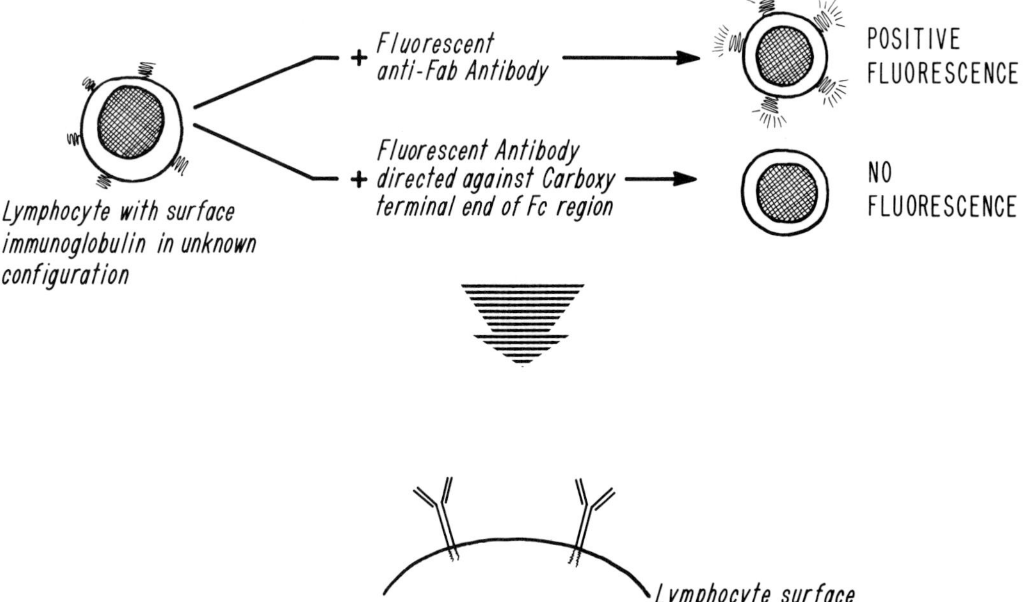

Fig. 3-2. Fluorescent antisera directed against the Fab portion of antibody will react with the surface immunoglobulin and stain the lymphocyte surface. Fluorescent antisera directed against the carboxy end of the Fc portion will not stain the lymphocyte surface, indicating that the carboxy terminal end of the immunoglobulin molecule is buried in the membrane and is inaccessible to the antisera.

face.[10] It was reported that IgM was present on about 65 per cent of Ig+ cells, IgG on up to 25 per cent and IgA on about 10 per cent.

More recent findings, however, differ from these earlier results.[11] These studies indicate that IgD is present on a very high percentage of immunoglobulin-bearing cells. This recently discovered immunoglobulin class, present in only very small amounts in the serum, may be the major surface immunoglobulin, present on up to 90 per cent of Ig+ cells. It has been further shown that most cells express *both* IgM and IgD on their surfaces.[12] What then of the many reports of surface IgG and IgA? Recent work on human peripheral blood lymphocytes suggests that many of the earlier studies may have been plagued by an artifact.[13] As we shall see later in this chapter, many lymphocytes are capable of binding serum IgG via surface receptors for the Fc part of the IgG molecule. These receptors would permit nonspecific binding of antisera to the lymphocyte surface with resultant false-positive fluorescence. If, instead of using intact antibody molecules as antisera, $F(ab)_2$ fragments of anti-immunoglobulin antisera are used as probes for surface immunoglobulin, one can be reasonably assured that there is no non-specific binding to the Fc receptors by the reagent. Using $F(ab)_2$ class-specific anti-immunoglobulin, very little IgG or IgA has been found on lymphocytes; IgD and IgM may comprise virtually all of the stainable surface immunoglobulin.

These findings are of great interest, but the basic premise of clonal restriction, the expression of immunoglobulin of a single antigen specificity on any clone of cells, remains without serious challenge. Burnet realized the importance of this observation and proposed the *clonal selection theory*, which today remains a cornerstone of immunology (Fig. 1-7).[14] According to this theory, any single cell or clone of cells is preprogrammed to be capable of synthesizing antibody molecules of *a unique antigenic specificity.* A lymphocyte expresses these molecules on its surface, where they function as the antigen receptors for that cell. When an appropriate antigen is bound by the $F(ab)_2$ portion of the surface-exposed antibody, a signal is transmitted to the cell interior and mechanisms are set into motion which ultimately lead to the proliferation and differentiation of the cell into active antibody-secreting cells. *The antibody that is produced and secreted has the same antigen-binding specificity as the surface immunoglobulin receptor*. Hence, the secreted antibody will be able to bind the antigen and carry out an effective immune response.

The clonal selection theory rests on three points, each of which has been supported by a considerable body of evidence: (1) surface immunoglobulin is the B-cell antigen receptor; (2) the surface immunoglobulin on each clone of B cells is of a single antigenic specificity; and (3) the secreted antibody is of the same antigenic specificity as the surface receptors.[7,15]

The T-Cell Antigen Receptor

The structure of the T-cell antigen receptor has proved to be extremely difficult to decipher. Indeed, until recently it was justifiably debated whether the T cell could be demonstrated to bind antigen at all. This particular issue, at least, has now been resolved. Autoradiographic techniques have demonstrated that T cells will bind antigen that has been labelled with radioactive iodine.[16] In addition, if the antigen presented to the T cells is so highly radioactive that it kills the T cells to which it attaches, the remaining T-cell population is no longer able to bind the labelled antigen.[17] This finding indicates not only that T cells are able to bind antigen, but that they do so specifically and with clonal restriction in that the receptors for a particular antigen are present on only a small percentage of the T-cell population.

The most obvious candidate for the role of T-cell receptor is the immunoglobulin molecule. However, standard immunofluorescent techniques using fluorescein-labelled anti-immunoglobulin have failed to detect immunoglobulin on the T-cell surface. Employing more sensitive techniques, some investigators have reported success.[18–20] The most commonly employed method has been to attach radioactive iodine to anti-immunoglobulin antiserum and to demonstrate by subsequent autoradiography that the T cells bind the iodine label. These studies indicate that the density of surface immunoglobulin on T cells appears to be many times less than that on B cells.

Utilizing another approach, several other workers have claimed to have found high densities of surface immunoglobulin on T cells. The enzyme lactoperoxidase is used to iodinate the tyrosine residues of exposed surface proteins (only surface molecules are labelled since the enzyme is too large to enter the cell).[18,21] The cells are then lysed and their membranes solubilized in a nonionic detergent. The product of this procedure can then be subjected to biochemical and immunologic analysis. The presence of the attached iodine label is a reasonable guaranty that the molecule under study is a surface molecule. With this technique, some investigators have reported detecting intact, monomeric IgM in considerable amounts in the T-cell membrane.[18] Other laboratories have not been able to confirm this finding[22] and the results remain extremely controversial.

There is evidence that T-cell immunoglobulin does not consist solely of cytophilic immunoglobulin randomly picked up from the serum, but that T cells can synthesize these molecules.[23,24] Nevertheless, the demonstration of surface immunoglobulin on T cells, even if it can be shown that it is made by the cells themselves, does not constitute proof that these molecules are the antigen receptors for those cells. Data to support such a view is still very limited.[24,26]

The recent development of still another technique has suggested a novel resolution to this problem. Several workers have been able to obtain antibody directed specifically against the idiotype of both the antibody produced in the humoral response to a given antigen and the T-cell receptor present on the T-cell clone proliferating against that same antigen. These workers have shown that the antigen-binding sites of the humoral antibody and of the T-cell receptors directed against the same antigen share immunologic identity. Thus the antigen-combining site of the T-cell receptor appears closely to resemble that of immunoglobulin.[27] It remains possible, however, that the remainder of the T-cell receptor molecule bears little resemblance to the constant regions of the immunoglobulin molecule.

In summary, the physical nature of the T-cell receptor is still in doubt. Although some investigators claim to have demonstrated immunoglobulin on the surface of T cells, in most studies it appears to be present in much lower density than on B cells, and there is little data at present to indicate that these molecules are the actual receptors for antigen. In addition, other laboratories have failed to confirm the existence of T-cell surface immunoglobulin. Recent work using anti-idiotype antisera strongly suggests that the antigen-binding region of the T-cell receptor is similar to that of immunoglobulin, but little can be said at present about the structural characteristics of the remainder of the molecule.

OTHER IMMUNE-RELATED SURFACE PHENOMENA

In addition to the presence of specific receptors for antigen, other functions have been attributed to the lymphocyte surface. Some of these receptor phenomena can also be found on other immune-related cells, such as the macrophage and the neutrophil.

The Formation of Spontaneous Erythrocyte Rosettes

In 1969 it was reported that sheep red blood cells (SRBC) would spontaneously attach to about 60 per cent or more of human peripheral blood lymphocytes, thus forming "erythrocyte rosettes" (Fig. 3-3).[28] Virtually 100 per cent of lymphocytes taken from the thymus and smaller percentages of spleen and lymph node cells exhibited this phenomenon.[29] These results suggested that rosette formation was a characteristic of T cells, and this conclusion was further supported by the failure to readily detect surface immunoglobulin on these cells.[30]

Not all T cells appear to be capable of rosette formation; it may be more charac-

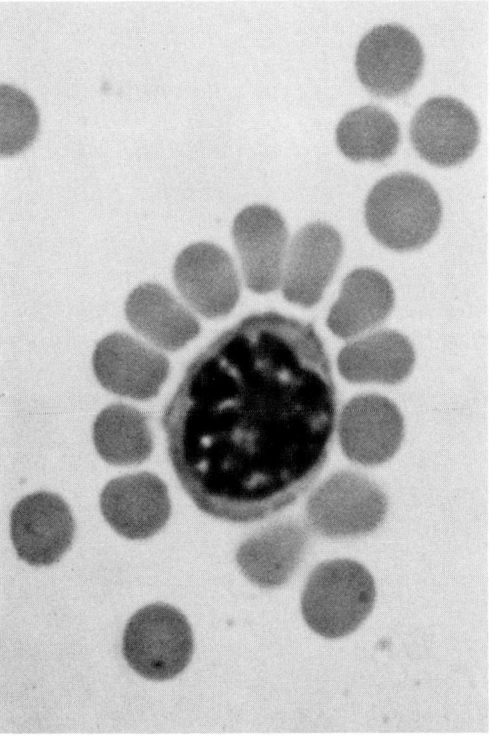

Fig. 3-3. A sheep erythrocyte rosette.

teristic of immature or young T cells.[31] Thus, whereas almost all thymic cells form spontaneous rosettes, a lesser, although still very high, percentage of peripheral T cells form rosettes. Peripheral T cells and thymic T cells also differ in their ability to form rosettes at varying temperatures.[31] Thymic cells form stable rosettes at both 4°C. and 37°C. Peripheral T cells form rosettes at 4°C., but most will dissociate from the erythrocytes when the temperature is raised to 37°C. This difference in temperature dependence becomes important in attempts to define the origin and state of maturation of the T cells in various T-cell malignancies (see below).

The major clinical importance of rosette formation derives from its use as a general marker for T cells. The biological significance of rosette formation, however, remains a total mystery. The nature of the lymphocyte receptor for SRBCs is unknown, except that it appears to be a surface glycoprotein. It does not seem to be immunoglobulin, and the antigenic determinants on the sheep erythrocytes do not appear to be the target for T-cell binding.

A modification of the normal procedure for obtaining spontaneous rosettes has been described, utilizing a much shorter incubation time. These rosettes are called "active" rosettes.[32] It has been suggested that the number of active rosette-forming T cells correlates well with T-cell activity both *in vitro* and *in vivo*.[33] Why spontaneous erythrocyte formation should reflect T-cell function is not understood.

Surface Receptors for Immunoglobulin: the Fc Receptor

In 1961, macrophages were shown to be able to bind immunoglobulin by the Fc portion of the molecule. This was the first demonstration of a cell-surface receptor for immunoglobulin (Fig. 3-4).[36,34] The macrophage can bind only immunoglobulin of the IgG class, primarily the IgG_1 and IgG_3 subclasses.[35] It is a weak interaction with a high rate of spontaneous dissociation. If the antibody has first bound antigen, the interaction of the antibody molecule with the cell is stabilized, although the binding energy of the Fc segment to the macrophage is still not great.[36] An antibody-coated red blood cell will adhere to a macrophage when about 10^3 to 10^4 antibody molecules are bound to the red-cell surface. Each macrophage has been calculated to possess more than 2,000,000 Fc receptors.[37] The most stable association occurs between aggregated 7S immunoglobulin and the macrophage, perhaps reflecting the stability afforded by multiple Fc attachment.

Fc receptors are present on monocytes, neutrophils and lymphocytes as well as on macrophages.[38] The standard assay for detecting Fc receptors employs aggregated IgG as the reagent. Another method for detecting these receptors utilizes IgG-coated red blood cells. Fc-receptor-bearing cells will bind the free Fc segments of the erythrocyte-bound antibody and form erythrocyte rosettes. Using this rosette technique, Fc+ monocytes may be distinguished from Fc+ lymphocytes. If the red cells are coated with a low density of IgG, rosettes will be preferentially formed with monocytes; lymphocytes bearing the Fc receptors will form rosettes only when the red cells are densely covered.

Fc receptors have been detected on at least two populations of human lymphocytes. Most (and possibly all) B cells, that is, cells bearing surface immunoglobulin, have Fc receptors.[39] A second population that is neither Ig+ nor spontaneous rosette-forming (T cell) has also been shown to bear Fc receptors.[40] These cells have been given a variety of names including "null cells" and "K cells." They are generally considered to be related to the B cell.[41] Because they have no detectable surface immunoglobulin, we will refer to them as "negative immunoglobulin lymphocytes" or "nil" cells. Human T

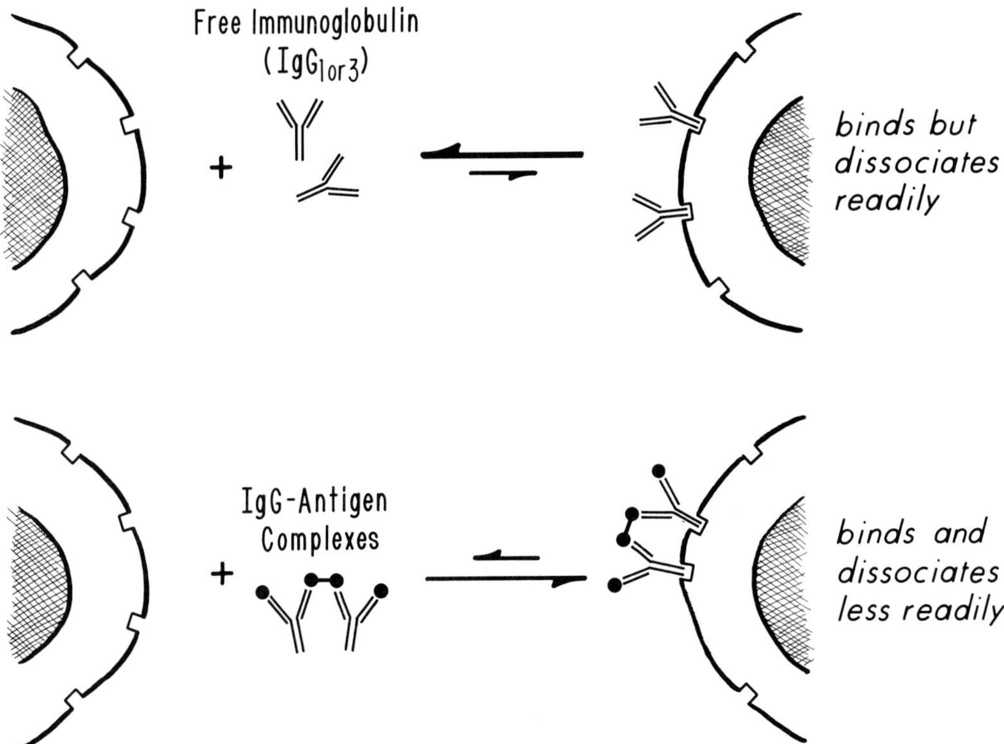

Fig. 3-4. Macrophages, monocytes, granulocytes and some lymphocytes possess receptors for the Fc portion of immunoglobulin. Antibody which has bound antigen can then bind with fair stability to the Fc receptors.

cells have not been demonstrated to carry the Fc receptor; in the mouse, however, *activated* T cells have been found to express the Fc receptor.[42]

The adherence of cytophilic antibody to macrophages via the Fc receptor plays an important part in the immune response. IgG that has bound antigen can attach to macrophages via these Fc receptors. This binding will lead to the rapid phagocytosis of the antigen-antibody complex.[43] The process by which a molecule facilitates the phagocytosis of antigen is called *opsonization*. Immune opsonization is one of the most important mechanisms by which the body handles potentially dangerous antigens.

The role of the Fc receptor on lymphocytes is currently being defined. Both B cells and nil cells bearing the Fc receptor have been implicated in the phenomenon of *antibody-dependent cell-mediated cytotoxicity* (ADCC); (see Chap. 6).[44] In this process, Fc+ lymphocytes can bind the Fc portion of antibody that has bound to a foreign cell and become activated to lyse that cell (Fig. 3-5). Thus, some of the Fc+ lymphocytes can function as killer lymphocytes.

The surface immunoglobulin receptors for antigen on B cells appear to be an integral part of the membrane and are not externally bound by the Fc receptors.[45] However, it has been suggested that anti-

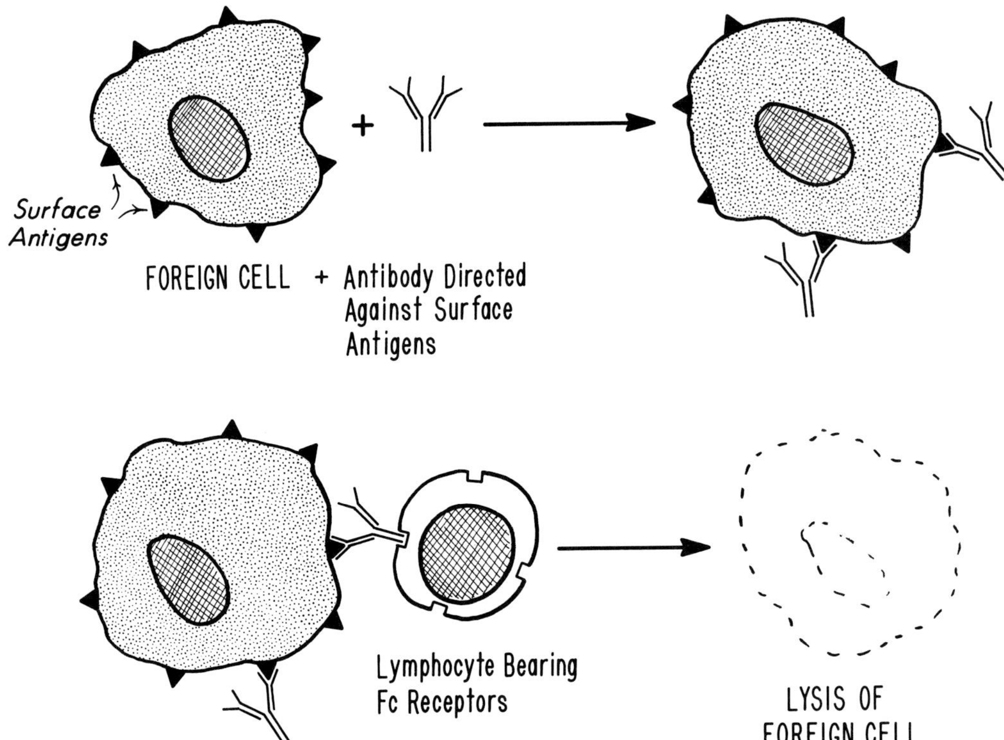

Fig. 3-5. Antibody-dependent cell-mediated cytotoxicity. Lymphocytes bearing Fc receptors can bind cell-bound antibody and lyse the target cell.

body produced and secreted during an immune response could be bound to B cells by the Fc receptors and in this way provide a signal to turn off further antibody production.[46] Such negative antibody feedback has been demonstrated, although this proposed mechanism is purely hypothetical.

The Complement Receptor

Lymphocytes, monocytes, macrophages and granulocytes all possess the ability to bind complement to their surfaces.[47] This phenomenon is commonly assayed by the use of a rosette technique. Antibody is attached to red cells in the presence of complement, thus forming erythrocyte-antibody-complement complexes. Cells with surface complement receptors will bind these complexes and form rosettes (Fig. 3-6).

Macrophages and granulocytes have receptors for the C3b component of complement.[48] Human lymphocytes can bind both C3b and C3d, a cleavage product of C3b.[49] The C3b and C3d receptors represent separate surface structures.[50] In addition, recent work suggests that several of these cell types can bind C4.[51] The relationship of the C4 receptor to the C3b receptor is still unknown.

Complement receptors are present on the majority of (and perhaps all) cells expressing easily detectable surface immunoglobulin.[52] Complement receptors also appear to be present on at least some nil cells. Thus, many cells with Fc receptors also possess receptors for complement. The complement receptor is believed to enhance processes that are mediated by the Fc receptor. For example, complement binding stabilizes the attachment of cytophilic IgG to macrophages and other phagocytes.[53] The bind-

Table 3-2. Cell Surface Markers

Marker	*B Cell*	*T Cell*	*Nil Cell*	*Monocyte/ Macrophage*
Surface Ig	+	−	−	−
SRFC	−	+	−	−
Fc	+	−	+	+
C3b	+	−	+*	+
C4	+	−	+*	+
C3d	+	−	+*	−
"T" antigen	−	+	−	−

*Not known for certain

ing of complement to the lymphocyte surface may also enhance the lymphocyte's capacity for antibody-dependent cell-mediated cytotoxicity.[54]

Complement binding to an antigen can itself cause an antigen to adhere to phagocytes bearing complement receptors. Whether such binding significantly opsonizes the antigen seems to vary for different antigens. Complement opsoniza-

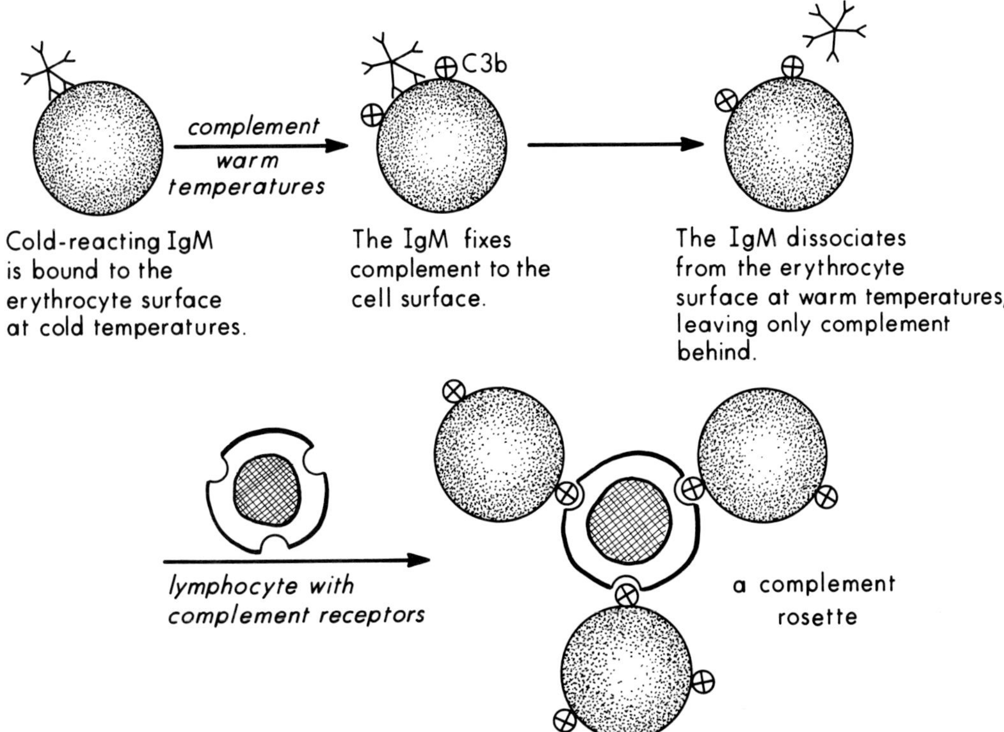

Fig. 3-6. A complement rosette. There are many mechanisms now employed to form complement rosettes. One of these is depicted here. Immunoglobulin is bound to the red-cell surface where it fixes complement. The immunoglobulin is removed from the cell surface, leaving only complement components on the cell surface. (One way to do this is to use antibodies that react with red cells only in the cold. If the cells are warmed after the immunoglobulin has been bound, the immunoglobulin will dissociate from the cell surface.) Erythrocyte rosettes will then form around lymphocytes possessing complement receptors.

tion has been shown to be capable of greatly enhancing the phagocytosis of certain bacteria (see Chap. 11), although complement-coated red cells do not seem to be targets for erythrophagocytosis.[55]

SURFACE MARKERS AS INDICATORS OF CELL TYPE

These surface receptor phenomena are now being used extensively to determine the functional identity of human lymphocytes in experimental and clinical settings. Thus, the finding of easily stainable immunoglobin, usually accompanied by the presence of Fc and complement receptors, indicates that the cell line under study is most likely of B-cell origin. The ability to form spontaneous sheep erythrocyte rosettes suggests a T-cell origin.

In some animal systems, especially the mouse, lymphocyte subpopulations can be distinguished by the presence or absence of cell-surface antigens that are detectable with specific antisera. For example, mouse T cells express a surface antigen called the θ antigen that is not present on B cells. Another class of antigens called the Ly antigens are also expressed exclusively on T cells. Therefore, in order to identify lymphocyte subpopulations in the mouse, one does not have to resort to complex assays of receptor phenomena, but can simply make use of identifying antisera.

Similar antigens specific for certain human lymphocyte subpopulations are in the process of being defined. Antiserum directed against human T-cell surface antigens has been prepared.[56] The target antigens have not been defined. This antiserum reacts with a greater number of cells than are identified by spontaneous rosette formation,[57] suggesting that only a subpopulation of T cells forms rosettes. Cell-surface antigens have also been detected that are present only on B cells and nil cells which also bear the complement receptor.[58] The antigen appears to be part of a protein complex that is found uniquely on these cells. The definition of human T-cell and B-cell-specific antigens would be a major step in simplifying the identification of lymphocyte subpopulations.

SURFACE MARKERS IN DISEASE

In recent years the various surface receptors have become of considerable clinical interest with the possibility that they may shed some light on the nature and origin of various diseases, notably the lymphoproliferative disorders. We must, however, emphasize the importance of a cautious approach to the interpretation of lymphocyte surface markers. Thus, some recent findings have suggested that there is a small subpopulation of human lymphocytes that expresses easily detectable surface immunoglobulin *and* can form spontaneous erythrocyte rosettes.[59] There are also reports of certain lymphocytes which form spontaneous rosettes and also bear either Fc or complement receptors. Therefore, although the surface phenomena we have just described are now commonly employed to classify immunocompetent cells along ontogenetic lines (that is, B cell vs. T cell), they are at present best used only as phenotypic markers of lymphocyte subsets. Because we know so little about the development of these cells in the human, we must approach the use of these receptors as labels of cellular origin with care. Finally, with specific regard to the lymphoproliferative diseases, it remains to be established that these markers, defined for normal cell populations, are equally applicable to malignant cells.

B-CELL MALIGNANCIES

Chronic Lymphocytic Leukemia

Chronic lymphocytic leukemia (CLL) is a proliferative disease of relatively mature lymphocytes. Between 80 and 90 per cent of cases involve a proliferation of B cells bearing surface immunoglobulin.[60] Immunoglobulin can be detected on more than 70 per cent of a patient's circulating lymphocytes and is homogeneous. About 10 per cent of patients with CLL possess an IgM monoclonal serum spike. In several instances, the IgM in the serum spike has been shown to be identical to the surface IgM of the proliferating clone of malignant cells.[61] However, there is no direct evidence that the malignant cells are secreting the serum immunoglobulin.

In 10 to 20 per cent of cases of CLL, the proliferating cells do not appear to express surface immunoglobulin, although some investigators have reported that most of these cells may have reduced amounts of surface immunoglobulin. The great majority of these cells express either Fc or complement receptors.[62] There are rare cases of CLL in which the lymphocytes bear no surface immunoglobulin, Fc or complement receptors but do form spontaneous erythrocyte rosettes. These few examples are considered to be cases of T-cell CLL.[62]

The C3b receptor on CLL lymphocytes may differ from the normal complement receptor with respect to its relative affinities for mouse and human complement.[63] Other abnormalities of the complement receptor have also been reported. These findings are particularly intriguing in light of recent work suggesting a role for complement as an immunoregulatory agent (see Chap. 5).

Lymphocytic Lymphoma

This is a primary malignancy of the small lymphocytes of the lymph node. Most lymphocytic lymphomas appear to be of the B-cell type.[64] In over 90 per cent of cases immunoglobulin can be detected on the surface of the lymphocytes in involved organs. In a given patient all of the cell-surface immunoglobulin appears identical, indicative of the monoclonal origin of the malignancy.[65] There are two patterns of surface immunoglobulin that have been observed on the surface of the malignant lymphocytes.[66] In diffuse, poorly differentiated lymphoma the cell surface is densely covered with a large amount of immunoglobulin. In the diffuse well-differentiated form of the disease the surface immunoglobulin is less densely distributed and more closely resembles the normal B-cell pattern, although the surface density is often less than that of the normal B cell. The amount of surface immunoglobulin varies from patient to patient, but any one patient's malignant cells all have a similar staining pattern. Most of the Ig+ cells have also been found to bear Fc receptors. Rarely, the cells of lymphocytic lymphoma have neither surface immunoglobulin nor Fc receptors; such cells instead form spontaneous rosettes and are presumably examples of T-cell lymphomas.[67]

Lymphosarcoma-Cell Leukemia

Lymphosarcoma-cell leukemia consists of a proliferation of a highly malignant, poorly differentiated population of lymphocytes in the lymph nodes, bone marrow and peripheral blood. Virtually all cases present with Ig+ lymphocytes and are thus presumably of the B-cell type.[68] These cells also display Fc receptors. The staining pattern is a very dense one, unlike that of CLL, and resembles the staining pattern of poorly differentiated lymphocytic lymphoma.[69] The meaning behind the distinction in surface immunoglobulin density between CLL and lymphosarcoma-cell leukemia is not known. Immunoglobulin density changes can be observed in animals in the normal course of cell development. Very young B cells have extremely sparse surface immunoglobulin, and there is a progressive increase in the surface density as the cells mature.[70] The correlation of increasing surface density with increasing maturity and differentiation is precisely the opposite of what we see in these malignancies if one considers lymphosarcoma-cell leukemia to represent the less differentiated of the two disorders as has been traditionally believed. We will discuss the relationship of the different lymphoproliferative diseases to normal lymphocyte differentiation in Chapter 12.

Hairy-Cell Leukemia

Hairy-cell leukemia (leukemic reticuloendotheliosis) is a systemic proliferative disorder, the classification of which has been quite controversial. It is characterized by splenomegaly without significant lymphadenopathy and the presence of a variable (often high) percentage of abnormal mononuclear cells in the bone marrow and peripheral blood. These cells contain a unique tartrate-resistant acid phosphatase isoenzyme. The name "hairy cell" derives from the many irregular villous projections of the cytoplasm of the proliferating mononuclear cells. A lymphocytic origin for the hairy cell has been gaining acceptance in recent years,[71] and several studies have indicated that the cells express readily stainable surface immunoglobulin.[72] These cells are generally unable to form spontaneous erythrocyte rosettes. Often the cells seem to lack Fc or C3 receptors, although the latter have occasionally been demonstrated.

Waldenström's Macroglobulinemia

Waldenström's macroglobulinemia is characterized by a pleomorphic lymphoid and plasma-cell-like proliferation in the bone marrow and the lymph nodes. Patients present with an IgM monoclonal serum immunoglobulin spike. In untreated patients, up to 80 per cent of the peripheral blood lymphocytes exhibit surface IgM identical to their serum spike.[73] When the disease is controlled by therapy only 10 per cent of the patient's lymphocytes display the monoclonal immunoglobulin. There characteristically is a variable staining pattern from cell to cell, specifically in terms of the density of surface immunoglobulin. Most of the lymphocytes that are IgM+ are also IgD+. Thus the disease appears to represent a proliferation of a single clone of B cells with maturation into immunoglobulin-secreting plasma cells. It is interesting that the IgD may disappear as the cells differentiate.

T-CELL MALIGNANCIES

The marked preponderance of B cells in the malignancies of the small lymphocyte discussed above is perplexing. Until we fully understand the controls regulating lymphocyte division and maturation we will not be able to understand the reasons for this proclivity. However, T-cell malignancies do exist, and include the following examples:

Acute Lymphocytic Leukemia

Acute lymphocytic leukemia (ALL) is a malignant proliferation of early cells of the lymphoid series, most commonly occurring in children. In several series, the leukemic cells in approximately 20 per cent of ALL patients have been demonstrated to form spontaneous erythrocyte rosettes.[74] Most patients' cells lack surface immunoglobulin as well as Fc receptors. Thus about 20 per cent of ALL patients present with what appears to be a T-cell proliferation. Very rarely, the malignant cells of ALL have stainable surface immunoglobulin. The majority of patients have cells lacking both B- and T-cell markers.[75]

There is some evidence that those cases of ALL with T-cell markers may represent a clinical entity distinct from those without any evidence of thymic origin.[76] In a small study of about 50 patients, T-cell ALL appeared to differ from the usual presentation of ALL in that it was a more aggressive disease and was associated with a thymic mass, higher white blood cell counts, and an older age group of children, affecting primarily males.

T-cell ALL may be related to a disease known as childhood lymphoblastic lymphoma, which is characterized by a thymic mass, lymphadenopathy and rapid progression. In childhood lymphoblastic lymphoma, the malignant cells eventually invade the marrow and peripheral blood. These cells have been felt to be histologically indistinguishable from the cells of ALL and also appear to be T cells. Further evidence for a relationship between these two disorders has been derived from studies of T-cell rosette formation in ALL. ALL lymphocytes form stable rosettes at both 4° C. and 37° C., a characteristic of thymic T cells.[77] This observation lends support to identifying this disorder with the thymic-associated lymphoblastic lymphoma. An alternate interpretation, however, is that rosette dissociation at 37° C. is a characteristic acquired with maturity by T cells, and the failure to demonstrate this in the ALL population may only reflect the immaturity of leukemic T cells.

Sezary's Syndrome

Sezary's syndrome is characterized by the clinical triad of pruritus, erythroderma and lymphadenopathy. Bizarre large lymphoid cells are present in the peripheral blood and the skin infiltrates. These cells exhibit neither surface immunoglobulin nor Fc receptors. Spontaneous rosette formation is a characteristic of 65 to 90 per cent of the abnormal lymphocytes, and up to 90 per cent are killed by anti-T-cell antiserum. Sezary's syndrome thus appears to involve a malignant proliferation of T cells.[78]

There are other malignant diseases of immune-related cells that manifest themselves in cutaneous infiltration. Mycosis fungoides and some uncommon forms of CLL are examples. There is evidence in many of these instances that the malignant cell has T-cell characteristics. This finding suggests a possible relationship between T-cell malignancies and skin involvement (see Chap. 12).

Lymphoproliferative Disorders and Cell-Surface-Marker Characteristics

CLL
- 90% of cases are Ig+.
- A small portion are Ig− and Fc+, C+.
- A few cases have been described in which the cells are SRFC+.

Lymphocytic lymphoma
- >90% are Ig+, Fc+.
- A small portion are SRFC+.

Lymphosarcoma-cell leukemia
- Almost all are Ig+, Fc+.

Hairy-cell leukemia
- Some studies indicate that the cells are Ig+.
- Usually lack Fc or C receptors.

Macroglobulinemia
- Ig+.

ALL
- 20% are SRFC+.
- Most lack Ig and Fc receptors.

Sezary's syndrome
- 65–90% are SRFC+.

REFERENCES

1. Raff, M. C.: Two distinct populations of peripheral lymphocytes in mice distinguished by immunofluorescence. Immunology, *19*:637, 1970.
2. Froland, S. S., and Natvig, J. B.: Surface-bound immunoglobulin on lymphocytes from normal and immunodeficient humans. Scand. J. Immunol., *1*:1, 1972.
3. Fu, S. M., and Kunkel, H. G.: Membrane immunoglobulin of B lymphocytes. J. Exp. Med., *140*:895, 1974.
4. Froland, S. S., and Natvig, J. B.: Identification of three different human lymphocyte subpopulations by surface markers. Transplant. Rev., *16*:114, 1973.
5. Roelants, G., Forni, L., and Pernis, B.: Blocking and redistribution of antigen receptors of T and B lymphocytes by anti-Ig antibody. J. Exp. Med., *137*:1060, 1972.
6. Raff, M. C., Feldmann, M., and dePetris, S.: Monospecificity of B lymphocytes. J. Exp. Med., *137*:1024, 1973.
7. Ada, G. L., and Byrt, P.: Specific inactivation of antigen reactive cells. Nature, *222*:1291, 1969.
8. Linthicum, D. S., and Sell, S.: Immunoelectron microscopic localization of allelic immunoglobulin determinants on the surface of rabbit lymphocytes. Fed. Proc., *34*:4620, 1975.
9. Pernis, B., Forni, L., and Amante, L.: Immunoglobulin spots on the surface of rabbit lymphocytes. J. Exp. Med., *132*:1001, 1970.

10. Froland, S. S., and Natvig, J. B.: Class, subclass and allelic exclusion of membrane-bound Ig of human B lymphocytes. J. Exp. Med., *136*:409, 1972.
11. Van Boxel, J. A., Paul, W. E., Terry, W. D., and Green, I.: IgD-bearing human lymphocytes. J. Immunol. *109*:648, 1972.
12. Fu, S. M.: Occurrence of IgM and IgD on human lymphocytes. J. Exp. Med., *139*:451, 1974.
13. Winchester, R. J., Fu, S. M., Hoffman, T., and Kunkel, H. G.: IgG on lymphocyte surfaces; technical problems. J. Immunol., *114*:1210, 1975.
14. Burnet, M.: The Clonal Selection Theory of Acquired Immunity. Cambridge, Cambridge University Press, 1959.
15. Cosenza, H., and Köhler, H.: Specific suppression of antibody response by antibody to receptor. Proc. Natl. Acad. Sci. U.S.A., *69*:2701, 1972.
16. Davie, J. M., and Paul, W. E.: Antigen-binding receptors in lymphocytes. Contemp. Top. Immunobiol., *3*:171, 1974.
17. Warner, N. L.: Membrane immunoglobulins and antigen receptors on B and T lymphocytes. Adv. Immunol., *19*:67, 1974.
18. Marchalonis, J. J.: Lymphocyte surface immunoglobulin. Science, *190*:20, 1975.
19. Bankhurst, A. D., Warner, N. L., and Sprent, J.: Surface immunoglobulins on thymus and thymic-derived lymphoid cells. J. Exp. Med., *134*:1005, 1971.
20. Nossal, G. J. V., *et al.*: Quantitative features of a sandwich radioimmune labelling technique for lymphocyte surface receptors. J. Exp. Med., *135*:405, 1972.
21. Marchalonis, J. J., Cone, R. E., and Santer, V.: Enzymic iodination. Biochem. J., *124*:921, 1971.
22. Grey, H. M., *et al.*: Ig on the surface of lymphocytes. J. Immunol., *109*:776, 1972.
23. Moroz, C., and Hahn, V.: Cell surface immunoglobulin of human T cells and its biosynthesis *in vitro*. Proc. Natl. Acad. Sci. U.S.A., *70*:3716, 1973.
24. Roelants, G., *et al.*: Active synthesis of Ig receptors for antigen by T lymphocytes. Nature, *247*:106, 1974.
25. Mason, S., and Warner, N. L.: The immunoglobulin nature of the antigen recognition site on cells mediating transplantation immunity and delayed hypersensitivity. J. Immunol., *104*:762, 1970.
26. Rouse, B. T., and Warner, N. L.: Suppression of graft-vs-host reaction in chickens by pretreatment of leukocytes with anti-light chain sera. Cell. Immunol., *3*:470, 1972.
27. Binz, H., and Wigzell, H.: Shared idiotypic determinants on B and T lymphocytes reactive against the same antigenic determinants. J. Exp. Med., *142*:197, 1218; 1231, 1975.
28. Coombs, R. R. A., Gurner, B. W., Wilson, A. B., Holm, G., and Lindgren, B.: Rosette-formation between human lymphocytes and sheep red cells not involving Ig receptors. Int. Arch. Allergy Appl. Immunol., *39*:658, 1970.
29. Bach, J. F.: Evaluation of T-cells and thymic serum factors in man using the rosette technique. Transplant. Rev., *16*:196, 1973.
30. Jondal, M., Holm, G., and Wigzell, H.: Surface markers on human T and B lymphocytes. J. Exp. Med., *136*:207, 1972.
31. Galili, U., and Schlesinger, M.: Subpopulations of human thymus cells differing in their capacity to form stable rosettes and in their immunologic reactivity. J. Immunol., *115*:827, 1975.
32. Wybran, J., Carr, M. C., and Fudenberg, H. H.: The human rosette-forming cell as a marker of a population of thymus-derived cells. J. Clin. Invest., *51*:2537, 1972.
33. Horowitz, S., Groshong, T., Albrecht, R., and Hong, R.: The "active" rosette test in immunodeficiency diseases. Clin. Immunol. Immunopathol., *4*:405, 1975.
34. Boyden, S., and Sorkin, E.: The absorption of antibody and antigen by spleen cells *in vitro*. Immunology, *4*:244, 1961.
35. Huber, H., and Fudenberg, H. H.: Receptor sites of human monocytes for IgG. Int. Arch. Allergy Appl. Immunol., *34*:18, 1968.
36. Phillips-Quagliata, J. M., Levine, B. B., Quagliata, F., and Uhr, J. W.: Mechanism underlying binding of immune complexes to monocytes. J. Exp. Med., *133*:589, 1970.
37. Arend, W., and Mannik, M.: The macrophage receptors for IgG. J. Immunol., *110*:1455, 1973.
38. Dickler, H. B., and Kunkel, H. G.: Interaction of aggregated γ globulin with B lymphocytes. J. Exp. Med., *136*:191, 1972.
39. Basten, A., Warner, N., and Mandel, T.: A receptor for antibody on B lymphocytes. J. Exp. Med., *135*:627, 1972.
40. Greenburg, A., Hudson, L., Shen, L., and Roitt, I.: Antibody dependent cell mediated cytotoxicity due to "null" lymphoid cell. Nature [New Biol.], *242*:111, 1973.
41. Chess, L., Levine, H., MacDermott, R., and Schlossman, S. F.: Immunologic functions of isolated human lymphocyte subpopulations. J. Immunol., *115*:1483, 1975.
42. Yoshida, T. O., and Anderson, B.: Evidence for a receptor recognizing antigen complexed immunoglobulin on the surface of activated mouse T lymphocytes. Scand. J. Immunol., *1*:401, 1972.
43. Berke, A., and Benacerraf, B.: Antibody cytophilic for macrophages. J. Exp. Med., *123*:119, 1965.
44. Forman, J., and Möller, G.: The effector cell in antibody-induced cell mediated immunity. Transplant. Rev., *17*:108, 1973.
45. Dickler, H. B.: Studies of the human lymphocyte receptor for heat aggregated or antigen-complexed immunoglobulin. J. Exp. Med., *140*:508, 1974.
46. Sinclair, N. R.: The role of the Fc portion in the regulation of immune responses by antibody. Cell. Immunol., *19*:162, 1975.
47. Sevach, E. M., Jaffe, E. S., and Green, I.: Receptors for complement and immunoglobulin on human and animal lymphoid cells. Transplant. Rev. *16*:3, 1973.
48. Ross, G. D., Polley, M. J., Rabellino, E. M., and

Grey, H. M.: Two different complement receptors on human lymphocytes. J. Exp. Med., *138*:798, 1973.

49. Eden, A., Miller, G. W., and Nussenzweig, V.: Human lymphocytes bearing membrane receptors for C3b and C3d. J. Clin. Invest., *52*:3239, 1973.
50. Ross, G. D., and Polley, M. J.: Specificity of human lymphocyte complement receptors. J. Exp. Med., *141*:1163, 1975.
51. ——: Human Lymphocyte and granulocyte receptors for the 4th component of complement and the role of granulocyte receptors in phagocytosis. Fed. Proc. *33*:759, 1974.
52. Ehlenbergen, A. G., *et al.*: Immunoglobulin bearing and complement receptor lymphocytes constitute the same populations in human peripheral blood. J. Clin. Invest., *57*:53, 1976.
53. Brown, D. L.: The behavior of phagocytic cell receptors in relation to allergic red cell destruction. Ser. Haematol., *7*:348, 1974.
54. Lustig, H. T., and Bianco, C.: Antibody-mediated cell cytotoxicity in a defined system: regulation by antigen, antibody and complement. J. Immunol., *116*:253, 1976.
55. Brown, D. L., Lachmann, P. J., and Dacie, J. V.: The *in vivo* behavior of complement-coated red cells. Clin. Exp. Immunol., *7*:401, 1970.
56. Bobrove, A. M., Strober, S., Herzenberg, A., and De Pamphilis, J. D.: Identification and quantitation of thymus-derived lymphocytes in human peripheral blood. J. Immunol., *112*:520, 1974.
57. Yata, J., Tsukimoto, I., Arimoto, T., Goya, N., and Tachibana, T.: Human thymus lymphoid tissue antigen, complement receptors and rosette formation with sheep erythrocytes of the lymphocytes from primary immunodeficiency diseases. Clin. Exp. Immunol., *14*:309, 1973.
58. Humphreys, R. E., *et al.*: Isolation and immunologic characterization of a human B-lymphocyte-specific, cell surface antigen. J. Exp. Med., *144*:98, 1976.
59. Dickler, H. B., Adkinsen, N. F., and Terry, W. D.: Evidence for individual human peripheral blood lymphocytes bearing both B and T cell markers. Nature, *247*:213, 1974.
60. Dickler, H. B., Siegal, F. P., Bentwich, Z. H., and Kunkel, H. G.: Lymphocyte binding of aggregated IgG and surface immunoglobulin staining in chronic lymphocytic leukemia. Clin. Exp. Immunol., *14*:97, 1973.
61. Fu, S. M., *et al.*: Idiotypic specificity of surface immunoglobulin and the maturation of leukemic bone marrow derived lymphocytes. Proc. Natl. Acad. Sci. U.S.A., *71*:4487, 1974.
62. Dickler, H. B., Siegal, F. P., Bentwich, Z. H., and Kunkel, H. G.: Lymphocyte binding of aggregated IgG and surface immunoglobulin staining in chronic lymphocytic leukemia. Clin. Exp. Immunol., *14*:97, 1973.
63. Ross, G. D., Rabellino, E. M., Polley, M. J., and Grey, H. M.: Combined studies of complement receptor and surface immunoglobulin bearing cells and sheep erythrocyte rosette-forming cells in normal and leukemic human lymphocytes. J. Clin. Invest., *52*:377, 1973.
64. Leech, J. H., *et al.*: Malignant lymphomas of follicular center cell origin in man. J. Natl. Cancer Inst., *54*:11, 1975.
65. Brouet, J. C., Labaune, S., and Seligmann, M.: Evaluation of T and B lymphocyte membrane markers in human non-Hodgkin's malignant lymphomata. Br. J. Cancer, *31* [Suppl. II]: 121, 1975.
66. Aisenberg, A. C., and Long, J. C.: Lymphocyte surface characteristics in malignant lymphoma. Am. J. Med., *58*:300, 1975.
67. Mann, R. B., *et al.*: Immunologic and morphologic studies of T cell lymphoma. Am. J. Med., *58*:307, 1975.
68. Aisenberg, A. C., and Bloch, K. J.: Immunoglobulin on the surface of neoplastic lymphocytes. N. Engl. J. Med., *287*:272, 1972.
69. Aisenberg, A. C., Bloch, K. J., and Long, J. C.: Cell-surface immunoglobulin in chronic lymphocytic leukemia and allied disorders. Am. J. Med., *55*:184, 1973.
70. Strober, S.: Immune function: cell surface characteristics and maturation of B cell subpopulations. Transplant. Rev., *24*:84, 1975.
71. Debusscher, J. L., *et al.*: Hairy cell leukemia: functional, immunologic, kinetic and ultrastructural characterization. Blood, *46*:495, 1975.
72. Catovsky, D., Pettit, J. E., Galetto, J., Okoss, A., and Galton, D. A. G.: The B-lymphocyte nature of the hairy cell of leukemic reticuloendotheliosis. Br. J. Haematol., *26*:29, 1974.
73. Seligmann, M., Preud'Homme, J. L., and Brouet, J. C.: B and T cell markers in human proliferative blood diseases and primary immunodeficiencies with special reference to membrane bound immunoglobulin. Transplant. Rev., *16*:85, 1973.
74. Catovsky, D., Goldman, J. M., Okoss, A., Frisch, B., and Galton, D. A. G.: T-lymphoblastic leukemia: a distinct variant of acute leukemia. Br. Med. J., *2*:673, 1974.
75. Davey, F. R., and Gottlieb, A. J.: Lymphocyte surface markers in acute lymphocytic leukemia. Am. J. Clin. Pathol., *62*:818, 1974.
76. San, L., and Borilla, L.: Clinical importance of lymphoblasts with T markers in childhood acute leukemia. N. Engl. J. Med., *292*:828, 1975.
77. Tsukimoto, I., Wong, K. Y., and Lampkin, B. C.: Surface markers and prognostic factors in acute lymphoblastic leukemia. N. Engl. J. Med., *294*:245, 1976.
78. Zucker-Franklin, D., Melter, J. W., and Quagliata, F.: Ultrastructural, immunologic and functional studies on Sezary cells. Proc. Natl. Acad. Sci. U.S.A., *71*:1877, 1974.

4 Between Recognition and Response

Lymphocytes first contact antigen by means of special surface receptors designed to interact specifically with antigen. However, simply knowing that antigen binds to a particular receptor does not tell us how that interaction leads to the activation of an immunocompetent cell. We have defined merely the first step in a long chain of complicated events, the ultimate product of which is a fully differentiated cell capable of carrying out immunologic effector functions with maximum efficiency and intensity. In this chapter we will study the events of lymphocyte activation. The relationship between recognition, activation and differentiation is depicted below (Fig. 4-1).

LYMPHOCYTE ACTIVATION

We must begin by defining what we mean by "activation." The typical small lymphocyte that one sees on a blood film is an inactive, quiescent cell. However, when such a cell is activated by an appropriate stimulus, it undergoes a series of radical alterations. These usually occur in a characteristic time sequence and are outlined in Figure 4-2.[1] Any one of these events can be assayed as an indication of activation. The most commonly employed assays measure (1) lymphokine production; (2) lymphocyte proliferation, usually by the incorporation of radiolabelled precursors into newly forming DNA; (3) antibody synthesis; or (4) cytotoxicity.

Lymphocyte activation is therefore defined functionally by means of one of these assays. Each of the assays measures only one aspect of lymphocyte activation, and they do not all give the same information about the state of activation. For example, antibody secretion is dependent upon both the proliferation and differentiation of lymphocytes into antibody-secreting cells. Under certain circumstances, lymphocytes may proliferate without maturing into cells capable of producing antibody. These cells could be readily demonstrated to be activated by measuring the incorporation of radiolabelled DNA precursors, whereas an assay for antibody production would fail to detect evidence of activation. Similarly, T-cell activation can be measured by assays for cytotoxicity and lymphokine production, but not by measuring antibody production.

THE INTRACELLULAR PROCESSES OF ACTIVATION[2]

The morphologic picture of lymphocyte activation is typical for a cell under stimulation.[3] There is progressive cellular

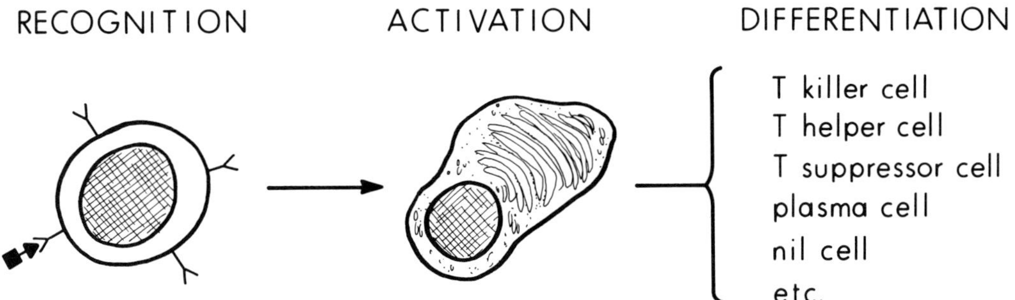

Fig. 4-1. The three basic events of the immune response are shown as they occur sequentially: *recognition*—the binding of antigen (discussed in Chap. 3); *activation*—the stimulation of a resting cell into an active cell (discussed in this chapter); *differentiation*—the production of the many different cell types that partake in an immune response (discussed in Chaps. 5 and 6).

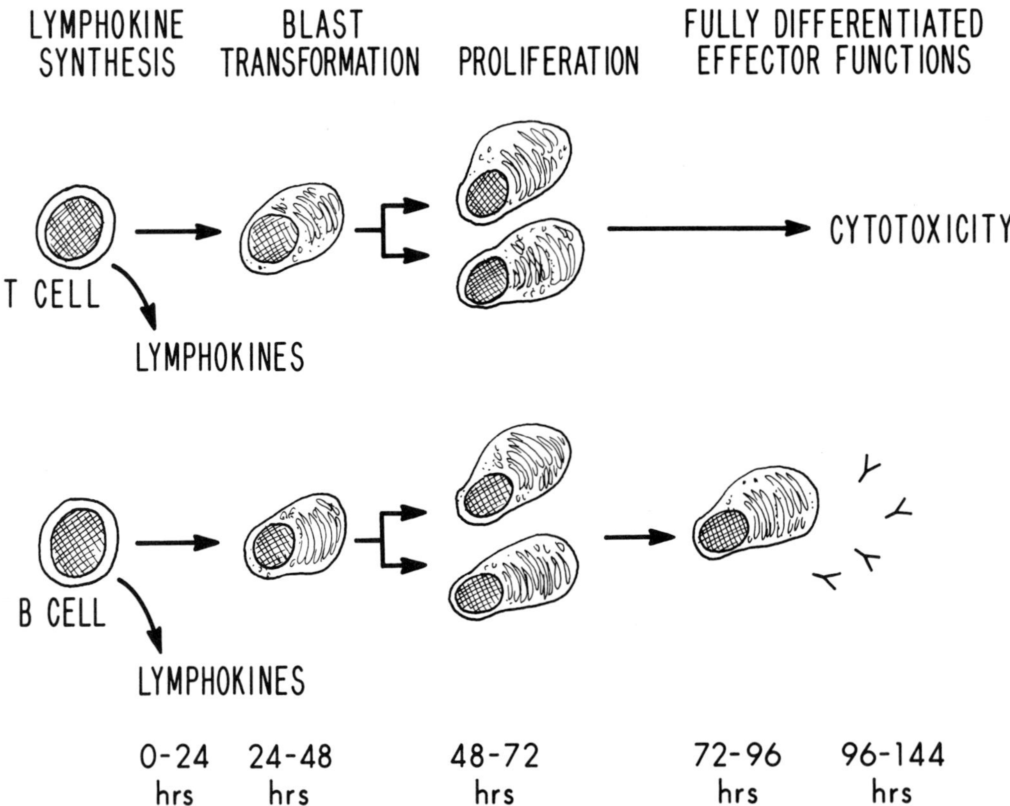

Fig. 4-2. The activation of immunocompetent cells can be measured by assaying any number of different cellular functions. These occur at different times during the activation sequence as shown. (Modified from Oppenheim, J. J., and Rosenstreich, D. L.: Signals regulating in vitro activation of lymphocytes. Prog. Allergy, *20*:65, 1976.)

enlargement, reflected by an increase in size of both the nucleus and cytoplasm, and the nuclear/cytoplasmic ratio decreases. The nuclear chromatin condenses so that by 48 to 72 hours following stimulation there is virtually no heterochromatin remaining. The nucleolus becomes more prominent. Ribosomes, aggregating as polysomes, rapidly fill the cytoplasm.[4] The Golgi apparatus, vacuoles and lysosomes all become pronounced, and there is a proliferation of mitochondria. Mitotic figures may appear by 40 hours, with mitosis occurring at a maximum rate 72 hours after activation. In activated B cells there is extensive development of the rough endoplasmic reticulum, and by 72 hours cells appear with some of the characteristics of plasma cells.[5]

The biochemical evidence of activation can be detected at every level of the cell's substructure. The cell membrane undergoes radical changes in its phospholipid and glycoprotein metabolism, and an increasing potassium and calcium influx can be measured. The uptake of nucleosides, amino acids and sugars is also increased.[6] Within the cytoplasm, the increase in the number of ribosomes is mirrored by a large increase in RNA.[7] Manufacture of new ribosomes may be essential for the production of DNA polymerase,[8] whereas more efficient use of the ribosome population in general (in one report, 70% of the ribosomes in an activated cell were engaged in protein synthesis, compared to 30% in a resting cell[9]) may be primarily responsible for the massive early increase in protein synthesis. Resting lymphocytes degrade 50 per cent of their rRNA before it ever reaches the cytoplasm[10]; this wastage is almost entirely eliminated in the activated cell. The synthesis of "protector proteins" may be one mechanism to prevent RNA breakdown following activation.[11]

Changes within the nucleus include an increased rate of acetylation of histones[12] and phosphorylation of nuclear proteins,[13] and the previously noted conversion of heterochromatin to euchromatin. All of these intracellular events are directed toward maximizing the ability of the transformed lymphocyte to act as a synthetic factory. Energy consumption is increased, its utilization made more efficient, and all aspects of the molecular mechanisms for protein synthesis are amplified.

STIMULI THAT CAN ACTIVATE A LYMPHOCYTE

There are two major categories of substances that can activate a lymphocyte, antigens and mitogens.

Antigens

The introduction of antigen into a population of lymphocytes *in vivo* or *in vitro* will result in the activation of those clones of cells able to recognize the antigen. Antigen-induced activation is very specific, and a given antigen will activate only a small fraction of a random population of lymphocytes. By utilizing ^{3}H-thymidine uptake and autoradiography as a measure of activation, it has been found that most antigens will activate fewer than 1 per cent of a random, unprimed population of cells.[14] It has therefore been difficult to study the cellular events of activation using antigens as the stimulating agents.

Mitogens

Mitogens, unlike antigens, possess the ability to activate a large percentage of the lymphocytes of many species of animals, including those of man. Mitogens have become important experimental tools and are used to activate large numbers of cells *in vitro*, in order to study the cellular events of activation. The first mitogen to be discovered, phytohemagglutinin (PHA), was isolated from the kidney bean in 1955.[15] Most mitogens are derived from plants or bacteria; those obtained from plants are often called phytomitogens, or lectins.[16]

As many as 80 per cent of cells may appear as lymphoblasts two to three days after mitogen stimulation. However, this figure reflects clonal amplification (the proliferation of activated clones of cells) of the stimulated population, and the actual percentage of lymphocytes activated by a mitogen probably ranges from 10 to 50 per cent.[17] The figure varies depending upon the particular mitogen used and the nature of the lymphocyte population.

A mitogen's stimulatory capacity is *not* a function of its antigenicity. Lymphocytes from individuals rendered tolerant to a particular mitogen (i.e., who will not mount a specific immune attack against that mitogen) nevertheless show the same high percentage of activated cells as those from "nontolerized" individuals.[18] Mitogens are *polyclonal* activators and will activate many clones of cells regardless of their antigenic specificity (Fig. 4-3). They do not bind to the antigen-specific receptors on lymphocytes, but bind instead to carbohydrate moieties present on all lymphocytes.[2] Nevertheless, most mitogens do not appear to be totally nonspecific in their actions, and some will preferentially activate T cells and others B cells.

T-Cell Mitogens. Some mitogens activate only T cells. B cells appear to be activated only indirectly, via the action of T helper cells which have been directly ac-

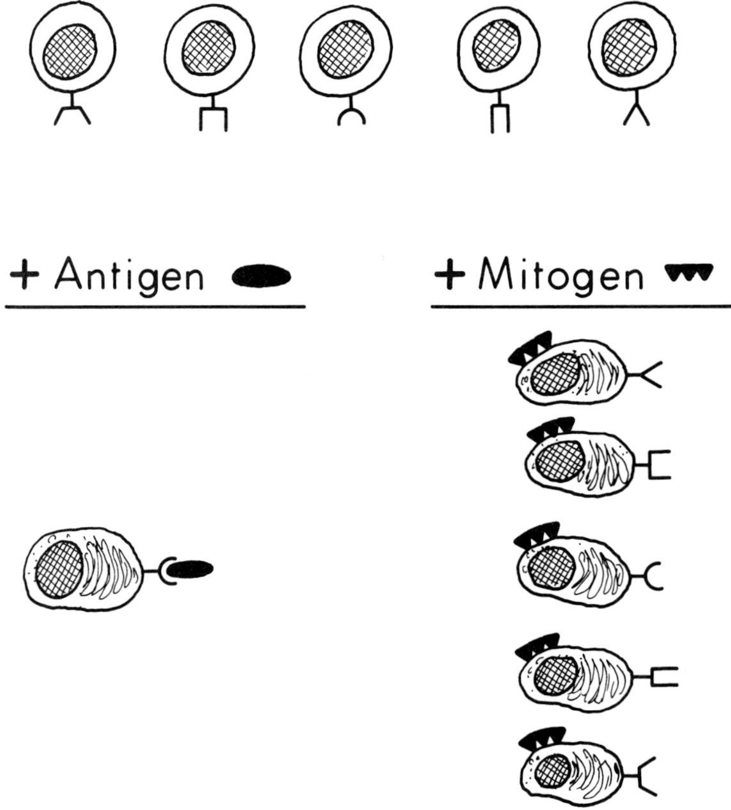

Fig. 4-3. Antigens are bound only by those cells bearing receptors specific for the given antigen. Mitogens bind to all or almost all lymphocytes, regardless of their antigenic specificity. Many, but not all, of the cells to which a mitogen binds will be activated.

tivated by the mitogen.[19,20] This is most clearly shown by the failure of purified B-cell populations to be activated by these mitogens.

The two most commonly employed T-cell mitogens are phytohemagglutinin (PHA) and concanavalin A (con A). PHA is a glycoprotein and con A is a pure protein. Almost all mammalian cell types will bind these mitogens, and PHA and con A have frequently been studied for their ability to agglutinate erythrocytes. PHA and con A bind equally well to both T and B lymphocytes.[21,22] Thus, the simple binding of a mitogen to a cell does not appear to be sufficient to activate that cell, and other surface processes may be involved (see below).

PHA and con A can induce a T lymphocyte to undergo a single cellular division. Repeated divisions require the persistence of the mitogen in the culture medium, presumably reflecting the need for continual stimulation in order to get a full response.[23,24]

B-Cell Mitogens. Several molecules have the ability to act as mitogens only for B cells. One of these is anti-immunoglobulin, that is, antibody directed against the B-cell-surface antigen receptors.[25] Most investigators have found that both intact antibody and $F(ab)_2$ fragments are equally effective as mitogens, but univalent Fab fragments are ineffective (Fig. 4-4).[25] This suggests that the ability to cross-link surface receptors may be important for the mitogenic activity of anti-immunoglobulin. In this regard it is

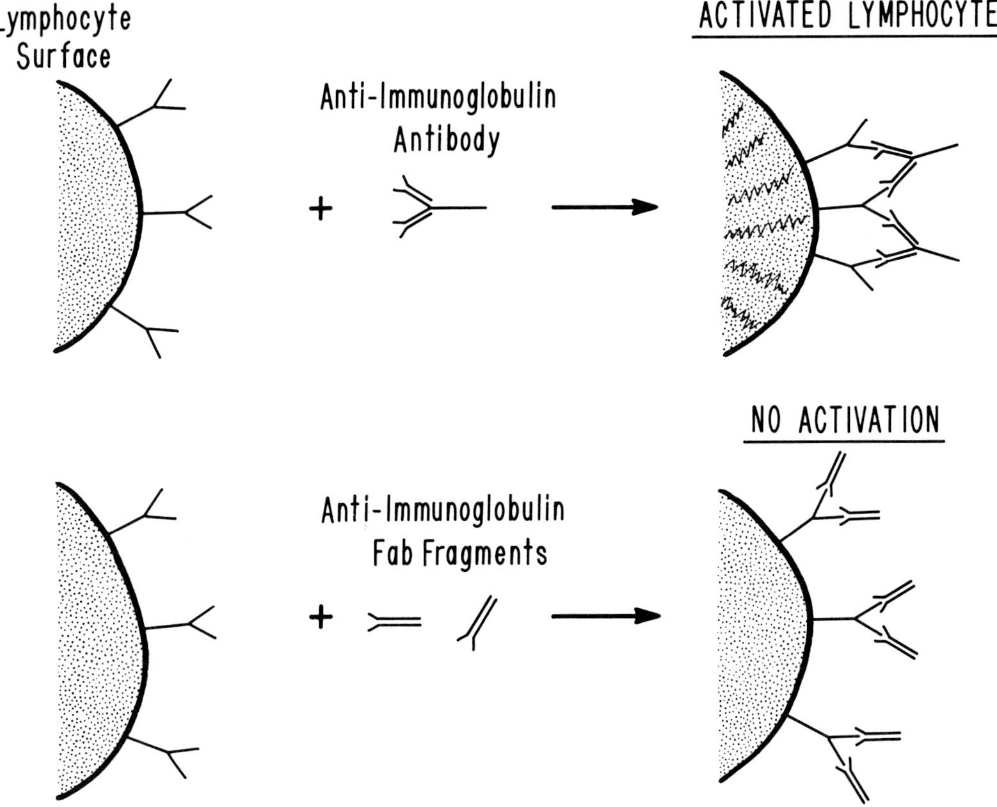

Fig. 4-4. Intact anti-immunoglobulin antibody is a B-cell mitogen. Anti-immunoglobulin Fab fragments are not mitogenic. This finding may reflect the ability of intact antibody to cross-link immunoglobulin molecules on the B-cell surface.

interesting that divalent antibody directed against histocompatibility antigens present on lymphocytes is also mitogenic, although for both B and T cells.

Lipopolysaccharide (LPS) is the prototype of a whole range of B-cell mitogens. These substances share several features: all are high molecular weight polymers and many are T-cell-independent antigens. All express many identical determinants in a repeating array on their molecular surface, and this observation has suggested that these substances might also be able to cross-link molecules which are part of the B-cell membrane.

Like the T-cell mitogens, these substances bind equally well to both T and B cells.[26] LPS is not mitogenic for human cells, although it is a potent B-cell mitogen in mice, rats and guinea pigs.[27]

Recently, there has been some question raised as to whether LPS is truly a pure B-cell mitogen. LPS seems to be able to enhance T-cell helper activity, and this may contribute in part to the polyclonal B-cell activation.

Mitogens for T and B cells. Pokeweed mitogen (PWM) has the capacity to activate both B and T cells. PWM can activate a pure T-cell population, and several reports have indicated that it can activate a pure B-cell population as well.[26,29]

Miscellaneous Mitogens. Many substances, including several metallic ions, sodium periodate and extracts of walnuts, also have the ability to activate a large percentage of lymphocytes.

The Mixed Lymphocyte Reaction (MLR).[30] The MLR shares many similarities with mitogen-induced activation. Lymphocytes cultured in the presence of allogeneic cells (that is, cells of a dissimilar genetic background) will respond with a profound degree of activation which can be assayed by measuring blastogenesis (Fig. 4-5). T cells appear to be the primary cell type that becomes activated. Up to a few per cent of cells may become activated (most estimates run in the neighborhood of 1 to 3%,[31] although there are reports that as many as 8% of lymphocytes may be activated in the MLR[17]). This is not as many as most mitogens will activate, but is far more than most antigens can activate. The MLR appears to be a clonally specific reaction involving recognition of antigens on the stimulating cell population by antigen-specific receptors.[32,33] It thus seems that many cells exist with the potential to recognize and respond to foreign tissue. In general, previous sensitization with the allogeneic cells is not required for extensive activation,[30] although sensitization may increase the number of activated cells.[17,31,34]

THE APPLICATION OF MITOGENS TO MEDICINE

Mitogenic stimulation has been widely employed for several years as a means of

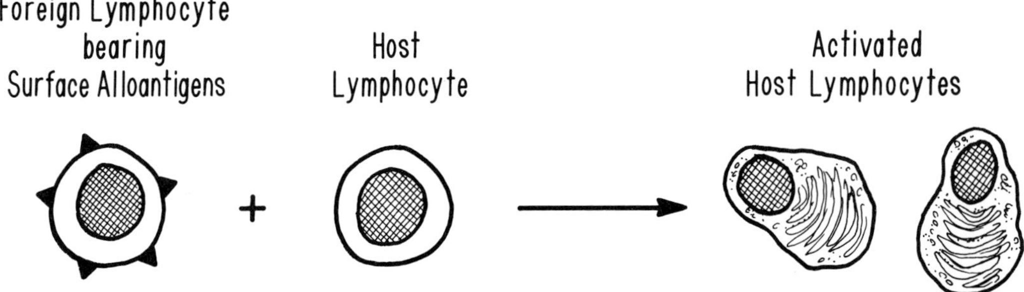

Fig. 4-5. The mixed lymphocyte reaction. Several per cent of lymphocytes will react to the presence of foreign cells and be stimulated to blastogenesis. The reaction is clonally specific despite the large number of cells that are activated.

assessing the competence of an individual's immune system. T-cell function is usually measured by reactivity to PHA or con A, and—because of the lack of a readily available mitogen that is specific for human B cells—PWM is often used to assay humoral competence. Diminished responsiveness to one of these mitogens indicates either a reduction in the number of cells in the appropriate population or else a functional impairment. For example, in patients with DiGeorge's syndrome in whom the thymus fails to develop properly and mature T cells are not produced, one can demonstrate a failure of the patients' lymphocytes to respond to the T-cell mitogens PHA and con A. Patients with severe combined immunodeficiency, an immunodeficiency disease that affects both the cellular and humoral limbs of the immune system, exhibit diminished reactivity *in vitro* to all mitogens. In both of these examples, the failure to respond is due to a reduction in the number of mature immunocompetent cells. On the other hand, diminished responsiveness to T-cell mitogens can occur in cancer, malnutrition, autoimmune diseases and aging,[35-37] and cannot always be attributed to a decrease in T-cell number. This decrease is frequently correlated with a depression in T-cell function *in vivo*, such as cutaneous anergy (i.e., the failure to react to skin test antigens). It is not immediately obvious why a cell's ability to react to a particular mitogen should be correlated with its normal *in vivo* function. Although many of the intracellular events of mitogenesis are almost certainly identical to those involved in antigen reactivity, there are differences in the two processes, the most obvious being the involvement of different cell-surface receptors. One must therefore be careful in drawing conclusions about immune reactivity *in situ* from the measurement of mitogen reactivity *in vitro*.

THE INTERACTION OF ANTIGENS AND MITOGENS WITH THE LYMPHOCYTE MEMBRANE

The interaction of externally bound molecules, including both antigens and mitogens, with lymphocyte receptors can initiate a dramatic series of surface events. These are called *patching, capping* and *internalization*, and describe the motion of lymphocyte receptors in the cell membrane (Fig. 4-6). Early views held that the cell membrane is a rigid and well-defined structure. More recent studies have evolved the picture of a fluid matrix structure, which has often been compared to a sea of lipid in which protein icebergs are able to move, although with certain restrictions. These lymphocyte surface phenomena further attest to the mobility of protein molecules within the surface membrane.[38]

Patching is a rapid process that results from the bridging of two or more receptors on the cell surface by an externally

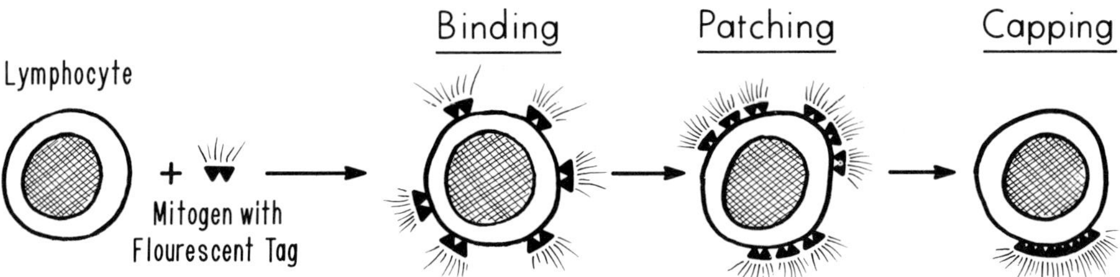

Fig. 4-6. Multivalent antigens and mitogens can cross-link surface molecules and induce lateral movement within the cell membrane. These events are called patching, capping and internalization (see text for further description).

bound molecule. Thus one basic requirement for this phenomenon is that the molecule be (at least) divalent.* The process derives its name from the small, fluorescent aggregates dotting the cell surface when the ligand is tagged with a fluorescent probe. *Capping* is an energy-dependent process, and describes the movement and localization of the scattered fluorescense to one pole of the cell. This reflects the multiple linking of all the bound surface receptors to each other. Following capping, the cell can *internalize* the polar aggregate of bound receptors.[38]

Most investigators have chosen to study mitogenesis in order to learn how the interaction of a molecule with the lymphocyte surface leads to activation. Since the binding of a mitogen with the appropriate receptor does not appear to be a sufficient explanation for activation, attempts have been made to determine whether mitogens have other effects on the lymphocyte membrane that might account for activation. The most obvious candidates are the events of patching, capping and internalization. However, no correlation has been found between a mitogen's ability to induce these surface changes and its ability to activate a cell.[21,39] Thus, con A can cap B cells but does not activate them.[21] One can also attach mitogens to sepharose beads, preventing their internalization by lymphocytes, without blocking their ability to activate those cells.[40]

Patching, as visualized with fluorescent techniques, also does not seem to correlate with activation. However, it has been suggested by a number of workers that the ability of a mitogen to cross-link only two receptors might be the basis of its activating capacity.[41,42] Such limited cross-linking might not be visualized by standard fluorescent techniques. This concept finds support in the mast-cell system, where it has been established that the bridging of two surface-bound IgE molecules by a divalent molecule can lead to mast-cell degranulation.[43] Although this hypothesis may explain the activating ability of multivalent mitogens

*There are circumstances where the requirement for divalency might not be necessary. For example, monovalent ligands could themselves be cross-linked by serum antibody, effectively creating a divalent molecule (Fig. 4-7).

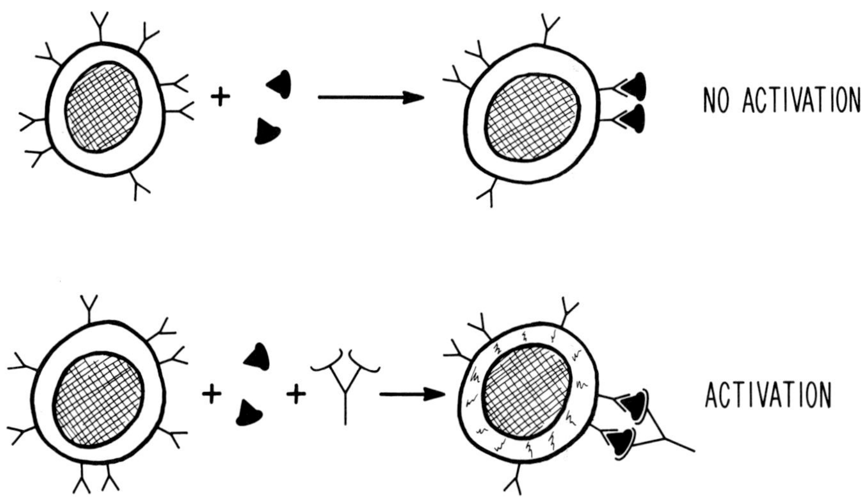

Fig. 4-7. Scheme for possible role of antibody in B-cell activation. Monovalent ligands could cross-link surface molecules if they were themselves externally bound by serum antibody.

(for example, native con A, PHA, LPS and anti-immunoglobulin), it cannot explain how univalent mitogens can activate a cell (for example, metallic ions and univalent con A).[44]

As further support for this limited cross-linking or "micropatching" hypothesis, it has been postulated that B cells may respond to a greater degree of surface cross-linking than T cells. Thus, although PHA is ordinarily a T-cell mitogen, if an insoluble matrix of PHA is formed on sepharose beads, its spectrum shifts toward that of a B-cell mitogen.[45] Similarly, when con A is chemically cross-linked to the bottom of a culture dish, it acquires the capacity to activate B cells.[46]

Even less is known about the surface events of antigen-induced activation. It is possible that the cross-linking mechanism may apply to some of the T-cell-independent antigens since these are large, multivalent molecules capable of bridging surface receptors.[47,48] On the other hand, because of the complex interaction of cells required to generate a response against T-cell-dependent antigens, very little is known about the direct effects of these antigens upon the lymphocyte surface.

INTRACELLULAR MESSENGERS

How are the triggering events on the lymphocyte surface communicated to the interior of the cell? Two candidates for the role of intracellular messenger have been suggested.

Calcium

A large calcium influx accompanies lymphocyte activation by both antigens and mitogens. Calcium has been shown to be essential for PHA-induced activation,[49] and calcium ionophores* can evoke cellular changes identical to those occurring with PHA stimulation.[50]. It has therefore been postulated that increasing intracellular levels of calcium are critical for the induction of nuclear and cytoplasmic processes associated with lymphocyte activation. Most interestingly, calcium has been shown to interact on many levels and in many different systems with the second group of proposed intracellular messengers, the cyclic nucleotides.[51, 52]

*Calcium ionophores are molecules—usually antibiotics—that intercalate into the cell membrane and increase calcium permeability.

The Cyclic Nucleotides

The importance of the cyclic nucleotides has been well established in a variety of systems. Cyclic AMP and, to a lesser degree, cyclic GMP have been found to mediate the effects of many hormones and to have clearly delineated roles in the regulation of cellular metabolism.

Most reports have indicated that cyclic AMP appears generally to inhibit the immune response.[53] PHA mitogenesis can be prevented by exogenously administered cyclic AMP and also by agents which, in other systems, are known to induce intracellular cyclic AMP synthesis by adenyl cyclase. These include the β-adrenergic catecholamines, histamine and the E-series prostaglandins.[54,55] Vibrio cholera toxin, which in virtually all mammalian cells produces a characteristic rise in cyclic AMP, and theophylline, which prevents the breakdown of cyclic AMP by a phosphodiesterase, are equally effective.[54] Exogenous cyclic AMP and cyclic-AMP-inducing agents maximally inhibit lymphocyte activation only if administered within the first few hours following stimulation, suggesting that cyclic AMP has its most potent regulatory effect early in the immune response.[56]

In order to understand the role of cyclic AMP in normal lymphocyte activation, many investigators have attempted to measure changes in endogenous cyclic AMP levels in cell cultures stimulated with PHA. The results have been conflicting, and both increases and decreases in cyclic AMP have been reported. One careful study found that PHA induces a rapid increase followed by a prolonged decrease in the intracellular concentration of cyclic AMP.[2] The complexity of these results has suggested that there may be several adenyl cyclase subsystems within each cell. This idea has been termed "compartmentalization."[2] If a given adenyl cyclase acts only locally within a specific subcellular compartment rather than pancellularly, cyclic AMP might play a stimulatory role in some compartments and an inhibitory role in others. The final cellular response would be determined by the interaction of these various local effects.

Two lines of evidence support the idea of compartmentalization in human lymphocytes:

1. When human lymphocytes were cultured with isoproterenol (a β-adrenergic agent), prostaglandin E1, and PHA, the effects of these agents on cyclic AMP levels were found to be additive, suggesting that each was affecting a separate pool of cyclic AMP.[2]

2. Immunofluorescence studies of human lymphocytes have revealed different patterns of subcellular cyclic AMP localization, depending upon the particular stimulatory agent used. PHA stimulation produces maximal staining along the plasma membrane; prostaglandin generates staining over the whole cytoplasmic matrix; isoproterenol evokes intense nuclear staining.[2]

The function of cyclic GMP in the immune response has also been investigated. There have been reports that acetylocoline augments lymphocyte effector functions and that this activity is mediated through a rise in intracellular cyclic GMP.[57-59] This cholinergic activity is inhibited by muscarinic blocking agents. Some investigators have observed large increases in intracellular cyclic GMP within minutes of PHA or con A stimulation.[60] All reports of cyclic GMP activity suggest a role opposite to that proposed for cyclic AMP, namely, that it is a stimulator of the immune response.[57,61,62] This idea has prompted an intracellular two-signal hypothesis of activation (Fig. 4-8).[63] It has been proposed that the binding of antigen to surface receptors stimulates adenyl cyclase to produce cyclic AMP. This blocks the immune response and may be one biochemical mechanism of tolerance (see Chap. 8). The addition of a second signal, such as might be provided by a T helper cell, provokes a rise in cyclic GMP. The ratio of cyclic GMP to cyclic AMP then determines whether or not the cell will be activated. Cyclic AMP alone paralyzes the cell, whereas both cyclic AMP and cyclic GMP are needed for activation. This hypothesis has been advanced on the basis of only the most preliminary data, and further investigation is clearly needed to elucidate the immunologic functions of the cyclic nucleotides.

With the discovery that histamine, prostaglandins, β-adrenergic agents, acetylcholine and insulin can bind to the lymphocyte surface and modulate lymphocyte activity, investigators have sought to determine the nature of the receptors for these substances. For several of these agents, the number of surface receptors rises during activation.[64] This observation has suggested the existence of a regulatory feedback mechanism on the immune response. For example, the cells activated in an immune response will express more and more histamine receptors on their surface while histamine accumulates in the accompanying inflammatory response. Histamine may bind to the activated lymphocytes and augment cyclic AMP production, thereby turning off the response.

Researchers have questioned whether receptors for hormones and other agents are present on all or only a subpopulation of lymphocytes. Lymphocytes can be passed over a column of insolubilized hormones and the nonadherent cells injected into an irradiated animal. When the animal is subsequently challenged with antigen, the immune response is increased over normal levels.[65] The implication is that the column has removed a population of suppressor cells (see Chap. 5) which express receptors for the hormones. Elution of these cells from the column and injection into the same animal decreases the response.[66] It is therefore possible that the hormone receptors are not randomly distributed throughout the entire lymphocyte population.

IMMUNOGLOBULIN SYNTHESIS

One of the consequences of the fervent biochemical activity occurring within activated B lymphocytes is the synthesis of immunoglobulin molecules. Immunoglobulin metabolism may comprise anywhere from 5 to 40 per cent of the total protein synthesis of an antibody-secreting cell.[67] This represents a major commitment on the part of the active cell.

There is still a great deal of uncertainty over which cells can and cannot synthesize and secrete immunoglobulin. The ability to *synthesize* immunoglobulin probably resides in peripheral blood lymphocytes as well as in fully differentiated plasma cells. This can be most readily shown by immunofluorescence studies demonstrating monoclonal immunoglobulin on the surface of these cells. The question of which cells can actively *secrete* immunoglobulin (versus the simple turnover of surface-bound immunoglobulin) is not yet resolved. When antigen activates a lymphocyte clone, the activated cells undergo a series of divisions, ultimately giving rise to a population of fully differentiated plasma cells. There is little doubt that plasma

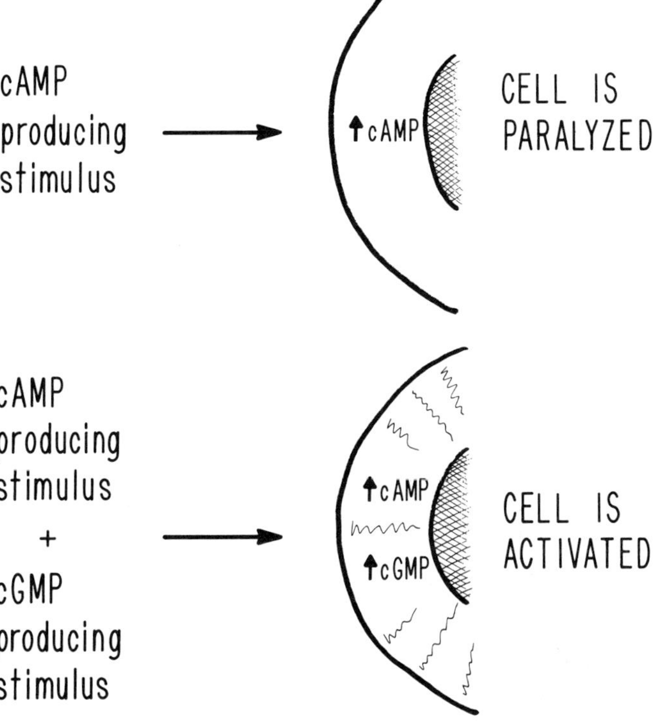

Fig. 4-8. The intracellular two-signal hypothesis of activation. Increasing cyclic AMP induces tolerance. Increasing cyclic AMP and cyclic GMP leads to immune activation.

cells are responsible for the bulk of immunoglobulin synthesis. However, it is not clear at what point in the pathway of differentiation cells first acquire the ability to actively secrete immunoglobulin. *In vitro* studies have not been very revealing since virtually the only human immunoglobulin-secreting cell lines which have been studied have been derived from patients with various lymphoproliferative disorders, and thus may or may not reflect normal lymphocyte functions.

The relation between cell division and immunoglobulin secretion is also a point of contention. There are some reports that immunoglobulin secretion can occur without cell division. However, the majority of data indicates that cell division and immunoglobulin secretion are intimately associated, and that cell division is probably requisite for immunoglobulin secretion.[68]

Immunoglobulin synthesis occurs in the late G1 and early S phases of the cell cycle (Fig. 4-9).[69] Translocation at the level of DNA may bring together the appropriate genetic regions coding for the

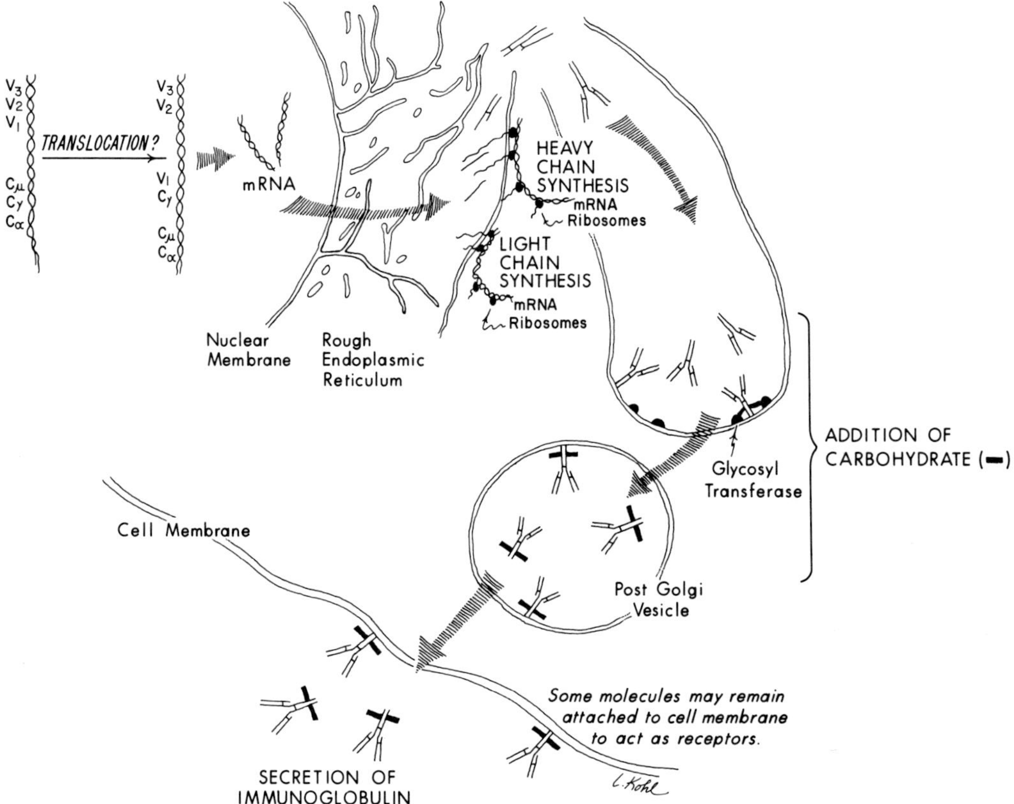

Fig. 4-9. The intracellular events of immunoglobulin synthesis. Following a (still hypothetical) process of translocation, mRNA strands bearing the genetic information for an intact polypeptide migrate to the rough endoplasmic reticulum, where the protein chains are synthesized. Assembly of the four-unit structure occurs in the RER, and the molecule is moved out toward the cell membrane. During this migration, carbohydrate is added to the immunoglobulin. Just before extrusion, the terminal carbohydrate groups are added. In the case of IgM, J chain is attached and the molecule now assumes its five-unit structure. Some of the molecules are then secreted as free antibody, others are bound to the cell membrane to serve as antigen receptors.

variable and constant domains of a given polypeptide chain so that a single mRNA molecule coding for an entire polypeptide can be formed. mRNA molecules have been isolated which can code for intact light chains in cell-free systems,[70,71] but at present it is still impossible to rule out the linear joining of separate mRNA strands which only together can code for the intact polypeptide.[72] Heavy and light chains appear to be coded for separately.[69]

Synthesis of the polypeptide chains takes only minutes.[73] Heavy and light chains are made on separate 300S and 200S membrane-bound polyribosomes, respectively. Heavy- and light-chain syntheses are carefully balanced, and either equal amounts or a slight excess of light chains are produced. It is not known how this balance is achieved.[74]

Some light chains may bind to heavy chains which are still attached to their polyribosomes, but the majority of the polypeptide chains are assembled into the complete four-chain immunoglobulin unit in the cisternae of the rough endoplasmic reticulum.[69] The order in which the chains are assembled has varied in different experimental systems; HL, H_2 and H_2L precursors have all been found.[75]

Once the polypeptide structure of the immunoglobulin is assembled, the molecule is moved into the smooth endoplasmic reticulum and out toward the cell surface. It can take from 30 minutes to several hours after assembly for the immunoglobulin to be secreted. During this migration, carbohydrate is added to the molecule in a stepwise and orderly fashion.[67] The most proximal carbohydrate groups may be added while the chains are still attached to the rough endoplasmic reticulum. The bulk of carbohydrate assembly occurs during the molecule's transit to the cell membrane, and a large percentage is added just prior to secretion. Many investigators have suggested that the attachment of carbohydrate may be required for immunoglobulin secretion, but experimental findings remain ambiguous on this point.[76] Pentamerization of IgM, with the addition of J chain, probably takes place just prior to secretion.[67]

The immunoglobulin molecule finally moves into a post-Golgi vesicle, although no true secretory granules are formed.[77] Some molecules are then secreted directly out of the cell, and others are inserted into the membrane, perhaps to act as cell-surface receptors. It is not understood how the fate of an individual immunoglobulin molecule is determined.

SUMMARY

Lymphocytes can be activated by antigens and mitogens. Because the latter group of molecules is capable of activating many clones of cells, mitogens have been used extensively to study the events of lymphocyte activation. The simple binding of a mitogen to the surface of a lymphocyte does not appear to be sufficient to activate a cell, and other surface phenomena may be involved. Both antigens and mitogens can induce receptor movement in the lymphocyte membrane, but the events of patching, capping and internalization cannot account for lymphocyte activation. A more limited surface process, such as the cross-linking of two surface receptors, may be the triggering event for some mitogens and antigens but cannot readily account for activation by many others of these substances. The surface events of activation must be communicated to the interior of the cell in order to induce the nuclear and cytoplasmic changes that characterize the activated cell. Both calcium and the cyclic nucleotides have been proposed to fulfill the role of intracellular messenger. Immunoglobulin synthesis is the most dramatic example of the synthetic potential of an activated lymphocyte, and reveals just one aspect of the profusion of intracellular processes involved in the phenomenon of lymphocyte activation.

REFERENCES

1. Oppenheim, J. J., and Rosenstreich, D. L.: Signals regulating in vitro activation of lymphocytes. Prog. Allergy, *20*:65, 1976.
2. Wedner, H. J., and Parker, C. W.: Lymphocyte activation. Prog. Allergy, *20*:195, 1976.
3. Douglas, S. D.: Electron microscopic and functional aspects of human lymphocyte response to mitogens. Transplant. Rev., *11*:39, 1972.
4. ——: Human lymphocyte growth in vitro: morphologic, biochemical, and immunologic significance. Int. Rev. Exp. Pathol., *10*:41, 1971.
5. Douglas, S. D., and Fudenberg, H. H.: In vitro development of plasma cells from lymphocytes following pokeweed mitogen stimulation: a fine structural study. Exp. Cell Res., *54*:277, 1969.
6. Cooper, H. L.: Effect of mitogens on the mitolic cycle: a biochemical evaluation of lymphocyte activation. In Zimmerman, A. M., Padilla, G. M., and Cameron, I. L. (eds.): Drugs and the Cell Cycle. p. 37. New York, Academic Press, 1973.
7. ——Studies on RNA metabolism during lymphocyte activation. Transplant. Rev., *11*:3, 1972.
8. Kay, J. E.: Leventhal, B. G., and Cooper, H. L.: Effects of inhibition of ribosomal RNA synthesis on the stimulation of lymphocytes by phytohaemagglutinin. Exp. Cell. Res., *54*:94, 1969.
9. Kay, J. E., Ahern, T., and Atkins, M.: Control of protein synthesis during the activation of lymphocytes by phytohemagglutinin. Biochim. Biophys. Acta., *247*:322, 1971.
10. Cooper, H. L.: Ribosomal ribonucleic acid wastage in resting and growing lymphocytes. J. Biol. Chem., *244*:5590, 1969.
11. Cooper, H. L., and Gibson, E. M.: Control of synthesis and wastage of ribosomal ribonucleic acid in lymphocytes: 1. The role of protein synthesis. J. Biol. Chem., *246*:5059, 1971.
12. Pago, B. G. T., Allfrey, V. G., and Musky, A. E.: RNA synthesis and histone acetylation during the course of gene activation in lymphocytes. *55*:805, 1966.
13. Kleinsmith, L. J., Aufrey, V. G., and Musky, A. E.: Phosphorylation of nuclear protein early in the course of gene activation in lymphocytes. Science, *154*:780, 1966.
14. Ada, G. L.: Antigen binding cells in tolerance and immunity. Transplant. Rev., *5*:105, 1970.
15. Rigas, D. A., and Osgood, E. E.: Purification and properties of the phytohemagglutinin of Phaseolus vulgaris. J. Biol. Chem., *212*:607, 1955.
16. Lis, H., and Sharon, N.: The biochemistry of plant lectins (phytohemagglutinins). Annu. Rev. Biochem., *42*:541, 1973.
17. Jones, G.: The number of reactive cells in mouse lymphocyte cultures stimulated by phytohemagglutinin, conconavalin A or histocompatibility antigen. J. Immunol., *111*:914, 1973.
18. Panzetta, P., Piroksky, B., and Rigas, D. A.: Mechanism of the mitogenic action of the phytohemagglutinin: 1. Induction of tolerance and lymphocyte transformation. J. Reticuloendothel. Soc., *13*:298, 1973.
19. Greaves, M., Janossy, G., and Doenhoff, M.: Selective triggering of human T and B lymphocytes in vitro by polyclonal mitogens. J. Exp. Med., *140*:1, 1974.
20. Janossy, G., Greaves, M. F., Doenhoff, M. J., and Snajdr, J.: Lymphocyte activation: V. Quantitation of the proliferative responses to mitogens using defined T and B cell populations. Clin. Exp. Immunol., *14*:581, 1973.
21. Greaves, M., and Janossy, G.: Elicitation of selective T and B lymphocyte responses by cell surface binding ligands. Transplant. Rev., *11*:87, 1972.
22. Andersson, J., Sjöberg, O., and Möller, G.: Mitogens as probes for immunocyte activation and cellular cooperation. Transplant. Rev., *11*:131, 1972.
23. Munakata, N., and Strauss, B.: Continued proliferation of mitogen-stimulated human peripheral blood lymphocytes: requirement for the stimulation of progeny. Cell. Immunol., *4*:243, 1972.
24. Jones, G.: Lymphocyte activation: III. The prolonged requirement for mitogen in phytohemagglutinin and concanavalin A-stimulated cultures. J. Immunol., *110*:1262, 1973.
25. Fanger, M. W., Hart, D. A., Wells, J. V., and Nisonoff, A.: Requirement for cross-linkage in the stimulation of transformation of rabbit peripheral lymphocytes by antiglobulin reagments. J. Immunol., *105*:1484, 1970.
26. Möller, G., Anderson, J., Pohlit, H., and Sjöberg, O.: Quantitation of the number of mitogen molecules activating DNA synthesis in T and B lymphocytes. Clin. Exp. Immunol., *13*:89, 1973.
27. Bona, C., *et al.*: Mitogenic effect of water-soluble extract of Nocardia opaca: a comparative study with some bacterial adjuvants on spleen and peripheral lymphocytes of 4 mammalian species. J. Immunol., *112*:2028, 1974.
28. Armerding, D., and Katz, D. H.: Activation of T and B lymphocytes in vitro: 1. Regulatory influence of bacterial lipopolysaccharide (LPS) on specific T-cell helper functions. J. Exp. Med., *139*:24, 1974.
29. Watson, J., Epstein, R., Nakoinz, I., and Ralph, P.: The role of humoral factors in the initiation of in vitro primary immune responses: II. Effects of lymphocyte mitogens. J. Immunol., *110*:43, 1973.
30. Bain, B., Vas, M. R., and Lowenstein, L.: The development of large immature mononuclear cells in mixed leukocyte cultures. Blood, *23*:108, 1964.
31. Wilson, D. B., and Nowell, P. C.: Quantitative studies on the mixed lymphocyte interaction in rats. V. Tempo and specificity of the proliferative response and the number of reactive cells from immunized donors. J. Exp. Med., *133*:442, 1971.
32. Marshall, W. H., Valentine, F. T., and Laurence, H. S.: Cellular immunity in vitro: clonal prolif-

eration of antigen-stimulated lymphocytes. J. Exp. Med., *130*:327, 1969.
33. Salmon, S. E., Krakauer, R. S., Whitmore, W. F.: Lymphocyte stimulation: selective destruction of cells during blastogenic response to transplantation antigens. Science, *172*:490, 1971.
34. Oppenheim, J. J., Whang, J., and Fui, E.: The effect of skin homograft rejection on recipient and donor mixed leukocyte cultures. J. Exp. Med., *122*:651, 1965.
35. Catalona, W. J., Sample, W. F., and Chretien, P. B.: Lymphocyte reactivity in cancer patients: correlation with tumor histology and clinical stage. Cancer, *31*:65, 1973.
36. McFarlane, H., and Hamid, J.: Cell-mediated immune response in malnutrition. Clin. Exp. Immunol., *13*:153, 1973.
37. Wheelock, E. F., Toy, S. T., and Stjernholm, R. L.: In Amos, D. B. (ed.): Progress in immunology. p. 787. New York, Academic Press, 1971.
38. Taylor, R. B., Duffus, P. H., Raff, M. C., and dePetris, S.: Redistribution and pinocytosis of lymphocyte surface Ig molecules induced by anti-Ig antibody. Nature [New Biol.], *233*:225, 1971.
39. Nossal, G. J. V., and Layton, J. E.: Antigen-induced aggregation and modulation of receptors on hapten-specific B lymphocytes. J. Exp. Med., *143*:511, 1976.
40. Greaves, M. F., and Bauminger, S.: Activation of T and B lymphocytes by insoluble phytomitogens. Nature [New Biol.], *235*:67, 1972.
41. Yahara, I., and Edelman, G. M.: The effects of concanavalin A on the mobility of lymphocyte surface receptors. Exp. Cell Res., *81*:143, 1973.
42. Edelman, G. M., Yahara, I., and Wang, J. L.: Receptor mobility and receptor-cytoplasmic interactions in lymphocytes. Proc. Natl. Acad. Sci. U.S.A., *70*:1442, 1973.
43. Ishizaka, K., and Ishizaka, T.: IgE and reagenic hypersensitivity. Ann. N.Y. Acad. Sci., *190*:443, 1971.
44. Sela, B. A., Wang, J. L., and Edelman, G. M.: Lymphocyte activation by monovalent fragments of antibodies reactive with cell surface carbohydrates. J. Exp. Med., *143*:665, 1976.
45. Greaves, M. F., and Bauminger, S.: Activation of T and B lymphocytes by insoluble phytomitogens. Nature [New Biol.], *235*:67, 1972.
46. Andersson, J., Edelman, G. M., Möller, G., Sjöberg, O.: Activation of B lymphocytes by locally concentrated concanavalin A. Eur. J. Immunol., *2*:233, 1972.
47. Sela, M., and Mozes, E.: The role of antigenic structure in B lymphocyte activation. Transplant. Rev., *23*:189, 1975.
48. Feldmann, M., Howard, J. G., and Desaymard, C.: Role of antigen structure in the discrimination between tolerance and immunity by B cells. Transplant. Rev., *23*:78, 1975.
49. Alford, R. H.: Metal cation requirements for phytohemagglutinin-induced transformation of human peripheral blood lymphocytes. J. Immunol., *104*:698, 1970.
50. Maino, V. C., Green, N. M., and Crumpton, M. J.: The role of calcium ions in initiating transformation of lymphocytes. Nature, *251*:324, 1974.
51. Rasmussen, H., and Goodman, D. B. P.: Calcium and cAMP as interrelated intracellular messengers. Ann.: N.Y. Acad. Sci., *253*:789, 1975.
52. Schultz, G., Hardman, J. G., Schultz, K., Baird, C. E., and Sutherland, E. W.: The importance of calcium ions for the regulation of guanosine 3′:5′ -cyclic monophosphate levels. Proc. Natl. Acad. Sci. U.S.A., *70*:3889, 1973.
53. Braun, W.: Regulatory factors in the immune response analysis and perspective. *In* Braun, W., Lichtenstein, L. M., and Parker, C. W. (eds.): Cyclic AMP, Cell Growth, and the Immune Response. P. 4. New York, Springer-Verlag, 1974.
54. Bourne, H. F., Melmon, K. L., Weinstein, Y., and Shearer, G. M.: Pharmacologic regulation of antibody release in vitro: effects of voasoactive amines and cyclic AMP. *In* Braun, W. Lichtenstein, L. M., and Parkef, C. W. (eds.): Cyclic AMP, Cell Growth and the Immune Response. P. 99. New York, Springer-Verlag, 1974.
55. Koopman, W. J., Gillis, M. H., and David, J. R.: Prevention of MIF activity by agents known to increase cellular cyclic AMP. J. Immunol., *110*:1609, 1973.
56. Bösing-Schneider, R., and Kolb, H.: Influence of cyclic AMP on early events of immune induction. Nature, *244*:224, 1973.
57. Hadden J. W.: Cyclic nucleotides in lymphocyte function. Ann. N.Y. Acad. Sci., *256*:352, 1975.
58. Kaliner, M., and Austen, K. F.: Hormonal control of the immunologic release of histamine and slow-reacting substance of anaphylaxis from human lung. *In* Braun, W., Lichtenstein, L. M., and Parker, C. W. (eds.): Cyclic AMP, Cell Growth and the Immune Response. P. 163. New York, Springer-Verlag, 1974.
59. Hadden, J. W., Johnson, E. M., Hadden, E. N., Coffey, R. G., and Johnson, L. D.: Cyclic GMP and lymphocyte activation. *In* Rosenthal, A. S. (ed.): Immune Recognition: Proc. of the 9th Leukocyte Culture Conference. Pp. 359–390. New York, Academic Press, 1975.
60. Hadden, J., Hadden, E. M., Haddox, M. K., and Goldberg, N. D.: Guanosine 3′:5′ -cyclic monophosphate: a possible intracellular mediator of mitogenic influences in lymphocytes. Proc. Natl. Acad. Sci. U.S.A., *69*:3024, 1972.
61. Hadden, J. W., Hadden, E., and Goldberg, N. D.: Cyclic GMP and cyclic AMP in lymphocyte metabolism and proliferation. *In* Braun, W., Lichtenstein, L. M., and Parker, C. W. (eds.): Cyclic AMP, Cell Growth and the Immune Response. Pp. 237–246. New York, Springer-Verlag, 1974.
62. Diamantstein, T., and Ulmer, A.: The antagonistic action of cyclic GMP and cyclic AMP on proliferation of B and T lymphocyte. Immunology, *28*:113, 1975.
63. Watson, J., Epstein, R., and Cohn, M.: Cyclic nucleotides as intracellular mediators of the

expression of antigen-sensitive cells. Nature, *246*:405, 1973.

64. Bourne, H. R., Lichtenstein, L. M., Melman, K. L., Henny, C. S., Weinstein, Y., and Shearer, G. M.: Modulation of inflammation and immunity by cyclic AMP. Science *184*:19, 1974.
65. Shearer, G. M., Melman, K. L., Weinstein, Y., and Sela, M.: Regulation of antibody response by cell expressing histamine receptors. J. Exp. Med., *136*:1302, 1972.
66. Shearer, G. M., Weinstein, Y., Melman, K. L., and Bourne, H. R.: Separation of leukocytes by their amine receptors: subsequent immunologic functions. *In* Braun, W., Lichtenstein, L. M., and Parker, C. W., (eds.): Cyclic AMP, Cell Growth, and the Immune Response. P. 135. New York, Springer-Verlag, 1974.
67. Melchers, F., and Andersson, J.: Synthesis, surface deposition and secretion of immunoglobulin M in bone marrow-derived lymphocytes before and after mitogenic stimulation. Transplant. Rev., *14*:76, 1973.
68. Bell, G. I.: B lymphocyte activation and lattice formation. Transplant. Rev., *23*:202, 1975.
69. Buxbaum, J. N.: The biosynthesis, assembly, and secretion of immunoglobulins Semin. Hematol., *10*:33, 1973.
70. Swan, D., Aviv, H., and Leder, P.: Purification and properties of biologically active messenger RNA for a myeloma light chain. Prac. Natl. Acad. Sci. U.S.A., *69*:1967, 1972.
71. Stavnezer, J., and Huang, R. C. C.: Synthesis of a mouse Ig light chain in a rabbit reticulocyte cell-free system. Nature [New Biol.], *230*:172, 1971.
72. Knopf, P. M.: Pathways leading to expression of immunoglobulins. Transplant. Rev., *14*:145, 1973.
73. Knopf, P. M., Parkhouse, R. M. E., and Lennox, E. S.: Biosynthetic units of an Ig heavy chain. Prac. Natl. Acad. Sci. U.S.A., *58*:2288, 1967.
74. Zolla, S., Buxbaum, J., Franklin, E. C., and Scharff, M. D.: Synthesis and assembly of Igs by malignant human plasmacytes: 1. Myeloma producing γ -chains and light chains. J. Exp. Med., *132*:148, 1970.
75. Baumal, R., and Scharff, M. D.: Synthesis, assembly and secretion of mouse Ig[1]. Transplant. Rev., *14*:163, 1973.
76. Melchers, F., and Knopf, P. M.: Biosynthesis of the carbohydrate portion of Ig chains: possible relation to secretion. Cold Spring Harbor Symp. Quant. Biol., *32*:255, 1967.
77. Vitetta, E. S., and Uhr, J. W.: Synthesis, transport, dynamics and fate of cell surface Ig and alloantigens in murine lymphocytes. Transplant. Rev., *14*:50, 1973.

5 Cellular Interactions and Controls

There are three major cell types that work together to generate an optimal immune response. These are the B lymphocyte, the T lymphocyte and the macrophage. Recent work has further subdivided these cellular classifications into a number of functional subpopulations which interact with each other and modulate each other's behavior. The picture of immunologic interactions and controls that is emerging is extraordinarily complex despite the fact that almost all of this work has been done in only the last ten to fifteen years. In this chapter we shall examine the ways in which the cells of the immune system communicate with each other, and how this extensive network of interactions affects the generation of an immune response.

THE T HELPER CELL

In the preceding chapter we saw how antigens and mitogens can interact with the lymphocyte surface and trigger cellular activation. Most of the work attempting to study the surface events of activation has employed mitogens and T-cell-independent antigens. However, many antigens—and possibly the great majority of antigens—are neither mitogenic nor T-cell-independent. In a classic experiment, Claman showed that the production of a humoral response against certain antigens required the participation of thymic-derived lymphocytes (Fig. 5-1).[1,2] These T cells do not make antibodies themselves, but rather act as *helper cells* for the humoral response. If T cells are not present, B-cell activation does not occur and little or no antibody is produced. We are therefore no longer considering only the way in which antigen interacts with the immunocompetent cells, but must look further at how the cells themselves interact. These two processes—antigen-cell interactions and cell-cell interactions—are closely interwoven.

The role of the T helper cell has been clarified to some extent by the discovery and elucidation of the hapten-carrier phenomenon (see Chap. 2). The ability to mount a humoral response against a given antigenic determinant (hapten) requires that it be conjugated to a larger molecule (carrier) which is recognized by the T helper cell. Carrier recognition induces the T helper cell to deliver some unspecified signal to the B cell which has bound the haptenic determinant. As a consequence, the B cell is activated and an antibody response is mounted against the hapten.

Many laboratories have devoted considerable attention to determining the na-

CELLS FROM ANIMAL IMMUNIZED WITH SHEEP RED BLOOD CELLS:

AFTER CHALLENGE WITH SHEEP RED BLOOD CELLS:

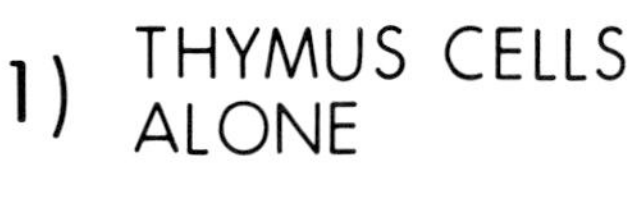

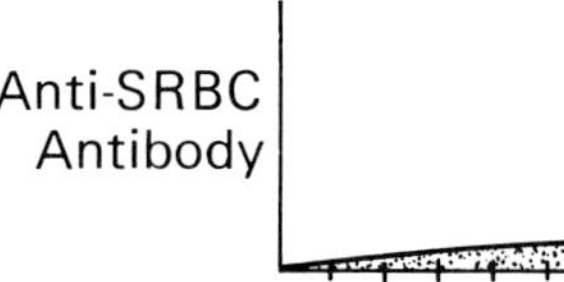

2) MARROW CELLS ALONE

Anti-SRBC Antibody

3) THYMUS AND MARROW CELLS

Anti-SRBC Antibody

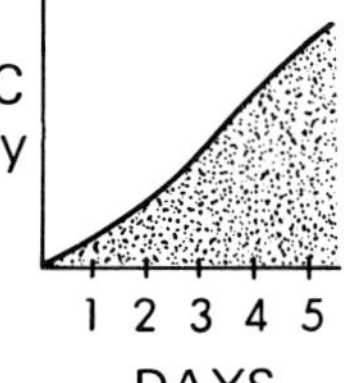

Fig. 5-1. The experiment that first demonstrated the requirement for T cells in the humoral response to an antigen. Both thymus cells (predominantly T cells) and marrow cells (containing a high percentage of B cells) independently produce an ineffective humoral response to sheep erythrocytes. Both cell types together produce a powerful anti-SRBC response.

ture of the T helper signal. The most basic question is whether direct T-cell-to-B-cell contact is required, or whether the T cell releases a soluble factor (or factors) which makes contact with the B-cell surface. Evidence for direct cell-to-cell contact has been difficult to obtain. On the other hand, a plethora of T-cell-derived soluble factors has been found, each factor capable of replacing T helper function in cultures depleted of T cells. These factors can be conveniently grouped into those whose actions are antigen-specific and those that are nonspecific.

Specific Helper Factors

The hapten-carrier phenomenon, as detailed in Chapter 2, indicates that T helper function is carrier-specific. In other words, in order to elicit a secondary anamnestic response to a hapten conjugated to a given carrier, the T-cell population must first have been primed to that specific carrier. It is therefore not surprising that several of the soluble helper factors that have been described are also carrier-specific.

Suppose we isolate a carrier-specific T-cell-derived soluble factor generated during an immune response to a particular hapten conjugated to carrier A. This factor can then be used in place of primed T cells to provide helper activity for a population of B cells responding against the hapten, but only if the hapten is conjugated to that same carrier A. The same soluble factor would be unable to provide helper activity for a humoral response against the hapten if it were conjugated to any other carrier.

Two specific helper factors have been most intensively studied:

One factor has been obtained from mouse T cells and appears to have the characteristics of an immunoglobulin molecule. It has been called "IgT."[3] The active factor appears to be a complex of "IgT" and antigen that is released from the T-cell surface. It has been proposed that the "IgT" molecule is cytophilic and that the "IgT"-antigen complex can be bound to a macrophage for presentation to a B cell. In the absence of macrophages, the "IgT"-antigen complex binds directly to B cells and is believed to induce tolerance.[4] Another "IgT"-like factor has been described which can restore an antigen-specific IgE response in neonatally thymectomized rats.[5]

A second antigen-specific helper factor does not seem to bear any resemblance to immunoglobulin.[6] Nevertheless, it appears to be able to bind antigen specifically. Immunologic analysis has shown that the factor itself bears antigenic determinants that appear to be coded for by genetic loci closely linked to the *major histocompatibility complex (MHC)*.[7] The MHC is a genetic region that codes for a number of molecules intimately associated with many immunologic functions. The best characterized of these is a group of antigens termed "histocompatibility antigens," that are expressed on cell surfaces and are important in transplantation both in animals and in man. Another region of the MHC has been named the I region and has been described in several animal species. Genes within the I region influence a variety of immunologic processes, including the level of immune responsiveness to particular antigens, the ability to stimulate a mixed lymphocyte reaction, and so on. Recently, loci within the I region have been implicated in the regulation of the interactions among immunocompetent cells. It is therefore of great interest that this particular helper factor bears determinants that are coded for by the I region of the mouse MHC. We will see throughout this chapter that the MHC, and the I region in particular, appears to be closely associated with the events of the immune response. A detailed discussion of the MHC in man will be presented in Chapter 9.

Nonspecific Helper Factors

The discovery that T cells can also secrete soluble factors which *nonspecifically* stimulate a heterogeneous population of antigen-primed B cells is, at first, surprising in light of the demonstration of T helper specificity in the hapten-carrier effect. One possible explanation is that the nonspecific stimulus is ordinarily overshadowed by a more powerful specific stimulation. A second possibility is that nonspecific stimulation is the result of the collective effects of many specific stimuli released from a heterogeneous population of T cells. Both of these suggestions are, however, pure speculation.

Two methods have been successful in the generation of nonspecific helper factors: (1) exposure of T cells to specific antigen, and (2) exposure of T cells to allogeneic cells. These factors are often referred to as *T-cell-replacing factors*, or TRFs. A TRF that is produced when T cells make contact with a given antigen can replace T cells *in vitro* in providing helper activity for antibody responses against many other unrelated antigens (Fig. 5-2).[8,9]

The production of a TRF upon T-cell exposure to allogeneic cells has been the most carefully studied example of nonspecific stimulation. This helper substance is called *allogeneic effect factor* (AEF) and is responsible for a phenomenon called the *allogeneic effect*.[10] Like the mixed lymphocyte reaction (MLR) (see Chap. 4), the allogeneic effect results

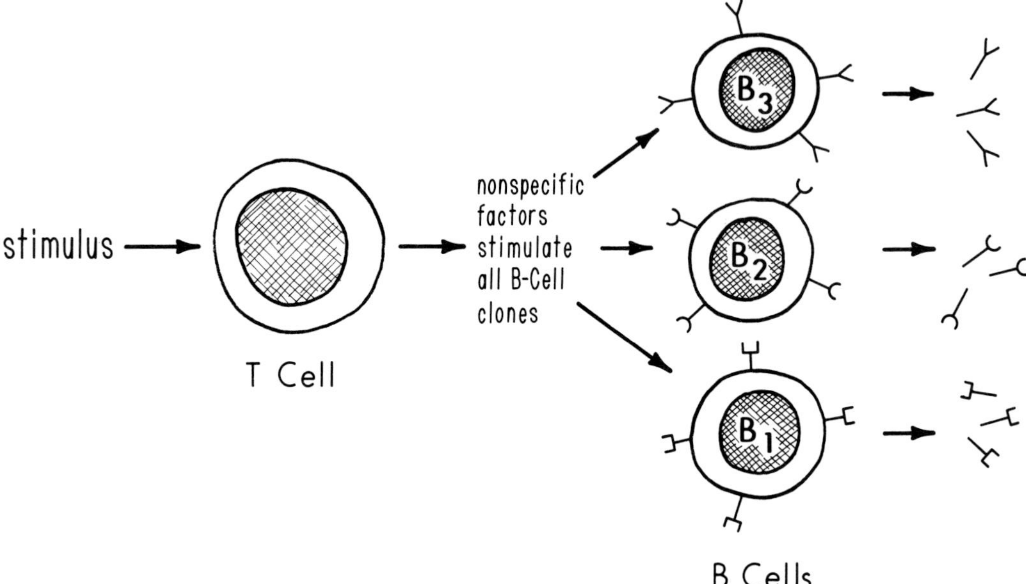

Fig. 5-2. T cells have been demonstrated to be able to secrete nonspecific factors which can stimulate many different B-cell clones.

from the recognition of foreign (allogeneic) cells by T cells. In the MLR, T cells cultured *in vitro* with allogeneic cells are stimulated to undergo blast transformation and acquire killer-cell potential. A similar phenomenon can be observed *in vivo.* In the latter case, lymphocytes are administered to a host of a dissimilar genetic background. The grafted cells will recognize the host cells as foreign and undergo the same sequence of changes as in the MLR. This phenomenon is termed a *graft-versus-host reaction* (GvHR) and is considered to be the *in vivo* correlate of the MLR.[11]

The allogeneic effect occurs within the setting of a GvHR. Thus, when allogeneic donor T lymphocytes are given to a host, the donor cells become activated. The activated donor cells are able to provide a powerful nonspecific T helper signal to the host B cells (Fig. 5-3). This has been demonstrated in the following way: the host is first sensitized to a particular hapten conjugated to carrier A. The host is then challenged with the hapten on carrier B in the presence of allogeneic T cells. Ordinarily, the host would be unable to mount a secondary response to the hapten presented on a new carrier. However, in the presence of the allogeneic donor T cells, a vigorous secondary response to the hapten ensues. Thus, the allogeneic effect can replace the need for antigen-specific T helper function by providing a powerful nonspecific stimulatory signal to the host B cells.

The magnitude of the host antibody production is proportional to the magnitude of the GvHR. If the allogeneic cells have been previously sensitized to the host tissue, a powerful GvHR will take place and host antibody production will be proportionally high. Similarly, if the genetic differences between the graft and the host are increased, the effect is also more pronounced.

The ability to mediate an allogeneic effect has been found to reside in a small soluble factor.[12,13] Allogeneic effect factor (AEF) is produced by the donor T cells and appears to act directly on the host B cells (Fig. 5-4).[13] Careful studies have shown that AEF bears antigenic determinants

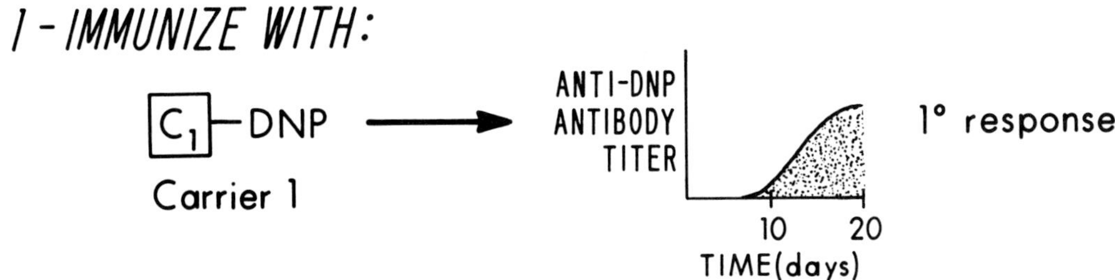

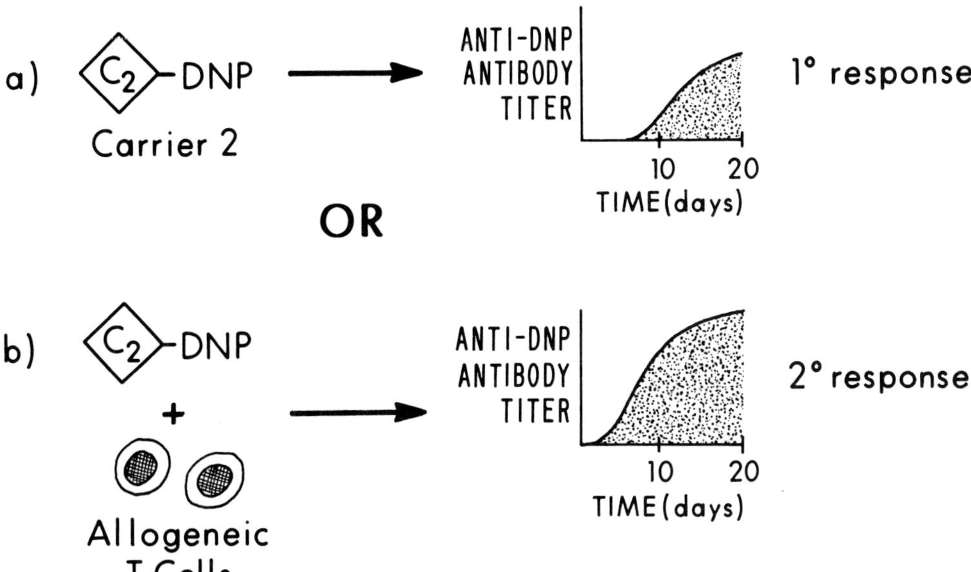

Fig. 5-3. The allogeneic effect. Ordinarily, rechallenge with a hapten on a new carrier will not evoke a secondary antihapten response. In the presence of allogeneic cells, however, a secondary response is evoked.

coded for by the I region of the mouse major histocompatibility complex.[14] Interestingly, although generated by an allogeneic confrontation and clearly able to act upon allogeneic cells, AEF is most effective in activating syngeneic B cells.

The Genetics of T-Cell–B-Cell Interactions

We have already seen that some specific and nonspecific T helper factors are at least partially coded for by genetic loci within the major histocompatibility complex. Some of the most exciting work in immunology at present is concerned with the attempt to unravel the genetic controls over T-cell–B-cell interactions. Most available evidence indicates that in order for antigen-specific T helper function to occur, the B and T cells involved must be genetically identical (syngeneic) at particular loci within the major histocompatibility complex.[15,16] Some very elegant work has localized the requirement for genetic identity to the I region of the MHC which contains the Ir genes.[17] These genes control the ability of an individual to respond to certain antigens, and

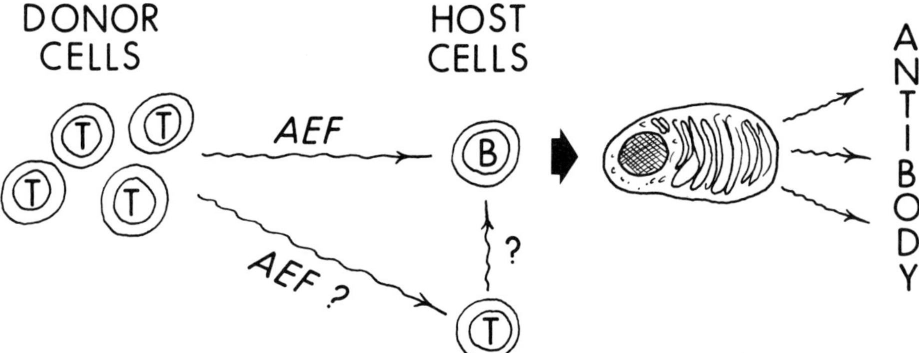

Fig. 5-4. The allogeneic effect is due to the secretion of a nonspecific factor by the donor T cells. This is a potent stimulant to the host B cells to secrete antibody.

may do so—at least in part—by controlling T-cell–B-cell interactions.

It was originally felt that the requirement for MHC identity reflected the necessity for T helper cells and B cells to make direct contact with each other. According to this view, cellular cooperation occurred as the result of mutually recognized surface gene products such that identical gene products on T and B cells would recognize and bind to each other. However, as we have seen, it is now clear that cell contact is not required for effective cellular cooperation. The association of I region gene products with several helper factors suggests that recognition of shared surface antigens may occur without direct cell-to-cell contact. However, the actual reason why T helper cells and responding B cells must share identical I region loci in order to produce an effective humoral response is not at all clear. In addition, some of the work exploring the behavior of certain of the soluble helper factors has produced results in apparent conflict with the requirement for I region identity. Thus, AEF, which bears I region determinants, is able to stimulate allogeneic cells. The lack of genetic restriction may be related to the nonspecific nature of AEF. However, the I-region-controlled specific helper factor also appears to be able to stimulate allogeneic cells. Thus, despite the requirement for genetic identity in most systems of T-cell–B-cell interactions, there are noted exceptions.

In summary, a great many antigens can induce a humoral response only in the presence of T cells. There is no evidence that these T helper cells must directly contact B cells in order to carry out their stimulatory function, and many soluble factors have been found which can mediate T helper activity. T cells can release antigen-specific factors and also nonspecific helper factors. We cannot at present assess the relative importance of each of these in the normal, *in vivo* humoral response. We cannot even be sure if one cell produces more than one type of factor, or if separate subpopulations are involved. At least one experiment has suggested that different subsets of T cells may be responsible for the elaboration of specific and nonspecific factors.[18]

SUPPRESSOR CELLS

The existence of cells which can suppress the immune response is currently under intensive investigation both in animals and in man. Suppressor cells are perhaps a logical addition to the existence of "helping" cells, and may represent another important regulatory component of the immune response.

T cells have been found to be able to

suppress humoral responses to T-cell-dependent and T-cell-independent antigens,[19] and may do so by suppression of B cells and/or T helper cells.[20–22] T suppressor cells can also inhibit T-cell functions such as proliferation and cytotoxicity in the mixed lymphocyte reaction.[23,24] Current evidence favors the view that T suppressor cells represent a subpopulation of T cells distinct from cells carrying out other T-cell functions (see below).

T suppressor cells appear to be most effective early in the course of an immune response, and can suppress primary humoral responses more readily than secondary humoral responses. They do not seem to act by blocking initiation of the immune response, but rather by preventing subsequent proliferation and expansion (and perhaps affinity maturation[25]; see Chap. 6) of the antigen-reactive clones.[26,27]

Most studies of T-cell-mediated suppression have indicated that it is antigen-specific.[28–30] Although it has not been convincingly demonstrated, it appears most likely that T suppressor cells are able to recognize specific antigens. An alternate suggestion is that T suppressor cells do not recognize antigen directly, but instead react against the proliferating clones of effector and helper cells.[31] This would produce the same effect as an antigen-specific suppressive response. At present there is little experimental support for this idea.

T-cell-derived antigen-specific soluble factors capable of mimicking T-suppressor-cell activity have been described. The best characterized of these is a small protein able to specifically inhibit IgE responses in rats.[30,32] This factor can specifically bind antigen although it does not appear to resemble immunoglobulin. Its activity can be blocked by antisera directed against antigens coded for by the rat major histocompatibility complex, and it is only effective in suppressing syngeneic cells.[33]

Nonspecific T-cell suppression has also been described, and soluble factors capable of mediating a generalized suppression have been reported.[26,34] One of the more interesting examples of nonspecific immune suppression is a phenomenon called *antigenic competition*.[35] Antigenic competition has been demonstrated in only a few experimental systems. It is defined as a process in which the induction of an immune response to one antigen or determinant reduces the ability of the immune system to respond to another antigen or determinant. The suppression is transient, lasting from days to weeks after the administration of the first antigen. During this period, the immune system is relatively refractory to other antigenic stimuli.

Competition can occur between separate antigens or between two determinants on a given antigen. With competition between *separate antigens* (Fig. 5-5), the antigens appear to be competing at the level of the T cell. In some situations of interantigenic competition, the first antigen may be nonspecifically activating suppressor cells which inhibit the response to any second antigen.[36,37] In others, the two antigens may be competing for a limited amount of T-cell help.[38] Competition between two determinants on the *same antigen* (Fig. 5-6) has been proposed to occur at the B-cell level.[39] In this case the binding of one B cell to its particular determinant probably blocks the access of B cells to other determinants on the same molecule.

T suppressor cells are being increasingly implicated in various animal and human diseases. The New Zealand Black (NZB) and the New Zealand Black/White (NZB/W) hybrid mice are excellent models for human autoimmune disease. These animals develop, among other things, antibodies against their own erythrocytes and nuclear antigens along with an immune complex nephritis. This abnormal production of antibodies

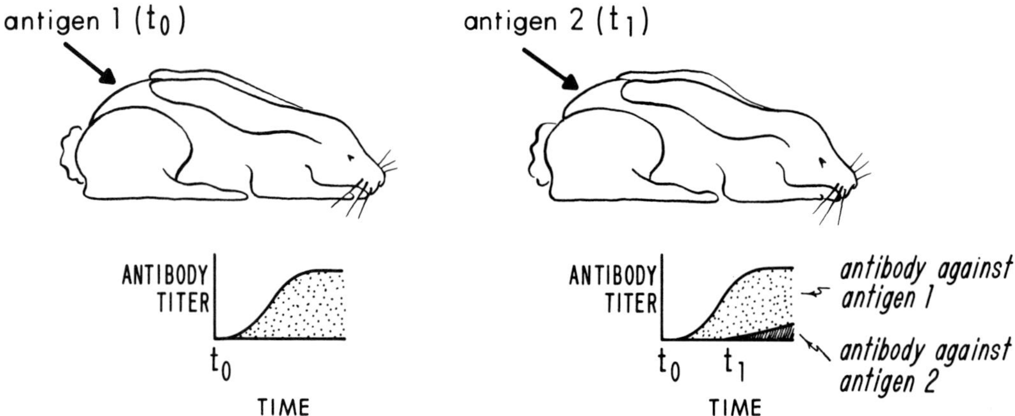

Fig. 5-5. Intermolecular antigenic competition appears to occur at the level of the T cell, either via the activation of suppressor cells or by tying up all of the available T-cell help.

against self-determinants has been attributed to a loss of T-suppressor-cell function.[40] We will explore in detail the immunology of the New Zealand mice as well as some examples of human autoimmune diseases where T-suppressor-cell activity may be decreased in Chapter 8.

T suppressor cells have also been implicated in the pathogenesis of the human disease, common variable hypogammaglobulinemia (see Chap. 10). In these patients an overactivity of T suppressor cells may be responsible for the greatly diminished production of immunoglobulin.

Other cell types in addition to T cells can mediate immune suppression. Macrophages have been demonstrated to be able to inhibit mitogen- and antigen-induced immunologic reactions.[41–43] It was originally felt that direct contact between suppressor macrophages and lymphocytes was required for suppression, but recent work has uncovered sol-

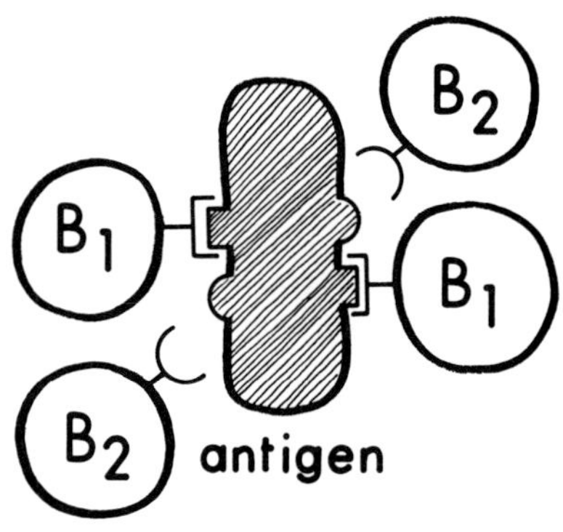

Fig. 5-6. Intramolecular antigenic competition occurs at the level of the B cell, perhaps by the steric inhibition of B cell binding to other determinants on the same molecule.

uble mediators derived from macrophages that are capable of immune suppression.[44–46]

T-CELL SUBPOPULATIONS AND T-CELL–T-CELL INTERACTIONS

From our discussion thus far it should be clear that T cells can perform a great many functions. These include effector functions such as cytotoxicity and accessory functions such as help and suppression. Do these functions represent the activity of a homogeneous, multifunctional population of T cells, or can specific functions be attributed to distinct subpopulations of T cells? There is a growing body of evidence supporting the view that T-cell subpopulations exist, each of which is capable of providing only one or a few of the functions attributable to the T-cell population as a whole.

T-cell subpopulations have been defined on the basis of physical properties, such as surface markers and circulatory patterns, and functional activities, such as helper function and suppressor function. It will become apparent in this brief discussion that some populations that were originally defined solely on a functional basis are now being associated with unique physical parameters, and vice versa. Establishing a correlation between physical and functional markers is an important step in achieving an understanding of subpopulation activities. We must emphasize, however, that most of this work has been done in animal systems, and the application of these concepts to man will require further work.

Classification of T-Cell Subpopulations by Physical Properties

In terms of understanding the development of immune competence within a given host, one of the most useful classifications involves the division of T cells according to their maturity. One example of a pattern of maturation within the mouse has been proposed (Fig. 5-7).[47] Stem cells enter the thymus and migrate to the cortex. These are actively dividing cells and are immunologically incompetent. They express a high concentration of θ antigen (a mouse T-cell marker) on their surface. Eventually these cells cease to divide, and move into the medulla. The medullary lymphocytes are more mature immunologically and express low surface concentrations of the θ antigen. These cells will ultimately leave the medulla to enter the periphery.

In the periphery two basic T-cell subpopulations are recognized:[48]

The first, often referred to as T_1, consists of a population of short-lived cells that is dependent upon the thymus for survival. This thymic dependency may simply reflect the rapid turnover of this pool of cells and the need for continual replacement. These cells are not part of the recirculating pool, home to the fixed lymphoid tissues such as the spleen, and are present in highest concentration in the spleen and thymus. They appear to be relatively resistant to the inhibitory effect of antilymphocyte serum (see Chap. 16).

The second subpopulation of T cells, or T_2, consists of long-lived cells. These form the recirculating pool and are found primarily in the peripheral blood, thoracic duct and lymph nodes. They are sensitive to antilymphocyte serum.

Other physical criteria have also been used to distinguish T-cell subpopulations:

Steroid Resistance. Most of the cells in the mouse spleen and thymus are steroid-sensitive (that is, they are lysed by high concentrations of hydrocortisone). However, the bulk of immunologic reactivity appears to reside in the small percentage of steroid-resistant cells.[49]

Surface Markers. Many antigenic markers have been detected on mouse T cells. One of them, θ, we have mentioned above. Another set of markers, the Ly antigens, consists of three markers each

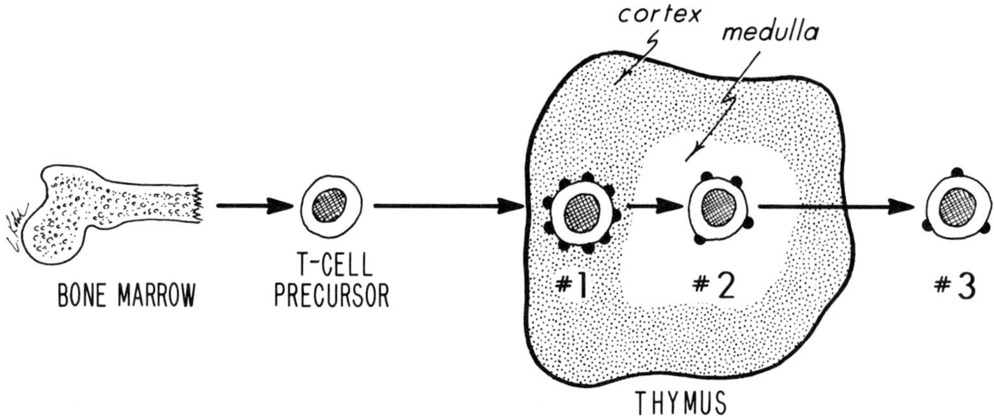

Fig. 5-7. One model of T-cell maturation within the mouse thymus. T-cell precursors pass through three distinguishable stages of differentiation as shown.

with two possible alleles.[50] These can be expressed in a variety of patterns which have in turn been associated with particular T-cell functions, such as helper and killer activity (see below).

Separation Techniques. Investigators have been able to subdivide T cells on the basis of their electrophoretic mobility and density characteristics.[47] These techniques may eventually prove to be especially valuable in isolating particular T-cell functional subpopulations.

Others. T cells have also been found to differ in their sensitivity to radiation and in their responsiveness to various T-cell mitogens.[47,51] It is likely that many other T-cell subdivisions will soon be defined on the basis of differing physical criteria.

Classification of T-Cell Subpopulations by Functional Activities

Analysis of T-cell subpopulations based on functional criteria revolves around three questions. Do killer and helper phenomena depend on two distinct cell populations? Are helper and suppressor functions the result of the activity of separate subpopulations? Are there helper cells for T-cell functions?

Helper Cell Versus Killer Cell. There is surprisingly little information on this important point. The best evidence that killer cells and helper cells are distinct comes from studies of the Ly antigens in the mouse. Killer-cell precursors have been shown to express predominantly Ly-2 and Ly-3 antigens; helper cells express primarily antigens of the Ly-1 locus.[50,52,53] Each subpopulation can be selectively removed by antiserum directed against the particular surface antigens, suggesting that these represent truly distinct cellular subsets.

Helper Cell Versus Suppressor Cell. Recent evidence favors the view that the T suppressor cell is physically separable from the helper cell.[54] Thus, for example, there is evidence that suppressor and helper cells from NZB/W mice can be separated by unit gravity sedimentation.[55] Suppressor functions also appear to be more susceptible to x-irradiation than helper function, an observation most easily explained by the existence of separate helper and suppressor populations.[56] Nevertheless, this conclusion remains to be confirmed. Finally, analysis of mouse T-cell populations bearing Ly antigens has revealed that suppressor cells bear the same antigens as the killer cell precursors, and hence are separable from the helper-cell population.[57,58] Suppressor cells may similarly be separable from T effector cells on the basis of a differential expression of surface antigens coded for by the I region of the MHC.[59]

Helper Cells for T Cells. The graft-versus-host reaction, as described earlier, involves the reaction of donor lymphocytes against an allogeneic host. It is generally believed to be a T-cell phenomenon. Two separate T-cell subpopulations appear to be involved.[60,61] One population is the precursors of the actual killer cells while the second population of cells acts primarily as amplifier cells. The precursors of the killer cells have been found to correlate with the T_1 subpopulation mentioned above, and the amplifier cells with the T_2 subpopulation.[48] The amplifier cells share many physical features with the T helper cells of the humoral response, and may, in fact, be the same population of cells. Similar T-cell subpopulations have been described to partake in the mixed lymphocyte reaction.[48,62]

THE MACROPHAGE AND THE IMMUNE RESPONSE

Within the past few years the macrophage has been recognized as an essential component of the immune system. Although its role as a phagocyte has long been known, the full scope of its activities has only recently been appreciated. In the following section we will examine the role of the macrophage as an immunologic cell, emphasizing its interaction with T and B lymphocytes.

With regard to immune processes, the macrophage performs two vital functions. First, it presents antigen to lymphocytes in such a way that it is able to elicit a maximal immune response. Second, the macrophage communicates with lymphocytes both by direct surface-to-surface contact and by soluble factors. These interactions can be either stimulatory or inhibitory to lymphocytes.

T-cell activation appears to have a definite requirement for macrophages. The situation is less certain for B cells; however, since in most cases B cells require T helper cells for activation, they have at least an *indirect* requirement for macrophages.[63] Recent work supports a *direct* role for macrophages in B-cell activation as well.[64]

Antigen Uptake and Processing

We shall begin our examination of the macrophage by looking at the ways in which it interacts with antigen. There is a strong association between macrophage uptake of antigen and immunogenicity.[65] Antigens which do not at some point interact with the macrophage population generally fail to elicit an immune response. Indeed, in one system, macrophage-associated antigen was able to induce T helper activity and a humoral response, whereas free, soluble antigen actually stimulated T suppressor activity.[65a] We must emphasize, however, that not all antigens that attach to macrophages are immunogenic, nor are all antigens that avoid interaction with macrophages unable to elicit immunologic responses. Macrophages can take up antigen in a variety of ways, including phagocytosis, pinocytosis and passive absorption. Cytophilic antibody may be important for antigen uptake when antigen is present in low concentrations, but at higher doses it does not appear to make a significant contribution.[66,67] Several workers have confirmed that macrophages can take up antigens without the intervention of antibody.[68,69]

The second stage of macrophage interaction with antigen has been termed "antigen processing." It has been thought for some time that an explanation for the powerful immunogenicity of macrophage-bound antigen might lie in the way that the macrophage modifies the antigen following antigen uptake. However, it has been exceedingly difficult to prove the existence of such a process, and many investigators now doubt whether it occurs at all.

Most of the antigen taken up by macrophages *in vitro* is rapidly degraded[70,71] and probably does not partake in the induction of an immune response. A small percentage of antigen persists in immunogenic form, perhaps for as long as several days.[72,73] Some of the immunogenic antigen is expressed on the cell surface following endocytosis.[74–76] There is little evidence that the internalized antigen is processed in any way in order to become a potent immunogen. There was much excitement when antigens were found to be able to complex with macrophage RNA, but the importance of "informational" RNA in immune induction has not been established. Investigation of this area continues.[77]

An alternative view to explain the potent immunogenicity of macrophage-bound antigen is that just the attachment of an antigen to the macrophage surface may by itself be sufficient for that antigen to be able to induce an immune response. There are two possible explanations why this might be, both of which seem to be correct: (1) macrophage binding protects the antigen from catabolism, and (2) the macrophage presents the antigen to the lymphocytes in such a way that immune induction is maximized. Antigen presentation is thus the next step in the macrophage's handling of antigen, and has been the focus of much experimental work.

Macrophage Presentation of Antigen to T Cells

We have already stated that T-cell activation requires the presence of macrophages. This has been clearly shown for activation by soluble antigens and allogeneic cells, although the requirement for macrophages in mitogenesis is still somewhat uncertain.[64,78–83] Most of the available evidence favors the view that macrophages are required for the *initial interaction* between T cells and antigen.

Although there is no convincing evidence for direct cell-to-cell contact in T-cell–B-cell interactions, T-cell–macrophage contact has been easy to demonstrate. Such direct contact appears to be required for T-cell activation when the antigen cannot be efficiently bound by the T cell alone. In this category we must consider most small, soluble antigens.[84] On the other hand, T cells appear to bind cell-surface antigens well, and macrophages may not be required for the presentation of cellular antigens to the T cell.[84] However, even in these circumstances, the macrophage is required for T-cell activation. We shall explore the possible reasons for this below.

When macrophages are incubated with soluble antigen, clusters of lymphocytes form around the macrophages (Fig. 5-8). These are composed of T and B lymphocytes[85–87] and have been observed with human cells as well as in other species.[88] If these clusters are artificially dispersed soon after formation, no immune response occurs.[89]

A series of experiments using the guinea pig as an experimental model has explored the events that occur within these clusters. This work has focused on T-cell–macrophage interactions. There

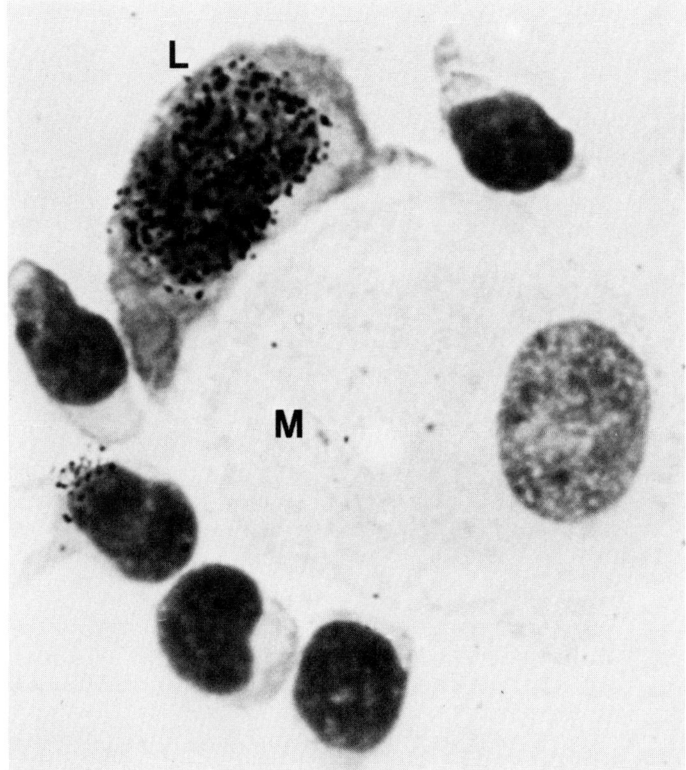

Fig. 5-8. The clustering of lymphocytes around a macrophage incubated with soluble antigen. Some of the lymphocytes have taken up ^{3}H-thymidine, and have therefore been activated. (Hanifin, J. M., and Cline, M. J.: Human monocytes and macrophages. J. Cell. Biol., *46*:97, 1970.)

appear to be two phases in the binding of lymphocytes to macrophages.

1. The first step occurs independently of the presence of antigen. Any T lymphocyte will bind to any macrophage. Binding is reversible and short-lived, and requires calcium and a healthy, metabolically active macrophage. If no antigen is present, the cells dissociate and the sequence proceeds no further than this.

2. If antigen is present, the lymphocyte and macrophage remain in contact provided the lymphocyte specifically recognizes the given antigen. As time goes on the antigen-specific clusters form a greater percentage of the total number of clusters. Within 72 hours of the introduction of antigen, the majority of bound lymphocytes have been activated and have begun to proliferate.[87]

The following interpretation of the above observations has been offered.[87,90] Lymphocytes will initially attach nonspecifically to the macrophage surface. The macrophage then "presents" the antigen to the lymphocyte. If the lymphocyte can bind the antigen, a second stable bond is formed between the lymphocyte and the macrophage using the antigen as a bridge (Fig. 5-9). If this second step is completed successfully, the lymphocyte is activated. The precise mechanism of triggering is unknown. Antigen recognition by the lymphocyte may be sufficient, or, alternatively, the macrophage may deliver an inductive signal to the lymphocyte. The requirement that macrophages must be metabolically active during induction argues against a completely passive process.

In order for macrophages and lymphocytes to interact efficiently in the guinea pig system, they must share MHC-related antigens.[87,90] However, this finding has

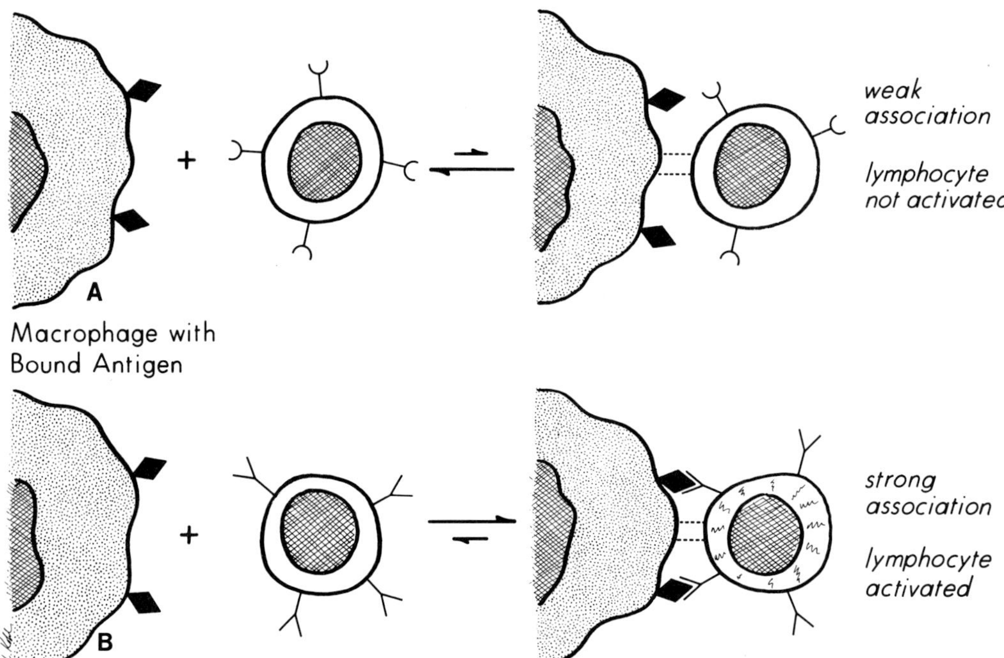

Fig. 5-9. A model for the interaction of T cells with macrophages in the guinea pig. Two events are postulated to be required for T-cell activation. (*A*) The nonspecific binding of lymphocytes to the macrophage. If only this phase of interaction takes place, activation will not occur. (*B*) The binding of the lymphocyte receptors to antigen presented by the macrophage. Activation can now occur.

not been confirmed in several other animal systems.[91] Part of the confusion may stem from the way in which the different experiments have been performed. When the ability to mount a secondary response has been studied, as in these experiments with the guinea pig, there appears to be a definite requirement for genetic identity between macrophage and T cell in all animal systems studied, whereas such a requirement does not hold for the generation of a primary response.[92] The region of the MHC involved in the genetic restriction on the secondary response is the I region.[93] The possibility that MHC-related antigens are involved in macrophage-lymphocyte interactions suggests another possible locus where genetic control of the immune response may be important.

Macrophage Presentation of Antigen to B Cells

Most investigators believe that the macrophage is required for the humoral response to T-cell-dependent antigens. However, it is not known whether the macrophage must directly interact with the B cell or is merely required for T-helper-cell activation. Evidence for the requirement for macrophages in the B-cell response to T-cell-independent antigens has been difficult to obtain.[94] A recent study, however, has shown that an antibody response to T-independent antigens can be diminished by employing very careful procedures to remove macrophages from cell cultures.[64] If it is true that macrophages are required for responses to T-cell-independent antigens, this is highly suggestive evidence that B cells interact with macrophages to produce a humoral response. Although B cells have been observed to form clusters around macrophages, the importance of *direct* macrophage contact (antigen presentation) for B-cell activation has not been established.[95]

Macrophage-Derived Soluble Factors

Macrophages can enhance responsiveness to some antigens without making direct contact with lymphocytes. The ability of the macrophage to release soluble mediators may explain why the T-cell response to cell-surface antigens requires the presence of macrophages but does not require macrophage presentation of the antigen. One soluble factor, lymphocyte-activating factor or LAF, is produced by both animal and human macrophages.[96] LAF can replace the requirement for macrophages in the T-cell response to allogeneic cells,[97] and can enhance the response to mitogens and soluble antigens.[96,98] It is a low molecular weight, heat-labile substance which can activate T cells.[99] LAF is not antigen-specific which befits a substance produced by the nonspecific macrophage. There are no histocompatibility constraints on its activity.

MODELS OF CELLULAR INTERACTIONS

In this and in the preceding chapters we have analyzed the ways in which the immune system prepares to deal with an antigen. We have considered these events in three time-related categories: (1) recognition, (2) activation, and (3) interaction and regulation. The fourth step is the immune response itself, and that will be the subject of Chapter 6. In this section we shall explore the theories and speculations which attempt to put the many ideas we have encountered thus far into a coherent explanation of the events of immune activation. The question around which we will center this discussion is: What are the signals that are generated by the presence of antigen which trigger the activation of an immunocompetent cell? There are almost as many hypotheses as there are experiments, and we shall attempt to confine this discussion to those theories which most simply and effectively incorporate the concepts we have been examining up to this point. A final understanding of the events of immune activation will entail a deeper understanding of cellular communication and surface phenomena than is available at present.

B-CELL ACTIVATION

There are two levels at which we must approach the question of B-cell activation. The first is the attempt to understand how many distinct signals are required to activate a B cell. The second is how the activating signals are generated and how they are communicated to the B cell.

How Many Signals Are Required to Activate a B Cell?[100,101]

Controversy currently surrounds the question of whether B-cell activation requires one or two discrete signals. The simplest view holds that antigen alone can provide the necessary signal to activate a B cell (a one-signal model). A second approach differs in that antigen is felt to be insufficient by itself to activate a B cell, and that a second signal must be delivered as well. The source of the second signal is generally considered to be the T helper cell (a two-signal model). Still a third idea is that antigen binding by the B cell does not deliver any signal at all, and it is only the extrinsic second signal that is required for B-cell activation (a one-signal model). These models are schematized in the diagram below (Fig. 5-10). We shall use these models to explore the various ideas concerning the nature of the activating signals.

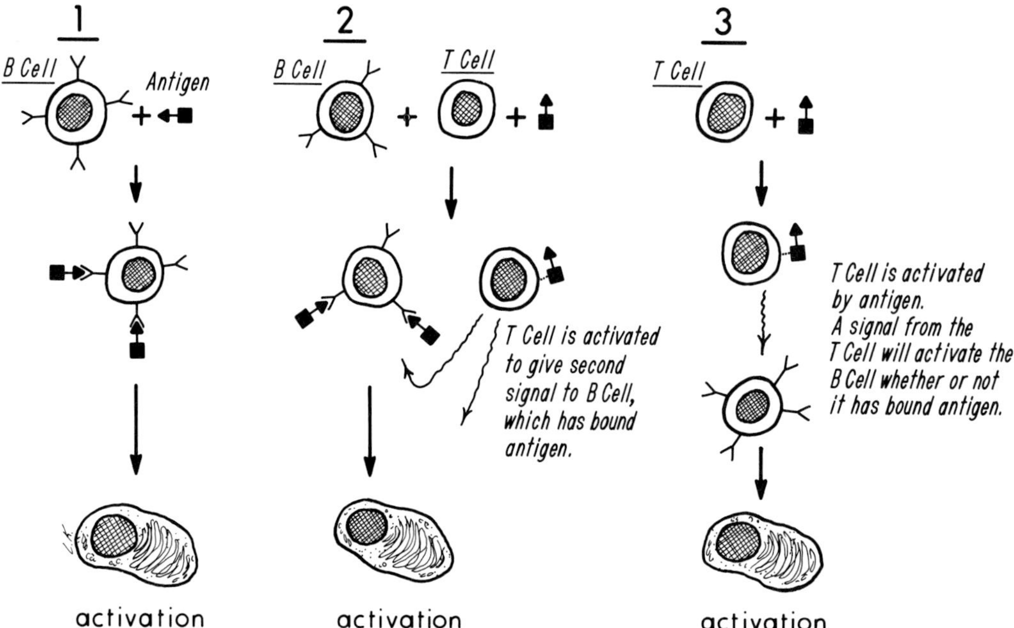

Fig. 5-10. Three models for B-cell activation. (1) Antigen binding by the B cell is sufficient for activation. (2) Antigen binding by the B cell plus a second signal, probably delivered by the T helper cell, is required for activation. (3) Delivery of a T-cell signal alone is required for activation.

How Are the Activating Signals Generated and Communicated to the B Cell?

The first model, that antigen alone can activate a B cell, is not widely accepted as it is shown in Figure 5-10. Although it can account for activation by T-cell-independent antigens and certain mitogens, it cannot explain why most antigens require the added presence of T cells in order to induce a humoral response. The necessity to account for thymic dependency has forced additional modifications in this otherwise simple picture. Two of the models which have emerged have excited a great deal of interest. They have been referred to as the *direct* and *indirect antigen-focusing* mechanisms of B-cell activation.

Direct Antigen Focusing.[102,103] This theory postulates that antigen attachment to the B cell is the only signal needed for activation, but that the T cell must present the antigen to the B cell in order to induce an immune response (Fig. 5-11). The T cell binds the carrier moiety in such a way that the hapten remains exposed on the T-cell membrane. The T cell therefore serves to focus these groups so that the B cell can bind the requisite number of haptenic determinants. One might speculate that the T cell, by binding and focusing several antigenic moieties, presents a multivalent haptenic structure to the B cell that can cross-link B-cell receptors (see Chap. 4). T-cell-independent antigens and mitogens might be able to create the necessary alterations in the B-cell surface without the aid of T-cell focusing.

Indirect Antigen Focusing. This model is built around the evidence for the "IgT" helper molecule discussed earlier in this chapter. According to this hypothesis (Fig. 5-12), T cells bear a surface immunoglobulin ("IgT") which binds carrier determinants. The "IgT"-antigen complex is shed from the T cell and binds cytophilically to macrophages by the Fc

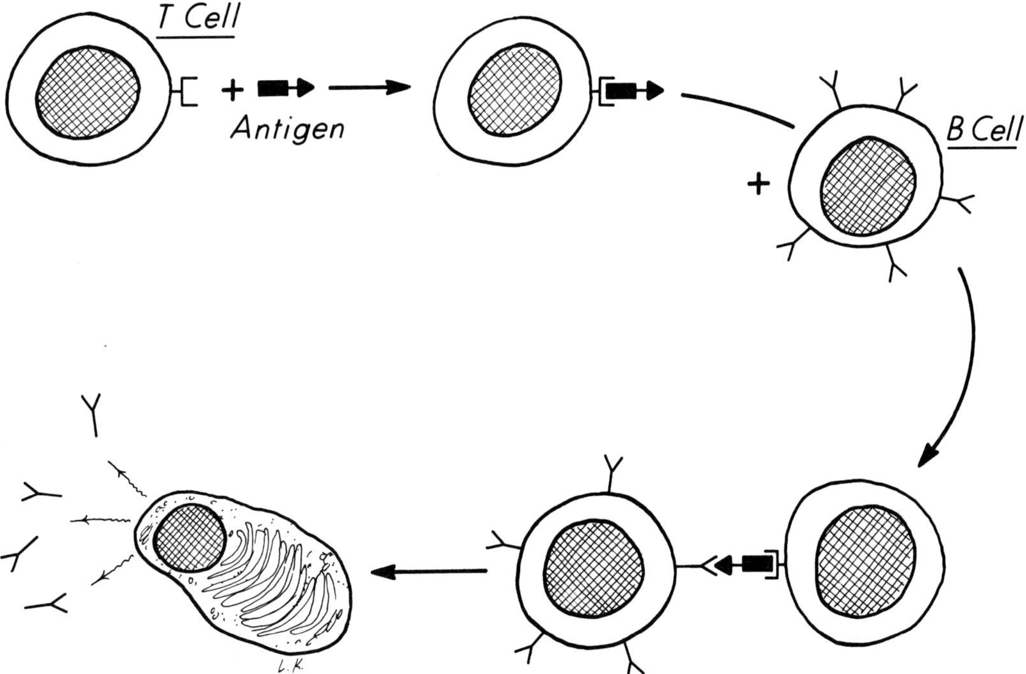

Fig. 5-11. The direct antigen-focusing theory. The T cell binds the carrier moiety and presents the hapten to the B cell. Binding of the hapten by the B cell leads to immune activation.

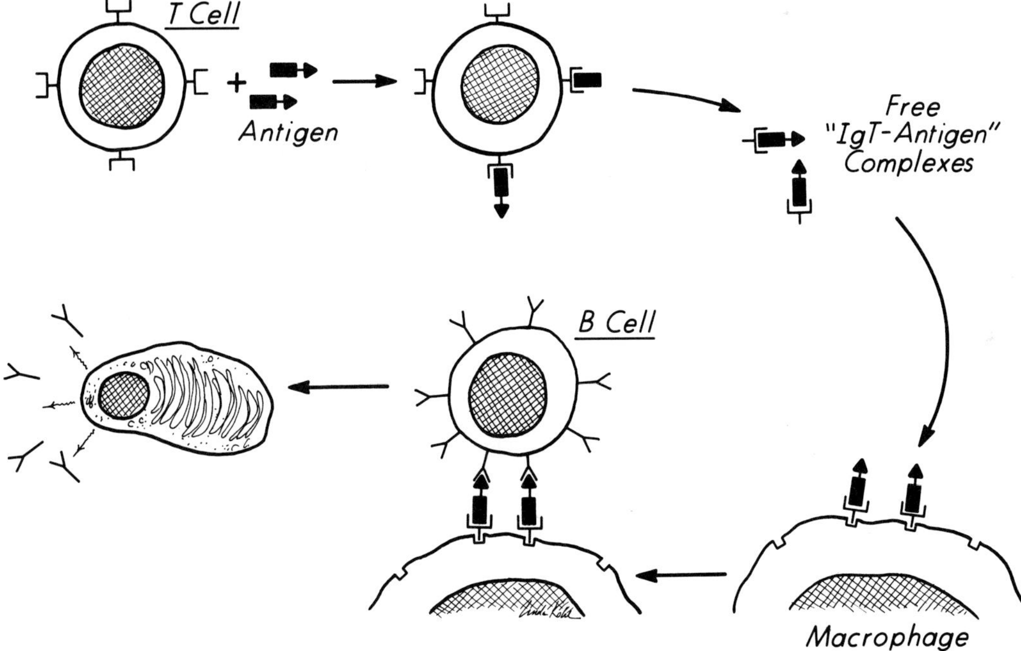

Fig. 5-12. The indirect antigen-focusing theory. The T cell binds the carrier, and the receptor-antigen complex is shed from the T-cell surface. The complex binds to the macrophage, leaving the haptenic determinant exposed. The B cell binds the hapten and is activated.

portion of the "IgT."[3,4,104,105] The B cell then binds the exposed haptenic groups just as in the direct focusing theory. This indirect model accounts not only for the requirement for T helper cells, but also for observations which indicate that the humoral response may require interaction between the macrophage and the B cell. Objections to this theory include the difficulty in detecting immunoglobulin on the surface of T cells (see Chap. 3) and the observation that anti-immunoglobulin antibody only partially blocks T-cell antigen binding.[106]

The two-signal hypothesis of B-cell activation attempts to account for thymic dependency in a more direct way. The two signals are (1) the binding of antigen to the B cell, and (2) a second signal delivered by the antigen-activated T helper cell. This second signal may be one of the soluble helper factors that we have described and thus could be antigen-specific or nonspecific. The existence of T-cell-independent antigens and mitogens is attributed to intrinsic properties of these molecules that allow them to generate their own second signal in addition to portions of those molecules that can bind to the antigen receptors and hence deliver the first signal. It has been suggested that a nonantigenic portion of T-cell-independent antigens and a particular component of mitogens can deliver a stimulatory signal to B cells.[107] For example, the stimulatory moiety of LPS has been reported to be the lipid A component.[108]

An especially intriguing approach has implicated complement as the stimulatory second signal.[109] The induction of a humoral response by mitogens and T-cell-independent antigens *in vitro* appears to require the presence of serum containing the C3 component. Many T-cell-independent antigens and several mitogens can activate C3, and active products of C3 have therefore been implicated as carrying second-signal-generating potential, perhaps by binding to the B-cell C3 receptor. However, not all T-cell-independent antigens or mitogens can activate complement, and the complement-activating ability of those that do is not always correlated with their B-cell-activating capacity.[110]

The C3 receptor of lymphocytes has been postulated to be related to B-cell activation in still another way. There is evidence in mice that the cells that respond to T-cell-dependent antigens bear C3 receptors while those cells without C3 receptors preferentially respond to T-cell-independent antigens.[111] It is certainly safe to say that the role of complement in immune activation remains highly uncertain at present.

The third postulated mechanism for B lymphocyte activation claims that antigen binding does not deliver a stimulatory message to the B cell. Instead, it is only the "second" signal (delivered by the T helper cell, the stimulatory component part of a mitogen, etc.) that is required for activation.[101] The role of the immunoglobulin receptors is to bind the antigen to the B cell so that the T helper cell, itself binding to the carrier moiety, is in a position to deliver the activating signal.

The Macrophage in B-Cell Activation

Finally, we must consider the role of the macrophage in B-cell activation. The macrophage could function in any of a number of ways to assist B-cell activation. These might include antigen focusing or cross-linking, and the release of stimulatory factors. One must also consider the possibility that the macrophage may have second-signal-generating capacity (Fig. 5-13). In addition, lymphocytes can potentiate the activity of macrophages by releasing several soluble factors, thereby establishing a positive feedback mechanism (Fig. 5-14). These lymphocyte-derived factors (lymphokines) will be discussed in Chapter 6.

THE MACROPHAGE IN B CELL ACTIVATION

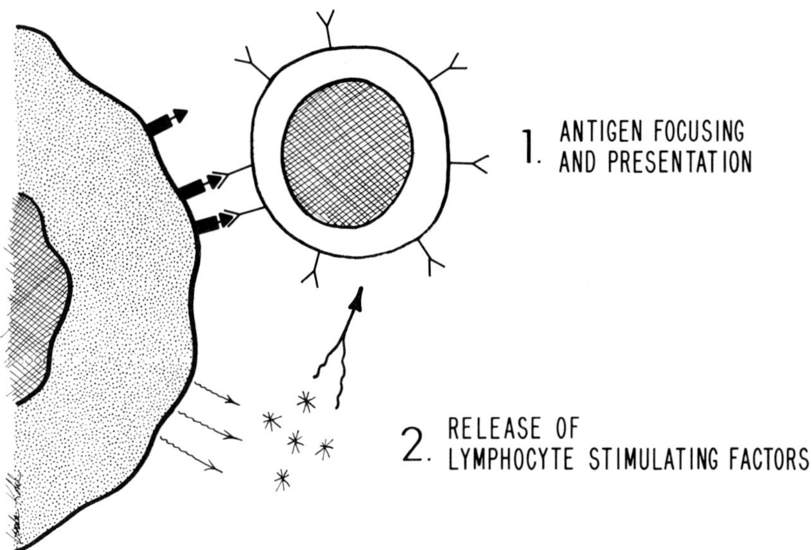

Fig. 5-13. The macrophage may be capable of delivering a second signal in much the same way as has been postulated for the T helper cell. One such model is shown here. The B cell binds macrophage-bound antigen (signal 1) and also receives an activating signal by the release of soluble factors from the macrophage (signal 2).

MACROPHAGE-LYMPHOCYTE FEEDBACK

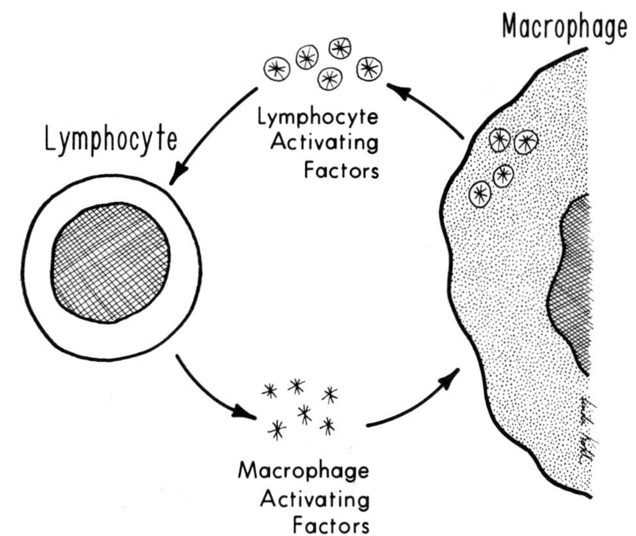

Fig. 5-14. Macrophages can release soluble factors capable of activating lymphocytes. Lymphocytes can in turn potentiate macrophage activity by releasing their own soluble substances. A positive feedback loop is thus established.

T-CELL ACTIVATION

In comparison to B-cell immune processes, much less is understood about T-cell recognition, activation and extrinsic regulatory controls. The one exception appears to be the requirement for macrophage assistance in T-cell activation. In the case of soluble antigens, T cells may have to make direct contact with macrophage-bound antigen in order to become activated. With cell-surface antigens, macrophage-derived soluble factors may be sufficient for activation, since the T cell appears capable of effectively binding the antigen on its own. The latter process is suggestive of a two-signal hypothesis (antigen binding and soluble factors), but it is not known whether the T cell requires one or two signals to be activated. Evidence for the existence of T amplifier cells suggests that T effector cells may be susceptible to signals in addition to that of antigen binding.

OTHER IMMUNOREGULATORY AGENTS

In the final section of this chapter, we shall focus our attention on three molecular species. The first is a group of substances secreted by the thymus and referred to as thymic hormones. These may exert a powerful influence on processes of immunologic maturation. The second group of substances is the lymphocyte chalones, inhibitors of lymphocyte proliferation. The third molecule is transfer factor. Although transfer factor has been at the center of much controversy, its effectiveness in treating several immunodeficiency states makes it worthy of our attention.

THYMIC HORMONES

The possibility that the thymus may influence immunologic maturation by the secretion of soluble factors has intrigued investigators for a number of years. One of the first experiments that firmly supported this view involved the implantation of diffusion chambers containing thymic tissue into the peritoneal cavities of thymectomized 7-day-old mice.[112] Thymectomized neonatal mice ordinarily will rapidly develop a wasting syndrome which culminates in death from massive infection. The mice given a thymic implant, however, did not develop a wasting syndrome. Their lymphocyte count remained slightly below normal, but significantly higher than thymectomized control mice. They were able to reject allogeneic skin grafts, and produced a nearly normal humoral response to sheep erythrocytes. The diffusion chamber did not allow the passage of cells, thereby indicating that the thymic tissue was coveying immunologic maturity via a soluble substance (or substances). The same diffusion chamber technique was later used in an attempt to restore immunologic function in a 10-week-old infant with DiGeorge's syndrome (an immunodeficiency disease characterized by the failure of the thymus to develop properly; see Chap. 10), the first clinical trial with a "thymic hormone."[113] The patient's T cells became responsive to mitogens *in vitro*, but she died before the treatment could be fully evaluated.

Several laboratories have now reported the isolation of thymic factors that appear to have significant effects on immunologic function. These include thymosin,[114] lymphocyte-stimulating hormone[115,116] (two separate extracts of LSH have been described, LSH_h and LSH_r), thymosterin,[117] thymin (or thymopoietin),[118] and thymic humoral factor.[119] All of these are proteins with the exception of thymosterin which is a lipid. Other thymic-derived factors have also been described but have not been as intensively investigated as those listed above. The thymus has also been reported to secrete a hypocalcemic factor and a hypoglycemic factor.[120]

The biological importance of these thymic hormones *in situ* has not yet been established, but they have been demonstrated to have profound effects in experimental systems. Probably the most carefully studied hormonal function is the ability of thymic extracts to induce immunologic maturity in lymphoid-cell populations. This has been shown by (1) the stimulation of the appearance of T-cell surface antigens in populations of cells lacking those markers[121–123] and (2) the ability to convey immune competence to immature cells.[124–126]

Much of the excitement in this field stems from initial reports of the use of thymic extracts in the successful treatment of certain immunodeficiency diseases (see Chap. 10). However, claims that thymic factors may prevent the decline in T-cell function and alter the course of the NZB/W mice,[127,128] animals whose disease process closely resembles human systemic lupus erythematosus, have been disputed.[129] Patients with systemic lupus have been reported to be deficient in serum thymic hormone.[130]

CHALONES

Chalones are inhibitors of cell mitosis, produced by the cells whose division they inhibit.[131] They are not species-specific but are specific for cell type. Thus there are epidermal chalones, fibroblast chalones, liver cell chalones, granulocyte chalones and lymphocyte chalones. The epidermal chalone has been the most intensively investigated. Chalones are not cytotoxic and their effects are reversible.[132]

The chalone concept was first applied to lymphocytes in 1969 when saline extracts of pig lymph nodes were found to be able to block PHA stimulation *in vitro*.[133] The active product had a molecular weight of between 30,000 and 50,000.[134] Only extracts of spleen, thymus and lymph nodes were effective.

Chalones derived from the thymus are more effective in suppressing T-cell function than B-cell function. Thymic chalones depress PHA stimulation, graft-versus-host reactivity and allograft rejection. The humoral response to T-cell-dependent antigens is considerably more suppressed than that to T-cell-independent antigens.[135,136]

The importance of these anti-mitotic agents in immune regulation has not been established. They have been offered as an explanation for the plateauing of cellular proliferation in certain lymphoproliferative disorders (see Chap. 12), but this remains to be proven.

TRANSFER FACTOR

Transfer factor is a small, dialyzable molecule which can convey specific immunologic reactivity to individuals previously unresponsive to a particular antigen.[137] Transfer factor is obtained by lysing sensitized lymphocytes and recovering and concentrating the dialyzable material. The chemical nature of transfer factor has not been established, but there are several indications that it may be at least partially composed of nucleotides.

Transfer factor seems to affect primarily—if not solely—cell-mediated immunity. The transfer of cellular immune reactivity by transfer factor has several distinguishing characteristics:

1. In most hands, the transferred immunity is antigen-specific. Reactivity is conveyed against only those antigens to which the lymphocytes from which the transfer factor is obtained have been previously sensitized. For example, in one report transfer factor prepared from lymphocytes sensitized to KLH transferred KLH reactivity to ten out of ten recipients.[138] Transfer factor obtained from individuals not responsive to KLH was unsuccessful in all of eleven trials in conveying KLH sensitivity. Transfer factor may, however, be able nonspecifically to augment immunologic reactions by acting as a chemotactic agent for polymor-

phonuclear leukocytes and monocytes and by augmenting monocyte/macrophage activity.[139]

2. The recipient demonstrates positive reactivity within hours to days, and may remain positive for years.

3. Transfer factor prepared from the lymphocytes of the recipient host will be equally reactive in serial transfers to other recipients.[140]

Perhaps the greatest puzzle surrounding transfer factor is how such a small molecule (its molecular weight is less than 10,000) can be endowed with such remarkable specificity that it conveys immunologic reactivity only against those specific antigens to which the donor has been sensitized. There is no adequate answer at present. One possibility is that transfer factor may act as an intracellular derepressor with specificity encoded within its postulated nucleotide sequence.

Transfer factor has been given in clinical trials where depression of the immune system is suspected. Too often the reports are either single-case studies or include too few patients to be of any interpretable value. In addition, the diseases under study run extremely variable courses and it is difficult to evaluate the effect of intervention with transfer factor. Still another problem in interpretation lies in the use of transfer factor as a last-ditch attempt to alter the course of a disease in its terminal stages. Intervention may therefore be too late to be of any benefit, and it is impossible to ascertain if transfer factor might have altered the patient's course if administered earlier.

Perhaps the greatest clinical success with transfer factor therapy has been in the treatment of chronic mucocutaneous candidiasis, a disease characterized by granulomatous lesions on the nails, skin, buccal and vaginal mucous membranes as well as variable involvement of other organs. These patients characteristically exhibit depressed or often no immune responsiveness to Candida. In 37 such patients described throughout the literature who were given transfer factor obtained from normal individuals with positive anti-Candida skin tests, 80 per cent converted to positive skin tests against Candida. Fifty per cent of the patients showed clinical improvement.[141] A success rate of 50 per cent has also been reported in reconstituting immunoreactivity and producing clinical improvements in patients with the Wiskott-Aldrich syndrome, an immunodeficiency disease with a well-documented depression of cell-mediated immunity.[142–144] The beneficial clinical response usually lasts for only a few months, and repeated injections of transfer factor have to be given.

The results of trials in other diseases are less impressive.[144] Often the conversion to positive skin tests and the observed *in vitro* stimulation of cellular immunity (the effects of transfer factor on cellular immunity are usually assayed by culturing a treated patient's lymphocytes with antigen and measuring RNA synthesis, rosetting or MIF production) are not associated with any improvement in the patient's clinical condition, indicating that the tests that are used to measure immunologic competence may not always correlate with the clinical reality. Trials of transfer factor administration in central nervous system fungal infections, multiple sclerosis,[145] subacute sclerosing panencephalitis (SSPE),[145] lepromatous leprosy,[146] and various neoplasms, particularly melanoma,[147,148] have not been clinically rewarding.

Since transfer factor does appear to have beneficial effects in several disorders, the failure of transfer factor to affect other diseases may be due either to the disease not being dependent upon cell-mediated immune processes, or to the improper choice of a transfer factor source. Indeed, the choice of a proper transfer factor donor and the development of an assay of transfer factor activity that will correlate with clinical efficacy are important areas of current research.

REFERENCES

1. Claman, H. N., Chaperon, E. A., and Triplett, R. F.: Thymus-marrow cell combinations: synergism in antibody production. Proc. Soc. Exp. Biol. Med., 122:1167, 1966.
2. Claman, H. N., and Chaperon, E. A.: Immunologic complementation between thymus and marrow cells—a model for the two-cell theory of immunocompetence. Transplant. Rev., *1*:92, 1969.
3. Feldmann, M., and Basten, A.: Specific collaboration between T and B lymphocytes across a cell impermeable membrane *in vitro*. Nature [New Biol.], *237*:13, 1972.
4. Feldmann, M.: Induction of B cell tolerance by antigen specific T cell factor. Nature [New Biol.], *242*:82, 1973.
5. Taniguchi, M., and Tada, T.: Regulation of homocytotropic antibody formation in the Rat X. IgT-like molecule for the induction of homocytotropic antibody response. J. Immunol., *113*:1757, 1974.
6. Taussig, M. J., and Munro, A. J.: Removal of specific cooperative T cell factor by anti-H-2 but not by anti-Ig sera. Nature, *251*:63, 1974.
7. Taussig, M. J., Munro, A. J., Campbell, R., David, C. S., and Staines, N. A.: Antigen-specific T-cell factor in cell cooperation. J. Exp. Med., *142*:694, 1975.
8. Schimpl, A., and Wecker, E.: Replacement of T-cell function by a T-cell product. Nature [New Biol.], *237*:15, 1972.
9. ——: Stimulation of IgG antibody response *in vitro* by T cell-replacing factor. J. Exp. Med., *137*:547, 1973.
10. Katz, D. H.: The allogeneic effect on immune responses: model for regulatory influence of T lymphocytes on the immune system. Transplant. Rev., *12*:141, 1972.
11. Elkins, W. L.: Cellular immunology and the pathogenesis of graft versus host reactions. Prog. Allergy, *15*:78, 1971.
12. Dutton, R. W., *et al.*: Is there evidence for a non-antigen specific diffusable chemical mediator from the thymus-derived cell in the initiation of the immune response. *In* Amos, B. (ed.): First International Congress of Immunology. P. 355. New York, Academic Press, 1971.
13. Armerding, D., and Katz, D. H.: Activation of T and B lymphocytes *in vitro*. II. Biological and biochemical properties of an allogeneic effect factor (AE) active in triggering specific B lymphocytes. J. Exp. Med., *140*:19, 1974.
14. Amerding, D., Sachs, D. H., and Katz, D. H.: Activation of T and B lymphocytes *in vitro*. III: Presence of Ia determinants on allogeneic effect factor. J. Exp. Med., *140*:1717, 1974.
15. Kindred, B., and Shreffler, D. C.: H-2 dependence of cooperation between T and B cells *in vivo*. J. Immunol., *109*:940, 1972.
16. Katz, D. H., Hamaoka, T., Dorf, M. E., and Benacerraf, B.: Cell interactions between histoincompatible T and B lymphocytes. The H-2 gene complex determines successful physiologic lymphocyte interactions. Proc. Natl. Acad. Sci. U.S.A., *70*:2624, 1973.
17. Katz, D. H., Graves, M., and Dorf, M. E., Dimuzio, H., and Benacerraf, B.: Cell interactions between histoincompatible T and B lymphocytes: VII. Cooperative responses between lymphocytes are controlled by genes in the I region of the H-2 complex. J. Exp. Med., *141*:263, 1975.
18. Marrack, P. C., and Kappler, J. W.: Antigen-specific and nonspecific mediators of T cell/B cell cooperation. 1. Evidence for their production by different T cells. J. Immunol., *114*:1116, 1975.
19. Gershon, R. K.: T cell control of antibody production. Contrib. Top. Immunobiol., *3*:1, 1974.
20. Basten, A., Miller, J. F. A. P., and Johnson, P.: T cell-dependent suppression of an anti-hapten antibody response. Transplant., *26*:130, 1975.
21. Tada, T., and Takemori, T.: Selective roles of thymus-derived lymphocytes in the antibody response. 1. Differential suppressive effect of carrier-primed T cells on Hapten-specific IgM and IgG antibody responses. J. Exp. Med., *140*:239, 1974.
22. Taniguchi, M., Tada, T., and Tokuhisa, T.: Properties of the antigen-specific suppressive T-cell factor in the regulation of antibody response of the mouse. J. Exp. Med., *144*:20, 1976.
23. Peavy, D. L., and Pierce, C. W.: Cell-mediated immune responses *in vitro* 1. Suppression of the generation of cytotoxic lymphocytes by concanavalin A and concanavalin A-activated spleen cells. J. Exp. Med., *140*:356, 1974.
24. Folch, H., and Waksman, B. H.: The splenic suppressor cell. II. Suppression of the mixed lymphocyte reaction by thymus-dependent adherent cells. J. Immunol., *113*:140, 1974.
25. Takemori, T., and Tada, T.: Selective roles of thymus-derived lymphocytes in the antibody response. J. Exp. Med., *140*:253, 1974.
26. Rich, R. R., and Pierce, C. W.: Biological expressions of lymphocyte activation. J. Immunol., *112*:1360, 1974.
27. Redelman, D., Scott, C. B., Sheppard, H. W., and Sell, S.: *In vitro* studies of the rabbit immune system. V. Suppressor T cells activated by concanavalin A block the proliferation, not the induction of antierythrocyte plaque forming cells. J. Exp. Med., *143*:919, 1976.
28. Basten, A., Miller, J. F. A. P., Sprent, J., and Cheers, C.: Cell-to-cell interaction in the immune response x. T-cell dependent suppression in tolerant mice. J. Exp. Med., *140*:199, 1974.
29. Weber, G., and Kölsch, E.: Transfer of low zone tolerance to normal syngeneic mice by theta-positive cells. Eur. J. Immunol., *3*:767, 1973.
30. Tada, T., Okumura, K., and Taniguchi, M.: Regulation of homocytotropic antibody formation in the rat. VIII. An antigen-specific T cell factor that regulates anti-hapten homocytotropic antibody response. J. Immunol., *111*:952, 1973.

31. Baker, P. J.: Homeostatic control of antibody responses. A model based on the recognition of cell-associated antibody by regulatory T cells. Transplant. Rev., *26*:3, 1975.
32. Okumura, K., and Tada, T.: Regulation of homocytotropic antibody formation in the rat. IX. Further characterization of the antigen-specific inhibitory T cell factor in hapten-specific homocytotropic antibody response. J. Immunol., *112*:783, 1974.
33. Takemori, T., and Tada, T.: Properties of antigen-specific suppressive T-cell factor in the regulation of antibody response of the mouse: 1. *In vivo* activity and immunochemical characterization. J. Exp. Med., *142*:1241, 1975.
34. Feldmann, M.: T cell suppression *in vitro*. 1. Role in regulation of antibody responses. Eur. J. Immunol., *4*:660, 1974.
35. Adler, F. L.: Competition of antigens. Prog. Allergy, *8*:41, 1964.
36. Gershon, R. K., and Kondo, K.: Antigenic competition between heterologous erythrocytes. 1. Thymic dependency. J. Immunol., *106*:1524, 1971.
37. Katz, D. H., Paul, W. E., and Benacerraf, B.: Carrier function in anti-hapten antibody responses. VI. Establishment of experimental conditions for either inhibitory or enhancing influences of carrier-specific cells on antibody production. J. Immunol., *110*:107, 1973.
38. Schrader, J. W., and Feldmann, M.: The mechanism of antigenic competiton. 1. The macrophage as a site of a reversible block of T-B lymphocyte collaboration. Eur. J. Immunol., *3*:711, 1973.
39. Taussig, M. J., Mozes, E., Shearer, G. M., and Sela, M.: Antigenic competition and genetic control of the immune response. A hypothesis for intramolecular competition. Cell. Immunol., *8*:299, 1973.
40. Talal, N., and Steinberg, A. D.: The pathogenesis of autoimmunity in New Zealand black mice. Curr. Top. Microbiol. Immunol., *64*:79, 1974.
41. Parkhouse, R. M. E., and Dutton, R. W.: Inhibition of spleen cell DNA synthesis by autologous macrophages. J. Immunol., *97*:663, 1966.
42. Kirchner, H., *et al.*: Inhibition of proliferation of lymphoma cells and T lymphocytes by suppressor cells from spleens of tumor-bearing mice. J. Immunol., *114*:206, 1975.
43. Yoshinaga, M., Yoshinaga, A., and Waksman, B. H.: Regulation of lymphocyte responses *in vitro*. 1. Regulatory effect of macrophages and thymus-dependent (T) cells on the response of thymus-independent (B) lymphocytes to endotoxin. J. Exp. Med., *136*:956, 1972.
44. Nelson, D. S.: Production by stimulated macrophages of factors depressing lymphocyte transformation. Nature, *246*:306, 1973.
45. Waldman, S. R., and Gottlieb, A. A.: Macrophage regulation of DNA synthesis in lymphoid cells: effects of a soluble factor from macrophages. Cell. Immunol., *9*:142, 1973.
46. Calderon, J., Williams, R. T., and Unanue, E. R.: An inhibitor of cell proliferation released by cultures of macrophages. Proc. Natl. Acad. Sci. U.S.A., *71*:4273, 1974.
47. Shortman, K., von Boehmer, H., Lipp, J., and Hopper, K.: Subpopulations of T-lymphocytes. Transplant. Rev., *25*:163, 1975.
48. Cantor., H., and Weissman, I.: Development and function of subpopulations of thymocytes and T lymphocytes. Prog. Allergy, *20*:1, 1976.
49. Claman, H. N.: Corticosteroids and lymphoid cells. N. Engl. J. Med., *287*:388, 1972.
50. Cantor, H., and Boyse, E. A.: Functional subclasses of T lymphocytes bearing different Ly antigens. 1. The generation of functionally distinct T-cell subclasses is a differentiative process independent of antigen. J. Exp. Med., *141*:1376, 1975.
51. Stobo, J. D., and Paul, W. E.: Functional heterogeneity of murine lymphoid cells. III. Differential responsiveness of T cells to phytohemagglutinin and concanavalin A as a probe for T cell subsets. J. Immunol., *110*:362, 1973.
52. Shiku, H., *et al.*: Expression of T-cell differentiation antigens on effector cells in cell-mediated cytotoxicity *in vitro*. J. Exp. Med., *141*:227, 1975.
53. Cantor, H., and Boyse, E. A.: Functional subclasses of T lymphocytes bearing different Ly antigens. II. Cooperation between sublcasses of Ly positive cells in the generation of killer activity. J. Exp. Med., *141*:1390, 1975.
54. Bash, J. A., Durkin, H. G., and Waksman, B. H.: *In* Rosenthal, A. S., (ed.): P. 829. New York, Academic Press, 1975.
55. Gerber, N. L., and Steinberg, A. D.: Physical separation of "suppressor" from "helper" thymocytes. J. Immunol., *115*:1744, 1975.
56. Cantor, H., and Simpson, E.: Regulation of the immune response by sublcasses of T lymphocytes. 1. Interactions between prekiller T cells and regulatory T cells obtained from peripheral lymphoid tissues of mice. Eur. J. Immunol., *5*:330, 1975.
57. Jandinski, J., Cantor, H., Tadakuma, T., Peavy, D. L., and Pierce, C. W.: Separation of helper T cells from suppressor T cells expressing different Ly components. I. Polyclonal activation: suppressor and helper activities are inherent properties of distinct T-cell subclasses. J. Exp. Med., *143*:1382, 1976.
58. Cantor, H., Shen, F. W., and Boyse, E. A.: Separation of helper T cells from suppressor T cells expressing different Ly components. II. Activation by antigen: after immunization, antigen-specific suppressor and helper activities are mediated by distinct T-cell subclasses. J. Exp. Med., *143*:1391, 1976.
59. Vadas, M. A., Miller, J. F. A. P., McKenzie, I. F. C., and Chism, S. E.: Ly and Ia antigen phenotypes of T cells involved in delayed-type hypersensitivity and in suppression. J. Exp. Med., *144*:10, 1976.
60. Cantor, H., and Asofsky, R.: Synergy among

lymphoid cells mediating the graft-versus-host response. III. Evidence for interaction between two types of thymus-derived cells. J. Exp. Med., *135*:764, 1972.

61. Tigelaar, R. E., and Asofsky, R.: Synergy among lymphoid cells mediating a graft-versus-host response. V. Derivation by migration in lethally irradiated recipients of 2 interacting subpopulations of thymus-derived cells from normal spleen. J. Exp. Med., *137*:239, 1973.
62. Cohen, L., and Howe, M. L.: Synergism between subpopulations of thymus-derived cells mediating the proliferative and effector phases of the mixed lymphocyte reaction. Proc. Natl. Acad. Sci. U.S.A., *70*:2707, 1973.
63. Oppenheim, J. J., and Rosenstreich, D. L.: Signals regulating *in vitro* activation of lymphocytes. Prog. Allergy, *20*:65, 1976.
64. Chused, T. M., Kassan, S. S., and Mosier, D. E.: Macrophage requirement for the *in vitro* response to TNP ficoll: a thymic independent antigen. J. Immunol., *116*:1579, 1976.
65. Unanue, E. R.: The regulatory role of macrophages in antigenic stimulation. Adv. Immunol., *15*:95, 1972.
66. Cohen, B. E., Rosenthal, A. S., and Paul, W. E.: Antigen-macrophage interaction. J. Immunol., *111*:820, 1973.
67. Cohen, B. E., and Paul, W. E.: Macrophage control of time-dependent changes in antigen sensitivity of immune T lymphocyte populations. J. Immunol., *112*:359, 1974.
68. Unanue, E. R., Schmidtke, J., Cruchard, A., and Grey, H. M.: *In* Miescher, P. A. (ed.): Proc. 6th Int. Symp. Immunopathol. P. 35. New York, Grune & Stratton, 1970.
69. Schmidtke, J. R., and Unanue, E. R.: Macrophage-antigen interaction: uptake, metabolism and immunogenicity of foreign albumin. J. Immunol., *107*:331, 1971.
70. Salmon, S. E., Morhenn, V. B., and Cline, M. J.: Uptake of radio-iodinated antigens by human monocytes. Clin. Exp. Immunol., *8*:409, 1971.
71. Ehrenreich, B. A., and Cohn, Z. A.: The uptake digestion of iodinated human serum albumin by macrophages *in vitro*. J. Exp. Med., *126*:941, 1967.
71a. Ishizaka, K., and Adachi, T.: Generation of specific helper cells and suppressor cells *in vitro* for the IgE and IgG antibody responses. J. Immunol., *117*:40, 1976.
72. Schechter, G. P., and McFarland, W.: Interaction of lymphocytes and a radioresistant cell in PPD-stimulated human leukocyte cultures. J. Immunol., *105*:661, 1970.
73. Unanue, E. R., and Cerottini, J.-C.: The immunogenicity of antigen bound to the plasma membrane of macrophages. J. Exp. Med., *131*:711, 1970.
74. ——: Fate and immunogenicity of macrophage associated hemocyanins. *In* Sterzl, J., and Riha, I. (eds.): Developmental Aspects of Antibody Formation and Structure. Ed. 2, vol. 2, p. 521. New York, Academic Press, 1970.
75. Rosenthal, A. S., Rosenstreich, D. L., Blake, J. T., Lipsky, P. E., and Waldron, J. A.: Mechanisms of antigen recognition by T lymphocytes. *In* Dagvillard, F. (ed.): Proc. 7th Leukocyte Culture Conference. P. 201. New York, Academic Press, 1973.
76. Calderon, J., and Unanue, E. R.: The release of antigen molecules from macrophages: characterization of the phenomena. J. Immunol., *112*:1804, 1974.
77. Schwartz, R. S., Ryder, R. J. W., and Gottlieb, A. A.: Macrophages and antibody synthesis. Prog. Allergy, *14*:81, 1970.
78. Waldron, J. A., Jr., Horn, R. G., and Rosenthal, A. S.: Antigen-induced proliferation of guinea pig lymphocytes *in vitro*: obligatory role of macrophages in the recognition of antigen by immune T-lymphocytes. J. Immunol., *111*:58, 1973.
79. Rosenstreich, D. L., and Rosenthal, A. S.: Peritoneal exudate lymphocytes, II. *In vitro* lymphocyte proliferation induced by brief exposure to antigen. J. Immunol., *110*:934, 1973.
80. Oppenheim, J. J., Leventhal, B. G., and Hersh, E. M.: The transformation of column-purified lymphocytes with nonspecific and specific antigenic stimuli. J. Immunol., *101*:262, 1968.
81. Levis, W. R., and Robbins, J. H.: Function of glass-adherent cells in human mixed lymphocyte cultures. Transplantation, *9*:515, 1970.
82. Rode, H. N., and Gordon, J.: The mixed leukocyte culture: a three component system. J. Immunol., *104*:1453, 1970.
83. Wagner, H., Feldmann, M., Boyle, W., and Schrader, J. W.: Cell-mediated immune responses *in vitro*. III. The requirement for macrophages in cytotoxic reactions against cell-bound and subcellular alloantigens. J. Exp. Med., *136*:331, 1972.
84. Rosenstreich, D. L., and Wilton, J. M.: The mechanism of action of macrophages in the activation of T-lymphocytes *in vitro* by antigens and mitogens. *In* Rosenthal, A. S. (ed.): Immune Recognition. P. 113. New York, Academic Press, 1975.
85. Weidelin, O., Braendstrüp, O., and Pedersen, E.: Macrophage-lymphocyte clusters in the immune response to soluble protein antigen *in vitro*. 1. Roles of lymphocytes and macrophages in cluster formation. J. Exp. Med., *140*:1245, 1974.
86. Hanifin, J. M., and Cline, M. J.: Human monocytes and macrophages: interaction with antigen and lymphocytes. J. Cell Biol., *46*:97, 1970.
87. Lipsky, P. E., and Rosenthal, A. S.: Macrophage-lymphocyte interaction. II. Antigen-mediated physical interactions between immune guinea pig lymph node lymphocytes and syngeneic macrophages. J. Exp. Med., *141*:138, 1975.
88. Cline, M. J., and Sweet, V. C.: The interaction of human monocytes and lymphocytes. J. Exp. Med., *128*:1309, 1968.
89. Mosier, D. E.: Cell interactions in the primary

immune response *in vitro*: a requirement for specific cell clusters. J. Exp. Med., *129*:351, 1969.

90. Rosenthal, A. S., Blake, J. T., Ellner, J. J., Greineder, D. K., and Lipsky, P. E.: The role of macrophages in T lymphocyte antigen recognition. *In* Rosenthal, A. S. (ed.): Immune Recognition. P. 39. New York, Academic Press, 1975.
91. Kapp, J. A., Pierce, C. W., and Benacerraf, B.: *In vitro* studies of the cellular interactions in an antibody response controlled by an immune response (Ir) gene. *In* Rosenthal, A. S. (ed.): Immune Recognition, New York, Academic Press, 1975.
92. Pierace, C. W., Kapp, J. A., and Benacerraf, B.: Regulation by the H-2 gene complex of macrophage and lymphoid cell interaction in secondary antibody responses *in vitro*. J. Exp. Med., *144*:371, 1976.
93. Erb, P., and Feldmann, M.: The role of macrophages in the generation of T-helper cells. J. Exp. Med., *142*:460, 1975.
94. Shortman, K., Diener, E., Russell, P., and Armstrong, W. D.: The role of nonlymphoid accessory cells on the immune response to different antigens. J. Exp. Med., *131*:461, 1970.
95. McIntyre, J. A., and Pierce, C. W.: Immune response *in vitro*. IX. Role of cell clusters. J. Immunol., *111*:1526, 1973.
96. Gery, I., and Waksman, B. H.: Potentiation of the T-lymphocyte response to mitogens. II. The cellular source of potentiating mediators. J. Exp. Med., *136*:143, 1972.
97. Bach, F. H., Alter, B. J., Solliday, S., Zoschke, D. C., and Janis, M.: Lymphocyte reactivity *in vitro*. II. Soluble reconstituting factor permitting response of purified lymphocytes. Cell Immunol., *1*:219, 1970.
98. Havemann, K., and Schmidt, W.: Potentiating effect of adherent cell supernatants on lymphocyte proliferation. *In* Proc. 8th Leukocyte Culture Conference. P. 181. New York, Academic Press, 1974.
99. Gery, I., and Handschumacher, R. E.: Potentiation of the T lymphocyte response to mitogens. III. Properties of the mediator(s) from adherent cells. Cell. Immunol., *11*:162, 1974.
100. Cohen, M., and Blomberg, B.: The self-nonself discrimination: one- or two-signal mechanism. Scand. J. Immunol., *4*:1, 1975.
101. Coutinko, A., and Möller, G.: Immune activation of B cells: evidence for "one nonspecific triggering signal" not delivered by the Ig receptors. Scand. J. Immunol., *3*:133, 1974.
102. Bretcher, P. A., and Cohn, M.: Minimal model for the mechanism of antibody induction and paralysis by antigen. Nature, *220*:444, 1968.
103. Rajewsky, K., Schirrmacher, V., Nase, S., and Jerne, N. K.: The requirement of more than one antigenic determinant for immunogenicity. J. Exp. Med., *129*:1131, 1969.
104. Feldmann, M., and Basten, A.: Cell interactions in the immune response *in vitro*. III. Specific collaboration across a cell impermeable membrane. J. Exp. Med., *136*:49, 1972.
105. Feldmann, M.: Cell interactions in the immune response *in vitro*. V. Specific collaboration via complexes of antigen and thymus-derived cell immunoglobulin. J. Exp. Med., *136*:737, 1972.
106. Hammerling, G. J., and McDevitt, H. O.: Antigen binding T and B lymphocytes. II. Studies on the inhibition of antigen binding to T and B cells by anti-immunoglobulin anti-H-2 sera. J. Immunol., *112*:1734, 1974.
107. Coutinko, A., and Möller, G.: B cell mitogenic properties of thymus-independent antigens. Nature [New Biol.], *245*:12, 1973.
108. Andersson, J., Melchers, F., Galanos, C., and Lüdevitz, O.: The mitogenic effect of lipopolysaccharide on bone marrow derived mouse lymphocytes: lipid A as the mitogenic part of the molecule. J. Exp. Med., *137*:943, 1973.
109. Dukor, P., *et al.*: Complement-dependent B cell activation by cobra venom factor and other mitogens. J. Exp. Med., *139*:337, 1974.
110. Feldmann, M., and Pepys, M. B.: Role of C3 in *in vitro* lymphocyte cooperation. Nature, *249*:159, 1974.
111. Lewis, G. K., Ranken, R., Nitecki, D. E., and Goodman, J. W.: Murine B-cell subpopulations responsive to T-dependent and T-independent antigens. J. Exp. Med., *144*:382, 1976.
112. Osaba, D., and Miller, J. F. A. P.: The lymphoid tissues and immune responses of neonatally thymectomized mice bearing thymus tissue in millipore diffusion chambers. J. Exp. Med., *119*:117, 1964.
113. Steele, R. W., *et al.*: Familial thymic aplasia: attempted reconstitution with fetal thymus in a millipore diffusion chamber. N. Engl. J. Med., *287*:787, 1972.
114. Goldstein, A. L., Slater, F. D., and White, A.: Preparation, assay, and partial purification of a thymic lymphocytopoietic factor (thymosin). Proc. Natl. Acad. Sci., U.S.A., *56*:1010, 1966.
115. Hand, T., Caster, P., and Luckey, T. D.: Isolation of a thymus hormone, LSH. Biochem. Biophys. Res. Commun., *26*:18, 1967.
116. Robey, G., Campbell, B. J., and Luckey, T. D.: Isolation and characterization of a thymic factor. Infect. Immunol., *6*:682, 1972.
117. Patop, I., and Milck, S. M.: Isolation of an antiblastic factor from the bovine thymus. Rev. Roum. Endocrinol., *7*:253, 1970.
118. Goldstein, G.: Isolation of bovine thymin: a polypeptide hormone of the thymus. Nature, *247*:11, 1974.
119. Trainin, N., and Small, M.: Studies on some physicochemical properties of a thymus humoral factor conferring immunocompetence on lymphoid cells. J. Exp. Med., *132*:885, 1970.
120. Pansky, B., House, E. L., and Cone, L. A.: An insulin-like thymic factor. Diabetes, *14*:325, 1965.

121. Sheid, M. P., *et al.*: Differentiation of T cells induced by preparations from thymus and by nonthymic agents. J. Exp. Med., *138*:1027, 1973.
122. Tourraine, J. L., Tourraine, F., Incefy, G. S., and Good, R. A.: Effect of thymic factors on the differentiation of human marrow cells into T-lymphocytes *in vitro* in normal and patients with immunodeficiencies. Ann. N.Y. Acad. Sci., *249*:335, 1975.
123. Tourraine, J. L., Incefy, G. S., Tourraine, F., Rho, Y. M., and Good, R. A.: Differentiation of human bone marrow cells into T lymphocytes by *in vitro* incubation with thymic extracts. Clin. Exp. Immunol., *17*:151, 1974.
124. Cohen, G. H., Hooper, J. A., and Goldstein, A. L.: Thymosin-induced differentiation of murine thymocytes in allogeneic mixed lymphocyte cultures. Ann. N.Y. Acad. Sci., *249*:145, 1975.
125. Rotter, V., Globerson, A., Nakamura, I., and Trainin, N.: Studies on characterization of the lymphoid target cell for activity of a thymus humoral factor. J. Exp. Med., *138*:130, 1973.
126. Bach, J. F., Dardenne, M., Pleau, J. M., and Bach, M. A.: Isolation, biochemical characteristics, and biological activity of a circulating thymic hormone in the mouse and in the human. Ann. N.Y. Acad. Sci., *249*:186, 1975.
127. Dauphinee, M. J., Talal, N., Goldstein, A. L., and White, A.: Thymosin corrects the abnormal DNA synthetic response of NZB mouse thymocytes. Proc. Natl. Acad. Sci., U.S.A., *71*:2637, 1974.
128. Gershwin, M. E., *et al.*: Correction of T cell function by thymosin in New Zealand mice. J. Immunol., *113*:1068, 1974.
129. Gershwin, M. E., Steinberg, A. D., Ahmed, A., and Derkay, C.: Study of thymic factors. Arthritis Rheum., *19*:862, 1976.
130. Bach, J. F., and Dardenne, M.: Absence d'hormone thymigue dans le serum de souris NZB et NZBxNZW et de malades atteints de lupus erythemateux dissemine. J. Urol. Nephrol., *78*:994, 1972.
131. Bullough, W. S., and Lawrence, E. B.: The control of epidermal mitotic activity in the mouse. Proc. Soc. Lond. [Biol], *151*:517, 1960.
132. Houck, J. C., and Dougherty, W. F.: Chalone: A Tissue-Specific Approach to Mitotic Control. P. 13., Medcom Press, 1974.
133. Moorhead, J. F., Paraskava-Tchernozenska, E., Pirrie, A. J., and Hayes, C.: Lymphoid inhibitor of human lymphocyte DNA synthesis and mitosis *in vitro*. Nature, *224*:1207, 1969.
134. Houck, J. C., and Irausguin, H.: Some properties of the lymphocyte chalone. Natl. Cancer Inst. Monogr., *38*:117, 1973.
135. Florentin, I., Kiger, N., and Mathé, G.: T lymphocyte specificity of a lymphocyte-inhibiting factor extracted from the thymus. Eur. J. Immunol., *3*:624, 1973.
136. Kiger, N., Florentin, I., and Mathé, G.: Some effects of a partially purified lymphocyte-inhibiting factor from calf thymus. Transplantation, *14*:448, 1972.
137. Laurence, H. S.: Transfer factor. Adv. Immunol., *11*:195, 1969.
138. Zuckerman, K. S., Neidhart, J. A., Balcezak, S. P., and LoBuglio, A. F.: Immunologic specificity of transfer factor. J. Clin. Invest., *54*:997, 1974.
139. Kirkpatrick, C. H.: Properties and activities of transfer factor. J. Allergy Clin. Immunol., *55*:411, 1975.
140. Lawrence, H. S.: Transfer factor and cellular immune deficiency disease. N. Engl. J. Med., *283*:411, 1970.
141. Grob, P. J., Franke, C. H., Raymond, J. F., and Frei-Wettstein, M.: Therapeutic use of transfer factor. Eur. J. Clin. Immunol., *5*:33, 1975.
142. Spittler, L. E., *et al.*: The Wiskott-Aldrich syndrome: results of transfer factor therapy. J. Clin. Invest., *51*:3216, 1972.
143. Wybran, J., Levin, A., Spittler, L. E., and Fudenberg, H. H.: Rosette-forming cells, immunologic deficiency diseases and transfer factor. N. Engl. J. Med., *288*:710, 1973.
144. Hitzig, W. H., and Grob, P. J.: Therapeutic uses of transfer factor. Prog. Clin. Immunol., *2*:69, 1974.
145. Graybill, J. R.: Transfer factor in diseases of the central nervous system. Adv. Neurol., *6*:107, 1974.
146. Bullock, W. E., Fields, J. P., and Brandeiss, M. W.: An evaluation of transfer factor as immunotherapy for patients with lepromatous leprosy. N. Engl. J. Med., *287*:1053, 1972.
147. LoBuglio, A. F., and Neidhart, J. A.: A review of transfer factor immunotherapy in cancer. Cancer, *34*:1563, 1974.
148. Spittler, L. E., *et al.*: Lymphocyte responses to tumor-specific antigens in patients with malignant melanoma and results of transfer factor therapy. J. Clin. Invest., *51*:1972.

6 The Effector Limb

In this chapter we shall examine the effector limb of the immune response. An active immune response is the final product of the complex recognition, activation and regulatory mechanisms that we have analyzed in the previous chapters. There is considerably more to an immune response than just the production of antibodies or the activation of cytolytic cells. The humoral response is a highly evolved, finely regulated phenomenon which contributes to the destruction and removal of antigen in many ways. T cells can function as killer cells, helper cells and suppressor cells, all with important contributions to the overall immune response. The macrophage can function both as an accessory cell and as a killer cell. A great variety of soluble factors play critical roles in the overall response by contributing directly to antigen elimination and by summoning inflammatory cells to the site of reactivity. All of these processes must then be balanced to produce an appropriate and effective immune response.

THE HUMORAL RESPONSE

THE PRIMARY RESPONSE

The first exposure to a given antigen elicits a characteristic pattern of antibody production termed a "primary response." Although the response will vary depending upon the nature of the antigen, the dosage and route of administration, and the immunologic competence of the host, it has been possible to define a "typical" primary response to which all primary responses are similar.[1]

Each clone of B lymphocytes appears to be preprogrammed to produce antibody of a unique specificity. With the introduction of antigen, those clones of cells which can recognize the intruder are stimulated to *proliferate* and *differentiate*. Both of these events contribute to the exponential rise in antibody production which typifies the early primary response. It has been estimated that an antigen-reactive cell undergoes approximately ten divisions by the end of the exponential rise, yielding approximately one thousand progeny cells.[2] It is not known what percentage of these are actively engaged in antibody production. As proliferation occurs, differentiation gives rise to a population of plasma cells with a greatly increased capacity for antibody production.

From the moment the antigen first enters the body, there is a lag period of several days before antibody can be detected (Fig. 6-1). When antibody does appear, it is of the 19S IgM class. IgM levels rise expo-

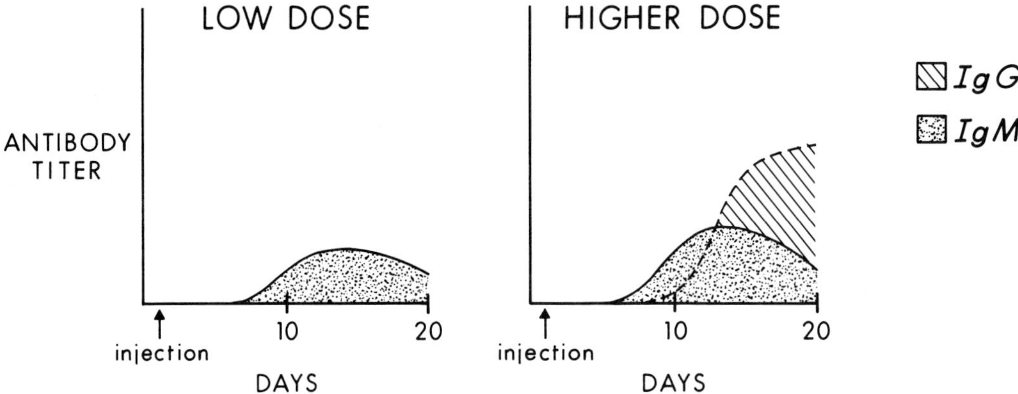

Fig. 6-1. The primary humoral response. Low-dose antigen stimulates IgM production. IgM appears about 7 days after antigen exposure and peaks at about 14 days. Higher doses of antigen will also evoke IgG production, appearing about day 10 and peaking several weeks out.

nentially, peak within several days, and then begin to fall. Little residual IgM antibody can be detected after a few weeks. When the antigen is given in low but still immunogenic doses, what we have just described may comprise the entire primary humoral response. However, as the antigen dose is increased, the amount of IgM that is produced increases as well, and, in addition, IgG can be detected.[3]

The kinetics of the primary IgG response are different than those of the IgM response. IgG production occurs after a greater lag period than IgM production, and IgG may first become detectable about the time that IgM levels peak. IgG levels peak later and in contrast to the rapid disappearance of IgM, may remain elevated for a long time.[4] The key distinction between the IgM and IgG responses is therefore a temporal one: IgG production builds just as IgM production begins to decline.

These observations have led investigators to explore the mechanisms by which this "switch" from IgM to IgG production occurs. Two major possibilities have been examined:

1. IgM-producing cells and IgG-producing cells represent distinct subpopulations, each with different kinetics of response.

2. IgM-producing cells switch during the course of an immune response to become IgG-producing cells.[5,6] This idea has been the more popular of the two, although there is only circumstantial evidence to support it. Some researchers have reported detecting a small subpopulation of cells that appear to be able to produce both IgM and IgG.[7] It has been suggested that these cells might be in the process of switching from one class to another. Others have shown that the injection of anti-μ anti-serum (which contributes to the elimination of cells bearing IgM on their surface) into neonatal mice suppresses their ability subsequently to produce IgG as well as IgM, suggesting that IgG-producing cells may be derived from IgM-bearing precursors.[8,9]

Affinity Maturation

Any antigen elicits a humoral response consisting of many antibody molecules with differing affinities for the target antigen. During the course of an immune response, the *average affinity* of the secreted antibody molecules increases with time.[10] This phenomenon has been termed *affinity maturation*. It is still uncertain whether the IgM response undergoes significant affinity maturation, but it is clear that the IgG response does, and there are reports of increases in IgG affinity of several hundredfold during the course of an immune response.[11,12] In addition, the affinity of the IgG produced in a given immune response appears to be consistently higher than the average affinity of the IgM produced at the same time.[11,13]

The following model has been proposed as an explanation for affinity maturation:[14] each B-cell clone is capable of producing a unique antibody molecule with a particular affinity for a given antigen. These antibody molecules are also expressed on the lymphocyte surface where they function as antigen receptors. The likelihood that a particular B-cell clone will be stimulated by an antigen is proportional to the probability that the antigen can be bound by the surface receptors. This probability depends upon the affinity of the surface receptors for the antigen. At the beginning of an immune response, a large amount of free antigen is present which will bind to B cells with a wide range of receptor affinities. As the response proceeds and antigen is cleared from the body, the concentration of free antigen falls. The B cells now compete for a diminishing supply of antigen, and only those cells with the highest affinity for antigen will be successful and thus continue to proliferate and produce antibody. One can demonstrate that the percentage of cells with low binding affinity for a given antigen diminishes as the supply of antigen declines, and the frequency of high-affinity antigen-binding cells increases.[15] The result is the progressive production of antibody molecules whose average affinity increases with time.

The basic premise of this model is that affinity maturation is driven by competition for decreasing amounts of antigen. Two observations support this view: (1) affinity maturation is delayed when the challenging antigen is present in very high doses, and (2) passively administered antibody directed against the inciting antigen accelerates the process of affinity maturation, presumably by hastening the removal of free antigen and thereby leading to a state of low antigen concentration.[14,16]

It is important to emphasize that there is no evidence that new affinities arise during the course of an immune response. Rather, it is only the increase in the ratio of high-affinity antibody to low-affinity antibody that leads to the overall affinity maturation.

T Helper Function

T helper function is required for a complete primary humoral response to many antigens. The obvious exception is the class of T-cell-independent antigens which can elicit strong antibody responses in thymic-deprived mice. However, these responses are predominantly restricted to the IgM class.[17–19] There are also several reports that even T-cell-dependent antigens can, under certain circumstances, elicit low IgM responses—but not IgG responses—in thymic-deprived animals.[19,20] These observations have led to the generally accepted view that *IgM production is relatively T-cell-independent, whereas IgG production is very much dependent upon T helper function*.[21] T cells appear to be required to mediate the switch from IgM to IgG during an immune response.[23,23] The way in which T cells affect this switch is not understood.

The relationship of T helper function to affinity maturation is uncertain. Some experiments have indicated that T helper function can accelerate the process of affinity maturation,[24] others that T helper function does not affect affinity maturation.[25] One way in which T cells might indirectly promote affinity maturation would be by amplifying the production of antibody and hastening the clearance of antigen from the host.

THE SECONDARY RESPONSE

Second exposure to an antigen elicits a humoral response which differs markedly from the primary response[26] in three major ways (Fig. 6-2): (1) there is a significantly shorter lag phase before antibody can be detected, (2) a much higher level of antibody is produced, and (3) there is an earlier and more pronounced bias toward IgG production.

The temporal relationship between the first and second doses of antigen influences the characteristics of the secondary response. In general, the longer the interval between doses, the more the secondary response will be biased toward only IgG production[27] and the smaller the challenge dose must be in order to elicit a given level of antibody production.[28]

The secondary response is thus "bigger and faster" than the primary response. It is called an *anamnestic* response because the immune system appears to carry the *memory* of previous antigenic exposure. In the broadest sense, immunologic memory can be viewed as the alteration of the immune response to an antigen resulting from previous exposure to that antigen. The phenomenon of immunologic memory is most readily demonstrated by the tremendous increase in IgG production upon second exposure to many antigens.[26] Increments in IgM production have also been described, although never of a magnitude equal to that of IgG.[29] Immunologic memory can be quite long-lived and mice have been shown to carry the memory for antigen-specific secondary responses for their full lifetimes.[30]

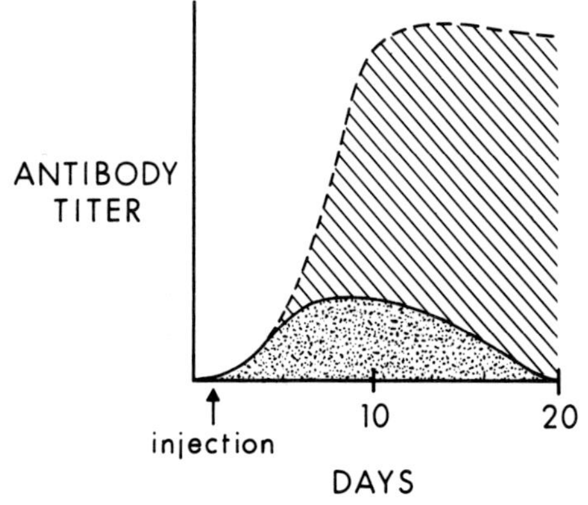

Fig. 6-2. The secondary humoral response. Both IgM and IgG appear early in the response. IgG titers may reach very high levels.

Both B- and T-cell populations are carriers of immunologic memory.[31,32] In the following discussion we will focus first on the role of the T helper cell in the secondary humoral response, and then look at the characteristics of B-cell memory.

T Helper Function in the Secondary Response

T helper function appears to be required for both the secondary IgM and IgG responses.[33] The classic example of T helper function and T-cell memory is the hapten-carrier phenomenon where carrier memory alone is often sufficient to produce a strong secondary antihapten response (see Chap. 2).[34–37] Carrier recognition, we will recall, is a T-cell function, and thus immunologic memory can clearly reside in the T cell.[38] It is believed that T-cell memory resides in a subpopulation of T cells referred to as "T memory cells."

It has been suggested that a secondary response results from a quantitative increase in the amount of helper signal compared to that produced in the primary response. Increased helper signal could theoretically result from an increase in either the number or activity of T helper cells following initial exposure to antigen. Two experiments provide at least suggestive evidence that an increased amount of T helper signal may be partially responsible for the secondary response:

1. Carrier moieties vary in their im-

munogenic potential. Hapten coupled to a poorly immunogenic carrier will elicit a low antihapten response; hapten coupled to a highly immunogenic carrier will elicit a strong response. Ordinarily, if we prime an animal with carrier A and then challenge with a hapten on carrier B, we will not elicit a secondary antihapten response. The classical hapten-carrier phenomenon demands that the homologous carrier (A) be used in the challenge in order to produce a secondary response. However, some investigators have shown that an antihapten response equal in magnitude to a secondary response can be elicited and the requirement for homologous carriers bypassed, if a heterologous carrier of high immunogenicity is used in the challenge.[39] The simplest interpretation of this finding is that increased T helper activity is responsible for the increased antibody production of the secondary response. A secondary-type response may therefore result either by priming and then challenging with the homologous carrier (the hapten-carrier phenomenon) or by simply stimulating intense T helper activity with a highly immunogenic carrier.

2. The allogeneic effect delivers a powerful T helper signal to antigen-primed B cells (see Chap. 5). The addition of allogeneic cells to an antigen-primed animal has been shown to enhance the secondary response to a rechallenge with that antigen.[40] This result can be most simply attributed to a large quantity of T helper signal delivered by the allogeneic cells.

B-Cell Memory

B-cell memory is considered to be hapten-specific. In most experiments, priming with hapten on a given carrier and then challenging with the same hapten conjugated to a heterologous carrier elicits only a primary response. However, in some experimental systems, a weak secondary-type response has been elicited.[41] This is evidence for a *quantitative* hapten memory akin to the T-cell carrier memory that we have already discussed. Another type of hapten memory has also been described.[42] Rechallenging an animal with hapten on a heterologous carrier has been shown to elicit antibody of greater affinity than that produced in the primary response, although the magnitude of the response may remain the same. This finding illustrates that B-cell memory can affect a *qualitatively* different and therefore anamnestic response.

Most observers feel that B-cell memory resides in a discreet subpopulation of B memory cells. B memory cells appear to differ from unprimed B cells in that they are longer-lived and recirculate.[43,44]

Whereas the T cell appears to be primarily responsible for the *magnitude* of the secondary response, the B cell appears to determine the *profile* of immunoglobulin that is produced. This conclusion has been most clearly demonstrated by the following experiment.[45,46] Animals were primed with the hapten-carrier complex sulf-BSA and the carrier moiety HGG. They were then challenged with sulf-HGG. This experimental design is a simple recapitulation of the hapten-carrier phenomenon, and a secondary anti-sulf antibody response was observed. The ratio of IgG and IgM produced in the secondary response could be varied by giving different priming doses of sulf-BSA but not by varying the dose of HGG. Thus, the profile of immunoglobulin produced depended upon the dose of hapten used for priming and was independent of the dose of priming carrier. This result is probably due to the generation of varying amounts of IgG B memory cells during the primary response. Thus, although T helper cells are required for the active production of IgG in an immune response (see above), the ratio of IgG to IgM produced is a function of the generation of different populations of B memory cells.

The study of the relationship of B

memory cells to other aspects of B-cell differentiation has led to the proposal that there are three functional B-cell types: (1) a precursor B cell, able to bind antigen in an unprimed host, (2) an antibody-forming cell which, in its most differentiated form, is the mature plasma cell, and (3) a B memory cell. Some reports indicate that these subpopulations can be physically separated.[47] By studying isolated clones of B cells in animal systems, it has been possible to evaluate the relationship between these three cell types.[48] Antigen-binding cells are present in very low numbers in the unprimed host. Introduction of antigen stimulates their proliferation.[49] Within several days, IgG memory cells can be detected (this is assayed by the ability of cell transfer to convey memory to unprimed syngeneic hosts).[50] The memory cell does not produce antibody but may be able to bind antigen.[51] The number of memory cells increases rapidly over the next three days. IgG antibody-forming cells can soon be detected.[52] After the peak in antibody production is attained, new memory cells may still be produced for several weeks or more.

IgG memory cells can be generated and induced to proliferate without the subsequent appearance of IgG antibody-forming cells. This may occur when T cells are absent or when the priming dose is extremely small.[11] Indeed, the lower the priming dose of antigen, the more likely is the secondary response to be comprised predominantly of IgM.[45] It has been postulated that memory cells may give rise directly to antibody-forming cells.[53] Thus, when memory cells are transferred to syngeneic hosts and restimulated with antigen, a secondary-type response occurs. IgG antibody-forming cells and more memory cells are generated in the process.

IgM memory cells have been described but these appear to be relatively short-lived. They may be generated earlier in a response than IgG memory cells.[54]

The final and perhaps the most critical question is how these memory cells are capable of producing a secondary-type response. The kinetics and magnitude of a secondary response are probably a result of the increased proliferative response of memory cells to antigen (a qualitative change) as well as simply an increased number of antigen-reactive cells available to respond (a quantitative change).[49,55]

CONTROLS OVER ANTIBODY PRODUCTION

We have now looked in some detail at the events contributing to the exponential rise in antibody production upon stimulation with antigen. But what limits the intensity of the immune response and ultimately terminates it? In this section we will examine some of the mechanisms that can inhibit the normal humoral response.

When an antigen is introduced into the body, antibody is formed and the antigen is cleared from the host. This process removes the stimulus to lymphocyte activation and might therefore be an adequate explanation for the subsequent decline in antibody production. However, a similar decline can be observed with antigens that are not readily cleared from the body,[56] suggesting that other factors may also be involved in limiting the humoral response. We will look at three of these.

Antibody Feedback

Many investigators have shown that passively administered antibody can suppress a primary humoral response[57] and that removal of antibody can lead to heightened levels of antibody production.[58] In most cases antibody inhibition appears to be specific; passively administered antibody inhibits production only of endogenous antibody with the same antigen specificity.[57]

The sooner antibody is passively administered following challenge with antigen, the greater is the extent of suppression.[59] The primary response can be readily inhibited by specific antibody,[60] whereas the secondary response is much more resistant to inhibition.[61] It has also been possible to block a primary humoral response in this manner without interfering with the generation of memory cells, so that subsequent challenge with antigen elicits a secondary response.[62]

Several groups of workers have shown that inhibition may result simply from the covering up of antigenic deteminants by the passively administered antibody,[63,64] but others feel that this explanation cannot adequately account for all of the experimental data.[65,66] Thus, although many workers have found that the F(ab) fragments of immunoglobulin can mediate inhibition,[67,68] others have shown that the Fc segment is required as well.[69–71] Consistent with the latter finding are the many reports (Fig. 6-3) that the characteristics of antibody feedback are dependent upon the class and subclass of the inhibiting antibody. Therefore, in certain circumstances IgG has been found to suppress antibody production, whereas IgM exerts an enhancing effect.[72,73] Others have found that IgG can also enhance antibody production,[74] and that the IgG subclasses may differ in their ability to enhance or suppress antibody production.[75]

We do not know how applicablc thc concept of antibody feedback may be to the normal *in vivo* immune response. Some investigators have suggested that IgG production inhibits IgM production and may be responsible for the rapid decline in IgM levels.[76] Although IgG has

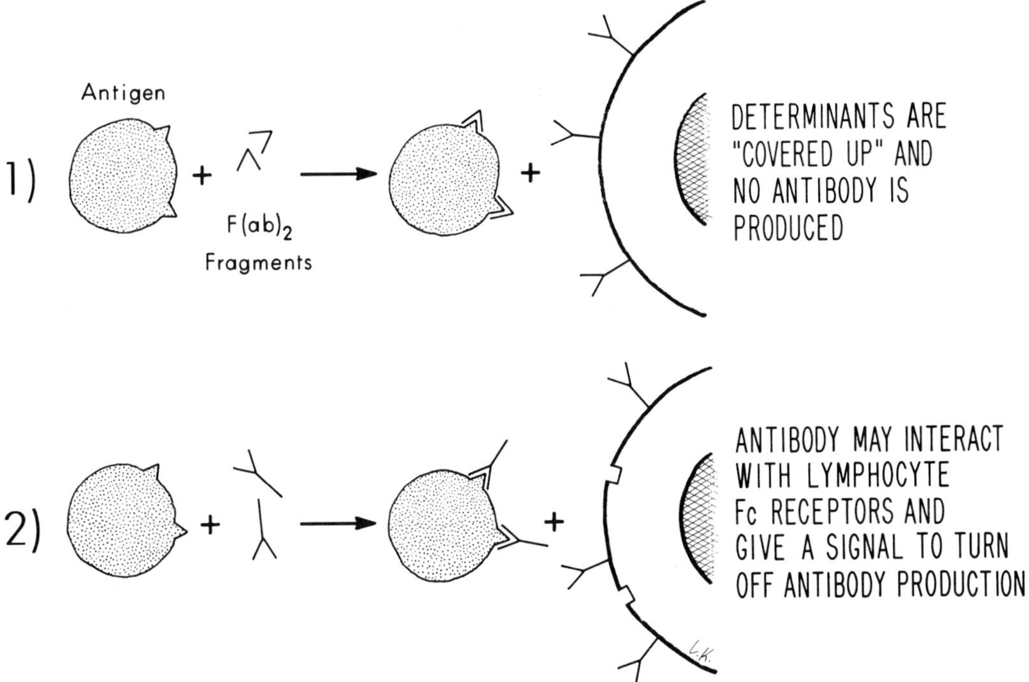

Fig. 6-3. Antibody feedback has been postulated to contribute to the termination of a humoral response. Two mechanisms have been suggested. (1) The covering up of antigenic sites and hence the effective removal of the stimulus to antibody production. Thus some observers have reported that Fab fragments alone can mediate antibody feedback. (2) Antibody may deliver an inhibitory signal to the responding cells, perhaps by binding to the cells' Fc receptors. Thus others have found that the Fc portion of antibody may be required for effective feedback.

been shown to be able to reduce IgM production,[77] its overall contribution to the decline of IgM in a normal immune response remains uncertain.

A very rewarding clinical application of antibody-mediated inhibition of antibody production has been in the prevention of sensitization to the Rh antigen due to Rh-incompatible pregnancies. Rh-negative mothers are now routinely given anti-Rh-antigen antibody within a few days of delivery of an Rh-positive baby. This procedure has proved to be extremely effective in preventing the production of anti-Rh antibody by the mother and has resulted in a dramatic decline in the incidence of erythroblastosis fetalis (see Chap. 14).

Antireceptor Antibody

"Idiotype" is the unique antigenic characteristic of an immunoglobulin molecule which most closely reflects the uniqueness of the antigen-binding site. According to the clonal selection theory, the clones of cells which proliferate in an immune response bear surface receptors with the same antigenic specificity and idiotype as the humoral antibody that is produced. A number of experimenters have been able to raise anti-idiotype antibody[78,79] which, upon injection into another animal, prevents the subsequent appearance of antibodies with the target idiotype.[80] Presumably, the anti-idiotype antibodies react against B cells bearing receptors with the appropriate idiotype.[81] It has been hypothesized that the appearance of anti-idiotype antibody in the course of a normal immune response may contribute to the inhibition of further antibody production and help bring the response to a halt.[82] This possibility is currently under investigation.

Allotype Suppression. If a pregnant animal is given antibody that is directed against a paternal immunoglobulin allotype, the offspring may subsequently fail to produce immunoglobulin bearing the target allotype.[83] Allotype suppression has been carefully studied in both the rabbit and the mouse, and is analogous to idiotype suppression by antireceptor antibody, although its mechanism may be quite different. Allotype suppression may be transient or may last for the lifetime of the animal. Immunoglobulin of the target paternal allotype may be totally or only partially suppressed in the offspring.[84]

It appears that more than one mechanism may be responsible for allotype suppression. In one murine system, chronic allotype suppression appears to be maintained by a population of T suppressor cells capable of specifically inhibiting production only of immunoglobulin bearing the target allotype.[85,86] The suppressor cells appear to act by removing those helper T cells which are required for the expansion of the clones of B cells committed to making immunoglobulin of the target allotype.[86a] The affected animals still possess B cells with surface immunoglobulin of the suppressed allotype.[87] It is not clear why perinatal injection of anti-allotype antibody should induce the appearance of anti-allotype suppressor cells.

A second mechanism of allotype suppression is suggested by experiments with allotype-suppressed rabbits. Unlike the mouse system above, these animals appear to lack B lymphocytes with surface immunoglobulin of the target allotype.[88] However, not all lymphocytes committed to synthesizing the target immunoglobulin seem to be eliminated.[89] The mechanism of allotype suppression in these animals remains a mystery.

Allotype suppression is an important phenomenon because it offers an excellent opportunity to study the way in which antibody can suppress the expression of specific lymphocyte products. Whether or not the suppression of allotypes per se is of any importance in more natural situations (that is, without requiring the experimental introduction of anti-allotype sera) is much less certain.

T Suppressor Cells

We have already discussed the phenomenon of the T suppressor cell in Chapter 5. Here we would like briefly to focus on its role in regulating the humoral response. Like their helper cell counterparts, suppressor cells are carrier-specific and can influence the magnitude and qualitative characteristics of an antibody response.[90] Both B cells and T cells can serve as suitable targets for T suppressor effects.[91]

Both the primary and secondary responses can be inhibited, although the primary response is more susceptible to the effects of T-cell suppression. T suppressor cells not only can reduce the magnitude of a humoral response, but it has been reported that they can also prevent the process of affinity maturation.[92] It is felt that the more dependent an aspect of the humoral response is upon T-cell help, the more vulnerable it is to T-cell suppression.

Examination of the effect of suppression at various times during a humoral response has yielded the following results:[93,94]

1. When suppressor T cells are added at the same time as the immunogen, the IgM response is slightly depressed and falls off rapidly, whereas the IgG response is greatly depressed.

2. When suppressor cells are added two days after the immunogen, the IgM response is further depressed, the IgG response less so.

3. When suppressor cells are given three days after immunization, IgG production is even less affected although still reduced below control levels.

These experiments show that the early IgM response is less sensitive to inhibition than the late IgM response, whereas IgG production can be most effectively suppressed early in the response. Unfortunately, we cannot generalize these observations about T suppressor cells to their possible relevance in the normal *in vivo* response.

THE IgA RESPONSE

Compared to IgG and IgM, little is known about the kinetics of production of this predominantly secretory immunoglobulin.[95] The route of antigen administration is the single most important determinant of how much IgA will be produced in a given response, and in this regard the oral route is the most favorable. In some experiments, IgA levels have been found to rise late in the course of a response,[96] often after IgG levels have already risen.[97] Some observers therefore feel that, in addition to the switch from IgM to IgG, there may be a second switch from IgG to IgA production.[98,99]

T helper function is required for both primary and secondary IgA responses.[100] Affinity maturation of IgA has been described[101] and IgA memory cells can be produced leading to a secondary-type IgA response.[102,103]

THE IgE RESPONSE

Development of Experimental Systems

Because of the unique role of IgE in the clinical settings of allergy and anaphylaxis, the expression and control of IgE production has been intensively investigated. However, IgE has proved to be extremely difficult to study experimentally. In most instances antigens do not elicit significant IgE responses.[104] In those situations where IgE production is stimulated, the response is of low magnitude and rapidly declines.[105] Rechallenge with the same antigen only succeeds in repeating the same brief burst of IgE secretion; no anamnestic response occurs.[106] Much work has therefore been directed at developing special experimental systems in which IgE responses are large enough to be carefully studied. From this work several ideas about what determines an antigen's ability to elicit an IgE response have emerged:

1. *The Nature of the Antigen.* Most

workers have found that helminthic antigens are potent IgE immunogens.[107] This finding is in agreement with the observation that IgE levels are characteristically elevated during the acute phase of parasitic infections.[108]

2. *The Manner of Antigen Administration*. Adjuvants, especially aluminum hydroxide ($AlOH_3$) gel, greatly enhance IgE responses.[109]

3. *Genetics*. Certain strains of animals produce higher IgE responses than others.[110] Genetically determined IgE responders are present in the human population as well (see below).

Utilizing helminthic antigens administered in adjuvants, it has been possible to study the characteristics of an IgE response in rodents. Both primary and secondary IgE responses have been observed, although IgE hapten-specific memory may be short-lived.[111] Affinity maturation has not been investigated.

IgE Production

IgE production requires T helper function.[112] The T helper cells are carrier-specific and the IgE B-cell line is specific for the hapten, just as with IgG.[113] However, there are several reasons for believing that the IgE B cells interact in a unique way with their helper cells.[114] First, they appear to be exquisitely sensitive to carrier-specific T helper function.[115] Secondly, they are relatively insensitive to nonspecific T-cell stimulation such as the allogeneic effect.[116] These observations indicate that IgE B cells are probably distinct from B cells committed to the production of other immunoglobulin classes.

There is further evidence that suggests a unique relationship between the IgE B cell and its T helper cell. For the IgM and IgG classes, the B cell appears to determine the profile of immunoglobulin classes that is produced whereas the T cells predominantly regulate the magnitude of the response. This may not be true for the IgE response.[117] Thus, if an animal is immunized with a particular hapten-carrier complex, the production of antihapten IgE depends upon the IgE immunogenicity of the *carrier*. An experiment illustrating this point is shown in Figure 6-4. Helminthic antigens, which can serve as powerful IgE-immunogenic carriers, are coupled to a hapten. A primary IgE antihapten response ensues, as do primary IgM and IgG responses. When the animal is now immunized with a second carrier that is not IgE-immunogenic, and rechallenged with the original hapten on this second carrier, one observes secondary antihapten IgM and IgG responses, but no IgE production. This result indicates that the helper T cells stimulated by the second carrier cannot interact with hapten-primed IgE B cells, although the T helper cells interact quite adequately with the IgM and IgG antihapten B cells. Only an IgE-immunogenic carrier is effective. Thus, only a specific subpopulation of T helper cells may be capable of stimulating IgE B cells.[118] Recently, a T-cell helper factor has been discovered which exclusively activates IgE B cells, and which has been physically separated from a helper factor for the IgM and IgG responses.[119,120]

Allergy in Humans

The basis of allergy in humans is far from completely understood, and it is likely that several factors are important in the production of the atopic state of allergic individuals. These factors include the predisposition to produce high levels of IgE against certain antigens and altered sensitivity to the humoral mediators of allergy. We will limit our discussion to the immunologic correlates of the first of these possible mechanisms, keeping in mind that it is likely that different mechanisms are operative in different atopic individuals.

Some atopic individuals produce a sustained IgE response when exposed to cer-

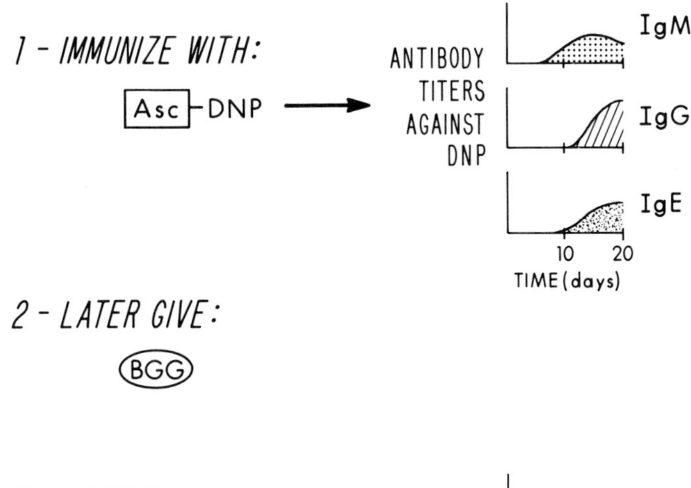

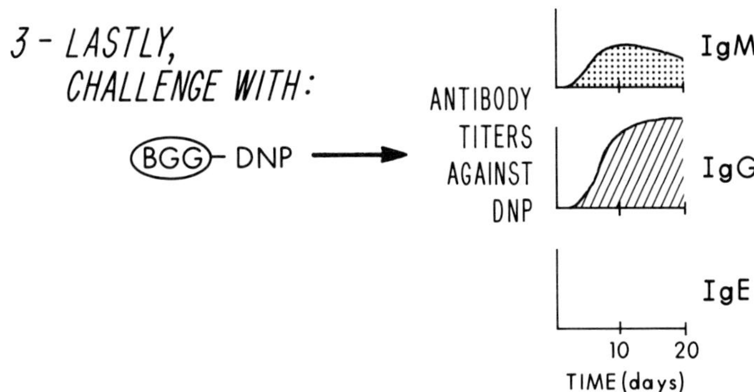

Fig. 6-4. An IgE response can be mounted against DNP when it is conjugated to Asc, whereas helper cells stimulated by BGG can not cooperate with the hapten-primed cells generated in step 1. Thus, only certain carriers appear to be immunogenic for IgE, suggesting that only a restricted subpopulation of T helper cells can stimulate IgE B cells.

tain antigens called allergens.[121–124] Different atopic individuals produce powerful IgE responses to different allergens. Atopic individuals not only produce a sizeable response against an allergen, but also display a secondary anamnestic IgE response upon rechallenge. Nonatopic people do not produce significant IgE responses against common allergens.

The most typical clinical result of antiallergen IgE production is allergy. Allergy is a consequence of the binding of IgE to basophils and mast cells. The combination of allergens with cytophilic IgE leads to cellular degranulation. The details and manifestations of this process are discussed at the end of this chapter.

In man, as in certain other animal strains, there is a genetic predisposition to atopy. It has long been a clinical dictum that allergy runs in families. Family studies have suggested that there is a chromosomal link between certain histocompatibility types and IgE responsiveness to the common ragweed allergen.[125] It has been postulated that human Ir genes may be involved in atopy and, more specifically, that these genes may control IgE production against specific antigens. There is evidence to suggest that allergic people are genetic responders to low doses of naturally occurring allergens while nonatopic people are not.[126] This heightened responsiveness may involve all classes of immunoglobulin, not just IgE.

One of the immunologic abnormalities in some atopic people may be the failure to normally abort IgE responses to specific allergens. Recent work in animal systems has strongly implicated the T suppressor cell in the experimental inhibition of IgE production.[127] Elimination of these T cells by a variety of procedures, including suppressive drugs, adult thymectomy or x-irradiation, results in a marked enhancement and prolongation of the normal IgE response.[128–130] The addition of carrier-specific suppressor T cells can terminate a sizeable and stable IgE response.[131] An antigen-specific suppressor substance has been isolated from these carrier-primed T cells.[132,133] These results have not yet been definitely extended to explain human atopy, but the similarity of the IgE kinetics in humans and in the experimental systems offers hope that this may soon be realized.

An antibody feedback mechanism has also been postulated to modulate IgE production. IgG has been shown to inhibit IgE production, and this inhibition is antigen-specific.[134,135] IgG feedback may contribute to the normal inhibition of the IgE response. Many atopic individuals, however, are able to maintain high levels of both IgG and IgE against their allergens.

Immunologic Intervention in Allergy

The clinical importance of the above work resides in the implications for possible manipulation of IgE responses in atopic individuals. At present, the treatment of allergy can essentially be broken down into two categories: (1) *pharmacologic* intervention that attempts to block the release of the chemical mediators of allergy or reduce their clinical effects; and (2) *immunologic* intervention that attempts to make an atopic person immunologically unreactive—with respect to IgE—to a particular allergen. This may be accomplished by a controlled program of allergen administration and is termed *hyposensitization*.

The latter approach has been shown to produce definite clinical benefits for many patients.[136] In some successfully treated patients there is a drop in IgE levels and a loss of their propensity to produce anamnestic IgE responses to their allergens.[137] The effectiveness of hyposensitization may derive from the activation of the normal IgE inhibitory mechanisms that are otherwise dormant in those atopic individuals who are producing large amounts of antiallergen IgE. These inhibitory mechanisms include:

IgG Feedback. Hyposensitization may produce a rise in antiallergen IgG titers. It has been proposed that this IgG may prevent the manifestations of allergy by (1) competing with IgE for allergen, or (2) feedback inhibiting IgE production. Neither of these mechanisms has been proved to be responsible for the clinical benefits. The rise in IgG titers is not strictly correlated with the decline in IgE during hyposensitization. In addition, most allergens gain entry to the body through the gastrointestinal or respiratory tracts where much of human IgE is produced, but where the importance of IgG has not been well established.[138]

Suppressor Cells. There is little evidence that hyposensitization induces an increase in IgE suppressor-cell activity. However, recent experimental observations employing a modification of the usual hyposensitization technique suggest that antigen-specific T suppressor cells may become activated. The common ragweed antigen, E, can be modified so that it no longer combines with antiallergen antibody, indicating that the relevant haptenic determinants have been destroyed.[139] However, it retains the ability to interact with T cells that recognize the native allergen, demonstrating the conservation of carrier determinants. Weekly injections of modified allergens to allergic mice cause a suppression of IgE levels, a diminished IgE anamnestic response to native ragweed, and often an increased IgG response.[140] Since the modified allergen only retains carrier determinants in common with the unmodified allergen, these results can be explained by either a selective inactivation of IgE T helper cells or an increase in IgE T-suppressor-cell activity.[141] Recent evidence supports the latter interpretation.[142] The results of this work may have great clinical implications for the treatment of allergic patients.

ANTIBODY EFFECTOR FUNCTIONS

Once antibody has been produced, it may have any of a number of effects upon the target antigen. These include:

Neutralization

The classic example of neutralization is the coating of a virus with antibody, rcsulting in a diminution of the infectiousness of the virus. Toxins and enzymes can also be neutralized by antibody (see Chap. 11).[143]

Clearance

The complexing of antibody with antigen enhances the clearance of the antigen by the reticuloendothelial system. This is due to the formation of antigen-antibody aggregates which are readily phagocytosed following their attachment to the Fc receptors on the phagocytes. Attachment of antigen-antibody complexes to Fc receptors present on monocytes, macrophages and granulocytes is called *opsonization.* IgG is the primary opsonizing immunoglobuin.

Cell Lysis

Antibody directed against target cells can induce cell lysis in two ways:

Complement-Dependent Lysis. Serum IgM and certain subclasses of IgG can fix complement. The details of complement-mediated cell lysis are discussed in Appendix A at the end of the text.

Antibody-Dependent Cell-Mediated Cytotoxicity (ADCC). Antibody-coated cells can bc attacked by host effector cells which attach to the Fc segment of the bound antibody and acquire the capacity to kill the target cells (see Fig. 3-5).[144] IgG appears to be the only class of immunoglobulin capable of mediating ADCC.[145] B lymphocytes, nil cells, monocytes and polymorphonuclear leukocytes all possess Fc receptors, and all have been implicated as the effector cell in ADCC.[146–148] Various types of target cells have been described, including microoganisms, allogeneic cells and tumor cells.[149–151]

ADCC is an energy-dependent process.[152,153] Within only a few minutes after attachment of the effector cell, the target cell begins to lose its ability to maintain a normal osmotic gradient across its membrane. Cell death occurs several hours later.[154]

Several investigators have suggested the involvement of ADCC in a variety of host defense phenomena, but the *in vivo* significance of ADCC remains to be confirmed. ADCC represents a crossroads between the humoral and cell-mediated limbs of the immune system, and illustrates the limitation of such a simple division of immunologic phenomena.

IgA Effector Functions

As the major secretory immunoglobulin, IgA serves as an initial protection against the entry of infectious and toxic agents into the body from the gastrointestinal and respiratory tracts. It is well suited to the harsh environment of the gastrointestinal secretions since it has been reported to be fairly resistant to the action of intestinal peptidases.[155] IgA neutralization of viruses at their site of entry is especially important in the prevention of local infections,[156] and IgA-deficient people often have an increased incidence of sinorespiratory infections (see Chap. 10).

IgE Effector Functions

High levels of IgE are present during helminthic infections. Mast-cell and basophilic infiltrates occur at the site of parasitic invasion (most often the gastrointestinal tract). It has been suggested that local anaphylaxis in the gastrointestinal tract due to IgE-mediated mast-cell degranulation may correlate with expulsion of the parasites.[157] The release of active amines may allow for the efficient diffusion of lymphocytes and other inflammatory mediators into the lumen of the gut where they can attack the worms.

The increased levels of IgE that accompany a helminthic infection reflect—at least partially—a nonspecific augmentation of IgE production. This has been most clearly demonstrated in rats.[158] The IgE molecules are directed not only against parasitic antigens, but against any antigens to which the host has previously made IgE.

IgE production always carries the potential danger of anaphylaxis, even when it assumes a presumed protective role in parasitic infections. Sudden death has been reported in African children infected with parasites, and is probably the result of systemic anaphylaxis.[159]

Despite these speculations upon the possible role of IgE in helminthic infections, the true importance of IgE in host defense remains unknown. It has been extremely difficult to demonstrate clearly any protective role for IgE. We are therefore left with the task of defining the *in vivo* function of a molecule whose destructive potential, ranging from allergy to systemic anaphylaxis, has been appreciated for several years. It is to be hoped that future work will resolve this difficulty.

CELL-MEDIATED IMMUNITY

Although it is now clear that cells are involved in all aspects of immunity, cell-mediated immunity has long been identified with T-cell-mediated responses. We can divide T-cell activity into three categories: (1) regulation of the immune response (see Chap. 5), (2) cytotoxicity, and (3) the production of bioactive factors (lymphokines).

CYTOTOXICITY

T killer cells recognize cell-surface antigens present on foreign cells (such as skin grafts and organ transplants), on altered host cells (cells infected by viruses and other microorganisms) and possibily on tumor cells. As a result, destruction of any of these cells by activated T cells is possible.

Much less is known about the details of the T-cell response than about the humoral response. This difficulty is primarily due to the lack of an easily quantifiable product of cellular activity, such as the immunoglobulin provides for the humoral response. Nevertheless, the generation of cytotoxic T lymphocytes has been found to bear many analogies to the production of antibody-forming cells.

Both primary- and secondary-type cell-mediated responses have been demonstrated.[160,161] The type and intensity of stimulation, as well as the experimental system under study, all affect the time course of the response. Injection of foreign cells into a mouse leads to the production of detectable cytotoxic lymphocytes within three days. Peak activity occurs around day ten and then declines over the ensuing weeks.[161] Rechallenge evokes a secondary response which is more rapid and of greater intensity (measured by the number of target cells lysed).[161] Memory cells for T-cell-mediated responses are long-lived, recirculating T cells.[162]

As we described in Chapter 5, two distinct T-cell subpopulations may contribute to the overall cytotoxic response. One consists of the actual effector cells, the other consists of amplifier cells which resemble the T helper cells of the humoral response.[163–165] There is evidence that the killer and amplifier cells recognize different cell-surface antigens, analogous to the hapten-carrier effect of the humoral response. The presence of an amplifier cell may not be absolutely required for cytotoxicity and may only enhance the response (see Chap. 9).

Following exposure to cell-surface antigen, two events take place: blast transformation and cellular proliferation.[166]

The precursor of the cytotoxic lymphocyte is a small, dense, quiescent T cell capable of recognizing antigen. Upon stimulation it transforms into a large, less dense blast cell which has cytotoxic potential.[167,168] This T lymphoblast is the earliest cell with killer potential to appear in the cell-mediated response.[169]

Peak blast response in a primary response occurs within a week and correlates with an increase in cytotoxicity. Peak proliferation occurs earlier than the peak in cytotoxic activity;[170] there is evidence that proliferation alone is insufficient to generate killer cells and some degree of differentiation is almost certainly required.[171] A major part of the proliferation appears to reflect activity in the amplifier-cell population.[172] Although proliferation is not sufficient for the generation of cytotoxic T lymphocytes, inhibition of proliferation markedly diminishes or may even prevent the cytotoxic response.[173] In a primary response, at least one round of cell division seems to be required in order to generate active killer cells.[174,175]

The large blast killer cell makes its appearance only transiently. It has been suggested that within several days it differentiates once more into a small, dense, circulating lymphocyte.[176] These small cells have been termed secondary lymphocytes and are believed to represent the memory cells that will effect the secondary cytotoxic response.[177,178] Upon antigenic challenge these cells rapidly give rise to blastlike killer cells. A round of DNA synthesis and cell division does not appear to be necessary for the generation of killer cells in a secondary response. (Fig. 6-5).[174]

The basis for the enhanced secondary response is probably both qualitative and quantitative, as with the humoral response.[179] There is evidence that the antigen receptors on the surface of sensitized T cells have a greatly increased ability to bind antigen compared to unsensitized precursor cells.[180] This may make the secondary lymphocyte both easier to stimulate and more efficient at target-cell killing. It has also been proposed that memory amplifier cells contribute to the increased cytotoxicity of the secondary response.[181] T-cell memory is long-lived although it may gradually decline without further antigenic challenge.[182]

Mechanism of T-Cell Cytotoxicity

Cytotoxic T lymphocytes must bind to their target cell in order to effect killing. Cytotoxicity does not seem to be mediated by soluble factors.[183] The best studies have been done with tumor allografts in mice and may not be applicable in general. However, the evidence from

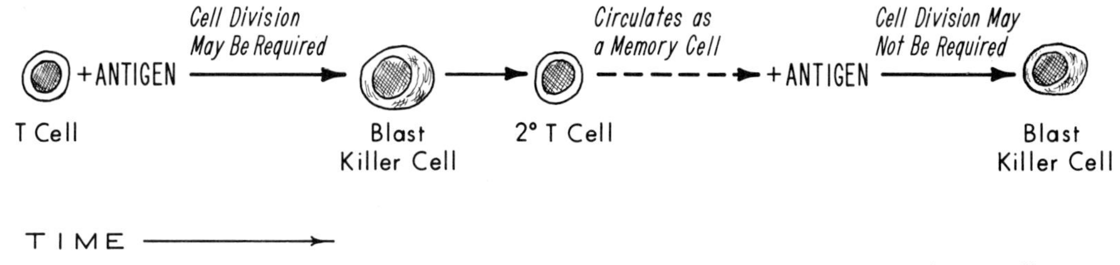

Fig. 6-5. The life cycle of a T cell. Upon initial exposure to antigen, the T cell is transformed into a large blast killer cell. This transformation requires at least one round of cell division. The T cell then circulates as a small memory cell until restimulation again induces blast transformation. Cell division may not be required this second time.

these systems suggests that killing occurs in two stages: a binding stage which is probably energy-independent and a killing stage which is energy-dependent. At some point after attachment, an irreversible lesion is created in the cell membrane of the target cell which leads to cell death. The lesion appears to be different than that caused by complement. In some systems, at least, the killer cell can be released from the target and can move on to kill additional target cells.[184,185]

LYMPHOKINES

Lymphokines are products of activated lymphocytes. It was originally thought that only T lymphocytes secreted lymphokines, but it is now clear that non-T lymphocytes can release lymphokines as well. Over the past several years an impressive array of soluble lymphokines has been reported,[186] although only a few of these have been well characterized.

Lymphocyte-Derived Chemotactic Factors (LDCF)

Activated lymphocytes release a factor which is chemotactic for macrophages.[187] The migration of macrophages to the site of reactivity is critical for the degradation and disposal of antigen. The macrophages can in turn enhance lymphocyte-antigen interactions (see Chap. 5). The resultant histologic lesion is that of the typical delayed hypersensitivity response, such as we see with a positive tuberculin skin test (see below).

There is some evidence that activated lymphocytes also produce a factor chemotactic for neutrophils. It is separable from the macrophage chemotactic factor and may be less potent.[188]

Macrophage Inhibition Factor (MIF) and Macrophage Activation

MIF prevents the migration of macrophages in various *in vitro* situations. It was therefore first believed that the *in vivo* function of MIF was to maintain macrophages at the site of antigen-lymphocyte interaction. More recent studies, however, have altered this view:[189] The ability of the macrophage to function as an efficient phagocyte can be greatly enhanced by the presence of activated lymphocytes.[190] This process is called *macrophage activation*. Specifically sensitized lymphocytes activate macrophages by secreting a lymphokine when challenged with the appropriate antigen.[191] By various physiochemical criteria, this activating factor appears to be identical to MIF. Thus MIF may primarily function as a macrophage-activating factor (MAF). We will refer to this lymphokine as MIF/MAF since these activities have not yet been separated.*

MIF/MAF enhances macrophage adherence to surfaces and increases ruffled membrane activity, the rate of glucose metabolism and the rate of phagocytosis.[192] Incubation of macrophages with MIF/MAF increases their ability to engulf bacteria by as much as tenfold.[193] The enhanced antibacterial activity is nonspecific and the activated macrophages will engulf antigens unrelated to the antigen that stimulated the release of the lymphokine in the first place. *In vitro* incubation of macrophages with MIF/MAF results in full activation within three days.[194] However, the process can be accelerated by incubating lymphocytes and antigen directly with the macrophages.[189]

MIF/MAF production by activated lymphocytes has long been considered to be a marker of T-cell activity. However, it has now been shown that B lymphocytes can also produce MIF/MAF,[195] and production of MIF/MAF should no longer be considered an indicator solely of T-cell function.

There are some reports which indicate

*It is important to mention that macrophages can also be activated by agents such as bacterial endotoxin which are not lymphokines.

that lymphocytes can specifically arm macrophages against specific antigens. The postulated lymphokine is called specific macrophage arming factor (SMAF).[196] Most experiments aimed at studying the activity of armed macrophages have focused on macrophage killing of specific target cells. This probably occurs by a process other than phagocytosis.[197] The biological significance of SMAF and its role in the normal immune response is still unclear.

Lymphocytotoxins

Sensitized lymphocytes can be stimulated by the appropriate antigen to release a lymphokine that will nonspecifically lyse target cells unrelated to the stimulating antigen.[198] Like MIF/MAF, this lymphocytotoxin was originally thought to be a product only of T cells, but B cells have now also been demonstrated to produce it.[199] Lymphocytotoxin has been reported in only a few *in vitro* systems, and it has not been established that it is involved in the *in vivo* killing of foreign cells.

Other Lymphokines

Listed below are other T-cell functions which have been attributed to the active secretion of soluble lymphokines (Table 6-1). These have not been nearly as well defined as those discussed above and it is still uncertain whether or not they represent uniquely defined soluble factors. The major exception to this qualification is the lymphokine interferon which will be discussed in detail in Chapter 11.

Table 6-1. Other Lymphokines

Buffy coat leukocyte migration inhibition factor (LIF)
Specific macrophage-arming factor (SMAF)
Additional chemotactic factors
Lymphocyte transforming factor (LTF)
Colony inhibitory factor (CIF)
Proliferation inhibition factor (PIF; possibly a chalone)
Interferon
Osteoclast activating factor (OAF)

THE HYPERSENSITIVITY STATES

Once the immune system has been primed to an antigen, rechallenge with that antigen will elicit a secondary response, the precise manifestations of which will depend upon (1) whether the antigen elicits a predominantly cellular or humoral response, (2) the class of antibody produced, and (3) whether the antigen is soluble, insoluble, cellular, and so on. Early investigators classified these responses into four basic reaction patterns and termed them the hypersensitivity states. The term "hypersensitivity" referred to the heightened response seen with the second challenge of antigen. These four reaction patterns were grouped according to the time course over which the reactions evolved; three of the hypersensitivity states were considered examples of *immediate hypersensitivity*, and the fourth was called *delayed hypersensitivity*. These distinctions are still used in clinical medicine today.

IMMEDIATE HYPERSENSITIVITY

Immediate hypersensitivity is mediated by the interaction of antigen with antibody and evolves rapidly over minutes to hours. The antibody molecules exist preformed in the host as a result of previous sensitization to the antigen. The ability to manifest an immediate hypersensitivity reaction against a given antigen can be transferred to a nonimmune host with serum from a sensitized host.

Type I: Anaphylactic Reactions

Type I reactions are mediated by the binding of antigen to preformed IgE molecules attached to mast cells and basophils, triggering the release of the intracellular stores of biologically active agents. Three of these substances are probably responsible for most of the varying manifestations of Type I reactions.[200]

Histamine exists preformed in the mast-cell granules and is thus capable of acting immediately upon cellular activation and release. Its most important biological effects include increasing vascular permeability, increasing airway resistance and reducing pulmonary compliance. The effects of histamine upon the respiratory system may be largely due to stimulation of vagal reflexes rather than a direct action on the lung itself.

Slow-reacting substance of anaphylaxis (SRS-A) does not exist preformed in the cell and must be both formed and released when the cell is activated. For this reason, the time course of SRS-A release is slower than that of histamine. SRS-A can contract smooth muscle and enhance vascular permeability.

Eosinophil chemotactic factor (ECF-A) exists preformed within the mast cell and is responsible for the accumulation of eosinophils at sites of Type I reactions. Eosinophils possess an aryl sulfatase that can deactivate SRS-A.

Ten to 20 per cent of the population in the United States manifest atopic (meaning "out of the ordinary") allergic reactions. There is a strong genetic predisposition to atopy, and genes within the major histocompatibility complex may be involved in the control of IgE responses.

Clinically, Type I reactions range from acute and often fatal vascular collapse with bronchial constriction to mild allergies such as hay fever. The different clinical manifestations of Type I reactions are due to the differing susceptibility of individuals to the various chemical mediators, the extent of antiallergen IgE production, the site of reaction, etc.

Hay fever (allergic rhinitis) is the most common clinically evident Type I response, and is primarily due to the effects of histamine released from mast cells located both in and under the nasal mucosa. Patients present with sneezing, nasal congestion, watery discharge, conjunctival itching, and occasionally cough and bronchoconstriction.

Asthma probably results from mast-cell release in the bronchial lumina. SRS-A may be the major chemical mediator producing smooth-muscle contraction with bronchial obstruction. Histamine may also contribute to the symptomatology of asthma by reducing lung compliance. Dyspnea and wheezing are the most common presenting symptoms. In occasional patients, attacks are precipitated by microbial infections.

Atopic eczema (atopic dermatitis) is a pruritic skin rash commonly first appearing in infancy although onset can occur at any age. The disease may spontaneously remit in childhood or persist throughout life. A high percentage of patients also have asthma or hay fever, and there is often a family history of atopy. Patients frequently have high IgE titers and an eosinophilia. However, the histology of the skin lesion is not typical of a Type I response (for example, eosinophils are present only transiently) and the cellular mechanisms of delayed hypersensitivity are probably involved as well.

Other IgE-mediated disorders include allergic bronchopulmonary aspergillosis (see Chap. 11), some forms of urticaria and anaphylactic reactions to certain drugs such as penicillin. However, most so-called drug allergies are not due to IgE-initiated processes.

The disorders described above are very common, and methods are continually being sought to determine if an individual is allergic to a particular allergen. At present, the two most commonly used tests are (1) a skin test where the suspected allergen is applied to the patient's skin, and (2) RAST (radio-allergo-absorbent test), a radioimmunoassay which measures the presence of free IgE to a given allergen.

Type II: Cytotoxic Reactions

Type II reactions are those which involve the binding of antibody, usually IgG or IgM, to cell-bound antigen. We have discussed the characteristics and importance of this type of response in this chapter.

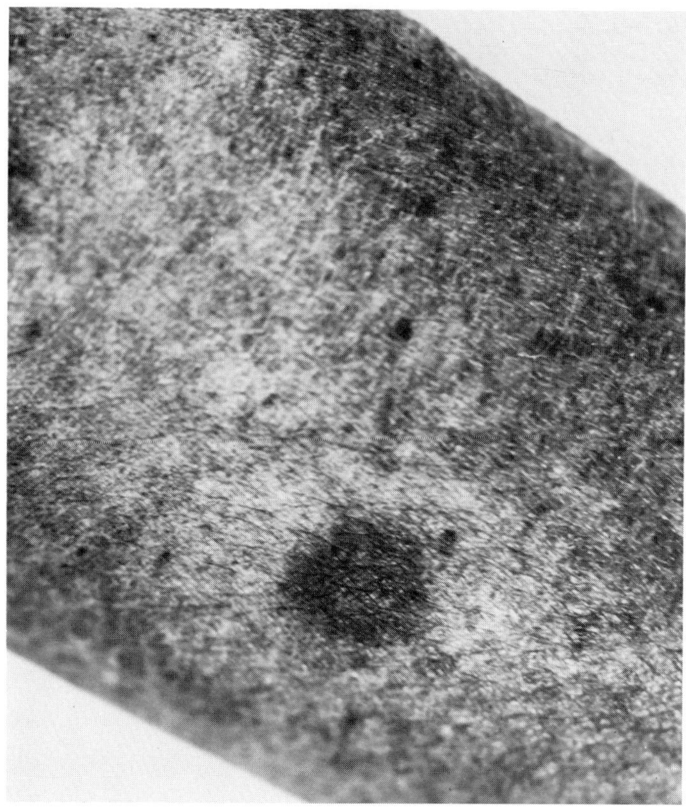

Fig. 6-6. A positive tuberculin skin test.

Type III: Immune Complex Formation

Antibody can interact with free antigen to form antigen-antibody complexes. Chapter 7 is devoted to a description of the formation and characteristics of immune complexes in the normal immune response, as well as their contribution to human pathology.

DELAYED HYPERSENSITIVITY

The intradermal injection of antigen elicits a characteristic host response which is visibly evident at the site of injection. The reaction evolves over hours to days and appears as a red, indurated area in the skin (see Fig. 6-6). This reaction pattern is termed delayed hypersensitivity and is employed clinically to measure the competence of an individual's cellular immunity. The correlation between delayed hypersensitivity and cellular immunity to a test antigen is not perfect (see Chap. 11), but in most situations the ability of an individual to produce a positive skin test to a given antigen is good evidence of that person's ability to mount a cellular immune response to the antigen.

Delayed hypersensitivity was first demonstrated by the injection of tuberculin into the skin of guinea pigs,[201] and has subsequently been shown for many antigens, including microorganisms, chemicals and proteins, and in many species of animals, including all vertebrates and man. The first visible cutaneous changes occur within several hours of the injection of antigen, and the size of the lesion usually peaks within 24 to 72 hours. If the antigen is diffusible there will be less elevation and induration than if it is poorly diffusible. Histologic studies reveal a mononuclear cell infiltrate in the dermis and surrounding tissues (see Fig. 6-7). The cells are heavily concentrated around the

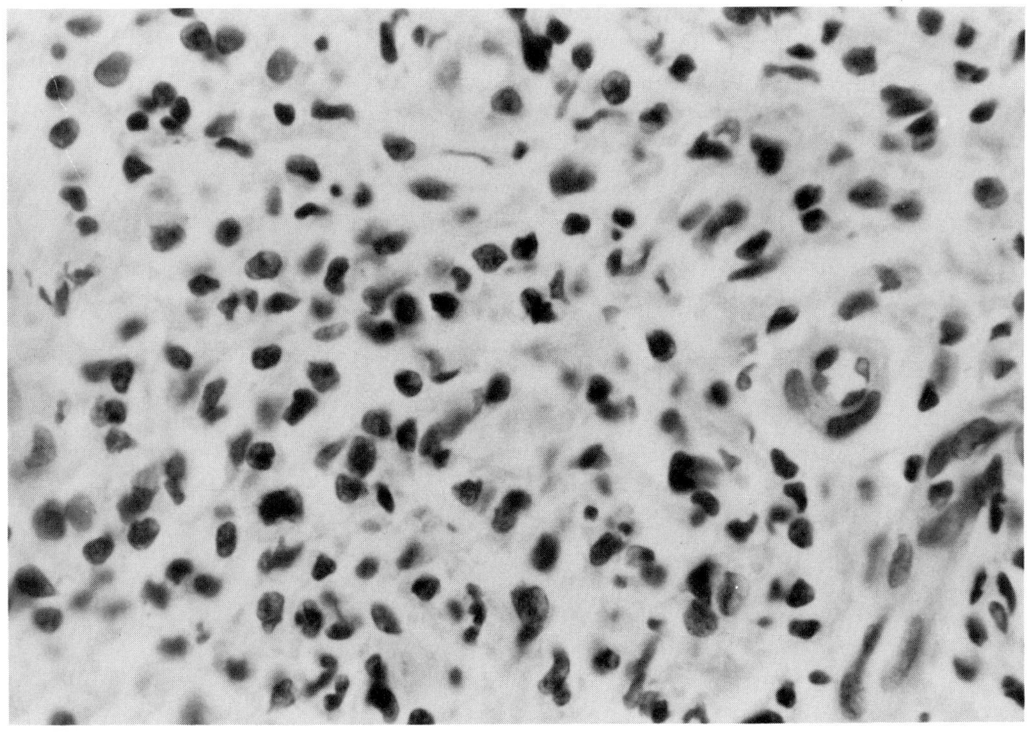

Fig. 6-7. The histology of a delayed hypersensitivity reaction. Note the mononuclear cell infiltrate in peri-vascular areas.

Fig. 6-8. The histology of a Jones-Mote lesion. (Dvorak, H.F. *et al.*: Cutaneous basophil hypersensitivity. IIA light- and electron microscopic study. J. Exp. Med., *132*:558, 1970.)

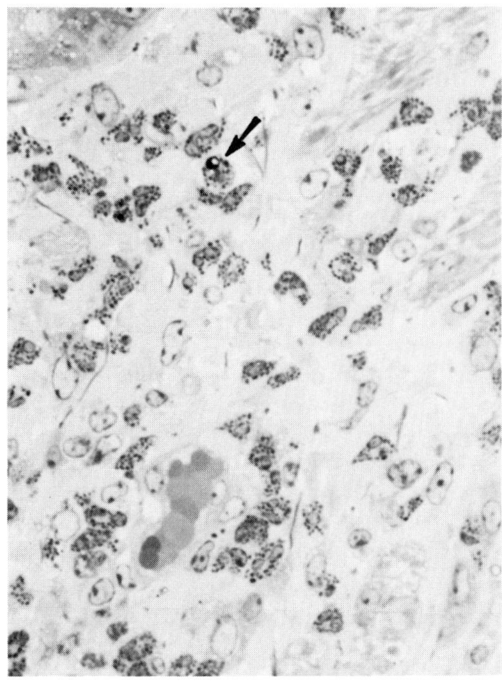

blood vessels. Polymorphonuclear leukocytes may or may not be present.

Delayed hypersensitivity is not transferrable by serum, but can be transferred with lymphocytes.[202] It has been definitively established that the T lymphocyte is the initiator of the response. The release of lymphokines serves to attract inflammatory cells to the site of reaction.

A second type of delayed hypersensitivity lesion has been defined, and is called cutaneous basophil hypersensitivity (or Jones-Mote sensitivity).[203] Some antigens elicit a profound basophilic infiltrate when given intradermally. The time course of this reaction is typically delayed, occurring after 6 to 24 hours. As many as 50 per cent of the infiltrating cells may be basophils (see Fig. 6-8). The mechanism of cutaneous basophil hypersensitivity appears to involve T-cell activation by antigen[204] with subsequent release of factors—as yet undefined—that are chemotactic for basophils. The basophils are thus nonspecific participants in the reaction. It is not known why certain antigens elicit this type of reaction; it is probably much less common than the classical delayed hypersensitivity reaction.

REFERENCES

1. Uhr, J. W., and Finkelstein, M. S.: Antibody formation. J. Exp. Med., *117*:457, 1963.
2. Makinodan, T., and Albright, J. F.: Proliferative and differentiative manifestations of cellular immune potential. Prog. Allergy, *10*:1, 1967.
3. Nossal, G. J. V., Austin, C. M., and Ada, G. L.: Antigens in immunity. Immunology, *9*:333, 1965.
4. Uhr, J. W., and Finkelstein, M. S.: The kinetics of antibody formation. Prog. Allergy, *10*:37, 1967.
5. Pierce, C. W., Solliday, S. M., and Asofsky, R.: Immune response *in vitro*. J. Exp. Med., *135*:675, 1972.
6. Cooper, M. D., Lawton, A. R., and Kincade, P. W.: A developmental approach to the biological basis of antibody diversity. Cont. Top. Immunobiol., *1*:33, 1972.
7. Greaves, M. F.: The expression of immunoglobulin determinants on the surface of antigen-binding lymphoid cells in mice. Eur. J. Immunol., *1*:186, 1971.
8. Lawton, A. R., Asofsky, N., Hylton, M. B., and Cooper, M. D.: Suppression of immunoglobulin class synthesis in mice. J. Exp. Med., *135*:277, 1972.
9. Manning, D. D., and Jutila, J. W.: Immunosuppression of mice injected with heterologous anti-immunoglobulin heavy chain antisera. J. Exp. Med., *135*:1316, 1972.
10. Eisen, H. N., and Siskind, G. W.: Variations in affinities of antibody during the immune response. Biochemistry, *3*:996, 1964.
11. Huchet, R., and Feldmann, M.: Studies on antibody affinity in mice. Eur. J. Immunol., *3*:49, 1973.
12. Voss, E. W., and Eisen, H. N.: Valence and affinity of IgM antibody to the 2,4-DNP group. Fed. Proc., *27*:684, 1967.
13. Pasanen, V. J.: Identification of direct hemolytic plaques as IgM or IgG plaques by hapten inhibition. Int. Arch. Allergy Appl. Immunol., *40*:171, 1971.
14. Siskind, G., Dunn, P., and Walker, J.: Studies on the control of antibody synthesis. J. Exp. Med., *127*:55, 1968.
15. Davie, J. M., and Paul, W. E.: Receptors on immunocompetent cells. J. Exp. Med., *135*:660, 1972.
16. Steiner, L. A., and Eisen, H. N.: Sequential changes in the relative affinity of antibody synthesized during the immune response. J. Exp. Med., *126*:1161, 1967.
17. Baker, J., and Stashak, P. W.: Quantitative and qualitative studies on the primary antibody response to Pneumococcal polysaccharides at the cellular level. J. Immunol., *103*:1342, 1969.
18. Humphrey, J. H., Parrott, D. M. V., and East, J.: Studies on globulin and antibody production in mice thymectomized at birth. Immunology, *7*:419, 1964.
19. Katz, D. H., and Benacerraf, B.: The regulatory influence of activated T cells on B cell responses to antigen. Adv. Immunol., *15*:1, 1972.
20. Gronowicz, E., and Möller, E.: Quantity and quality of anti-hapten antibodies in normal and in T-cell deprived mice studied at the cellular level. Scand. J. Immunol., *1*:371, 1972.
21. Taylor, R., and Wortis, H.: Thymus dependence of antibody response: variation with dose of antigen and class of antibody. Nature, *220*:927, 1968.
22. Romano, T. J., and Thorbecke, G. J.: Thymus influence on the conversion of 19S to 7S antibody formation in the response to TNP-Brucella. J. Immunol., *115*:332, 1975.
23. Davie, J. M., and Paul, W. E.: Role of T lymphocytes in the humoral immune response. J. Immunol., *113*:1438, 1974.
24. Gershon, R. K., and Paul, W. E.: Effective thymus-derived lymphocytes on amount and affinity of anti-hapten antibody. J. Immunol., *106*:872, 1971.
25. Sanfillipo, F., and Scott, D. W.: The effect of carrier specific helper T-cell tolerance on anti-

body avidity in the antihapten response. Cell Immunol., *21*:112, 1976.
26. Celada, F.: The cellular basis of immunologic memory. Prog. Allergy, *15*:223, 1971.
27. Tao, T.: Antibody response to bacteriophage ΦX174 *in vitro*: demonstration of immunologic memory in terms of IgM and IgG responses. Eur. J. Immunol., *2*:332, 1972.
28. Bullock, W., and Rittenberg, M.: *In vitro* initiated secondary anti-hapten response. J. Exp. Med., *132*:926, 1970.
29. Wigzell, H.: The rise and fall of 19S immunological memory against sheep red cells in the mouse. Med. Exp. Fenn., *44*:209, 1966.
30. Celada, F.: Quantitative studies of the adoptive immunologic memory in mice. J. Exp. Med., *125*:199, 1967.
31. Strober, S., and Dilley, J.: Biological characteristics of T and B memory lymphocytes in the rat. J. Exp. Med., *137*:1275, 1973.
32. Mitchell, G., M., *et al*.: Immunologic memory in mice. J. Exp. Med., *135*:165, 1972.
33. Stavitsky, A. B., and Cook, R. G.: *In vitro* anamnestic response of rabbit lymph node cells. J. Immunol., *112*:583, 1974.
34. Mitchison, N. A.: The carrier effect in the secondary response to hapten-carrier conjugates. Eur. J. Immunol., *1*:10, 1971.
35. ———: The carrier effect in the secondary response to hapten-carrier conjugates. Eur. J. Immunol., *1*:18, 1971.
36. Rajewsky, K., Schirrmacher, V., Nase, S., and Jerne, N. K.: The requirement of more than one antigenic determinant for immunogenicity. J. Exp. Med., *129*:1131, 1969.
37. Katz, D. H., Paul, W. E., Goidl, E. A., and Benacerraf, B.: Carrier function in anti-hapten immune responses. J. Exp. Med., *132*:261, 1970.
38. Paul, W. E., Katz, D. H., Goidl, E. A., and Benacerraf, B.: Carrier function in anti-hapten immune responses. J. Exp. Med., *132*:283, 1970.
39. Havas, H., and Packard, A.: The effect of the immunogenicity of the heterologous carrier on the early secondary anti 2,4-DNP response of Balb/c mice. J. Immunol., *109*:791, 1972.
40. Elfenbein, G., Green, I., and Paul, W.: The allogeneic effect: increased affinity of serum antibody produced during a secondary response. Eur. J. Immunol., *3*:640, 1973.
41. Klinman, N.: The secondary immune response to a hapten *in vitro*. J. Exp. Med., *133*:963, 1971.
42. Paul, W., Siskind, G., Benacerraf, B., and Ovary, Z.: Secondary antibody responses in haptenic systems: cell population selection by antigen. J. Immunol., *99*:760, 1967.
43. Hunt, S. V., Ellis, S. T., and Gowans, J. L.: The role of lymphocytes in antibody formation. Proc. R. Soc. Lond. [Biol.], *82*:211, 1972.
44. Strober, S., and Dilley, L.: Maturation of B lymphocytes in the rat. J. Exp. Med., *138*:1331, 1973.
45. Schirrmacher, V., and Rajewsky, K.: Determination of antibody class in a system of cooperating antigenic determinants. J. Exp. Med., *132*:1019, 1970.
46. Kishimoto, T., and Ishizaka, K.: Regulation of antibody response *in vitro*. J. Immunol., *109*:612, 1972.
47. Schlegel, R., Von Boehmer, H., and Shortman, K.: Antigen-initiated B lymphocyte differentiation. Cell Immunol., *16*:203, 1975.
48. Williamson, A., McMichael, A., and Zitron, I.: B memory cells in the propagation of stable clones of antibody forming cells. *In* Sercarz, E., Williamson, A., and Fox, C. (eds.): The Immune System. P. 387. New York, Academic Press, 1974.
49. Davie, J. M., and Paul, W. E.: Receptors on immunocompetent cells. J. Exp. Med., *135*:643, 1972.
50. Askonas, A., Williamson, A., and Wright, B.: Selection of a single antibody-forming cell clone and its propogation in syngeneic mice. Proc. Natl. Acad. Sci. U.S.A., *67*:1398, 1970.
51. Ada, G.: Antigen binding cells. Transplant. Rev., *5*:105, 1970.
52. McMichael, A., and Williamson, A.: Clonal memory. J. Exp. Med., *139*:1361, 1974.
53. Secarz, E., and Byers, V.: The X-Y-Z scheme of immunocyte maturation. J. Immunol., *98*:836, 1967.
54. Black, S., and Inchley, C.: Characteristics of immunological memory in mice. J. Exp. Med., *140*:333, 1975.
55. Farrar, J., and Nordin, A.: Cellular requirements for the expression of IgM immunological memory *in vitro*. Cell. Immunol., *12*:102, 1974.
56. Weigle, W. O.: Cyclic production of antibody as a regulatory mechanism in the immune response. Adv. Immunol., *21*:87, 1975.
57. Uhr, J. W., and Möller, G.: Regulatory effect of antibody on the immune response. Adv. Immunol., *8*:81, 1968.
58. Bystryn, J., Graf, M. W., and Uhr, J. W.: Regulation of antibody formation by serum antibody. J. Exp. Med., *132*:1279, 1970.
59. Horibata, K., and Uhr, J. W.: Antibody content of single antibody-forming cells. J. Immunol., *98*:972, 1967.
60. Wigzell, H.: Antibody synthesis at the cellular level. J. Exp. Med., *124*:953, 1966.
61. Rowley, D. A., and Fitch, F. W.: Homeostasis of antibody formation in the adult rat. J. Exp. Med., *120*:987, 1964.
62. Uhr, J. W., and Baumann, J. B.: Antibody formation. J. Exp. Med., *113*:959, 1961.
63. Cerottini, J., McConahey, P. J., and Dixon, F. J.: The immunosuppressive effect of passively administered antibody-IgG fragments. J. Immunol., *102*:1008, 1969.
64. Chang, H., Schneck, S., Brody, N. I., Deutsch, A., and Siskind, G. W.: Studies in the mechanism of the suppression of active antibody synthesis by passively administered antibody. J. Immunol., *102*:37, 1969.
65. Henney, C. S., and Ishizaka, K.: Studies on the

immunogenicity of antigen-antibody precipitates. J. Immunol., *104*:154, 1970.

66. Kappler, J. W., Van der Hooven, A., Dharmarajan, V., and Hoffmann, M.: Regulation of the immune response. J. Immunol., *111*:1228, 1973.
67. Tao, T., and Uhr, J. W.: Capacity of pepsin-digested antibody to inhibit antibody formation. Nature, *212*:208, 1966.
68. Feldmann, M., and Diener, E.: Antibody-mediated suppression of the immune response *in vitro*. J. Immunol., *108*:93, 1972.
69. Gordon, J., and Murgita, R. A.: Suppression and augmentation of the primary *in vitro* immune response by different classes of antibody. Cell. Immunol., *15*:392, 1975.
70. Chan, P. L., and Sinclair, N. R.: Regulation of the immune response. Immunology, *21*:967, 1971.
71. Sinclair, N. R.: Regulation of the immune response. J. Exp. Med., *129*:1183, 1969.
72. Henry, G. C., and Jerne, N. K.: Competition of 19S and 7S antigen receptors in the regulation of the primary immune response. J. Exp. Med., *128*:133, 1968.
73. Dennert, G.: The mechanism of antibody-induced stimulation and inhibition of the immune response. J. Immunol., *106*:951, 1970.
74. Pearlman, D. S.: The influence of antibody on immunologic responses. J. Exp. Med., *126*:127, 1967.
75. Murgita, R. A., and Vas, S. I.: Specific antibody-mediated effect in the immune response. Immunology, *22*:319, 1972.
76. Sahiar, K., and Schwartz, R. S.: Inhibition of 19S antibody synthesis by 7S antibody. Science, *145*:395, 1964.
77. Finkelstein, M. S., and Uhr, J. W.: Specific inhibition of antibody formation by passively administered 19S and 7S antibody. Science, *146*:67, 1964.
78. Rodkey, L. S.: Studies of idiotypic antibody. J. Exp. Med., *139*:712, 1974.
79. Eichmann, K.: Idiotypic identity of antibody to streptococcal carbohydrate in inbred mice. Eur. J. Immunol., *3*:301, 1972.
80. Hart, D. A., Wang, A., Pawlah, L. L., and Nisinoff, A.: Suppression of idiotypic specificities in adult mice by administration of anti-idiotype antibody. J. Exp. Med., *135*:1293, 1972.
81. Nisinoff, A., and Bargasser, S. A.: Immunological suppression of idiotypic specificities. Transplant Rev., *27*:100, 1975.
82. Kluskens, L., and Kohler, H.: Regulation of immune response by autogenous antibody against receptor. Proc. Natl. Acad. Sci. U.S.A., *71*:5083, 1974.
83. Dray, S.: Effect of maternal isoantibodies on the quantitative expression of two allelic genes controlling γ -globulin allotypic specificities. Nature, *195*:677, 1962.
84. ——: Allotype suppression. *In* Ontogeny of Aquired Immunity. Amsterdam. Ciba Foundation Symposium, Ass. Sci. Pub., 1972.
85. Jacobson, E., Herzenberg, L. A., Riblet, R. J., and Herzenberg, L. A.: Active suppression of immunoglobulin allotype synthesis. J. Exp. Med., *135*:1163, 1972.
86. Herzenberg, L. A., Chan, E. L., Ravitch, M. M., Riblet, R. J., and Herzenberg, L. A.: Active suppression of immunoglobulin allotype synthesis. J. Exp. Med., *137*:1311, 1973.

86a. Herzenberg, L. A., *et al.*: T-cell regulation of antibody responses: demonstration of allotype-specific helper T cells and their specific removal by suppressor T cells. J. Exp. Med., *144*:330, 1976.

87. Herzenberg, L. A., Okumura, K., and Metzler, C. M.: Regulation of immunoglobulin and antibody production by allotype suppressor T cells in mice. Transplant. Rev., *27*:57, 1975.
88. Harrison, M. R., Mage, R. G., and Davie, J. M.: Deletion of 65 immunoglobulin-bearing lymphocytes in allotype-suppressed rabbits. J. Exp. Med., *137*:254, 1973.
89. Adler, L. T.: Studies on allotype suppression and its abrogation in cultured rabbit spleen cells. Transplant. Rev., *27*:3, 1975.
90. Tada, T., Taniguchi, M., and Takemori, T.: Properties of primed suppressor T cells and their products. Transplant, Rev., *26*:106, 1975.
91. Gershon, R. K.: T cell control of antibody production. Cont. Top. Immunobiol., *3*:1, 1974.
92. Tada, T.: *In* Katz, D., and Benacerraf, B. (eds.): Immunologic Tolerance. P. 471. New York, Academic Press, 1974.
93. Tada, T., and Takemori, T.: Selective roles of thymus-derived lymphocytes in the antibody response. J. Exp. Med., *140*:239, 1974.
94. Okumura, K., and Tada, T.: Suppression of hapten-specific antibody response by carrier-specific T cells. Nature [New Biol.], *245*:180, 1973.
95. Tomasi, T. B., and Grey, H. M.: Structure and function of immunoglobulin A. Prog. Allergy, *16*:81, 1972.
96. Tokumaru, T.: A possible role of IgA in Herpes simplex virus infection in man. J. Immunol., *97*:248, 1966.
97. Ogra, P. L., Karzon, D. T., Righthand, F., and MacGillivray, M.: Immunoglobulin response in serum and secretions after immunization in live and inactivated polio vaccine and natural infections. N. Engl. J. Med., *279*:893, 1968.
98. Rudders, R. A., and Ross, R.: Partial characterization of the shift from IgG to IgA synthesis in the clonal differentiation of human leukemic bone marrow-derived lymphocytes. J. Exp. Med., *142*:549, 1975.
99. Lamm, M. E.: Cellular aspects of immunoglobulin A. Adv. Immunol., *22*:223, 1976.
100. Benner, R., Meima, F., and Van der Meulen, G. M.: Antibody formation in mouse bone marrow. Cell. Immunol., *13*:95, 1974.
101. Makela, O., Kostiainen, E., Koponen, T., and Ruoslahti, E.: *In* Killander, J. (ed.): Gamma Globulin Structure and Control of Biosynthesis. P. 505. New York, Interscience Publication, 1967.

102. Klinman, N. R., Rockey, J. H., Frauenberger, G., and Karosh, F.: Equine anti-hapten antibody. J. Immunol., *96*:507, 1966.
103. Robertson, P. W., and Cooper, G. N.: Immune response in intestinal tissues to particulate antigen. Aust. J. Exp. Biol. Med. Sci., *51*:575, 1973.
104. Revoltella, R., and Ovary, Z.: Reaginic antibody production in different mouse strains. Immunology, *17*:45, 1969.
105. Tada, T., Okumura, K., and Taniguchi, M.: Cellular and humoral controls of reaginic antibody synthesis in the rat. *In* Goodfriend, L., Sehon, A. H., and Orange, R. P. (eds.): Mechanisms in Allergy. P. 43. New York, Marcel Dekker, 1973.
106. Ishizaka, K., and Kishimoto, T.: Cellular basis of reaginic antibody formation *in vitro*. *In* Goodfriend, L., Sehon, A. H., and Orange, R. P. (eds.): Mechanisms in Allergy. P. 63. New York, Marcel Dekker, 1973.
107. Strejan, G., and Campbell, D. H.: Hypersensitivity to ascaris antigens. J. Immunol., *98*:893, 1967.
108. Ogilvie, B. M.: Reagin-like antibodies in animals immune to helminth parasites. Nature, *204*:91, 1964.
109. Levine, B. B., and Vaz, N. M.: Effect of combination of inbred strain, antigenic dose on immune responsiveness of reagin production in the mouse. Int. Arch. Allergy, *39*:156, 1970.
110. ——: Genetic control of reagin production in mice. Fed. Proc., *30*:469, 1972.
111. Ishizaka, K., and Kishimoto, T.: Regulation of antibody response *in vitro*. J. Immunol., *109*:65, 1972.
112. Hamaoka, T., Katz, D. H., Block, K. J., and Benacerraf, B.: Hapten-specific IgE antibody responses in rat. J. Exp. Med., *138*:306, 1973.
113. Strejan, G. H., and Marsh, D. G.: Hapten-carrier relationship in the production of rat homocytotropic antibody. J. Immunol., *107*:306, 1971.
114. Hamaoka, T., Newburger, P. E., Katz, D. H., and Benacerraf, B.: Hapten-specific IgE antibody responses in mice. J. Immunol., *113*:958, 1974.
115. Hamaoka, T., Katz, D. H., and Benacerraf, B.: Hapten-specific IgE antibody responses in mice. J. Exp. Med., *138*:538, 1973.
116. Katz, D. H., Hamaoka, T., Newburger, P. E., and Benacerraf, B.: Hapten-specific IgE antibody responses in mice. J. Immunol., *113*:974, 1974.
117. Kishimoto, T., and Ishizaka, K.: Regulation of antibody response *in vitro*. J. Immunol., *109*:612, 1972.
118. ——: Regulation of antibody response *in vitro*. J. Immunol., *111*:720, 1973.
119. ——: Regulation of antibody response *in vitro*. J. Immunol., *112*:1685, 1974.
120. ——: Immunologic and physiochemical properties of enhancing soluble factors for IgG and IgE antibody responses. J. Immunol., *114*:1177, 1975.
121. Berg, T., and Johansson, S. G. O.: *In vitro* diagnosis of atopic allergy. Int. Arch. Allergy, *41*:452, 1971.
122. Ishizaka, K., and Ishizaka, T.: Human reaginic antibody and IgE. J. Allergy, *42*:330, 1968.
123. Osler, A. G., Lichtenstein, L. M., and Levy, D. A.: *In vitro* studies of human reaginic allergy. Adv. Immunol., *8*:183, 1968.
124. Yunginger, J. M., and Gleich, G. J.: Seasonal changes in IgE antibody to ragweed antigen E. J. Allergy, *49*:118, 1972.
125. Levine, B. B., Stember, R. H., and Fotino, M.: Ragweed hay fever: genetic control and linkage of HLA haplotypes. Science, *178*:1201, 1972.
126. Platts-Mills, T. A. E., *et al.*: IgA and IgG anti-ragweed antibodies in nasal secretions. J. Clin. Invest., *57*:1041, 1976.
127. Tada, T., Okumura, K., and Taniguchi, M.: Cellular and humoral controls of reaginic antibody synthesis in the rat. *In* Goodfriend, L., Sehon, A. H., and Orange, R. P., (eds.): Mechanisms in Allergy. V. p. 43. New York, Marcel Dekker, 1973.
128. Taniguchi, M., and Tada, T.: Regulation of homocytotropic antibody formation in the rat. J. Immunol., *107*:579, 1971.
129. Okumura, K., and Tada, T.: Regulation of homocytotropic antibody formation in the rat. J. Immunol., *106*:1019, 1971.
130. Tada, T., Taniguchi, M., and Okumura, K.: Regulation of homocytotropic antibody formation in the rat. J. Immunol., *106*:1012, 1971.
131. Okumura, K., and Tada, T.: Regulation of homocytotropic antibody formation in the rat. J. Immunol., *107*:1682, 1971.
132. Tada, T., Okumura, K., and Taniguchi, M.: Regulation of homocytotropic antibody formation in the rat. J. Immunol., *111*:952, 1973.
133. Okumura, K., and Tada, T.: Regulation of homocytotropic antibody formation in the rat. J. Immunol., *112*:783, 1974.
134. Ishizaka, K., and Okudaira, H.: Reaginic antibody formation in the mouse. J. Immunol., *109*:84, 1972.
135. Tada, T., and Okumura, K.: Regulation of homocytotropic antibody formation in the rat. J. Immunol., *106*:1002, 1971.
136. Sadan, N., *et al.*: Immunotherapy of pollinosis in children. N. Engl. J. Med., *280*:623, 1969.
137. Evans, R., Pence, H., Kaplan, H., and Rocklin, R. E.: The effect of immunotherapy on humoral and cellular responses in ragweed hayfever. J. Clin. Invest., *57*:1378, 1976.
138. Tada, T., and Ishizaka, K.: Distribution of IgE-forming cells in lymphoid tissues of the human and monkey. J. Immunol., *104*:377, 1970.
139. Ishizaka, K., Kishimoto, T., Delespesse, G., and King, T. P.: Immunogenic properties of modified antigen E. J. Immunol., *113*:70, 1974.
140. Ishizaka, K., Okudaira, H., and King, T. P.: Immunogenic properties of modified antigen E. J. Immunol., *114*:110, 1975.

141. Takatsu, K., Ishizaka, K., and King, T. P.: Immunogenic properties of modified antigen E. J. Immunol., *115*:1469, 1975.
142. Takatsu, K., and Ishizaka, K.: Reaginic antibody formation in the mouse. J. Immunol., *116*:1257, 1976.
143. Groth, S. F., and Notkins, A. L.: Neutralization of virus by antibody. Prog. Immunol., *2*:1215, 1971.
144. Scornik, J. C., Cosenza, H., Lee, W., Kohler, H., and Rowley, D. A.: Antibody dependent cell-mediated cytotoxicity. J. Immunol., *113*:1510, 1974.
145. MacLennan, I. M., Howard, A., Gotch, F. N., and Quie, P. G.: Effector activity determinants on IgG. Immunology, *25*:459, 1973.
146. Forman, J., and Möller, G.: The effector cell in antibody-induced cell-mediated immunity. Transplant. Rev., *17*:108, 1973.
147. Ralph, P., Prichard, J., and Cohn, M.: Reticulum cell sarcoma: an effector cell in antibody-dependent cell-mediated immunity. J. Immunol., *114*:898, 1975.
148. Gale, R. P., and Zighelboim, J.: Polymorphonuclear leukocytes in antibody dependent cellular cytotoxicity. J. Immunol., *114*:1047, 1975.
149. Weissman, I., Lammin, D., Jerabek, L., and Barcelay, T.: Cellular immunity to heterologous erythrocytes *in vitro*. Cell Immunol., *7*:222, 1973.
150. Pollack, S., and Nelson, K.: Effects of carrageenan and high serum dilutions on synergistic cytotoxicity to tumor cells. J. Immunol., *110*:1440, 1973.
151. Diamond, R. D.: Antibody-dependent killing of Cryptococcus neoformans by human peripheral blood mononuclear cells. Nature, *247*:148, 1974.
152. Trinchieri, G., and deMarchi, M.: Antibody-dependent cell-mediated cytotoxicity in humans. J. Immunol., *115*:256, 1975.
153. Gelfand, E. W., Morris, S. A., and Resch, K.: Antibody dependent cytotoxicity: modulation by cytochalasins and microtubule-disruptive agents. J. Immunol., *114*:919, 1975.
154. Scornik, J. C.: Antibody dependent cell mediated cytotoxicity. J. Immunol., *113*:1519, 1974.
155. Tomasi, T. B., and Grey, H. M.: Structure and function of immunoglobulin A. Prog. Allergy, *16*:81, 1972.
156. Smith, C. B., Purcell, R. H., Bellanti, J. A., and Chanock, R. M.: Protective effect of antibody to parainfluenza type 1 virus. N. Engl. J. Med., *275*:1145, 1966.
157. Murray, M., Miller, H. R. P., Sanford, J., and Jarrett, W. F. H.: 5-Hydroxytryptamine in Intestinal immunological reactions. Int. Arch. Allergy, *40*:236, 1971.
158. Jarrett, E. E. E., and Stewart, D. L.: Potentiation of rat reaginic antibody by helminthic antigen E. Immunology, *23*:749, 1972.
159. Odunjo, E. O.: Helminthic anaphylactic syndrome in children. Pathol. Microbiol., *35*:220, 1970.
160. Rollinghoff, M.: Secondary cytotoxic tumor immune response induced *in vitro*. J. Immunol., *112*:1718, 1973.
161. Canty, T. G., Wunderlich, J. R., and Fletcher, F.: Qualitative and quantitative studies of cytotoxic immune cells. J. Immunol., *106*:200, 1971.
162. Sprent, J., and Miller, J. F. A. P.: Interaction of thymus lymphocytes with histoincompatible cells. Cell. Immunol., *3*:385, 1972.
163. Cantor, H., and Asofsky, R.: Synergy among lymphoid cells mediating the graft versus host reaction. J. Exp. Med., *131*:235, 1970.
164. Tigelaar, R. F., and Asofsky, R.: Synergy among lymphoid cells mediating the graft versus host reaction. J. Exp. Med., *135*:1059, 1972.
165. Wagner, H.: Synergy during *in vitro* cytotoxic allograft responses. J. Exp. Med., *138*:1379, 1973.
166. Andersson, L. C., Hayry, P.: Clonal isolation of alloantigen-reactive T-cells and characterization of their memory function. Transplant. Rev., *25*:121, 1975.
167. Shortman, K., Brunner, K. T., and Cerottini, J.: Separation of stages in the development of the T cells involved in cell-mediated immunity. J. Exp. Med., *135*:1375, 1972.
168. Cerottini, J., Engers, H. D., MacDonald, H. R., and Brunner, K. T.: Generation of cytotoxic T lymphocytes *in vitro*. J. Exp. Med., *140*:703, 1974.
169. Greenberg, A. H.: Fractionation of cytotoxic T lymphoblasts in ficoll gradients by velocity sedimentation. Eur. J. Immunol., *3*:793, 1973.
170. Wagner, H., Rollinghoff, M., and Nossal, G. J. V.: T-cell-mediated immune responses induced in vitro. Transplant. Rev., *17*:3, 1973.
171. Alter, B. J., *et al.*: Cell-mediated lympholysis. J. Exp. Med., *137*:1303, 1973.
172. Bach, F. H., et al.: Cell-mediated immunity: separation of cells involved in cognitive and destructive phases. Science, *180*:403, 1973.
173. Howe, M., Berman, L., and Cohen, L.: Relationship between proliferation and effector phases of the mixed lymphocyte reaction and the graft versus host reaction. J. Immunol., *111*:1243, 1973.
174. Nedrud, J., Tooton, M., and Clark, W. R.: The requirement for DNA synthesis and gene expression in the generation of cytotoxicity *in vitro*. J. Exp. Med., *142*:960, 1975.
175. Cantor, H., and Jandinski, J.: The relationship of cell division to the generation of cytotoxic activity in mixed lymphocyte cultures. J. Exp. Med., *140*:1710, 1974.
176. Andersson, L. C., and Hayry, P.: Specific priming of mouse thymus-dependent lymphocytes to allogeneic cells *in vitro*. Eur. J. Immunol., *3*:595, 1973.
177. Andersson, L. C.: Size distribution of killer cells during allograft response. Scand. J. Immunol., *2*:75, 1973.
178. Wagner, H., and Rollinghoff, M.: Secondary cytotoxic allograft responses *in vitro*. Eur. J. Immunol., *6*:15, 1976.
179. MacDonald, H. R., Engers, H. D., Cerottini, J.,

and Brunner, J.: The generation of cytotoxic T lymphocytes *in vitro*. J. Exp. Med., *140*:718, 1974.
180. Kimura, A. K., and Clark, W. R.: Functional characteristics of T cell receptors during sensitization against histocompatibility antigens *in vitro*. Cell. Immunol., *12*:127, 1974.
181. Hayry, P., and Andersson, L. C.: T cells in mixed lymphocyte culture-induced cytolysis. Transplant. Proc., *5*:1697, 1973.
182. Andersson, L. C., and Hayry, P.: Clonal isolation of alloantigen-reactive T-cells and characterization of their memory function. Transplant. Rev., *25*:121, 1975.
183. Henney, C. S.: On the mechanism of T-cell mediated cytolysis. Transplant. Rev., *17*:37, 1973.
184. Wagner, H., and Rollinghoff, M.: T cell-mediated cytotoxicity: Discrimination between antigen recognition, lethal hit and cytolysis phase. Eur. I. Immunol., *4*:745, 1974.
185. Berke, G., and Amos, D. B.: Mechanism of lymphocyte-mediated cytolysis: the lymphocyte-mediated cytotoxicity cycle and its role in transplantation immunity. Transplant. Rev., *17*:71, 1973.
186. David, J. R., and David, R. R.: Cellular hypersensitivity and immunity. Prog. Allergy, *16*:300, 1972.
187. Ward, P. A., Remold, H. G., and David, J. R.: Leukotactic factor produced by sensitized lymphocytes. Science, *163*:1079, 1969.
188. ———:The production of antigen-stimulated lymphocytes of a leukotactic factor distinct from MIF. Cell. Immunol., *1*:162, 1970.
189. David, J. R.: *In* Bellanti, J. A., and Dayton, D. H. (eds.): Phagocytic Cell in Host Resistance. P. 143. New York, Raven Press, 1974.
190. Mackaness, G. B., and Blanden, R. V.: Cellular immunity. Prog. Allergy, *11*:89, 1967.
191. Mackaness, G. B.: The influence of immunologically committed lymphoid cells on macrophage activity *in vivo*. J. Exp. Med., *129*:973, 1969.
192. Nathan, C. F., Karnofsky, M. L., and David, J. R.: Alterations of macrophage function by mediators from lymphocytes. J. Exp. Med., *133*:1356, 1971.
193. Fowles, R. E., Fajardo, I. M., Leibowitch, J. L., and David, J. R.: The enhancement of macrophage bacteriostasis by products of activated lymphocytes. J. Exp. Med., *138*:952, 1973.
194. Nathan, C. F., Karnovsky, M. L., and David, J. R.: Alterations of macrophage functions by mediators from lymphocytes. J. Exp. Med., *133*:1356, 1971.
195. Rocklin, R. E., MacDermott, R. P., Chess, L., Schlossman, S. F., and David, J. R.: Studies on mediator production by highly purified human T and B lymphocytes. J. Exp. Med., *140*:1303, 1974.
196. Evans, R., Grant, C. K., Cox, H., Steele, K., and Alexander, P.: Thymus-derived lymphocytes produce an immunologically specific macrophage-arming factor. J. Exp. Med., *136*:1318, 1972.
197. Lohmann-Matthes, M. L., and Fischer, H.: T-cell cytotoxicity and amplification of the cytotoxic reaction by macrophages. Transplant. Rev., *17*:150, 1973.
198. Ruddle, N. H., and Waksman, B. H.: Cytotoxicity mediated by soluble antigen and lymphocytes in delayed hyposensitivity. J. Exp. Med., *128*:1267, 1968.
199. Granger, G. A., *et al*.: Production of lymphocytotoxins and MIF by established human lymphocyte cell lines. J. Immunol., *104*:1476, 1970.
200. Austen, K. F.: Reaction mechanisms in the release of mediators of immediate hypersensitivity from human lung tissue. Fed. Proc., *33*:2256, 1974.
201. Zinsser, H.: Studies on the tuberculin reaction and on specific hypersensitiveness in bacterial infection. J. Exp. Med., *34*:495, 1921.
202. Landsteiner, K., and Chase, M. W.: Experiments on transfer of cutaneous sensitivity to simple compounds. Proc. Soc. Exp. Biol. Med., *49*:688, 1942.
203. Richerson, H. B., Dvorak, H. F., and Leskowitz, S.: Cutaneous basophil hypersensitivity: a new interpretation of the Jones-Mote reaction. J. Immunol., *103*:1431, 1969.
204. Stadecker, M. and Leskowitz, S.: Genetic control of cutaneous basophil hypersensitivity. J. Exp. Med., *143*:206, 1976.

7 Immune Complexes and Immune Complex Disease

Immune complexes are the products of the binding of antibody to antigen. They play an essential role in the clearance and destruction of many antigens, but may, under certain circumstances, cause significant disease in tissues and organs throughout the body. In this chapter we shall explore the composition, function and pathophysiology of immune complexes.

COMPOSITION OF IMMUNE COMPLEXES

Immune complexes can range from large, insoluble aggregates to small, soluble structures. The *size* of an immune complex is the single most important physical parameter that determines its ability to be cleared from the circulation and its ability to cause significant tissue damage. We must begin, therefore, by examining the factors that determine the size of an immune complex. These include: (1) the ratio of antibody to antigen in the complex, (2) the molecular weight of the component parts, and (3) the affinity of the antibody for the antigen.

Antibody/Antigen Ratio

The classical precipitin reaction illustrates the effect of the ratio of antibody to antigen on the size and solubility of the resultant immune complex. To demonstrate this reaction, increasing amounts of antigen are added to a given quantity of antibody and the size of precipitable and soluble complexes is examined at various ratios of antibody to antigen.

The results of a typical precipitin reaction are shown in Figure 7-1. The antigens are usually proteins or carbohydrates and are thus multideterminant. Multivalency is essential for obtaining the type of curve seen in Figure 7-1.

We begin with a solution of antibodies; no precipitate is present. With the addition of small amounts of target antigen, the excess of free antibody rapidly saturates all the antigen valencies (Fig. 7-2). The result is a small complex the precise size of which is determined by the valency of the antigen, and which precipitates out of solution. Rarely, complexes formed in this region of *antibody excess* can remain soluble.[1]

As we increase the amount of antigen and hence the ratio of antigen to antibody, it becomes increasingly likely that a given antibody molecule will cross-link two separate antigen molecules. This allows the formation of a lattice, producing a large, insoluble complex. At last a point is reached where lattice formation is optimal, no more free antibody remains in solution, and the largest complexes are formed (Fig. 7-2). This point is called *equivalence*. With the further addition of

A

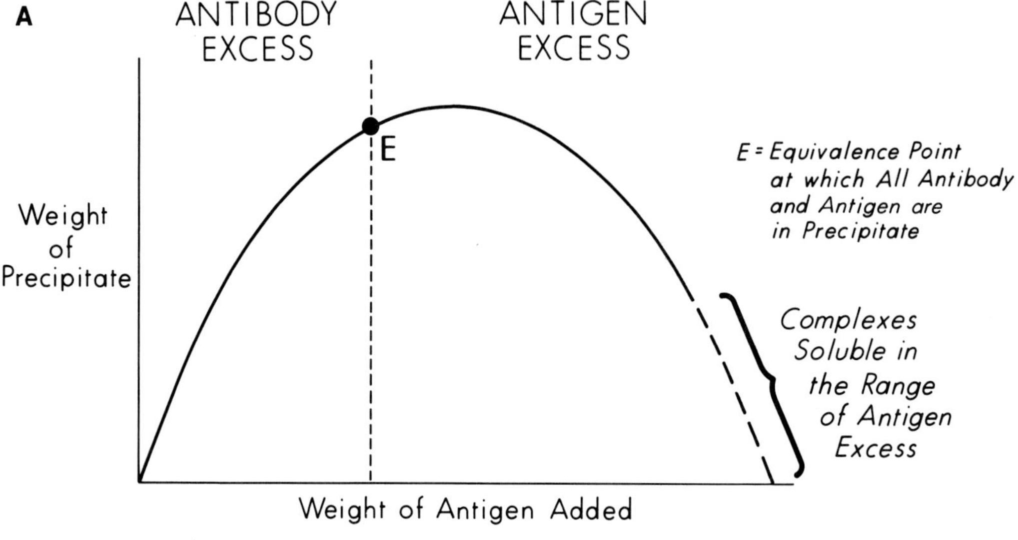

B

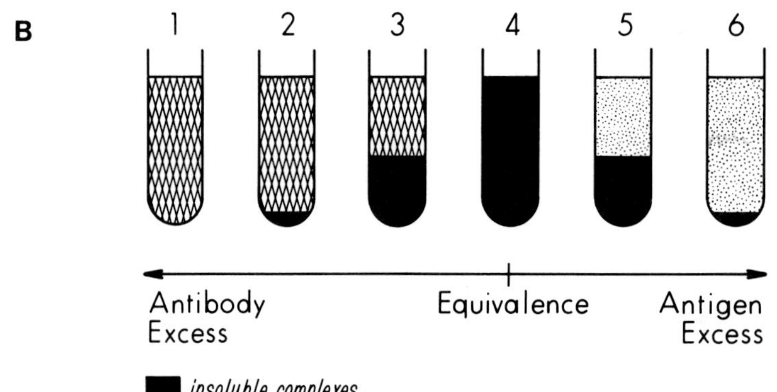

Fig. 7-1. (*A*) The precipitin curve. (*B*) As antigen is added to a solution of antibodies, a precipitate begins to form which achieves a maximum weight near equivalence. The addition of further antigen produces small, soluble complexes and the size of the precipitate declines.

antigen, free unbound antigen is detectable in the supernatant for the first time.

Past the zone of equivalence, as more and more antigen is added, it becomes increasingly unlikely that a single antigen molecule will be bound by many antibody molecules. Optimal lattice formation is thus no longer possible, and the large, cross-linked complexes give way to smaller complexes (Fig. 7-2). This is the region of *antigen excess*. As we move toward extreme antigen excess, the complexes achieve minimum size. Unlike the complexes formed in antibody excess or at equivalence, these complexes are soluble.

The complexes formed in a precipitin reaction with a univalent antigen are also depicted in Figure 7-2. It is readily apparent that large cross-linked structures cannot form since only one antibody can combine with any given antigen.

The actual immune response to a circulating antigen essentially recreates the precipitin reaction, but in reverse. Several days after the appearance of antigen, antibody begins to appear and increases rapidly. At first, small soluble complexes in antigen excess are formed. These gradually give way to the larger, less soluble complexes of equivalence and antibody excess.

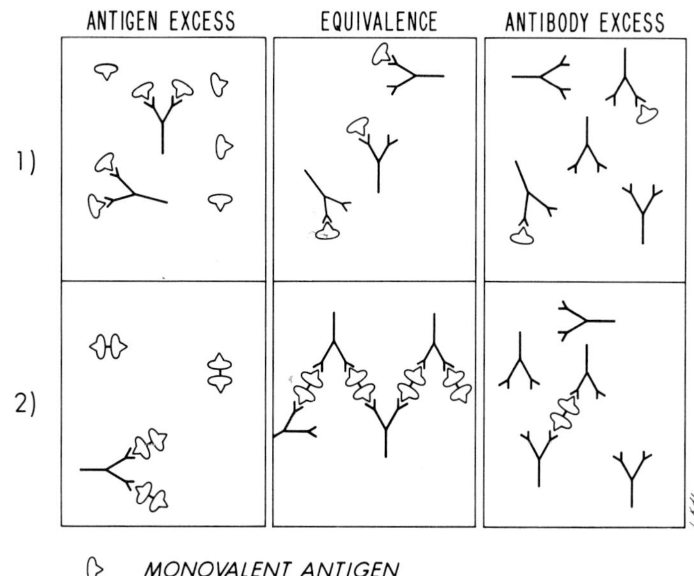

Fig. 7-2. The complexes formed with monovalent and divalent antigen at different ratios of antigen to antibody. Note that large, cross-linked complexes cannot form at equivalence when monovalent antigen is used.

We have seen that the size of immune complexes is affected by the relative concentrations of antigen and antibody as well as the valency of the antigen. The valency of the binding antibody is also a factor. IgM, with its pentavalency, allows for extensive cross-linking. Hence the ratio of antigen to antibody must be much higher in order to exceed equivalence and begin to produce the small soluble complexes of antigen excess than with IgG.

Molecular Weight

The molecular weight of both antigen and antibody is clearly a factor in determining the size of an immune complex. For a given antibody-to-antigen ratio, a high molecular weight antigen will form a larger complex than will a low molecular weight antigen. The same is true of antibody class: since IgM is roughly five times larger than IgG, this can be a major factor in determining the size of the complex. Additional factors which can increase the molecular weight of an immune complex include (1) the binding of complement to the complex, and (2) the presence of antibodies directed against and reacting with the antibody already within the complex. These anti-immunoglobulin antibodies are called rheumatoid factors and they can convert soluble complexes into larger, insoluble complexes (see below).[2]

Affinity

Large complexes will be stable only if the antibody has a high affinity for the antigen. If antibody is raised against a given antigen and then complexed with a crossreacting antigen for which the antibody has less affinity, the ready dissociation of the crossreacting antigen will produce smaller, more soluble complexes at any given antibody-to-antigen ratio than if the original antigen were used.

FUNCTION OF IMMUNE COMPLEXES

The effects of antibody upon antigen are legion, ranging from functional neutralization and clearance to the initiation of lymphocyte killing and, via complement activation, evocation of an inflammatory response.

Clearance

Figure 7-3 depicts the disappearance of an antigen injected directly into the vas-

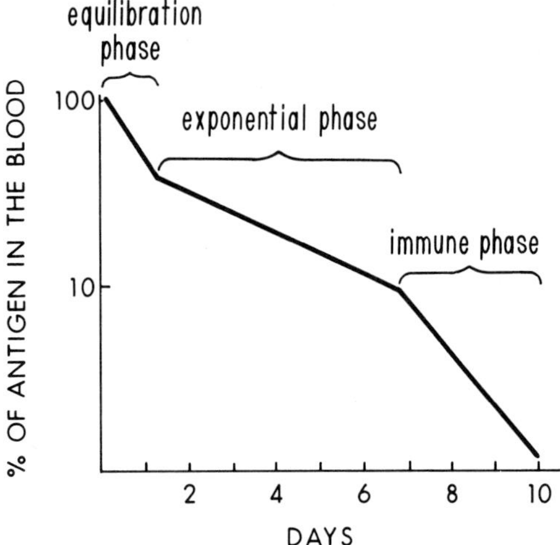

Fig. 7-3. The three phases of antigen elimination from the vascular space. The equilibration phase reflects the movement of antigen between the intravascular and extravascular spaces. The exponential phase is due to host catabolism of the antigen. The immune phase results from the production of antibody and the clearance of the antigen as an immune complex. (Adapted from Weigle, W. O.: Fate and biological action of antigen-antibody complexes. Adv. Immunol., *1*:283, 1961.)

cular space. Three phases of elimination can be detected.[3] (1) *Equilibration phase*: the initial decline in antigen concentration results from the equilibration of antigen between the intravascular and extravascular spaces. (2) *Exponential phase*: following equilibration, the antigen now undergoes normal catabolism by the host. The rate of decline is variable, depending upon the chemical and physical properties of the antigen. (3) *Immune phase*: after several days, antibody against the antigen begins to be produced. Immune complexes form and the rate of antigen disappearance is greatly accelerated.

The clearance of immune complexes is carried out primarily by the reticuloendothelial system. Its efficiency in this regard is, in part, dependent upon the size and solubility of the immune complex. The complexes formed in antibody excess are cleared most rapidly from the circulation and are rarely associated with any pathologic lesions. The small, soluble complexes formed in antigen excess are phagocytosed least well by the reticuloendothelial system.[4] The greater the antigen excess, the smaller and more soluble are the complexes and the longer they will persist in the circulation.

Macrophages, monocytes, neutrophils and possibly all the cells of the phagocytic system express surface receptors for the Fc portion of immunoglobulin molecules (Fc receptors).[5] These receptors contribute greatly to the adherence of immune complexes to the reticuloendothelial system, eventuating in their phagocytosis and clearance.[6] Fc receptors bind antibody which has itself bound antigen. The valency of the antigen exerts a powerful regulatory influence on this process. Univalent haptens do not markedly enhance immunoglobulin binding. Divalent antigens promote binding and multivalent antigens are better still. These findings may reflect the fact that complexes containing more than one antibody increase the strength of binding through multiple attachment. We would therefore predict that those complexes with many antibody molecules bound per antigen would bind most favorably to Fc-receptor-containing cells and thus be cleared most efficiently. Such complexes exist on the antibody-excess side of equivalence and indeed have been found to bind optimally to macrophages.[7] Complexes formed at extreme antigen excess do not demonstrate significantly enhanced binding. These observations correlate well with the clearance data in the preceding paragraph.

Another factor which may also contribute to determining immune complex clearance is the ability of the complex to bind complement. Complement can mediate immune complex attachment to phagocytic cells via complement receptors present on these cells, and also enhance complex binding to Fc receptors. Complement is required for IgM complex binding to phagocytic cells.[8]

Complement Activation

The binding of complement by immune complexes initiates the complement cascade. Immune complexes can bind $C1_q$ and activate the classical pathway; this activity is restricted to those immunoglobulin classes capable of fixing $C1_q$ (IgM, IgG_1, IgG_3 and, to a lesser extent, IgG_2). All immune complexes can activate the properdin pathway.[9]

Whereas a single molecule of IgG binds complement poorly, aggregates of IgG bind complement very well.[10] It is therefore not surprising that the large complexes formed near equivalence bind complement most efficiently.[11]

Because of its pentameric structure, a single molecule of IgM which has bound antigen can bind complement.[12] Extreme lattice formation is not required and may even block access to certain complement-binding sites on the IgM molecules. IgM-containing complexes formed in antibody excess bind complement most effectively.[11]

The consequences of complement activation were discussed in Chapter 1. The ability to activate complement imparts a tremendous biological potential to immune complexes. This potential can be appropriately directed toward antigen elimination, but can also lead to considerable tissue destruction in immune complex diseases.

Other Functions

Immune complexes can trigger the release of a number of other bioactive substances.[13] These include the vasoactive constituents of basophils and mast cells which are released by the binding of antigen to cell-bound IgE,[14] or indirectly via the activation of complement-derived anaphylatoxins. Also, the attachment of immune complexes to neutrophils induces a degranulation reaction in which the contents of the neutrophil lysosomes are released into the immediate environment.[15,15a] Many of these biochemically active materials may be important in the pathogenesis of several types of immune complex disease, but more importantly are probably essential to an adequate host defense against many pathogens.

PATHOGENESIS OF IMMUNE COMPLEX DISEASE

Immune complex disease results when immune complexes are not properly cleared by the reticuloendothelial system and are deposited in the body's tissues. As we have just seen, clearance is largely determined by the size and solubility of the complex. Thus the complexes formed in antigen excess are most likely to evade the reticuloendothelial system and be deposited in tissues. Large complexes formed nearer to equivalence can also contribute to disease. Only those complexes formed in antibody excess do not appear to contribute to human pathology. Their rapid clearance by the reticuloendothelial system protects the body from tissue deposition and hence from disease. It is important to emphasize that simply because complexes are not cleared disease will not necessarily ensue.

TISSUE DEPOSITION OF IMMUNE COMPLEXES

How do immune complexes gain entry to the body's tissues? The simplest hypothesis is that immune complexes are *passively* deposited beneath the vascular endothelium. However, this does *not* appear to be true. It is difficult to induce tissue deposition in animals by passive injection of preformed immune complexes.[16] However, immune complexes can be made to deposit within vessel walls by the simultaneous infusion of substances that cause the release of vasoactive amines from mast cells.[17] Antihistamines can prevent deposition. These findings suggest that tissue deposition is an *active* process requiring increased vascular permeability (Fig. 7-4).

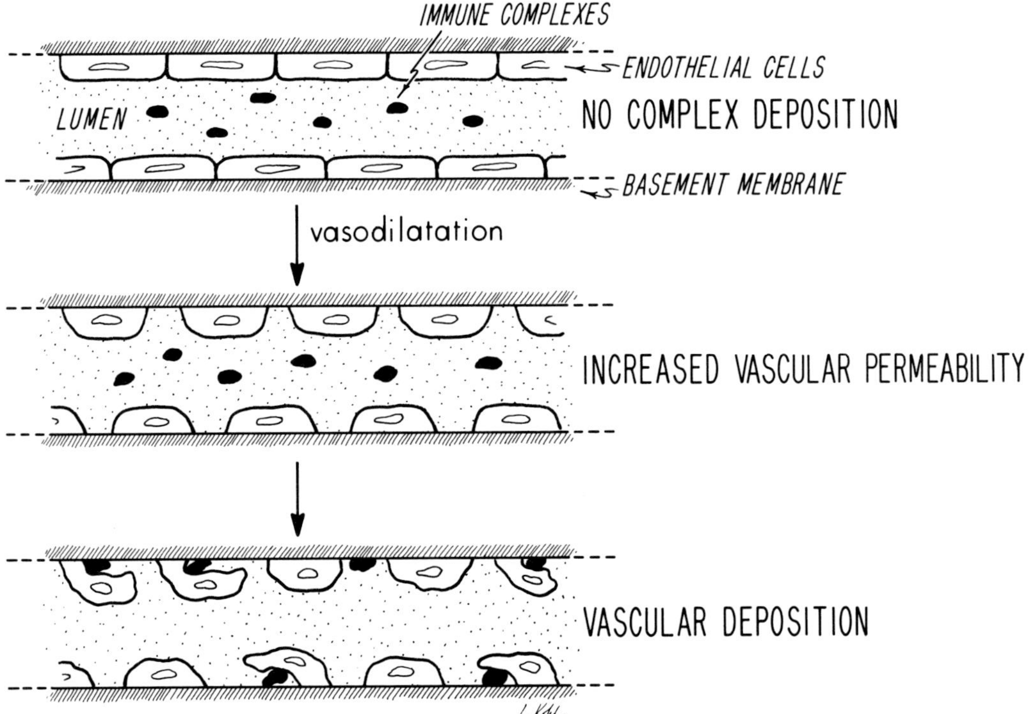

Fig. 7-4. Tissue deposition of immune complexes appears to be an active phenomenon, requiring increased vascular permeability for immune complex deposition to occur.

In the body there are two ready sources of vasoactive amines: basophils (and mast cells) and platelets. If IgE exists with specificity for the circulating antigen, histamine release from basophils can ensue. Immune complexes can also lead to basophil degranulation via the activation of complement resulting in the production of the C3a and C5a anaphylatoxins which can degranulate leukocytes.[18,19] Not only might direct basophil release of histamine lead to the required permeability changes, but the release of platelet-activating factor (PAF) contained within basophils could result in platelets releasing their contingent of vasoactive amines.[20]

It is known that immune complexes can induce platelet degranulation in animals in the presence of complement.[21,22] This may occur via the activation of the properdin pathway by immune complexes adsorbed nonspecifically to platelet surfaces.[23] This mechanism may not be important *in vivo* since immune complexes can be deposited in animals depleted of complement.[24]

The precise site of deposition of immune complexes within the vascular system is determined by the hemodynamics of blood flow and the concentration of circulating complexes. The sites with the most marked predilection for complex deposition are areas of great flow and turbulence. These include the branch points of the arteries from the aorta and the heart valves. Hypertension augments immune complex deposition.[25] In general, it seems that areas under hydrodynamic stress will be the most permeable to the passage of immune complexes.

The concentration of circulating im-

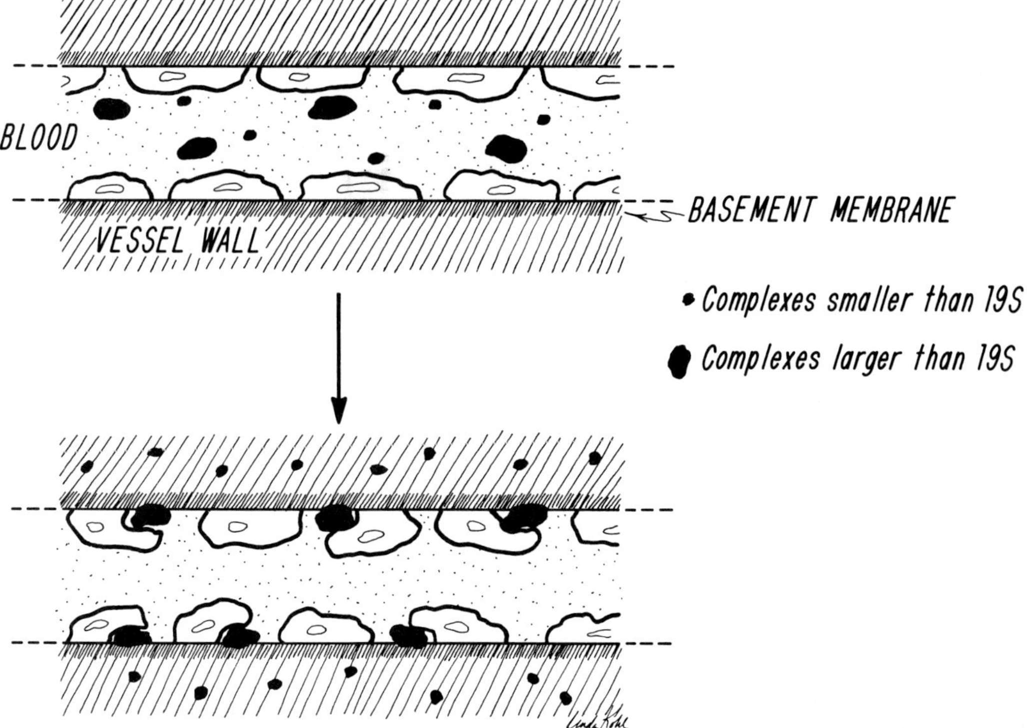

Fig. 7-5. The basement membrane acts as a filter, allowing complexes smaller than 19S to pass through while retaining larger complexes on the vascular side.

mune complexes also contributes to determining the site of deposition. It appears that a much higher concentration of circulating complexes is required to produce generalized vasculitis than is needed to produce glomerulonephritis (see below).

The localization of immune complexes within the subendothelium is largely determined by the size of the complex. The basement membrane acts as a filter, trapping large complexes while allowing smaller complexes to pass through (Fig. 7-5).[26] The approximate cutoff size for entrapment by the basement membrane is 19S;[27] complexes larger than 19S cannot pass through the membrane whereas smaller complexes can. In the glomerulus, small complexes filter across the glomerular basement membrane and are seen as subepithelial deposits (Fig. 7-6). Larger complexes localize within the endothelium or mesangium. Whether a complex passes through or is retained by the basement membrane is a significant determinant of the type of lesion that results.

The renal glomeruli are prime targets of immune complex deposition. One might suspect that this is due to the unusual hydrodynamic stresses to which the renal glomerulus is subject. An alternative explanation has been suggested by recent reports of the presence of receptors for the C3b component on normal glomerular endothelial cells.[27a] The deposition of complement-containing immune complexes may therefore be furthered by adherence to this complement receptor. It will certainly be of interest to learn whether similar receptors are also present in other areas of the vasculature where immune complexes and complement tend to localize.

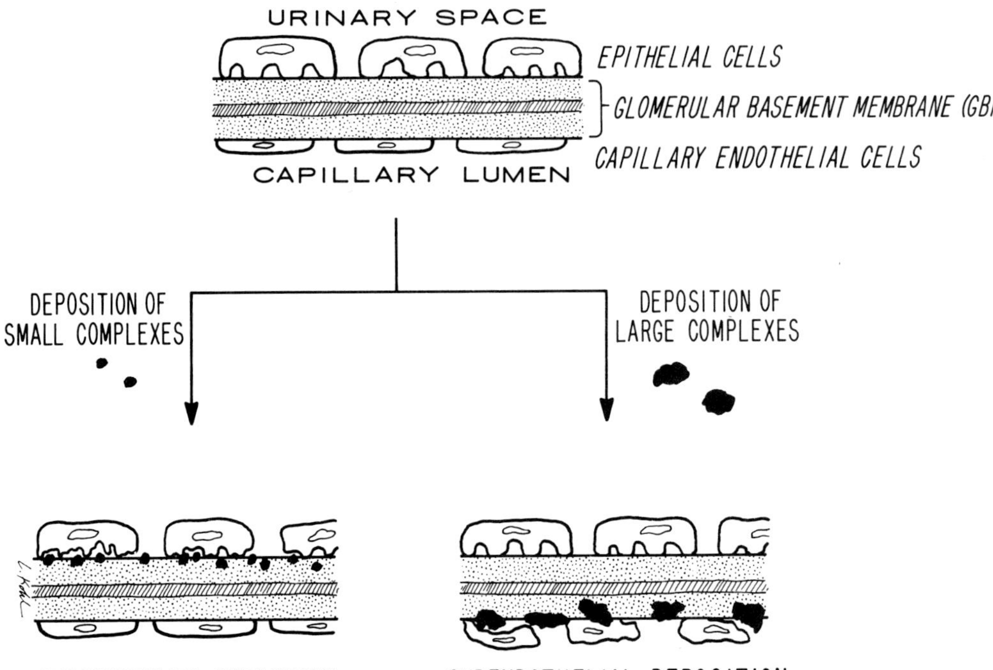

Fig. 7-6. Immune complex deposition in the glomerulus. Small complexes pass through the basement membrane and are deposited in the subepithelium; large complexes are retained and deposit subendothelially.

TISSUE DESTRUCTION BY IMMUNE COMPLEXES

The deposition of immune complexes can cause injury in two ways: (1) by the physical disruption of a tissue's integrity due to infiltration by immune complexes, and (2) as a result of the biological potency of immune complexes, especially the ability to activate complement, degranulate infiltrating leukocytes, and release vasoactive substances from platelets and basophils. Of these two mechanisms, the biological potency of immune complexes is probably the more significant.

From the preceding discussion we can conclude that the immune complexes most likely to result in tissue pathology are those formed on the antigen-excess side of equivalence. This is probably because (1) these complexes are not readily cleared, and (2) they are capable of activating the mediators of inflammation.

ACUTE SERUM SICKNESS

The classical model for studying the pathogenesis of immune complex disease is experimental serum sickness.[28] There are both acute and chronic forms of serum sickness. Serum sickness can be induced in a rabbit by injecting it with bovine serum albumin (BSA); one injection can produce acute serum sickness, while daily injections can produce chronic serum sickness. Acute serum sickness illustrates the complicated interplay of immunologic and inflammatory factors that produces the lesions of immune complex disease.

When a single injection of BSA is given to rabbits who have never experienced this antigen before and therefore have no preformed anti-BSA antibodies, we can observe the three phases of antigen elimination described above. During the immune phase (8 to 15 days after injection),

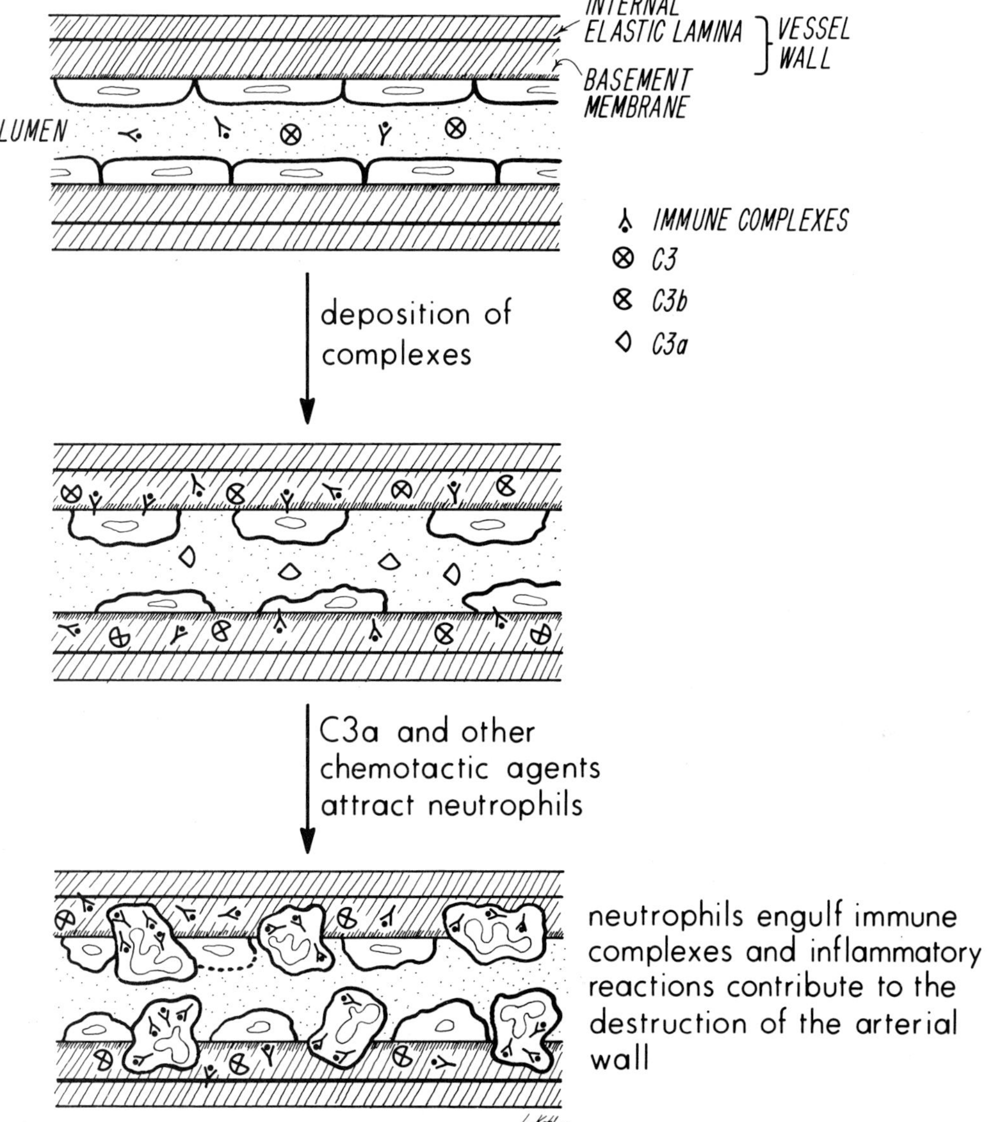

Fig. 7-7. The pathogenesis of immune complex arteritis.

immune complexes can be detected. Also at this time the animal develops lesions of acute serum sickness involving the arteries, renal glomeruli and joints. These lesions are due to immune complex deposition in these tissues.

Vasculitis in Acute Serum Sickness

A vasculitis results only with high levels of circulating complexes; low levels do not produce vascular lesions. The vasculitis is most prominent at the branches of the aorta, the coronary outflow tract and the pulmonary arteries. Immune complexes are deposited around the area of the internal elastic lamina and can be stained by immunofluorescence. IgG, antigen and C3 can all be detected. The first microscopic lesions are swelling and lifting of the endothelial cells (Fig. 7-7). Within the next day or so neutrophils are attracted to the site of deposition presumably as a result of complement-derived chemotactic factors activated by the immune complexes. The neutrophils release their store of hydrolytic enzymes and are responsible for the destruction of the arterial wall. However, these active phagocytes also rapidly consume the immune complexes, thereby eliminating the initiating force behind the destruction. Finally, fibrinoid necrosis of the arterial wall develops, with scarring of the damaged vessel.

During these events the serum complement levels are depressed. This is felt to be due to the rapid activation and fixation of complement by the immune complexes both within the circulation and at their site of deposition. The importance of complement and neutrophils in causing the arterial destruction is evidenced by the complete absence of pathology when the animals are first depleted of polymorphonuclear leukocytes and/or complement.[29,30]

Glomerulonephritis in Acute Serum Sickness

The glomeruli are profoundly affected during acute serum sickness. The lesions appear at the same time as the vasculitis. As with the arteritis, immunofluorescence reveals the deposition of antigen, antibody and C3 (Fig. 7-8). The pattern of deposition is granular and diffuse throughout each glomerulus. Light microscopy reveals a diffuse proliferative glomerulonephritis that is characterized by a widespread proliferation and hypertrophy of the glomerular endothelial and mesangial cells. Electron microscopy re-

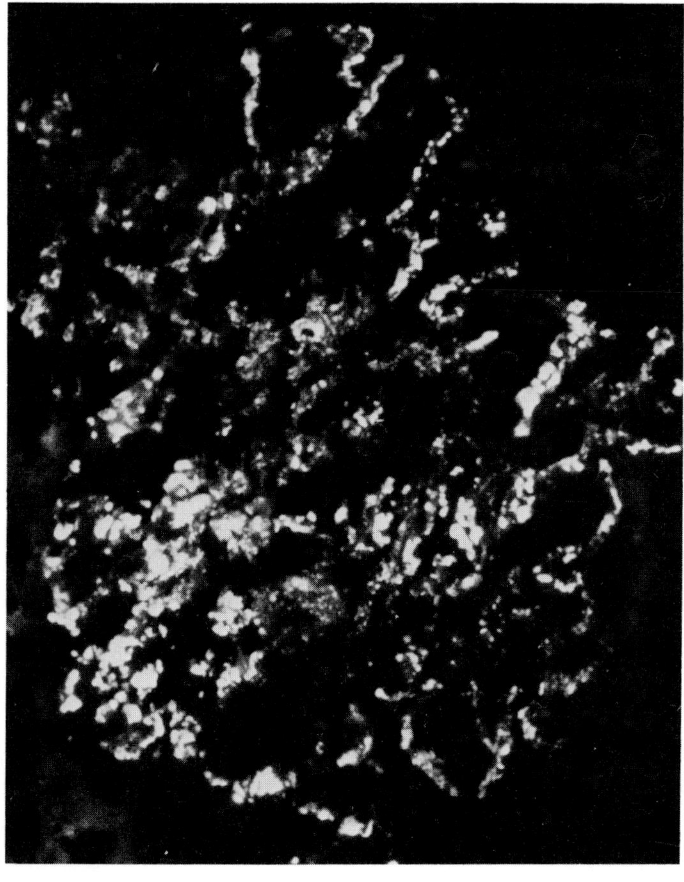

Fig. 7-8. Immunofluorescent study showing the lumpy-bumpy deposition of immune complexes in the glomerulus. (Burkholder, P. M.: Atlas of Human Glomerular Pathology. New York, Harper and Row, 1974.)

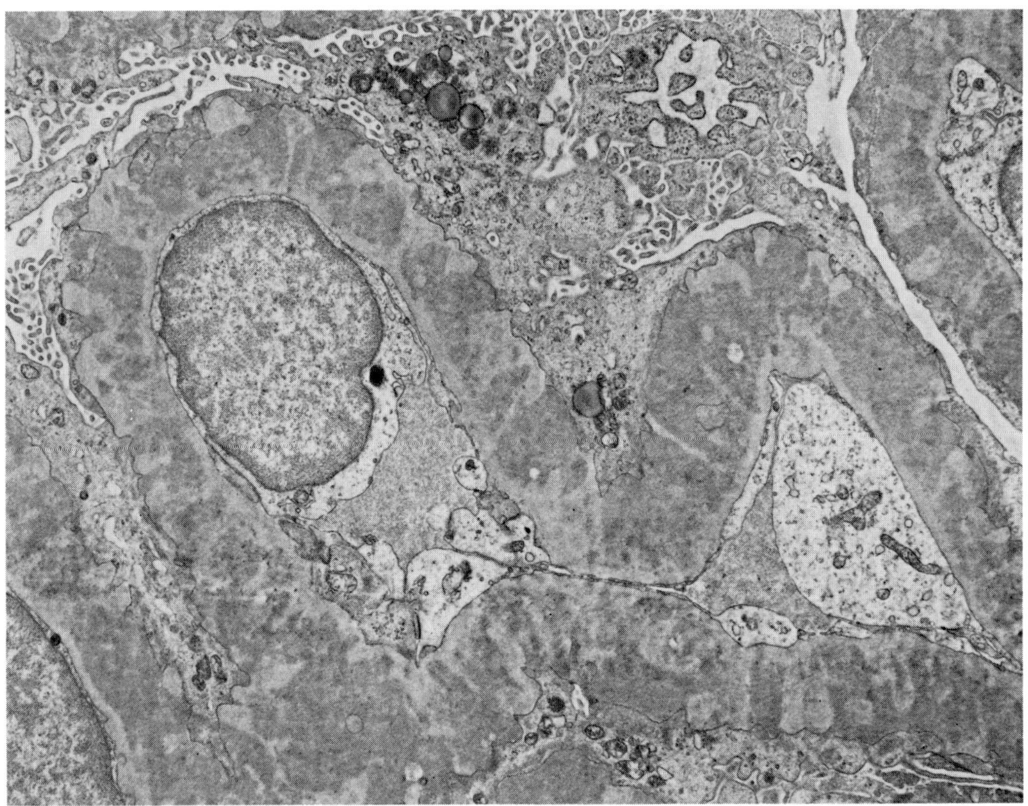

Fig. 7-9. Electron microscopy reveals dense deposits in the subepithelium which are believed to represent the localization of immune complexes in the glomerulus. (Burkholder, P. M.: Atlas of Human Glomerular Pathology. New York, Harper and Row, 1974.)

veals lumpy electron-dense deposits in a subepithelial distribution (Fig. 7-9). These electron-dense deposits are believed to correlate with the localization of the immune complexes.

There are several differences between the destructive mechanisms involved in the vasculitis and those active in the glomerulonephritis. In the vasculitis neutrophils are requisite for the tissue destruction and the major role of complement is largely to attract these cells to the region of complex deposition. On the other hand, a neutrophilic infiltrate in the glomerulus is quite variable. The presence of these inflammatory cells does not seem to be necessary for glomerular damage by immune complexes.

The glomerulonephritis of acute serum sickness is always transient. It is characterized by proteinuria and hematuria. Nitrogen retention may be seen, but within several weeks renal function returns to normal. Serial biopsies reveal a resolution of whatever inflammatory infiltrates may have occurred as well as a diminution in the extent of proliferation and hypertrophy of the glomerular cells. Mesangial-cell hypertrophy is often the last change to resolve. Along with this morphologic resolution is a loss of stainable immune complexes. These complexes are eventually eliminated and not replaced as the single antigenic dose is cleared from the body.

A consistent pattern of resolution can

Table 7-1. Renal Lesions of Chronic Serum

Group	Level of Antibody Production	Type of Immune Complex	Immunofluorescence
1	None	———	———
2	Low-level responders		
A	Low concentration	Antigen excess	Regular deposition of IgG and C3
B	Higher concentration	Antigen excess	Irregular deposition of IgG and C3
3	Intermediate responders	Near equivalence	IgG and C3 throughout the glomerulus
4	High-level responders	Antibody excess	———

be seen with immunofluorescence. The BSA antigen is only detected early in the formation of the glomerular lesions. As the antigen becomes unstainable, IgG and complement increase in the glomeruli. It is possible that the trapped antigen becomes progressively covered with free antibody and is hidden from visulization.[31] It is interesting to note that, as the amount of tissue-bound IgG and complement increases, the glomerulonephritis is healing and renal function is returning to normal indicating that it is primarily during initial deposition that circulating immune complexes are toxic. Following deposition they are bound by increasing amounts of antibody and, for some reason, lose their toxic potential.

The size of the complexes causing the glomerulonephritis of acute serum sickness has been studied.[32] They are almost entirely IgG-containing complexes and have a molecular weight of about 500,000. These characteristics are consistent with IgG-BSA complexes formed in slight antigen excess with an antibody-to-antigen ratio of about 2 to 3. From our previous discussion we would expect that these complexes could be highly destructive. Certain animals only produce IgM in this experimental system and have circulating complexes with a molecular weight of 1,000,000.[33] They display distinctive glomerular lesions with a marked mesangial-cell proliferation at the glomerular tuft and much more prominent necrosis than occurs in the IgG-producing animals. Their glomerulonephritis is focal rather than diffuse.

Summary

Acute serum sickness demonstrates many of the basic facets of immune complex disease. Deposition is site-specific, resulting in (1) a vasculitis (which can be manifest as a dermatitis from deposition in the vascular walls of cutaneous vessels, a pneumonitis from deposition in the pulmonary vasculature, an arthritis perhaps from deposition in joint vessels, etc.), and (2) a glomerulonephritis. The type and severity of the lesions are a function of the nature of the immune complex. Acute serum sickness beautifully illustrates the role of complement and inflammatory cells in forming the lesions of at least one particular type of immune complex disease. It is an excellent model for certain human diseases, notably poststreptococcal glomerulonephritis (see below). However, human immune complex disease can express itself in a great variety of ways, many of which cannot be adequately explained by the events of acute serum sickness. For these we must turn to the second experimental model, chronic serum sickness.

CHRONIC SERUM SICKNESS

Glomerulonephritis in Chronic Serum Sickness

Daily injections of BSA can produce a chronic immune complex disease in rab-

Sickness in Rabbits Injected with BSA

Electron Microscopy	Renal Histology
---	No lesions
Subepithelial deposits	Membranous glomerulonephritis
Subepithelial and trans-basement-membrane deposits	Diffuse proliferative glomerulonephritis
Deposits within the basement membrane and subendothelium	Benign mesangial hypertrophy and proliferation can progress to membranoproliferative glomerulonephritis.
---	No lesions

bits that stands in contrast to the acute, self-limiting lesions of acute serum sickness. Animals differ in their response to chronic BSA injections. Four general groups have been recognized on the basis of differing levels of antibody produced against BSA (Table 7-1).[33]

Group 1. Animals in this group produce no antibody. They have free circulating antigen but no immune complexes. These animals are free from disease.

Group 2. These animals produce a persistent low level of anti-BSA antibody, and are called "low-level responders." Immune complexes are formed at antigen excess, and therefore it is not surprising that these animals develop diffuse glomerular lesions much like the animals with acute serum sickness. More specifically, these small, antigen-excess complexes can produce two types of glomerular pathology, depending upon the concentration of circulating complexes.

Group 2A. When the level of circulating complexes is low, the histopathology is one of diffuse thickening of the basement membrane, *a membranous glomerulonephritis* (Fig. 7-10A). The low concentration of immune complexes induces very little cellular proliferation. Clinically this presents as a nephrotic syndrome with proteinuria but no significant azotemia.

Immunofluorescence reveals IgG and C3 throughout the glomerulus. The pattern of staining is one of a regular array of finely granular material (unlike the more irregular distribution in acute serum sickness). Electron microscopy reveals subepithelial deposits which are believed to correspond to immune complex deposition.

If the antigenic challenge is stopped, the basement-membrane thickening may decrease. The electron-dense deposits will resolve and immune complexes will no longer be detectable by immunofluorescence. The proteinuria may resolve to varying degrees, depending upon the extent of glomerular damage.

Group 2B. With a high level of circulating complexes, the histologic picture is a *diffuse glomerulonephritis* (Fig. 7-10B). This is a more destructive lesion, characterized by proliferation of endothelial and mesangial cells with a varying amount of inflammatory infiltrate. There will often be necrotizing changes, with resultant scarring and fibrosis. The greater destruction in this situation is probably attributable to the higher load of toxic substances. Azotemia results when renal function is significantly impaired.

Immunofluorescence shows a diffuse, somewhat irregular, coarsely granular or globular deposition of IgG and C3. Electron microscopy reveals "lumpy" subepithelial deposits. In both this situation and the one described above, subepithelial deposition reflects filtration of small, antigen-excess complexes through the basement membrane. However, here we can also see large aggregates extending across the thickness of the basement

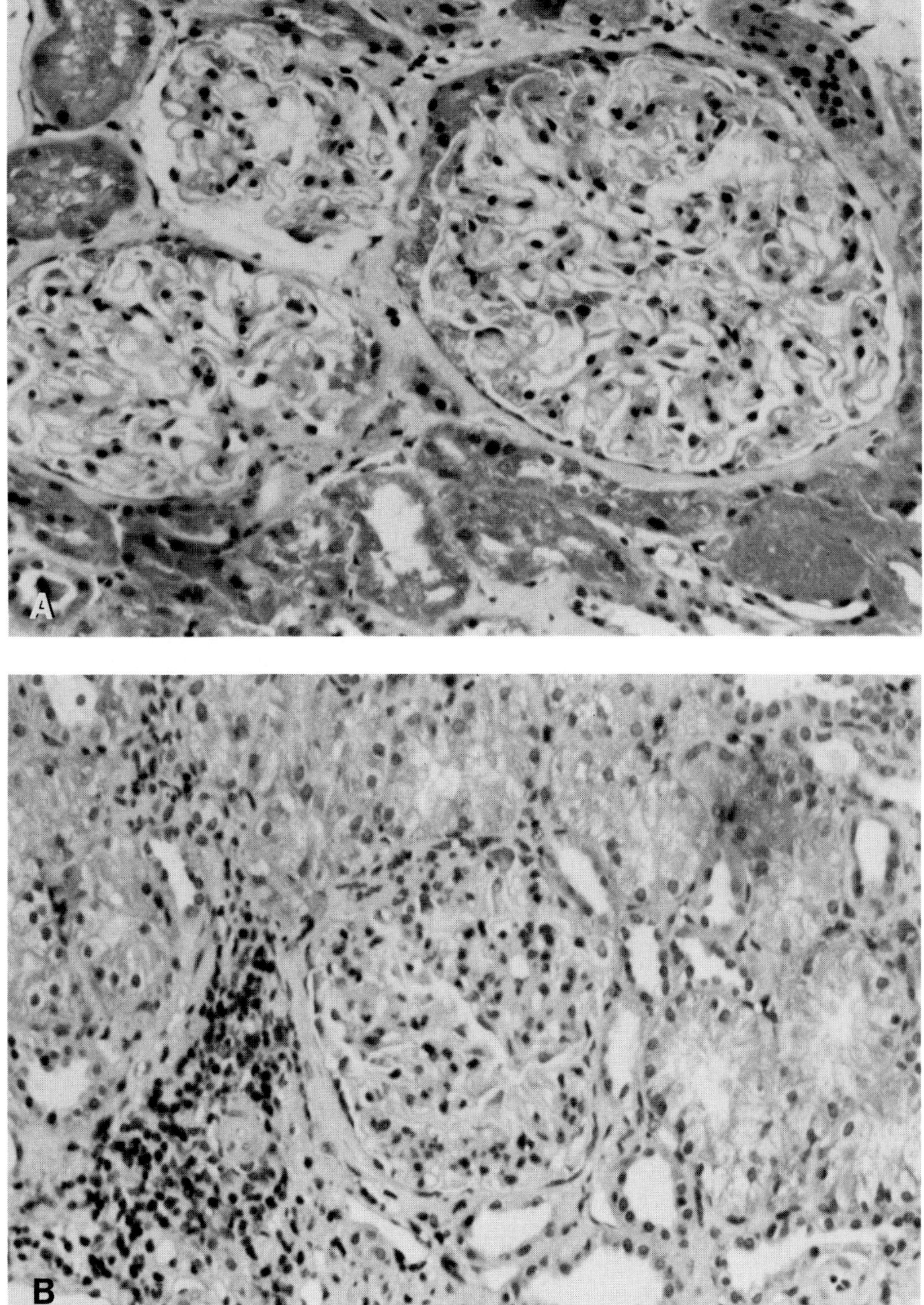

Fig. 7-10 A, B. The various immune complex nephritides. (*A*) Membranous glomerulonephritis; (*B*) diffuse proliferative glomerulonephritis. (*Continued opposite*)

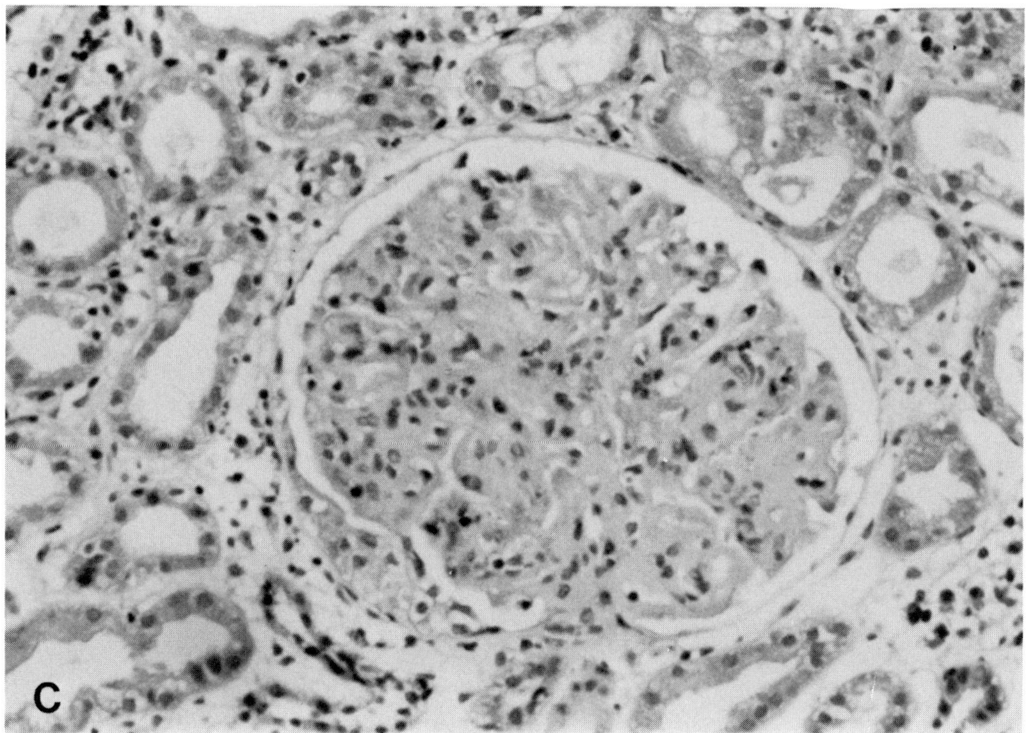

Fig. 7-10 C. Membranoproliferative glomerulonephritis.

membrane from the epithelial to the endothelial side.

Group 3. The animals in this group produce a greater anti-BSA antibody response and are called "intermediate responders." The complexes are formed closer to equivalence and are thus more rapidly cleared, usually within five hours of injection. The renal histology consists of *mesangial hypertrophy* and *proliferation*. Electron microscopy shows the deposits to be within the mesangium and basement membrane. The lesion is not destructive to the kidney and is relatively benign, presumably reflecting the successful handling of deposited material by the mesangial cells, the phagocytic guardians of the glomerulus. Mesangial hypertrophy and proliferation most likely reflect the intense activity of these cells.

It has been proposed, but not proved, that trouble can arise if the mesangium cannot handle the load of immune complexes delivered to it. Some investigators have suggested that this can occur with continued antigen presence. They believe that the mesangium (and the reticuloendothelial system in general) becomes exhausted from chronic stimulation. With mesangial failure, complexes are allowed to deposit in the rest of the glomerulus.[33] Because these are large complexes they will be found only within the glomerular basement membrane and subendothelially. Proliferation of other elements of the glomerulus may produce the picture of *membranoproliferative glomerulonephritis* (Fig. 7-10C). This may occur focally, depending upon the extent of antigenic overload and the health of the mesangium.

Group 4. Animals that fall into this group produce the greatest antibody response and are called "high responders."

Complexes are formed at antibody excess and are rapidly cleared. No disease results.

Vasculitis in Chronic Serum Sickness

In the models of chronic serum sickness, vasculitis is rarely encountered.[34] If the antigen dose is considerably raised, however, the high concentrations of immune complexes will produce a significant necrotizing vasculitis. The concentration of the complexes, rather than their composition, appears to be the major determinant of general vascular deposition.

Early in the development of a vasculitis, IgG, antigen and C3 can be seen deposited along the internal elastic lamina. They are distributed in the expected granular pattern of immune complex deposition. Soon after the arrival of the neutrophils, however, the complexes are no longer detectable.[35] Later, with necrosis of the vessel wall, immunofluorescence may reveal immunoglobulin and complement throughout the vessel wall, but these findings cannot be distinguished from the nonspecific transudation of plasma components. Because of this extensive destruction, it is often difficult to determine whether many vasculitides are immune complex in nature.

The vascular lesions in acute serum sickness and chronic serum sickness are usually identical, consisting of a necrotizing, inflammatory vasculitis with a prominent neutrophilic infiltrate. However, in some animals given repeated antigenic doses, a different lesion is observed in the renal arteries. These exceptional animals can develop a granulomatous arteritis replete with mononuclear epithelioid cells. This last finding is interesting as a possible model for a variety of the human vasculitides that are characterized by granulomatous arterial lesions, including Wegener's granulomatosis, temporal arteritis and others.

SUMMARY

The above animal models allow us to correlate the pathologic changes of glomerulonephritis with the size and concentration of circulating immune complexes.

1. The *size* of immune complexes, largely a function of the ratio of antibody to antigen, determines the localization of the complexes within the glomerulus. Complexes smaller than 19S can filter through the membrane and be deposited subepithelially. Larger complexes are localized to the mesangium and subendothelium.

2. The *concentration* of circulating complexes can determine the kidney's response to complex deposition. For the group of low-level antibody responders, low immune complex concentrations provoke a *membranous glomerulonephritis*. Higher levels induce proliferation of the endothelium and mesangium, producing a *diffuse, proliferative glomerulonephritis*. Among the intermediate responders, pathology results only with high levels of circulating complexes. This chronic load of immune complexes to the kidneys may exhaust the normal mesangial defenses and culminate in a *membranoproliferative glomerulonephritis*.

It appears that high concentrations of circulating complexes are required to generate a vasculitis in both the models of acute and chronic serum sickness. The destructive nature of the vascular lesions often makes it difficult to prove that immune complexes are responsible for the vascular damage.

SPECIAL TYPES OF IMMUNE COMPLEXES

In order to fully understand human immune complex disease, we need to discuss two special types of immune complexes which may have considerable importance in human disease: (1) rheumatoid factor, and (2) cryoglobulins.

RHEUMATOID FACTOR

Rheumatoid factor is a name used to describe any antibody that has specificity for IgG.[36] The existence of anti-immunoglobulin antibodies has been known for some time. Rheumatoid factor represents a fascinating example of what appears to be an autoimmune phenomenon. Although rheumatoid factor is associated with a variety of human diseases, its name is derived from its closest association with rheumatoid arthritis. The titer of rheumatoid factor has been qualitatively correlated with the extent and severity of rheumatoid arthritis. Rheumatoid factor can also be seen in many nonrheumatoid diseases,[37] including infections with viruses and parasites, tuberculosis, leprosy and subacute bacterial endocarditis. In subacute bacterial endocarditis the presence of rheumatoid factor correlates with the activity of the infection.[38] The majority of renal-transplant recipients develop rheumatoid factor postimplantation,[39] as do patients receiving blood transfusions. The probability of a transfusion recipient possessing rheumatoid factor is proportional to the number of transfusions.[40]

The classical rheumatoid factor is a 19S IgM molecule. Recently, however, it has been found that IgG, IgA and even 7S to 8S IgM can have anti-IgG activity. Each of these complexes has different physical properties, and hence different clinical effects. For example, several patients with IgG-IgG complexes have been described with the clinical manifestations of hyperviscosity syndrome, whereas this is not a major problem in patients with IgM rheumatoid factor.

The effect of rheumatoid factor on the clearance of antigen-antibody complexes has not been well studied. It has been suggested that when rheumatoid factor combines with soluble immune complexes, it renders them less soluble and thus presumably increasingly susceptible to phagocytosis.[2] Rheumatoid factor complexes are able to fix complement, although there are examples of complement-fixing immune complexes that lose their ability to activate complement when rheumatoid factor is added.[41,42]

Rheumatoid factor is directed against the Fc portion of the IgG molecule. IgG-IgG dimers have been described in which each molecule serves as both antibody (rheumatoid factor) and antigen (Fig. 7-11).[43] For some time there has been controversy over whether native IgG is the natural antigen or if an altered IgG molecule is the target. Using a precipitin assay, aggregated IgG has been demonstrated to serve as a better antigen than native IgG.[44] However, this conclusion has not been confirmed with other techniques.[45]

What induces the formation of anti-immunoglobulin antibodies? Chapter 8

Self-Associated Dimer of IgG Rheumatoid Factor

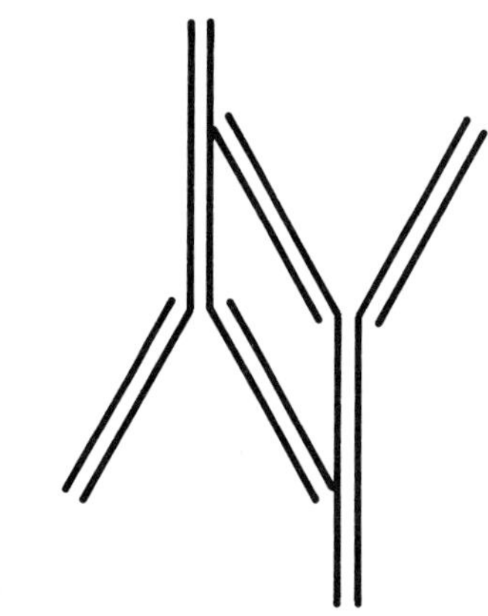

Fig. 7-11. IgG-IgG rheumatoid factor dimer. Each molecule acts as both antigen and antibody.

will explore the genesis of autoimmunity in detail, but several features stand out as peculiar to rheumatoid factor formation and will be addressed here. The suggestion has been made that a powerful or chronic antigen stimulation provides the necessary setting for rheumatoid factor production. This association has been convincingly illustrated in animals.[46] Also of relevance is the finding of antibody directed against IgA in a few patients with chronic respiratory infections.[44] There are several ways in which an antigenic stimulus could provoke rheumatoid factor production:

1. Antigen-antibody binding may lead to conformational shifts and exposure of new antigenic determinants on the antibody, thereby stimulating rheumatoid factor production. However, rheumatoid factor can bind native monomeric uncomplexed IgG and Fc segments. In addition it has been difficult to identify changes in the Fc region of an antibody molecule caused by antigen binding (see Chap. 2).

2. Chronic antigenic stimulation will lead to high levels of antibody production (and even, at times, a polyclonal hypergammaglobulinemia). Degraded products of these immunoglobulins may present immunogenic determinants that crossreact with native nonimmunogenic IgG. Consistent with this view is a report that the binding strength of rheumatoid factor for native IgG is relatively low.[47] This would be expected if native IgG represents only a crossreacting antigen and not the original immunogen.

3. The production of rheumatoid factor may not necessarily be an abnormal event. It has been postulated that low levels of rheumatoid factor may be produced in the course of a normal immune response, although little evidence has been offered in support of this idea. Rheumatoid factor is not always associated with disease and is present in 1 to 5 per cent of healthy individuals.[48] These rheumatoid factors may bind to immune complexes and facilitate their clearance. Chronic antigenic stimulation may merely represent an exaggeration of this phenomenon as the body attempts to eliminate the persistent antigenic load.

CRYOGLOBULINS

A *cryoprotein* is any serum protein or protein complex that precipitates from solution on cooling. The resulting cryoprecipitate may be a gelatinous mass or a flocculent or occasionally crystalline precipitate. The precipitation is reversible and upon rewarming the cryoprecipitate returns to solution. Several types of cryoproteins have been described (including cryofibrinogens), but the most common cryoprotein found in significant amounts is immunoglobulin or immunoglobulin complexes. These are called *cryoglobulins*.

Types of Cryoglobulins

Three types of cryoglobulins are now recognized. A patient with cryoglobulinemia will have one of these three types:[49]

Type 1. These cryoglobulins consist of a single monoclonal immunoglobulin. They are most often IgM or IgG, although IgA and Bence Jones monoclonal cryoglobulins do occur. Type 1 cryoglobulins are often found in high concentrations, frequently exceeding 5 mg. per ml.

Type 2. Unlike type 1, both type 2 and type 3 consist of mixed cryoglobulins; that is, they are complexes composed of immunoglobulin (the antigen) and anti-immunoglobulin (the antibody). Type 2 cryoglobulins are immune complexes composed of polyclonal antigen and monoclonal antibody. Polyclonal IgG is generally the antigen and monoclonal IgM is most frequently the antibody. IgA and IgG rheumatoid factors have also been observed. These cryoglobulins occur in moderate to high concentration, 80 per cent of the time exceeding 1 mg. per ml.

Type 3. Type 3 complexes differ from type 2 in that both the antigen and the antibody are polyclonal. IgM-IgG complexes are by far the most common. In addition, three-component (IgG, IgM, IgA) cryoglobulins have been described. Various complement components are often found in type 3 complexes. Type 3 cryoglobulinemia accounts for about half of the cases of cryoglobulinemia. These cryocomplexes are often present in very low levels (usually less than 1 mg./ml.) and have been difficult to study.

Mechanism of Cryoprecipitation

No one really knows what makes these proteins precipitate in the cold. The concentration of precipitable proteins appears to be the most important determinant of the temperature at which precipitation will occur. High concentrations can lead to precipitation at temperatures as high as 35°C.; at lower concentrations precipitation may not occur above 5°C. The pH and ionic strength of the solution also influence precipitability.

No particular structural abnormality has been described which can account for the cold precipitability of these immunoglobulin molecules. In some studies predispositions toward light-chain type (κ) or heavy-chain subclass (γ_2) have been noted, but these have not provided much insight into the mechanism of cryoprecipitation. Probably the simplest hypothesis, and one held by many investigators, is that cryoprecipitability is due to weak noncovalent interactions between the precipitating proteins. Some investigators have pointed to what they believe to be an increased number of hydrophobic residues in cryoglobulins,[50,51] which could account for poor protein-solvent interactions inducing precipitation in a slightly altered (cold) environment. Such findings have not been universally supported, and at present we have little understanding of the physicochemical requirements for cryoprecipitation.

Occurrence of Cryoglobulins

Cryoglobulins occur in a variety of conditions. The type of cryoglobulin seen in any particular disease setting may reflect the nature of the underlying disease process.[49] Cryoglobulins containing a monoclonal component (types 1 and 2) are found in immunoproliferative disorders, including multiple myeloma, Waldenström's macroglobulinemia, leukemia and lymphoma. It has been estimated that as many as 5 per cent of patients with multiple myeloma and an even higher percentage of patients with macroglobulinemia have type 1 cryglobulins.[49,52] Mixed cryoglobulins (types 2 and 3) can be seen with autoimmune diseases, and transient low levels can occur in chronic and acute infections and chronic liver disease. It is not surprising that cryoglobulins with rheumatoid factor activity arise in association with diseases noted for rheumatoid factor production. Presumably, these cryoprecipitable rheumatoid factor complexes share a similar mode of pathogenesis with "normal" rheumatoid factor. Almost one third of cryoglobulins occur without any underlying disease and are considered cases of *essential cryoglobulinemia.* Cryoglobulinemia without any other signs or symptoms has been reported to precede the overt manifestations of a malignancy or autoimmune disease by as much as 10 years.[49] Lastly, approximately 50 per cent of healthy people have detectable cryoglobulins in their sera, although in very low levels (less than 80 μg./ml.).

Symptoms Associated with Cryoglobulinemia

Cryoglobulinemia is associated with a unique set of symptoms which arise from the special physical and chemical characteristics of the cryoglobulins.[49] Most clinical findings in this disorder are attributable to (1) the proclivity of these proteins to precipitate in the cold, (2) hyperviscosity caused by circulating complexes, and (3) complex deposition in tissues.

Clinical Manifestations of Cryoglobulinemia

1. Cold precipitability
   - Raynaud's phenomenon
   - Acrocyanosis
   - Skin necrosis
   - (Cold urticaria)
2. Hyperviscosity
   - Vascular occlusion
   - Peripheral neurologic deficits
   - Renal involvement
3. Immune complex disease
   - Renal involvement (glomerulonephritis)
   - Cutaneous involvement (purpura)
   - Arthralgias
4. Other (probably related to 1, 2 and 3 above)
   - Hemorrhage
   - Abdominal crises
   - Arterial thrombosis
   - (Cold agglutinin disease)

1. Cold Precipitability. Many of the cutaneous and vasomotor symptoms seen in cryoglobulinemia appear to be related to the cold precipitability of the protein. Raynaud's phenomenon, acrocyanosis, the exacerbation of purpuric lesions, and skin necrosis especially on the tip of the nose, fingers and toes are all cold-induced phenomena. The limb involvement can be severe, progressing from distal necrosis to gangrene. These severe changes usually occur in patients with type 1 cryoglobulins which circulate in very high concentrations. Patients with mixed cryoglobulins generally pursue a more chronic course without sudden exacerbations. Cryoglobulins are also found in 20 per cent of patients with cold urticaria.[53]

2. Hyperviscosity is responsible for the sludging seen in the conjunctival and retinal vessels, and occurs most commonly with type 1 cryoglobulins. Vascular occlusion and sludging may also account for peripheral neurologic findings in these patients. Some aspects of the renal involvement seen in these patients may be due to cryoprecipitation and the effects of hyperviscosity in the capillary vessels. The concentration of serum proteins normally rises at the end of the renal capillary loops. This phenomenon enhances cryoglobulin deposition since high concentrations raise the temperature at which these proteins will precipitate.

3. Immune Complexes. Severe vasculitis and glomerulonephritis most commonly are seen in patients with mixed (type 2 and 3) cryoglobulinemia. Deposition of cryoglobulin complexes in these patients causes the same pathologic consequences as we have described for noncryoprecipitable immune complexes. Purpuric lesions of the skin occur most commonly in the lower extremities, and are exacerbated by standing, physical effort and often by cold, viral infections and certain drugs.

Over 20 per cent of patients with cryoglobulins, aside from those patients who also have systemic lupus erythematosus, have renal disease. This most commonly takes the form of a diffuse proliferative glomerulonephritis. Immunofluorescence reveals immunoglobulin and complement deposited in a granular pattern. Severe renal disease is usually limited to those patients with type 2 cryoglobulins, and is probably a function of their high circulating concentrations and immune complex nature. No correlation has been made between the type of cryoglobulin and the renal histopathology. Thus even type 1 cryoglobulins, although not of an immune complex nature, can cause a diffuse nephritis.

Other complications of cryoglobulinemia that may be the result of circulating immune complexes include joint symptoms, characteristically arthralgias. Joint disease is rarely seen with monoclonal cryoglobulins but is not uncommon with the mixed (especially type 3) cryoglobulins.

Miscellaneous Symptoms. Cases of hemorrhage, abdominal crises and arterial thrombosis in patients with cryoglobulinemia have been reported. There are also reports that cryoglobulins may be associated with cold agglutinin disease (see Chap. 14).[54,55]

Perhaps the best way of assessing the direct effects of cryoglobulins on the body is to look at the clinical manifestations in patients with essential cryoglobulinemia, since the clinical picture in other patients may be complicated by their underlying disease. Patients with essential cryoglobulinemia have been found to express any and all of the symptoms we have just described. Findings may range from mild involvement to disabling vascular and skin involvement to renal and neurologic disease. Thus, cryoglobulins can clearly be responsible for a wide range of clinical symptomatology.

Recent work has implicated cryoglobulins in a number of human immune complex diseases. We have mentioned the high frequency of renal disease in patients with cryoglobulinemia. The frequency of cryoglobulinemia in patients with immune complex renal disease has also been examined. In one extensive study it was found that virtually every patient with acute proliferative glomerulonephritis (poststreptococcal and other causes) had detectable serum cryoglobulins.[56] The serum precipitates included IgG and usually IgM and/or complement. Cryoprecipitable IgA was also detected in a significant number of patients. Antigens that might have served as targets for these cryoglobulins were not found, although antistreptococcal activity was detected in occasional patients. This study demonstrated the prognostic value of measuring cryoglobulins in patients with certain forms of immune complex glomerulonephritis. The presence of cryoglobulins was closely correlated with active disease, and the persistence of cryoglobulins with chronic disease. The disappearance of cryoglobulins was often associated with recovery or progression to end-stage renal disease.

HUMAN IMMUNE COMPLEX DISEASE

GLOMERULONEPHRITIS IN HUMAN IMMUNE COMPLEX DISEASE

The animal models of acute and chronic serum sickness have contributed greatly to our understanding of immune complex glomerulonephritis, and have been fruitfully applied as model systems for human immune complex disease. However, a strong word of caution is necessary. Individual cases of immune complex glomerulonephritis in man have not been nearly as carefully studied in order to define the molecular characteristics of the deposited immune complexes as have the complexes in the experimental animals. Thus, one cannot assume that similar histologic pictures necessarily imply similar causative immune complexes. At best we can use these animal studies to predict what we may eventually find when further work is done to elucidate the nature of the immune complexes in human disease. In the following discussion we shall examine several human immune complex glomerulonephritides both to illustrate the various types of lesions that can occur and to compare, by analogy, the histologic pictures with those observed in the experimental systems.

Acute Poststreptococcal Glomerulonephritis[57]

Poststreptococcal glomerulonephritis is an acute form of glomerulonephritis that follows infection with certain nephritogenic strains of streptococcus. The onset of renal disease is usually about 10 to 14 days after the infection and presents as a nephritic picture with azotemia. The histopathology is one of a diffuse proliferative glomerulonephritis with a variable inflammatory infiltrate. Immunofluorescence reveals the presence of IgG and C3 in an irregular granular pattern.[58] In the great majority of cases, electron microscopy shows subepithelial deposits.

Table 7-2. Glomerulonephritis in Human Immune Complex Disease

Disease	*Renal Lesion*	*Immunofluorescence*	*Electron Microscopy*
Acute poststreptococcal glomerulonephritis	Diffuse proliferative glomerulonephritis	Irregular deposition of IgG and C3	Subepithelial deposits
SLE	Focal proliferative glomerulonephritis	Deposition of IgG and C3 in the mesangium	Mesangial deposits
	Diffuse proliferative glomerulonephritis	Irregular deposition of IgG, IgM, C3 and properdin in the mesangium and subendothelium	Large deposits in the endothelium and mesangium
	Membranous glomerulonephritis	Regular deposition of IgG and C3	Subepithelial deposits
Subacute bacterial endocarditis	Focal proliferative glomerulonephritis	Diffuse deposition of IgG and C3	Deposits in the mesangium and subendothelium
	Diffuse proliferative glomerulonephritis	Diffuse deposition of IgG and C3	Subepithelial deposits, *or* mesangial-subendothelial deposits
Syphilis	Membranous glomerulonephritis	Deposition of IgG and C3	Subepithelial deposits

In most affected children, the renal lesions resolve both morphologically and clinically.

In virtually all respects the renal disease appears identical to the lesions seen in acute serum sickness nephritis. The subepithelial localization suggests that relatively small immune complexes are involved. However, it has been difficult to demonstrate the antigen in these lesions. Some investigators have reported being able to stain involved glomeruli with antisera raised against streptococcal antigen,[59] but others have not been able to confirm this finding.

As mentioned above, complement is deposited along with immunoglobulin in the glomeruli, and it is likely that complement activation contributes to the renal damage. When the profile of complement activity is examined, the properdin complement pathway appears to be primarily involved.[60] Thus, only C3 through C9 are depleted in the circulation, whereas the serum levels of C1, C4 and often C2 are normal or only slightly decreased. Why the immune complexes formed in this disease preferentially activate the properdin pathway is not known.

Systemic Lupus Erythematosus (SLE)

This is a disease in which several autoimmune phenomena have been documented (see Chap. 9). Prominent among these are antibodies directed against various cellular components, including nucleoproteins, double-stranded DNA and cytoplasmic constituents. Immune complex nephritis is a common and often serious complication of SLE. Investigators have analyzed the immune complexes deposited in the affected glomeruli in an attempt to learn the nature of the antibody and antigen constituents.[61] Several of the circulating autoantibodies can be eluted from involved kidneys. These include antibodies directed against DNA, soluble nuclear antigens and ribosomes. Furthermore, in some patients, DNA (presumably the antigen) can be demonstrated to be deposited within the glomeruli by immunofluorescence. Thus it appears that the autoantibodies present in the serum of patients with SLE may comprise the offending antibodies in the renal immune complex disease.

Renal lesions in lupus erythematosus have been divided into three basic histologic types:[62]

Focal Proliferative Glomerulonephritis. Only certain glomeruli are involved. Within each affected glomerulus only a few capillary loops appear abnormal by light microscopy. These areas show mesangial- and endothelial-cell proliferation and often include a neutrophilic infiltrate.

The focal involvement revealed by light microscopy is not borne out by immunofluorescence. Immunoglobulin (predominantly IgG) and C3 are deposited diffusely in all glomeruli although confined to the mesangium. Electron-dense deposits are likewise seen in the mesangium.

The clinical presentation of this lesion is usually hematuria and mild proteinuria without the full nephrotic syndrome. Renal function is usually good and this has been considered to be a relatively benign lesion. Recently it has been reported that up to one third of these patients will progress to the more aggressive diffuse form of the disease.[63]

Diffuse Proliferative Glomerulonephritis. This lesion bears the worst prognosis with an often rapid progression to azotemic renal failure. Histologic changes involve virtually all glomeruli and consist of irregular proliferation of both mesangial and endothelial cells. There is some increase in basement-membrane thickening, leading to a "wire loop" appearance of the capillaries. A neutrophilic infiltration can be observed.

Immunofluorescence reveals an irregular, globular, heavy deposition of IgG, C3, early components of the classical complement pathway and properdin. Thus both the classical and properdin complement pathways are activated by the deposited immune complexes. The deposits are distributed throughout the mesangium and in the subendothelium. IgM is also prominently deposited in this lesion. Electron-dense deposits may be very large and are localized to the endothelial-mesangial region.

Membranous Glomerulonephritis. In this form of renal involvement there is little cellular proliferation, but rather a diffuse hypertrophy of the glomerular basement membrane. The hypercellularity that does develop is confined to the mesangial cells. This lesion is frequently associated with the nephrotic syndrome and generally follows a slowly progressive course.

Immunofluorescence shows a diffuse, finely granular pattern of IgG and complement throughout the glomeruli. Electron-dense deposits are found on the epithelial side of the basement membrane.

Each of these three types of renal involvement in SLE has its histologic analogue in the experimental models of chronic serum sickness. The membranous lesion in SLE is similar to the lesion formed in chronic serum sickness when low concentrations of small immune complexes are deposited. The complexes in both instances are deposited in the subepithelium. Deposition in the focal and diffuse forms of lupus nephritis is localized to the mesangium and mesangium-endothelium and can therefore be compared to the glomerulonephritis of chronic serum sickness seen with large-sized immune complexes. The focal lesion may represent a situation in which the mesangium is able to remove the majority of deposited complexes with only minimal damage to the endothelium. The diffuse lesion may be due to an antigenic overload of the mesangial apparatus with subsequent diffuse deposition of the toxic complexes. The not infrequent progression of the focal to the diffuse form supports a close relationship between the two.

Patients with systemic lupus erythematosus may have a necrotizing vasculitis as well. Some studies have demonstrated the deposition of immunoglobulin and complement as well as DNA within the walls of affected blood vessels.[64]

Infectious Diseases

Glomerulonephritis is a complication of several infectious diseases. This is not unexpected since immune complex formation plays a role in the defense against many infectious agents. We will discuss a few examples.

Bacterial Endocarditis. The development of renal glomerular lesions during the course of bacterial endocarditis is not unusual. However, renal failure is rarely encountered. Both focal and diffuse proliferative glomerulonephritis may occur. The pathogenesis of these lesions has long been debated but recent evidence supports the notion that both of these lesions may be the result of immune complex deposition.[65,66]

The focal lesions can be stained for IgG, IgM and C3 in a diffuse granular pattern. Electron-dense deposits are localized to the mesangial-subendothelial areas.[66] The active deposition of immune complexes in both the focal and diffuse forms leads to the activation and deposition of complement and may be responsible for the depression in the total hemolytic complement titer that may occur.

Analysis of the diffuse proliferative glomerulonephritis reveals two types of lesions.[65] In one, immunofluorescence and electron microscopy show diffuse subepithelial deposition suggestive of small immune complexes. In the other, large complexes are implicated by the presence of mesangial-subendothelial deposits. It has been suggested that the subepithelial deposits (presenting a picture very much like acute poststreptococcal glomerulonephritis) are seen with acute infections[67] while the diffuse subendothelial deposition occurs later and in more chronic infections of subacute endocarditis.[68] In fact, the latter lesion can be seen when the blood is sterile.

It is tempting to view these two forms of diffuse nephritis in terms of the experimental models of serum sickness. An acute streptococcal infection may well represent a situation of antigen excess with the formation of small complexes. The subepithelial deposition that is observed may be due to filtration of these small complexes through the basement membrane. On the other hand, one would expect a chronic infection to be associated with greater antibody production and a higher ratio of antibody to antigen. The complexes would therefore be larger and we might predict that they would preferentially localize in the mesangium-subendothelium. This is what is observed. This simple scheme is speculative, and it has been emphasized that the distinction between the patterns of localization is not always clear-cut.

Syphilis. Renal disease in syphilis is a relatively rare occurrence, but may occasionally be seen in both secondary[69] and congenital syphilis.[70] The majority of patients with renal disease present with a transient nephrotic syndrome, although nephritis with azotemia has also been reported. The renal lesions in patients with the nephrotic picture are characterized by mesangial hypertrophy and basement-membrane thickening with some cellular proliferation. Subepithelial electron-dense deposits are seen under the electron microscope.[71]

Recently, a patient with syphilis whose renal disease illustrates some of the principles of immune complex deposition has been described.[72] The patient presented with an acute onset of nephrotic syndrome. Renal biopsy revealed the expected mild mesangial hypertrophy with a diffuse, finely granular deposition of IgG and C3 throughout the glomeruli. Subepithelial deposits were apparent under the electron microscope. However, this patient also had focal endothelial-cell hyperplasia and basement-membrane thickening, with IgM deposition restricted to the mesangial areas. This patient therefore had a combined glomerular lesion, possibly resulting from two distinct immune complexes. Arguing by analogy with the models of chronic serum sickness, the subepithelial deposition of low levels of IgG complexes most probably gave rise to the membranous glomerulonephritis while the mesangial deposition of large IgM complexes may have led to the focal proliferative lesion.

Many other infections have been associated with glomerulonephritis. We will not discuss these in any detail since they do not, in general, enlarge upon the immunologic principles of immune complex disease that we have been considering. A brief list of these infectious processes includes hepatitis,[73] quartan malaria,[74] fungal endocarditis,[75] infected atrioventricular shunts,[76] and numerous viral infections.[77-79] There are also many noninfectious situations in which immune complexes are formed and lead to glomerular lesions. A nephrotic syndrome has been seen in association with various nonrenal malignancies.[80] Patients with sickle cell anemia will, on rare occasions, develop a membranoproliferative glomerulonephritis.[80a] One study reported four such patients whose glomeruli could be stained for immunoglobulin and complement. It was suggested that the antigen was derived from the renal tubular epithelial cells that were damaged by ischemia secondary to the sickle cell disease. Renal tubular material was then released into the circulation where immune complexes formed which eventually deposited in the kidneys.

VASCULITIS IN HUMAN IMMUNE COMPLEX DISEASE

The Arteritis of Rheumatoid Arthritis

Many patients with rheumatoid arthritis have evidence of widespread vasculitis at autopsy. These patients usually have severe arthritis with high titers of circulating rheumatoid factor and rheumatoid factor immune complexes. The existence of high titers of potentially toxic circulating complexes as well as depressed serum complement levels in patients with a necrotizing arteritis has supported the idea that the vascular disease is due to immune complex deposition.[81]

The deposition of IgG, IgM and C3 in a granular pattern has been demonstrated in the walls of necrotic arteries.[82] The composition of the complexes is not known and no antigen has been detected.

It is interesting that patients with rheumatoid arthritis rarely develop renal immune complex disease. Thus, if immune complexes are the cause of the vasculitis, they do not appear to be harmful to the glomeruli. Investigators have found IgG or 7S IgM rheumatoid factor in the majority of patients with arteritis.[83] Perhaps the explanation for renal sparing lies in this unique nature of the rheumatoid factors causing the vasculitis.

Henoch-Schönlein Purpura

This is a disease of young people, characterized by a clinical triad of rash, abdominal pain and joint symptoms.[84] The basic lesion is a widespread vasculitis that involves the skin, joints and gastrointestinal tract. Acute attacks are frequently preceded by an upper respiratory infection. Although the existence of a necotizing vasculitis suggests a possible immune complex etiology, this has not been easy to demonstrate.

One indicator that the syndrome may involve immune complexes is provided by an examination of the renal lesions that occur in about half of the patients.[85] Most patients with renal involvement display hematuria and some proteinuria but rarely have impaired renal function. Examination of the kidneys most often shows a mesangial proliferation with IgG, IgA and C3 staining in the mesangium. Some patients with renal impairment have been shown to have a mesangial proliferative lesion. In these patients, immunoglobulin and complement appear to be distributed in both the mesangium and subendothelial area. This evidence for immune complex renal disease is suggestive of a role for such complexes in the vasculitis.

Other Forms of Vasculitis

There are several forms of vasculitis, including polyarteritis nodosa and hypersensitivity angititis, whose pathologic pictures reiterate those seen in the models for experimental vasculitis. An interesting recent development in our understanding of the pathogenesis of polyarteritis nodosa has been the finding that 30 to 40 per cent of affected patients possess the surface antigen of the hepatitis B virus (HB_s Ag; see Chap. 11).[85a] Circulating immune complexes containing the hepatitis antigen are present and IgM, IgG, C3 and HB_s Ag can all be stained within the vessel walls. The clinical course of these patients may be somewhat different from the course of patients with polyarteritis nodosa without HB_s Ag complexes.[85b]

JOINT INVOLVEMENT IN HUMAN IMMUNE COMPLEX DISEASE

Joint involvement, either in the form of arthralgias or arthritis, is associated with a variety of settings in which circulating immune complexes are present. These include rheumatoid arthritis, systemic lupus erythematosus, serum sickness, viral diseases and the arteritides. Nevertheless, the precise contribution of immune complexes to joint disease has been difficult to establish.

The most popular view is that circulating immune complexes deposit in the walls of synovial blood vessels. A study of synovial tissue taken from patients with various acute arthritides (including rheumatoid arthritis, systemic lupus erythematosus, hypersensitivity angiitis, and acute transient synovitis associated with undiagnosed febrile illnesses) disclosed the presence of small vessel disease, primarily affecting the venules, in virtually all patients.[86] The morphology of the vascular lesions ranged from thrombosis and occlusion to an inflammatory vasculitis. The vasculitis resembled that caused by immune complexes, but electron microscopy failed to detect electron-dense deposits in the vessel walls. However, we should emphasize again the great difficulty in demonstrating complex deposition in vascular lesions.

Vascular permeability may explain the proclivity for circulating immune complexes to localize in the synovia. Several studies have suggested that the synovial vasculature is leaky to a variety of substances including whole bacteria.[87] One study has further localized the leakiness to the venules.[88]

Rheumatoid arthritis is a chronic inflammatory disease that primarily affects the joints. It can occasionally present as a wide-spread disease with systemic vasculitis (see above) but more commonly it is clinically limited to the joints. The arthritis of rheumatoid arthritis can be very severe, and complete joint destruction may be the end result of a devastating inflammatory process. Typically, there are circulating immune complexes composed of rheumatoid factor and target IgG. The synovium is infiltrated by lymphoid cells, and lymphoid follicles may form. Local plasma cells secrete IgG and rheumatoid factor.[89] The synovial fluid contains several types of immune complexes,[90] including IgG-rheumatoid factor complexes ranging in size from 7S to 30S.[91] Immune complexes in which the antigen is a nucleoprotein have also been detected.[92] Cryoglobulins can be detected in the synovial fluid of almost all affected joints. These cryoprecipitates are composed of IgG and IgM—some of which have rheumatoid factor activity—fibrinogen, and DNA.[93] Some of the cryo-IgG may have anti-DNA activity.[94]

Immune complexes are present in higher concentrations in the synovial fluid than in the circulation. The characteristics of the synovial and serum complexes may also differ. Thus the synovial complexes tend to be larger than the circulating complexes.[95] The dominant rheumatoid factor in the joint appears to be IgG, whereas that found in the serum is most often IgM. Cryoglobulins may be present solely in the synovial fluid.

The immune complexes present in the joint can fix complement, the larger complexes fixing complement most efficiently. A large percentage of the complement-fixing activity may reside with the cryoprecipitable fraction. Both the classical and properdin pathways are activated,[96,97] and this is reflected in lowered levels of complement components in the synovial fluid; serum complement levels are usually normal.

Complement activation contributes greatly to the destructive potential of the immune complexes in rheumatoid arthritis. Complement-derived chemotactic factors attract phagocytes to the joint and neutrophils often comprise the majority of cells present in the synovial fluid. Once localized to the joint, these cells ingest the immune complexes, aided by the binding of the complexes to their Fc receptors. Neutrophils that have ingested immune complexes form the characteristic RA cells.[98] The cytoplasmic inclusions that give these cells their distinct morphology are composed of immunoglobulin, rheumatoid factor and complement.

Neutrophils, especially those which have ingested immune complexes, leak their lysosomal enzymes into the joint.[99] These enzymes may be the primary mediators of joint destruction. The level of intra-articular lysosomal enzymes has been correlated with the degree of joint inflammation.[100]

INNOCENT BYSTANDER DESTRUCTION

The destructive potential of immune complexes is not limited to the fixed tissues. Circulating complexes can nonspecifically adhere to the circulating elements of the blood and initiate their destruction. Such a process is called the *innocent bystander mechanism*[101] and appears to primarily affect erythrocytes and platelets (Fig. 7-12).

A significant percentage of cases of immune hemolytic anemia are related to the administration of drugs (see Chap. 14). Possibly the most common cause of this drug-induced syndrome arises out of the adsorption of circulating drug-antibody complexes onto the red-cell surface.[101,102] The exact mechanism of this adsorption is not known. The antibody involved is often IgM which can readily activate complement. Complement fixation on the red-cell membrane can result in the intravascular destruction of these cells. The immune complex is usually poorly bound to the red cell and easily dissociates, leaving only the complement components behind. When these complexes dissociate they are free to bind to other cells, fix complement, dissociate, bind to still more cells, and so on. For this reason this form of drug-induced hemolysis can occur with very low concentrations of the drug. Some of the more common drugs involved in innocent bystander erthrocyte destruction are quinidine, phenacetin, the sulfonamides and p-aminosalicylic acid.

Many examples of platelet destruction have also recently been traced to immune mechanisms (see Chap. 14). The antigenic target need not be a platelet antigen; rather, the platelets may be the innocent victims of the adsorption of immune complexes.[103] The target antigens may be drugs or other molecules. Platelet damage by an innocent bystander mechanism appears to be initiated by complement activation, either by the classical or properdin

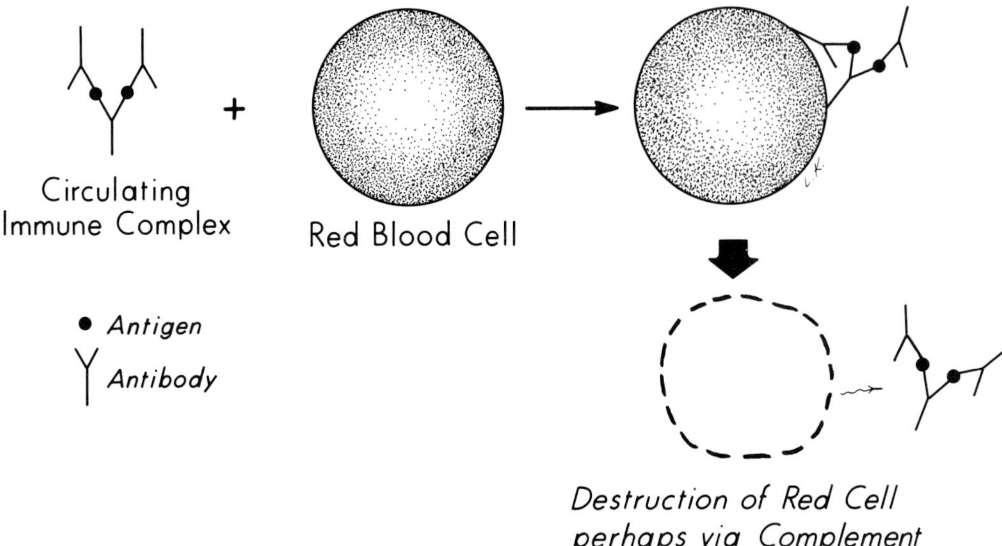

Fig. 7-12. The innocent bystander mechanism of destruction. Circulating immune complexes can nonspecifically attach to red cells (or platelets), activate complement, and thereby initiate the intravascular destruction of the cell.

pathway. Platelet destruction then ensues either by direct lysis, platelet aggregation and release reactions, or by phagocytosis of the coated platelets by the reticuloendothelial system.

REFERENCES

1. Forster, O., and Weigle, W.: The formation of soluble complexes in the region of antibody excess with protein antigen and their rabbit antibodies. J. Immunol., *90*:935, 1963.
2. Tesar, J., and Schmid, F.: Conversion of soluble immune complexes into complement fixing aggregates by IgM rheumatoid factor. J. Immunol., *105*:1206, 1970.
3. Weigle, W.: Fate and biological actions of antigen-antibody complexes. Adv. Immunol., *1*:283, 1961.
4. Germuth, F., Senterfit, L., and Dreesman, G.: Immune complex disease. Johns Hopkins Med. J., *130*:344, 1972.
5. Uhr, J., and Phillips. J.: In vitro sensitization of phagocytes and lymphocytes by antigen-antibody complexes. Ann. N.Y. Acad. Sci., *129*:793, 1966.
6. Patterson, R., and Susyko, I.: Passive immune elimination and in vitro phagocytosis of antigen-antibody complexes and relation to species origin of antibody. J. Immunol., *97*:138, 1966.
7. Phillips-Quagliata, J., Levine, B., Quagliata, F., and Uhr, J.: Mechanisms underlying binding of immune complexes to macrophages. J. Exp. Med., *133*:589, 1971.
8. Wellek, B., Hahn, H., and Opferkuch, W.. Quantitative contributions of IgG, IgM, and C3 to erythrophagocytosis and rosette formation by peritoneal macrophages. Eur. J. Immunol., *5*:378, 1975.
9. Osler, A., and Sandberg, A.: Alternate complement pathways. Prog. Allergy, *17*:51, 1974.
10. Ishizaka, K., Ishizaka, T., and Banovitz, J.: Biologic activity of soluble antigen-antibody complexes. J. Immunol., *93*:1001, 1964.
11. Ishizaka, T., Tada, T., and Ishizaka, K.: Fixation of C′ and C′1a by rabbit γG and γM antibody with particulate and soluble antigen. J. Immunol., *100*:1145, 1968.
12. Borsos, T., and Rapp, H.: Hemolysin titration based on fixation of the activated first component of complement: evidence that one molecule of hemolysin suffices to sensitize an erythrocyte. J. Immunol., *95*:559, 1965.
13. Becker, E.: Nature and classification of immediate-type allergic reactions. Adv. Immunol., *13*:267, 1971.
14. Ishizaka, K., Ishizaka, T.: Induction of erythema-wheal reaction by soluble antigen-γE antibody complexes in humans. J. Immunol., *101*:68, 1968.
15. Weissmann, G., Zurier, R., Spieler, P., and Goldstein, I.: Mechanisms of lysosomal enzyme release from leukocytes exposed to immune complexes and other particles. J. Exp. Med., *134*:149s, 1971.

15a. Henson, P. M.: Interaction of cells with immune complexes: adherence, release of constituents, and tissue injury. J. Exp. Med., *134*:114s, 1971.

16. Fish, A., Michael, A., Vernier, R., and Good, R.:

Acute serum sickness nephritis in the rabbit. Am. J. Pathol., *49*:997, 1966.

17. Cochrane, C.: Studies on the localization of circulating antigen-antibody complexes and other macromolecules in vessels. J. Exp. Med., *118*:503, 1963.
18. Hook, W. A., Siraganian, R. P., and Wahl, S. M.: Complement-induced histamine release from human basophils. J. Immunol., *114*:1185, 1975.
19. Siraganian, R., and Hook, W.: Complement-induced histamine release from human basophils. J. Immunol., *116*:639, 1976.
20. Siraganian, R., and Osler, A.: Destruction of rabbit platelets in the allergic response of sensitized leukocytes. J. Immunol., *106*:1244, 1971.
21. Gocke, D., and Osler, A.: In vitro damage of rabbit platelets by an unrelated antigen-antibody reaction. J. Immunol., *94*:236, 1965.
22. Henson, P., and Cochrane, C.: Antigen-antibody complexes, platelets, and increased vascular permeability. *In* Movat, H. Z. (ed.): Cellular and Humoral Mechanisms of Anaphylaxis and Allergy. P. 129. Basel, Karger, 1969.
23. Siraganian, R., Secchi, A., and Osler, A.: The allergic response of rabbit platelets. J. Immunol., *101*:1148, 1968.
24. Henson, P., and Cochrane, C.: Acute immune complex disease in rabbits. J. Exp. Med., *133*:554, 1971.
25. Fisher, E. R., and Bark, J.: Effect of hypertension on vascular and other lesions of serum sickness. Am. J. Pathol., *39*:665, 1961.
26. Cochrane, C.: Studies on the localization of circulating antigen-antibody complexes and other macromolecules in vessels. J. Exp. Med., *118*:489, 1963.
27. Cochrane, C., and Hawkins, D.: Studies on circulating immune complexes. J. Exp. Med., *127*:137, 1967.

27a. Gelfand, M. C., Frank, M. M., and Green, I.: a receptor for the third component of complement in the human renal glomerulus. J. Exp. Med., *142*:1029, 1975.

28. Dixon, F. J., Feldman, J. D., and Vazquez, J. J.: Experimental glomerulonephritis. J. Exp. Med., *113*:899, 1960.
29. Kniker, W. T., and Cochrane, C. G.: Pathogenic factors in vascular lesions of experimental serum sickness. J. Exp. Med., *122*:83, 1965.
30. Henson, P. M. and Cochrane, C. G.: Acute immune complex disease in rabbits. J. Exp. Med., *133*:554, 1971.
31. Wilson, C. B., and Dixon, F. J.: Antigen quantitation in experimental immune complex glomerulonephritis. J. Immunol., *105*:279, 1970.
32. Dreesman, G. R., and Germuth, F. G.: Immune complex disease. Johns Hopkins Med. J., *130*:335, 1975.
33. Germuth, F. G., and Rodriguez, E.: Immunopathology of the Renal Glomerulus. Boston, Little, Brown & Co., 1973.
34. Heptinstall, R. H., and Germuth, F. G.: Experimental studies on the immunologic and histologic effects of prolonged exposure to antigen. Bull. Johns Hopkins Hosp., *100*:71, 1957.
35. Cochrane, C. G., and Koffler, D.: Immune complex disease in experimental animals and man. Adv. Immunol., *16*:185, 1973.
36. Walter, M.: Present status of the rheumatoid factor. CRC Crit. Rev. Clin. Lab. Sci., *2*:173, 1971.
37. Bartfeld, H.: Distribution of rheumatoid factor activity in nonrheumatoid states. Ann. N.Y. Acad. Sci., *168*:30, 1969.
38. Williams, R. C., and Kunkel, H. G.: Rheumatoid factor, complement and conglutinin aberrations in a patient with subacute bacterial endocarditis. J. Clin. Invest., *41*:666, 1961.
39. Bravo, J. F., Herman, J. H., and Smyth, C. J.: Musculoskeletal disorders after renal homotransplantation. Ann. Intern. Med., *66*:87, 1966.
40. Allen, J. C., and Kunkel, H. G.: Antibody versus γG after repeated blood transfusions in man. J. Clin. Invest., *45*:29, 1966.
41. Tanimoto, K., Cooper, N. R., Johnson, J. S., and Vaughan, J. H.: Complement fixation by rheumatoid factor. J. Clin. Invest., *55*:437, 1974.
42. McDuffie, F. C., and Brumfield, H. W.: Effect of rheumatoid factor on complement mediated phagocytosis. J. Clin. Invest., *51*:3007, 1972.
43. Pope, R. M., Teller, D. C., and Mannik, M.: The molecular basis of self-association of antibody to IgG (rheumatoid factor) in rheumatoid arthritis. Proc. Natl. Acad. Sci. U.S.A., *71*:517, 1974.
44. Eggert, R. C., Brauer, D. J., and Caperton, E. M.: Anti-IgA antibodies in rheumatic and pulmonary disease. Ann. Rheum. Dis., *32*:41, 1973.
45. Normansell, D. E.: Anti-γG in rheumatoid arthritis sera. Immunochemistry, *8*:593, 1971.
46. Abruzzo, J. L., and Christian, C. L.: The induction of rheumatoid factor-like substance in rabbits. J. Exp. Med., *114*:791, 1961.
47. Cerottini, J., and Grey, H. M.: Binding properties of monoclonal γG-antiglobulin factor with human γG. Ann. N.Y. Acad. Sci., *168*:76, 1969.
48. Vaughan, J. H.: Summary: rheumatoid factors and their biological significance. Ann. N.Y. Acad. Sci., *168*:204, 1969.
49. Brouet, J. C., *et al.*: Biologic and clinical significance of cryoglobulins. Am. J. Med., *57*:775, 1974.
50. Saha, A., Edwards, M. A., Sargent, A. U., and Rose, B.: Mechanism of cryoprecipitation. I. Characteristics of a human cryoglobulin. Immunochemistry, *5*:341, 1968.
51. Sargent, A. O., Saha, A., Klassen, G. K., and Rose, B.: Studies of cryoprecipitation. Am. J. Med., *48*:54, 1970.
52. Osserman, E. F.: Plasma cell myeloma, II. Clinical aspects. N. Engl. J. Med., *261*:952, 1959.
53. Houser, D. D. Arbesman, C. E., Ito, K., and Wicker, K.: Cold urticaria: immunologic studies. Am. J. Med., *49*:23, 1970.
54. Christenson, W. N., Dacie, J. V., and Groucher,

B. E. E.: Electrophoretic studies on sera containing high titre cold hemagglutinins: identification of the antibody as the cause of an abnormal γ_1 peak. Br. J. Haematol., *3*:262, 1957.

55. Macris, N. T., *et al.*: A λ light chain cold agglutinin-crymacroglobulin occurring in Waldenström's Macroglobulinemia. Am. J. Med., *48*:524, 1970.
56. McIntosh, R. M., *et al.*: Cryoglobulins III. Q. J. Med., *44*:285, 1975.
57. Schwartz, W. B., and Kassirer, J. P.: Clinical aspects of acute post-streptococcal glomerulonephritis. *In* Strauss, M. B., and Welt, L. G. (eds.): Diseases of the Kidney. Ed. 2, Boston, Little, Brown & Co. p. 419, 1971.
58. Michael, A. F., Drummond, K. N., Good, R. A., and Vernier, R. L.: Acute poststreptococcal glomerulonephritis: immune deposit disease. J. Clin. Invest., *45*:237, 1966.
59. Seegal, B. C., Andres, G. A., Hsu, K. C., and Zabriskie, J. B.: Studies on the pathogenesis of acute and progressive glomerulonephritis in man by immunofluorescein and immunoferriten techniques. Fed. Proc., *24*:100, 1965.
60. Gewurz, H., Pickering, R. J., Mergenhagen, S. E., and Good, R. A.: The complement profile in acute glomerulonephritis, systemic lupus erythematosus, and hypocomplementemic chronic glomerulonephritis. Int. Arch. Allergy Appl. Immunol., *34*:557, 1968.
61. Koffler, D., Schur, P. H., and Kunkel, H. G.: Immunological studies concerning the nephritis of SLE. J. Exp. Med., *126*:607, 1967.
62. Baldwin, D. S., *et al.*: The clinical course of the proliferative and membranous forms of lupus nephritis. Ann. Intern. Med., *73*:929, 1970.
63. Zimmerman, S. W., *et al.*: Progression from minimal or focal to diffuse proliferative lupus nephritis. Lab. Invest., *32*:665, 1975.
64. Grishman, F., and Chung, J.: Ultrastructure of dermal lesions in SLE. Lab. Invest., *22*:189, 1970.
65. Gutman, R. A., Striker, G. E., Gilliland, B. C., and Cutler, R. E.: The immune complex glomerulonephritis of bacterial endocarditis. Medicine, *51*:1, 1972.
66. Boulton-Jones, J. M., Sissons, J. G. P., Evans, G. T., and Peters, D. K.: Renal lesions of subacute infectious endocarditis. Br. Med. J., *2*:11, 1974.
67. Tu, W. H., Shean, M. A., and Lee, J. L.: Acute diffuse glomerulonephritis in acute staphylococcal endocarditis. Ann. Intern. Med., *71*:335, 1969.
68. Heptinstall, R. H. (ed): *In* Pathology of the Kidney. Ed. 2, p. 456. Boston, Little, Brown & Co., 1974.
69. Bhorade, M. S., *et al.*: Nephropathy of secondary syphilis. J.A.M.A., *216*:1159, 1971.
70. Kaplan, B. S., Wiglesworth, F. W., Marks, M. I., and Drummond, K. N.: The glomerulopathy of congenital syphilis—an immune deposit disease. J. Pediatr., *81*:1154, 1972.
71. Braunstein, G. D., *et al.*: The nephrotic syndrome associated with secondary syphilis. Am. J. Med., *48*:643, 1970.
72. Gamble, C. N., and Reardon, J. B.: Immunopathogenesis of syphilitic glomerulonephritis. N. Engl. J. Med., *292*:449, 1975.
73. Combes, B., *et al.*: Glomerulonephritis with deposition of Australian antigen-antibody complexes in the glomerular basement membrane. Clin. Res., *19*:389, 1971.
74. Ward, P. A., and Kjbukamusoke, J. W.: Evidence for soluble immune complexes in the pathogenesis of the glomerulonephritis of quartan malaria. Lancet, *1*:283, 1969.
75. Roberts, W. C., and Rabson, A. S.: Focal glomerular lesions in fungal endocarditis. Ann. Intern. Med., *56*:610, 1962.
76. Stickler, G. B., *et al.*: Diffuse glomerulonephritis associated with infected ventriculoatrial shunt. N. Engl. J. Med., *279*:1077, 1968.
77. Yuceoglu, A. M., Berkovich, S., and Minkewitz, S.: Acute glomerulonephritis as a complication of Varicella. J.A.M.A., *202*:879, 1967.
78. ——: Acute glomerulonephritis associated with ECHO virus type 9 infection. J. Pediatr., *69*:603, 1966.
79. Burch, G. E., and Colcolough, H. L.: Progressive Coxsackie viral pericarditis and nephritis. Ann. Intern. Med., *71*:963, 1969.
80. Lewis, M. G., Loughridge, L. W., and Phillips. T. M.: Immunological studies in nephrotic syndrome associated with extrarenal malignant disease. Lancet, *2*:134, 1971.

80a. Pardo, W., *et al.*: Nephropathy associated with sickle cell anemia. Am. J. Med., *59*:650, 1975.

81. Mongan, E. S., Cass, R. M., Jacox, R. F., and Vaughan, J. H.: A study of the relation of seronegative and seropositive rheumatoid arthritis to each other and to necrotizing vasculitis. Am. J. Med., *47*:23, 1969.
82. Conn, D. L., McDuffie, F. C., and Dyck, P. J.: Immunopathologic study of sural nerves in rheumatoid arthritis. Arthritis Rheum., *15*:135, 1972.
83. Theofilopoulos, A. N., Bartonboy, G., LoSpalluto, J. J., and Ziff, M.: IgM rheumatoid factor and low molecular weight IgM. Arthritis, *17*:272, 1974.
84. Taylor, J. R., *et al.*: Immunologic Diseases. Ed. 2, p. 964. Boston, Little, Brown & Co., 1971.
85. Urizar, R. E., Michael, A., Sisson, S., and Vernier, R. L.: Anaphylactoid purpura. Lab. Invest., *19*:437, 1968.

85a. Gocke, D. J., *et al.*: Association between polyarteritis and Australia antigen. Lancet, *2*:1149, 1970.

85b. ——: Extrahepatic manifestations of viral hepatitis. Am. J. Med. Sci., *270*:49, 1975.

86. Schumacher, H. R., and Kitrodou, R. C.: Synovitis of recent onset. Arthritis Rheum., *15*:465, 1972.
87. Shaffer, M. F., and Bennett, G. A.: The passage of type III rabbit virulent Pneumococci from the vascular system into joints and certain other body cavities. J. Exp. Med., *70*:293, 1939.
88. Schumacher, H. R.: The microvasculature of the synovial membrane of the monkey: ultra-

structural studies. Arthritis Rheum., *12*:387, 1969.

89. Smiley, J. D., Sachs, C., and Ziff, M.: In vitro synthesis of immunoglobulin by rheumatoid synovial membrane. J. Clin. Invest., *47*:624, 1968.
90. Zvaifler, N. J.: The immunopathology of joint inflammation in rheumatoid arthritis. Adv. Immunol., *16*:265, 1973.
91. Winchester, R. J., Agnello, V., and Kunkel, H. G.: Gamma globulin complexes in synovial fluids of patients with rheumatoid arthritis. Clin. Exp. Immunol., *6*:689, 1970.
92. Elling, P., Graudal, H., and Faber, V.: Granulocyte-specific antinuclear factors in serum and synovial fluid in rheumatoid arthritis. Ann. Rheum. Dis., *27*:225, 1968.
93. Marcus, R. L., and Townes, A. S.: The occurrence of cryoproteins in synovial fluid; the association of a complement-fixing activity with cold-precipitable protein. J. Clin. Invest., *50*:282, 1971.
94. ———: Partial dissociation of rheumatoid synovial fluid cryoprotein: micro-complement fixation by IgG or IgG and IgM containing fractions and denatured calf thymus DNA. J. Immunol., *106*:1499, 1971.
95. Winchester, R. J., Kunkel, H. G., and Agnello, V.: Occurrence of γ-globulin complexes in serum and joint fluid of rheumatoid arthritis patients: use of monoclonal rheumatoid factors as reagents for their demonstration. J. Exp. Med., *134*:286s, 1971.
96. Ruddy; S., and Austen, K. F.: The complement system in rheumatoid synovitis. Arthritis Rheum., *13*:713, 1970.
97. Götze, O., Zvaifler, N. J., and Müller-Eberhard, H. J.: Evidence for complement activation by the C3 activator system in rheumatoid arthritis. Arthritis Rheum., *15*:111, 1972.
98. Hollander, J. L., McCarty, D. J., Astorga, G., and Castro-Murillo, E.: Studies on the pathogenesis of rheumatoid joint inflammation. Ann. Intern. Med., *62*:271, 1965.
99. Weissmann, G., Zurier, R. B., Spieler, J., and Goldstein, I. M.: Mechanisms of lysosomal enzyme release from leukocytes exposed to immune complexes and other particles. J. Exp. Med., *134*:149s, 1971.
100. Chayen, J., and Bitensky, L.: Lysosomal enzymes and inflammation. Ann. Rheum. Dis., *30*:522, 1971.
101. Croft, J. D., *et al.*: Coombs'-test positivity induced by drugs. Ann. Intern. Med., *68*:176, 1968.
102. Harris, J. W.: Studies on the mechanism of drug-induced hemolytic anemia. J. Lab. Clin. Med., *47*:760, 1956.
103. Karpatkin, S.: Drug-induced thrombocytopenia. Am. J. Med. Sci., *262*:69, 1971.

8 Tolerance and Autoimmunity

Just as immunity can be defined as the state of specific reactivity to an antigen resulting from prior exposure, *tolerance* is the state of specific unresponsiveness to an antigen following initial exposure to that antigen. The initial paralyzing dose of antigen is said to *tolerize* the recipient. The immune system can be experimentally rendered unresponsive to many antigens, as we shall see below. The ability to induce tolerance to foreign materials may be of great significance in transplantation. Even more important, however, is the critical requirement for selective immunologic unresponsiveness to the body's own tissue components. Paul Ehrlich first imagined the consequences of unrepressed immunologic reactivity against the body's own tissues, a phenomenon he aptly termed "horror autotoxicus." In this chapter, we will explore the characteristics and mechanisms of tolerance, as well as the realization of Ehrlich's horror autotoxicus—autoimmunity.

TOLERANCE

Tissue grafts between genetically nonidentical individuals are almost always unsuccessful. The recipient recognizes antigens on the donor tissue that are not present on his own cells (alloantigens) and produces an immune response that ultimately leads to the rejection of the graft. This observation had been known for a long time. However, in 1945, it was noted that genetically dissimilar cattle twins which had exchanged blood in fetal life by placental fusion grew up to possess two distinct populations of blood cells, one expressing the animal's own antigens and the other expressing antigens of his twin *without inciting immunologic rejection*.[1] Furthermore, skin grafts could be exchanged between these twins with good tissue acceptance.[2] The exposure of each animal's immune system to the alloantigens of his twin during fetal life had tolerized each animal to his twin's antigens.

This experiment of nature in fetal tolerization was duplicated in the laboratory when mouse spleen cells were transferred to embryonic mice of an unrelated strain. Subsequent grafting of donor tissue to the now adult recipients evoked no rejection in the majority of animals.[2] Animals who had not received the fetal or neonatal injections responded normaly to a challenge of allogeneic adult cells.

These early experiments illustrate two basic principles of tolerance:

1. *Tolerance to a particular antigen is something that the immune system learns.* In the experiments above, tolerance to *foreign* antigens was acquired by

means of some natural or laboratory manipulation. This work does not, however, allow us to make any conclusions about the genetic or acquired basis of tolerance to *self*-antigens.

2. In both examples, tolerance to foreign antigens was achieved by fetal or neonatal exposure to the antigenic material. In general, *the less immunologically mature the host, the easier it is to tolerize him to a particular antigen.*[3,4] However, many experiments have shown that adults can also be rendered tolerant to a great variety of antigens.

Another series of experiments demonstrated a third principle of tolerance. Investigators found that the administration of high doses of pneumococcal polysaccharide could induce unresponsiveness to that substance in individuals who previously had demonstrated the ability to respond to smaller doses.[5,6] Since these early observations, the ability to induce tolerance to an antigen by administering it in special dosage regimens has been seen with a great number of antigens. In general, *very high doses of antigen induce tolerance, whereas lower doses are immunogenic.*[4] Other dosage regimens such as the multiple injections of small doses of antigen may also be tolerogenic in certain circumstances.[7]

Some antigens display two distinct and separate dose ranges at which they can induce tolerance.[8] Both very high and very low concentrations of these molecules will induce tolerance, while at intermediate doses they will stimulate an immune response. These two levels of tolerance are called high zone and low zone tolerance. This phenomenon has been demonstrated for very few antigens and only under specific circumstances.[9]

TOLERANCE IN T AND B CELLS

Both T and B cells can be rendered specifically tolerant to an antigen.[10] The humoral response against those antigens requiring T helper function can be inhibited if either the B- or T-cell population is made tolerant. *In vivo* studies have demonstrated certain differences in the characteristics of B- and T-cell tolerance (Fig. 8-1).[11]

1. T-cell tolerance has a briefer induction period, occurring within 24 hours of antigen administration. B-cell tolerance can take weeks to become established. This distinction is much less marked *in vitro*, and may simply reflect the more complex *in vivo* situation where antigen availability to the different cell populations may vary significantly, rather than an intrinsic difference in the two cell types.

2. T-cell tolerance is more durable. Whereas B-cell unresponsiveness is lost within several weeks, T cells may remain unreactive for many months.

3. Tolerance is easier to induce in T cells, sometimes requiring antigen doses 100 to 10,000 times less than those needed to induce B-cell tolerance. This is an extremely important observation, for it suggests that low tolerogenic concentrations of certain antigens may induce tolerance solely in the T-cell population. In these situations the B cells would be capable of responding and would lack only the necessary T-cell helper signal.

There are several examples in the literature of carrier-specific tolerance occur-

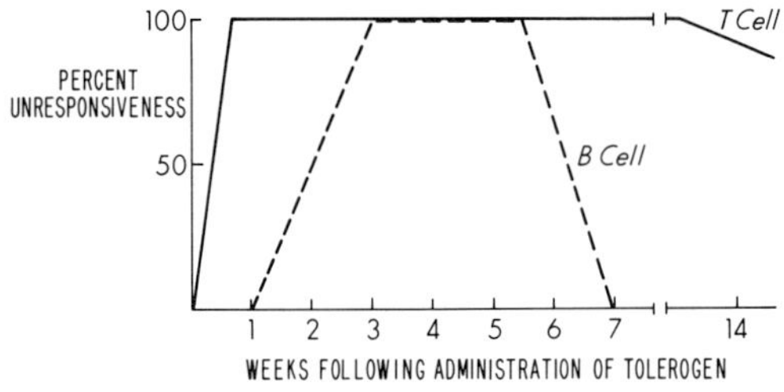

Fig. 8-1. Differences in the characteristics of T- and B-cell tolerance. T-cell tolerance is easier and quicker to induce and lasts longer than B-cell tolerance. (Adapted from Weigle, W. O.: Immunological unresponsiveness. Adv. Immunol., *16*:61, 1973.)

ring without concomitant hapten-specific tolerance. For example, animals rendered tolerant to the carrier moiety sheep gammoglobulin (ShIg) show a marked diminution in their ability to respond against the hapten TNP when it is conjugated to ShIg. However, they will respond perfectly well to TNP conjugated to rabbit gammaglobulin.[12] Thus, hapten-reactive cells exist and it is only the carrier-specific T cells that are tolerant in these instances.

The establishment of a state of tolerance usually includes both the ability to mount a humoral response and the capacity for cell-mediated immune processes directed against the tolerogen. Such complete tolerance would be expected whether T and B cells or just T cells were unresponsive to the antigen. However, several instances of unresponsiveness affecting only one of the limbs of the immune system have been reported. The injection of certain antigens into guinea pigs can prevent the delayed hypersensitivity response to the tolerogen while sparing the humoral response.[13,14] Others have been able to selectively abrogate the humoral response to a particular antigen while sparing the cellular response.[15] This phenomenon is termed *split unresponsiveness*; it is uncommon and as yet incompletely understood.

THE MACROPHAGE AND THE RETICULOENDOTHELIAL SYSTEM

The macrophage may play a decisive role in determining the balance between immunogenicity and tolerogenicity. Immunity is enhanced whenever an antigen is presented in a form susceptible to macrophage phagocytosis (see Chap. 5). Particulate aggregates of antigen are readily cleared from the circulation by the reticulo-endothelial system and are usually potent immunogens. Small, soluble antigens are not easily cleared and are often tolerogenic.[16] The RES of the Balb/c mouse is exceptionally efficient at clearing material—even when it is deaggregated—from the circulation and is remarkably resistant to tolerance induction.[17,18] It has been further suggested that the relative ease of inducing tolerance in neonates may be the result of the immaturity of the neonatal macrophages.[19]

These observations have led to the hypothesis that an antigen must interact with a macrophage in order to be able to induce an immune response. Those antigens which fail to do so behave as tolerogens. Thus, one might speculate that high concentrations of many antigens induce tolerance because the large number of particles overwhelms the ability of the macrophage population to deal with each and every particle. Some molecules therefore remain free to interact directly with the lymphocyte population where they induce tolerance. This rather uncomplicated view of the role of the macrophage in determining immunogenicity versus tolerogenicity may be an oversimplification since there is evidence that macrophages can present antigens to lymphocytes in either an immunogenic or a tolerogenic form.[20]

The clearance of antigen from the host circulation may be important in still another way in determining immunogenicity versus tolerogenicity. Once tolerance to an antigen is induced, the maintenance of tolerance requires the persistence of the tolerizing antigen in the host.[21] If the RES can effectively remove the antigen from the body, tolerance is lost. Thus tolerance to metabolizable antigens is often short-lived, whereas nonmetabolizable antigens which persist in the host can maintain a state of unresponsiveness for a long time.[22,23]

The failure of the RES to remove antigen completely from the body can result in a situation that can mimick tolerance but is not an example of true tolerance. This phenomenon has been termed *treadmill neutralization*.[24] The noncatabolizable antigen continually leaks back into the circulation where it binds to serum antibody. Measurements of free antibody will therefore fluctuate depending upon the amount of free antigen able to remove antibody from the circulation. Thus, at certain times following antigenic challenge, serum antibody titers may be very low, and a state of true tolerance may be mistakenly assumed.

MODELS FOR THE INDUCTION OF TOLERANCE

We have seen that, under certain circumstances, an antigen can induce a state of specific unresponsiveness. The ability to induce tolerance is a function of the nature and dose of antigen as well as the immunologic status of the host. Just as we explored the possible mechanisms by which an antigen can activate a cell to produce an immune response, so we can examine the ways in which an antigen can render a cell unreactive, that is, tolerant. Two points need to be emphasized beforehand:

1. It is generally believed that any cell that can effect an immune response can be tolerized. If this is so, then a competition exists between tolerance and immunity at the level of the antigen-sensitive cell. Tolerance and immunity can therefore be viewed as merely alternate states of immunologic activity.

2. There are many models which postulate mechanisms of tolerance induction. At present it is impossible to say which of these—if any—are significant *in vivo*.

Clonal Deletion

Burnet first proposed the concept of clonal deletion (Fig. 8-2) in order to explain the development of self-tolerance.[25] He theorized that during development those clones of cells which are capable of reacting against self-components are destroyed and thus eliminated from the body. This idea was later refined by Lederberg, who proposed that lymphocytes pass through various stages of maturation.[26] In the first stage, the lymphocyte (or lymphocyte precursor) is capable of recognizing specific antigens

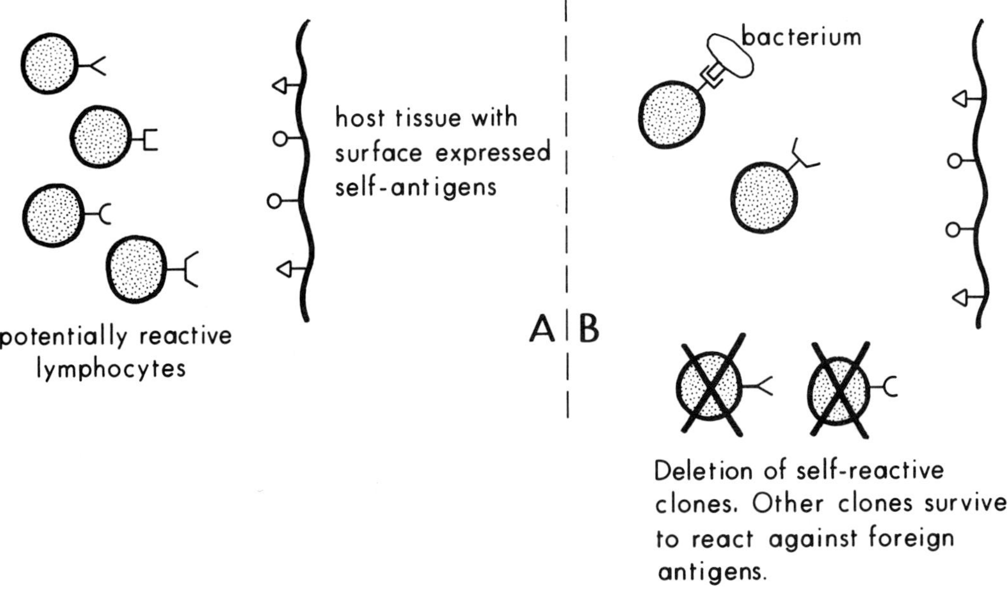

Fig. 8-2. The clonal deletion hypothesis.

but cannot be stimulated by those antigens. "Clonal abortion"[27] is postulated to take place when the antigen-sensitive cell interacts with its specific antigen during this susceptible stage (Fig. 8-3). Self-reacting clones will be unable to avoid contact with self-determinants during this initial period and will be inactivated (although not necessarily destroyed). Other lymphocytes may avoid contact with antigen during their tolerogenic phase, and will pass into the second stage where interaction with antigen provides an immunogenic stimulus.

Several intricate hypotheses have been recently advanced which are essentially modifications of this maturation hypothesis. One of the more intriguing of these revolves around the growing interest in surface IgD (Fig. 8-4).[28] It has been suggested that the different surface immunoglobulin classes appear sequentially on the lymphocyte's surface during development. According to this theory, IgM is the first immunoglobulin receptor to appear on the cell surface. Interaction of antigen with the IgM receptors induces tolerance. In the natural course of their differentiation, lymphocytes next acquire IgD. IgD is the postulated "triggering" receptor. Interaction of antigen with this receptor induces differentiation of the stimulated cell into an immunoglobulin-secreting plasma cell. This model attributes tolerance to a specific tolerogenic receptor, IgM, that is present early in development. No attempt is made to explain adult-acquired tolerance. The model's appeal lies in its explanation of early-acquired self-tolerance and in its ability to account for the presence of IgD on most peripheral lymphocytes (see Chap. 3). Nevertheless, it remains highly speculative at this time.

The concepts of clonal deletion and abortion are attractive for several reasons. First, they provide a very simple explanation for the elimination of self-reacting clones. Second, they can account for the increased susceptibility of neonates to tolerance induction.

These models cannot explain the induction of tolerance in adults nor do they account for the many documented in-

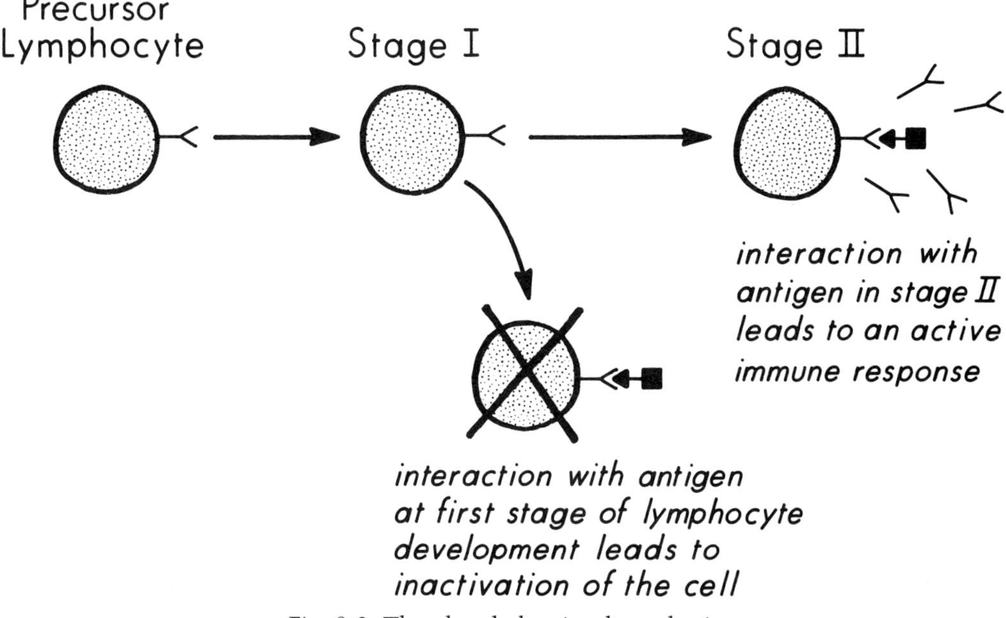

Fig. 8-3. The clonal abortion hypothesis.

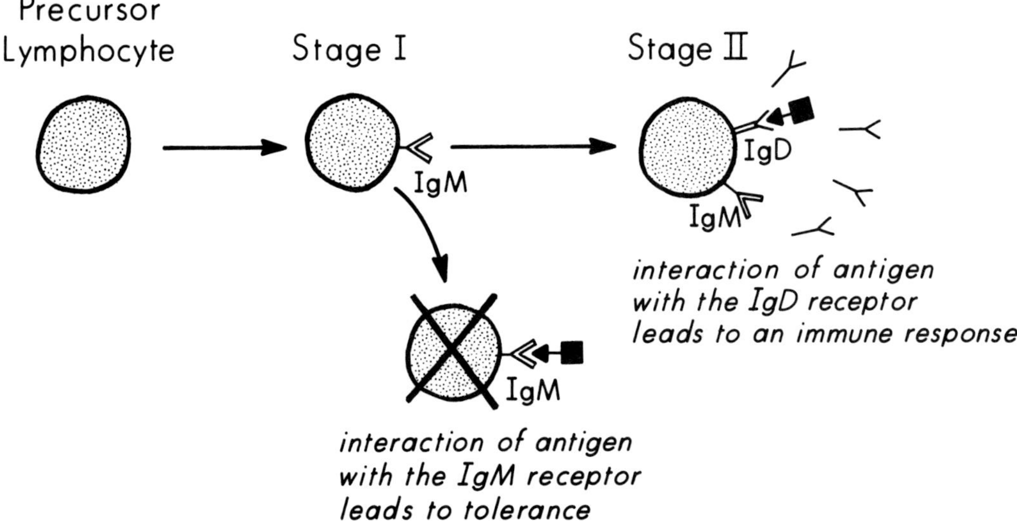

Fig. 8-4. One variant of the clonal abortion hypothesis (see text).

stances of fetal immunity. There is little evidence that clones of self-reacting lymphocytes are preferentially destroyed during development. Further, the existence of lymphocytes capable of recognizing and responding to self-determinants in the adult host has now been amply demonstrated.[29-31] Thus, although clonal elimination schemes may provide a first step toward self-tolerance, clearly other mechanisms must exist to render many self-reacting cells unresponsive. If clonal deletion (or abortion) does contribute to self-tolerance, it is not the universal mechanism it was originally believed to be. With the proliferation of alternative models of both neonatal and adult tolerance, the emphasis on clonal elimination has considerably lessened.

Surface Receptor Cross-Linking: the B Cell

In Chapter 4 we saw that *limited* cross-linking of surface molecules has been postulated as one way to activate a lymphocyte. Similar types of experiments have led to the suggestion that *extensive* cross-linking may inactivate a cell (Fig. 8-5). T-cell-independent antigens have been employed in the study of surface inactivation, a choice necessitated by the enormous complexity of cellular events involved in the response to T-cell-dependent antigens. The discussion that follows therefore pertains only to B cells and to a limited class of antigens.

B cells can be either irreversibly or reversibly inactivated. Irreversible inactivation is often taken to mean cell death, and may be reflected in a decrease in the number of specific antigen-binding cells following administration of a tolerogen. Such a decrease has been observed in several experimental systems.[32,33] Reconstitution of immune responsiveness to the tolerizing antigen occurs only when new B cells arise with the proper antigenic specificity.[34]

Reversible inactivation of immunocompetent cells has also been described,[34a,35] and may occur via the temporary blocking of B-cell receptors by the tolerogen. These cells are not eliminated from the host.[33] The ability to regain responsiveness is considered to be a function of the ability of the cells to clear the tolerogen from their surface and express new receptors. It has been suggested that

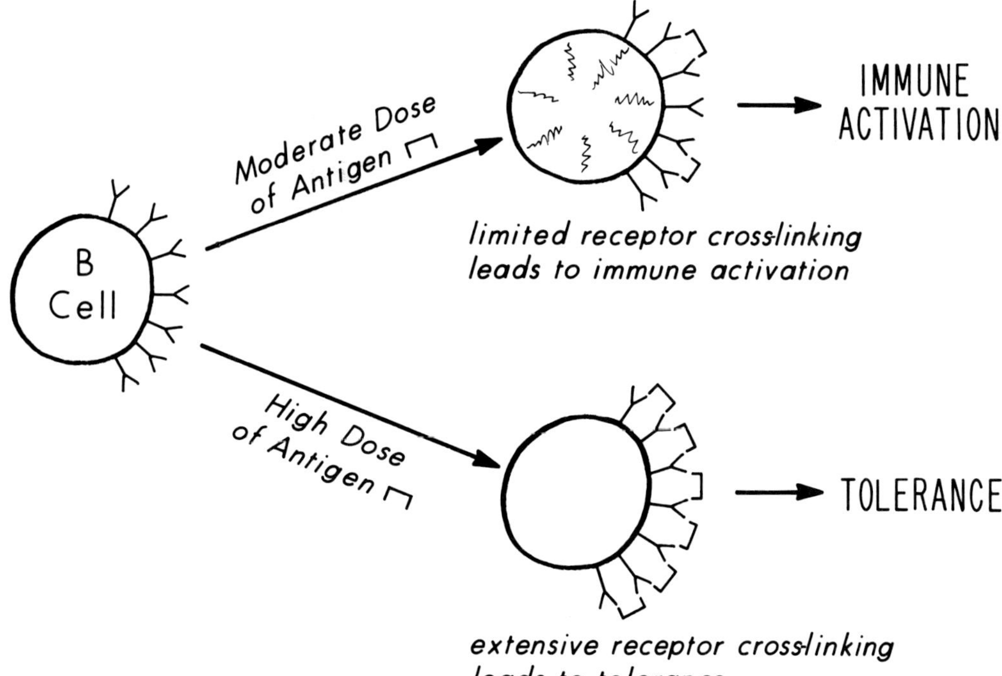

Figure 8-5. Extensive surface receptor cross-linking (for example, by high doses of a divalent antigen), has been postulated as one mechanism for inducing B-cell tolerance. Less extensive cross-linking may lead to immune activation.

the intensity of interaction of the tolerogen with the B-cell surface receptors, as well as the ability of the B-cell to clear the tolerogen from its surface, determines the extent of reversibility of the tolerant state.[36] The intensity of interaction may be, in part, a measure of the degree of receptor cross-linking by the tolerogen. The model for surface inactivation by extensive receptor cross-linking implies certain special characteristics of the tolerogens involved. Clearly, only those antigens capable of cross-linking surface receptors could induce tolerance in this way.

One example of a tolerogen that may irreversibly inactivate a cell is the hapten-carrier conjugate DNP-D,GL. This molecule is a nonmetabolizable, T-cell-independent, B-cell tolerogen, capable of inducing tolerance in thymic-deprived mice.[36] It is immunogenic only at very low doses.[37] DNP-D,GL binds avidly to B cells, persists on their surface for a long time, and is poorly internalized.[38] One report indicates that those cells to which DNP-D,GL binds do not re-express their antigen receptors despite long incubation in culture.[38] Once tolerance has been established in these cells it cannot be overridden even by a powerful immunologic stimulus such as the allogeneic effect.[39]

DNP-D,GL possesses certain properties which may be critical to its role as an irreversible tolerogen:[36]

1. *DNP-D,GL is a highly repeating structure* and displays many identical determinants on its surface. The number of repeating determinants present on a molecule is called its *epitope density*, and thus DNP-D,GL is said to possess a high epitope density.

2. *DNP-D,GL is nonmetabolizable.*

DNP-D,GL thus possesses features

which would enable it both to persist on the cell surface for a long time and to extensively cross-link surface receptors. The tolerance may be irreversible because: (1) the surface binding is very tight and the antigen cannot be cleared from the cell; (2) as a result, the cell is unable to express new antigen receptors; (3) the antigen itself is nonmetabolizable and cannot be cleared from the body; (4) nonspecific T-cell help cannot override this tolerance; (5) those cells rendered unreactive will be removed from the body by phagocytes.

Proteolysis can remove the DNP-D,GL from the surface of the cell and reverse the effect of the tolerogen within several days of tolerance induction.[36] The failure of proteolytic treatment to have an effect if attempted more than two days after induction is evidence that irreversible inactivation does eventually occur. Similar findings have also been reported with other antigens.[40]

The importance of epitope density in tolerance induction has been explored with several other T-cell-independent antigens, notably DNP-flagellin.[41] This hapten-carrier complex can be structured to have either high or low epitope density by controlling the amount of DNP conjugated to the flagellin molecule. At low levels of conjugation the antigen is immunogenic, while at higher densities the antigen can be tolerogenic. Thus there is a correlation between the ability of this molecule to cross-link surface molecules and its tolerogenic capacity.

Blocking Factors

Serum blocking factors may play a role in maintaining self-tolerance. Some investigators have reported that donor T cells cultured *in vitro* with self-antigens will respond against those antigens. They have termed this phenomenon *autosensitization*.[42] Addition of autologous serum to the culture medium prevents this response. This observation suggests the existence of an active blockade that prevents *in vivo* sensitization. Antigen-antibody complexes are known to be able to mediate blocking effects (see Chap. 13), but it has not yet been shown whether this particular serum blocking effect is due to low levels of circulating antigen-antibody complexes. This phenomenon has not yet been confirmed by other investigators.

Exhaustive Immunization

It has been hypothesized that the administration of an overwhelming antigenic load might elicit a unique type of response from the immune system.[43] In order to cope with the excess antigen, all of the antigen-reactive cells would differentiate to become short-lived antibody-secreting cells. No memory cells would be produced. Thus all of the antigen-specific B cells would be depleted and the host would be unable to respond to a subsequent challenge with the original antigen. There is little evidence to support an *in vivo* role for this mechanism.

Suppressor Cells

With the recent demonstrations that suppressor cells exist that are capable of profoundly inhibiting the immune response (see Chap. 5), many investigators have sought to attribute certain examples of tolerance to active immune suppression. Immune suppression has been called "infectious tolerance" because the transfer of lymphocytes from an animal rendered tolerant to a particular antigen by suppression produces a similar state of unresponsiveness in a recipient animal.[44]

The contribution of suppressor cells to the overall tolerance of an individual is still uncertain, but recent work suggests an important place for suppression among the many other mechanisms available for achieving selective unresponsiveness. In particular, tolerance associated with low doses of antigen may prove to be primarily a T-suppressor-cell phenomenon and would account for the observation that low-dose tolerance resides solely in the T-cell population. The primary motivation behind this belief is the observation that some experimental and naturally occurring autoimmune diseases have been associated with a loss of suppressor cells and the subsequent expression of "forbidden clones." We shall return to this point in the section on autoimmune disease.

SUMMARY

Tolerance is a learned response. The ability of an antigen to induce a state of specific unresponsiveness is a function of: (1) the nature of the antigen, e.g., soluble versus aggregate, and epitope density; (2) the dosage of administration; in general, high doses of antigens are tolerogenic, low doses immunogenic; and (3) the immunologic status of the host, e.g., immunologic maturity, and reticuloendothelial system activity.

Most tolerogens elicit an across-the-board unresponsiveness including both cellular and humoral immunity. Humoral unresponsiveness can result from tolerance of either the B- or the T-cell populations, or both.

T-cell tolerance is easier to induce, occurs more rapidly and at lower antigen doses, and lasts longer than B-cell tolerance. It therefore appears that tolerogens present in low concentrations may tolerize only T cells, whereas tolerogens circulating in high concentrations may tolerize both B and T cells.

Many models have been proposed to explain the mechanisms of tolerance induction. Early emphasis on finding a single mechanism of tolerance has given way to a more generalized view that there may be several ways to induce tolerance. Among the more widely studied possibilities are clonal deletion and abortion, direct surface inactivation by extensive receptor cross-linking, blocking factors, and suppressor cells.

AUTOIMMUNITY

Autoimmunity can be defined as the expression of immunologic reactivity against host self-constituents. It is the realization of Ehrlich's "horror autotoxicus," the activation of cells that, under normal circumstances, are quiescent and unresponsive. As common as autoimmune diseases are, autoimmune phenomena, without any clinical manifestations, are even more prevalent. More than 50 per cent of people in their seventh decade have at least one type of autoantibody readily detectable in their serum.[45]

The existence of autoimmune phenomena is a major reason for believing that clonal deletion and/or clonal abortion may not be able to account for the full expression of tolerance. Cells *do* exist which can react against self-constituents, and they must therefore be actively maintained in a state of unresponsiveness throughout life. The development of autoimmunity can thus be viewed as an escape from the mechanisms by which self-tolerance is maintained.

We have already seen that tolerance can reside in both the B- and T-cell populations. Humoral as well as cellular unresponsiveness to most antigens can result from paralysis of both B and T cells or just the T-cell population alone. Most experimental work examining tolerance induction to foreign antigens has led to the view that T cells are easier to render tolerant than B cells. Thus, T cells can be tolerized by low doses of antigen that are ineffectual in tolerizing B cells. By analogy, we could predict that tolerance to some *self*-antigens might reside in both B- and T-cell populations, while tolerance to other self-constituents would reside only in the T-cell. Thus, it has been suggested that tolerance to self-antigens which circulate in high concentrations, such as albumin, may be the result of unresponsiveness of both B and T cells. On the other hand, tolerance to antigens present in low concentrations, for example, thyroglobulin, may reside solely in the T-cell population.[29] Consistent with this hypothesis are several reports of the detection of thyroglobulin-binding B cells in normal individuals, whereas similar studies have failed to detect albumin-binding B cells.[29]

At present it is still uncertain how applicable the distinction between "B- and T-cell" versus "T-cell-only" tolerance is for self-antigens. Nevertheless, this concept has proven extremely useful in attempting to understand how the tolerant state can be broken and result in autoimmunity. Some of the most satisfying models for the induction of autoimmunity involve situations in which it seems that the T-cell population carries the full burden for the maintenance of tolerance.

If tolerance to a particular self-antigen resides only in the T cells, antigen-reactive B cells should exist that are capable of producing antibody against the self-antigen. The B cells would fail to respond only because they lack the appropriate T helper signal. However, there are several ways in which the T-helper-cell block could be *bypassed* that would result in the activation of autoreactive B cells. We will call this mechanism for breaking tolerance *bypassing the T-cell block*. A second way to break tolerance would be to *remove the T-cell block*. We shall discuss each of these mechanisms in turn (Fig. 8-6).

BYPASSING THE T-CELL BLOCK

Crossreactivity

It has been known for some time that the injection of an antigen that crossreacts with a molecule to which a host is tolerant can elicit antibody production against the tolerogen. We can put this concept in more concrete terms. For example, rabbits can be readily tolerized to bovine serum albumin (BSA). Subsequent administration of human serum albumin (HSA), which crossreacts to a small extent with BSA, can elicit the production of antibodies that react with BSA, the original tolerogen (Fig. 8-7). Hence tolerance to BSA is effectively broken and an anti-BSA response is observed.[46]

We can explain this result in the following way: let us say that the T-cell population is tolerant to all of the antigenic determinants on BSA, but that the B cells are potentially responsive to these determinants. These include determinants found only on BSA (BSA-specific) as well as those BSA determinants shared with HSA (BSA-crossreactive). The host T cells will clearly be tolerant to those determinants on HSA that are shared with BSA since HSA-crossreactive = BSA-crossreactive. However, the T cells are perfectly responsive to those determinants on HSA that are uniquely its own (HSA-specific) since tolerance to BSA will not affect a response against these determinants. This situation is depicted in Figure 8-8.

Because we are dealing with a situation of T-cell-only tolerance, the B cells are potentially responsive to all of these determinants, even those on BSA, and merely await the proper T-cell stimulation. In the animal tolerant to BSA this stimulation never arrives. With the injection of HSA, however, the situation is altered. Because the T cells can recognize and respond to at least some part of the HSA molecule (which can functionally be viewed as the carrier portion), they can effectively function as T helper cells for a humoral response against all the determinants on HSA, including those unique to HSA *and* those it shares with BSA. Antibody is therefore produced against all of these determinants, and we observe an anti-BSA response. *The antibodies that are produced against BSA react only against those determinants on BSA that crossreact with determinants on HSA.* If we absorb out the antisera with HSA, no reactivity remains against BSA (see diagram, Fig. 8-9).[4]

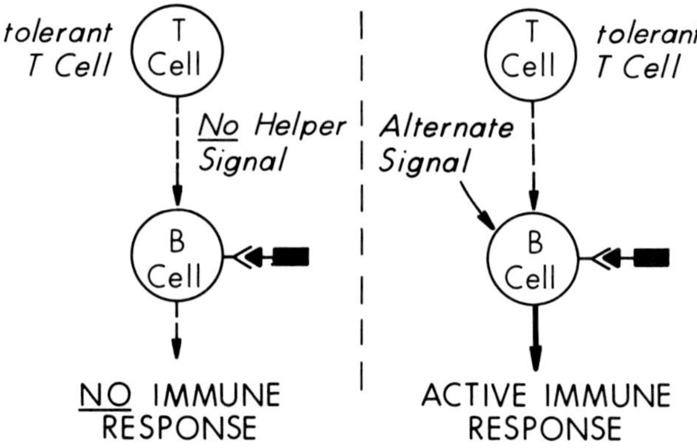

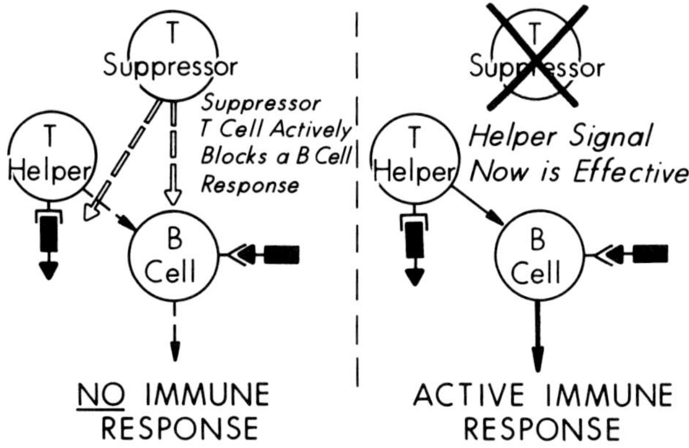

Fig. 8-6. In situations where tolerance to an antigen resides solely in the T-cell population, tolerance can be broken either by bypassing or removing the T-cell block.

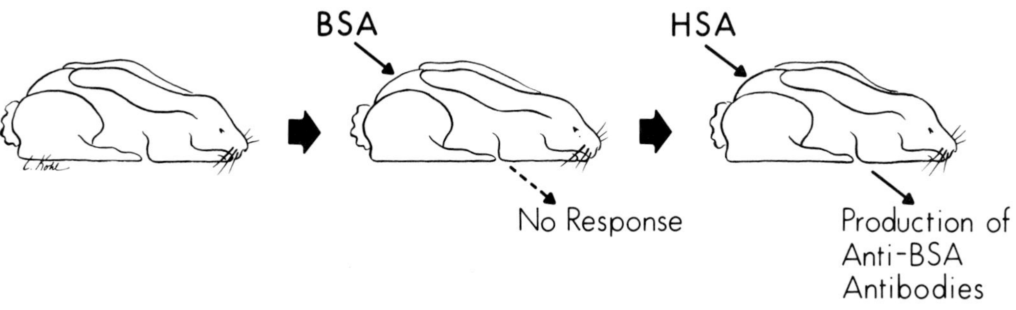

Fig. 8-7. Tolerance to BSA can be broken by injecting HSA, an antigen that crossreacts with BSA.

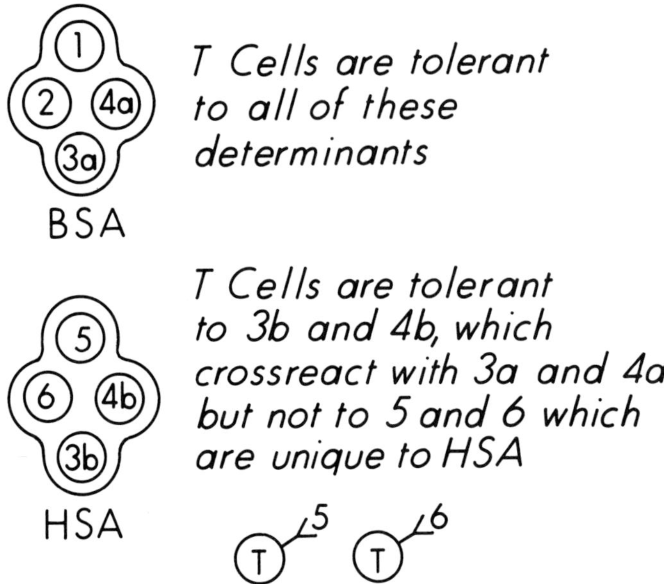

Fig. 8-8. BSA and HSA are each represented as expressing 4 antigenic determinants. Determinants 1 and 2 are unique to BSA, and 5 and 6 are unique to HSA; 3a and 4a on BSA crossreact with 3b and 4b on HSA.

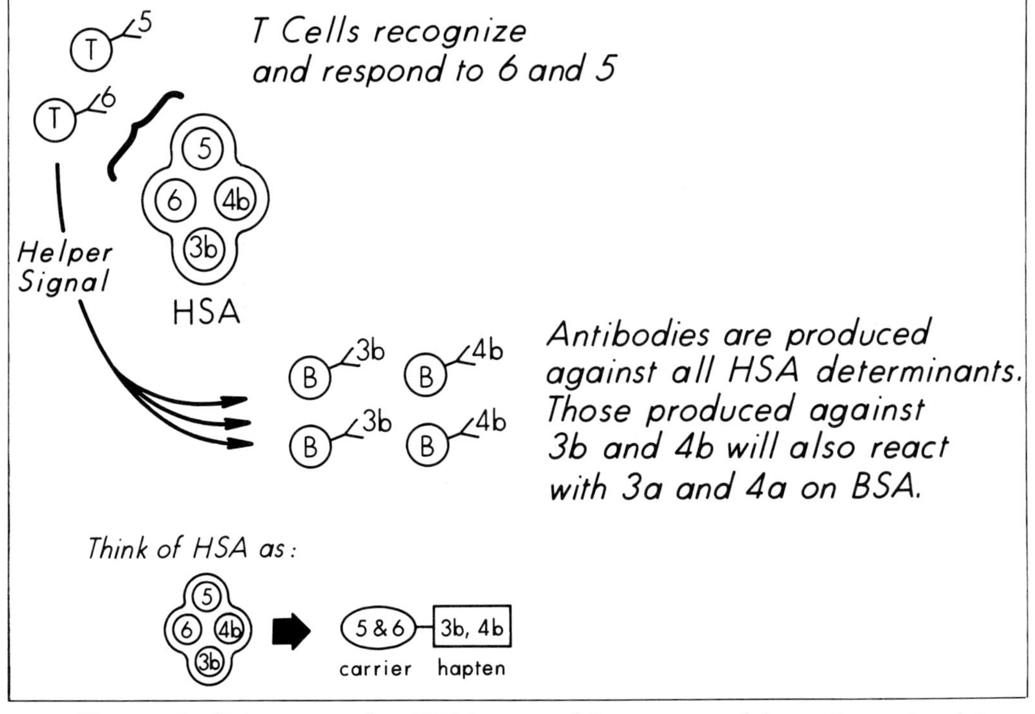

Fig. 8-9. T cells can respond to HSA because of the presence of determinants 5 and 6 which can serve as an effective carrier unit. B-cell clones reactive against 3b and 4b are thus stimulated. The antibody produced against 3b and 4b will also react with 3a and 4a of BSA.

When sheep serum albumin (SSA), which crossreacts to a very great extent with BSA, is used to try to break tolerance to BSA, no anti-BSA response is observed.[47] This is because SSA possesses such great crossreactivity with BSA that it is viewed as BSA-identical (and hence tolerogenic) by the T-cell population, and SSA therefore cannot trigger T helper activity. Hence, the second challenging molecule must be sufficiently different from the tolerogenic molecule to elicit a response. Such extensive crossreactivity with host antigens could permit a microorganism to persist in a host. If the organism is viewed by the immune system as very similar to a component of self, no response will be initiated against it. Such biological mimicry has been suggested for certain species of Salmonella, *E. coli*, streptococci, and other microorganisms in certain mammalian hosts.[48,49]

The essential point of our discussion thus far is that if the T-cell population can be induced to respond to a particular carrier moiety, a humoral response can be mounted against any hapten attached to that carrier, provided the hapten-specific B cells are potentially responsive. Thus, if host determinants are displayed on an immunogenic carrier, tolerance to those determinants can be broken. Such a situation could occur in several ways *in vivo*.[50-52] (1) Host determinants could become incorporated in the capsid of a virus which would serve as the immunogenic carrier. (2) Part of a host antigen could become altered, and thus appear as a new, immunogenic carrier for unaltered associated determinants. (3) A host determinant could bind to an exogenously administered carrier such as a drug (Fig. 8-10).

The model best exemplifying these principles as they might apply to autoimmunity is experimental autoimmune thyroiditis.[29] The induction of thyroiditis in the mouse resembles the breaking of tolerance to BSA in several ways. Thyroglobulin ordinarily circulates in very low levels and B cells can be detected which are capable of specifically binding thyroglobulin. These observations suggest, although they do not prove, that tolerance

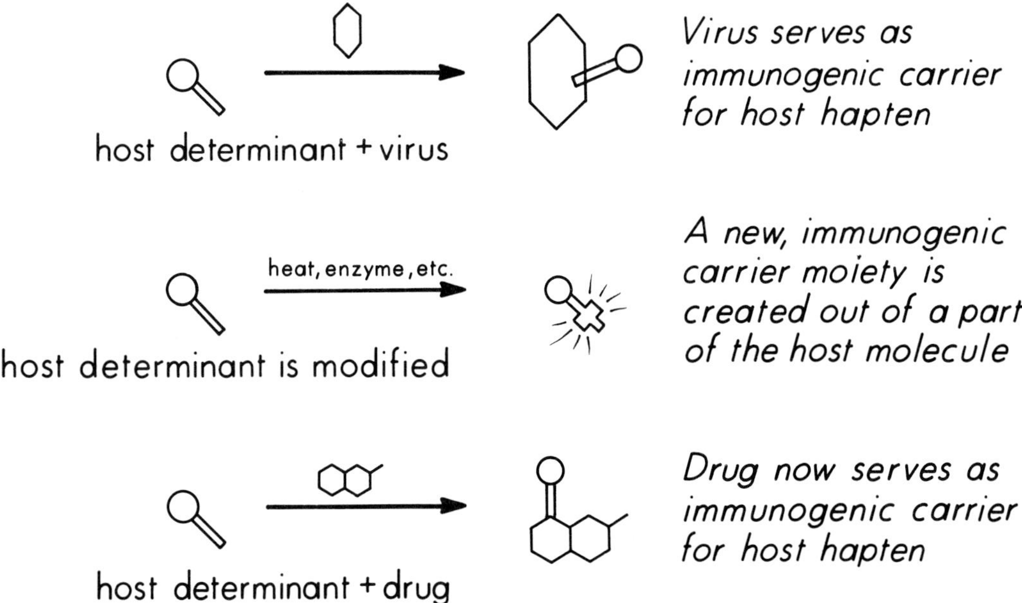

Fig. 8-10. Three *in vivo* mechanisms by which a host determinant could be expressed on an immunogenic carrier and thus become the target for autoreactivity.

to thyroglobulin might reside solely in the T-cell population. Autoimmune thyroiditis can be established by injecting heterologous thyroglobulin into such animals. This is presumably due to the crossreactivity of heterologous thyroglobulin with the autologous molecule. As with the breaking of tolerance to BSA with HSA, the resultant anti-autologous thyroglobulin antisera can be completely absorbed out with the heterologous thyroglobulin, indicating that autoantibody production is directed solely against those determinants identical to, or crossreactive with, those on the heterologous molecule.

It appears from our discussion thus far that there are a number of ways in which T-cell tolerance can be bypassed and result in the induction of autoimmune phenomena. However, there may be mechanisms by which T cells are *actively* maintained in a state of unresponsiveness in addition to, or instead of, tolerance resulting from just the passive paralysis of specific T-cell clones. One such mechanism may be the existence of T suppressor cells specific for self-antigens.[52] If such cells do exist in the normal host, they may act as a secondary defense against the breaking of autotolerance. Thus, the introduction of crossreacting antigens or the exposure of new determinants may not only stimulate T helper cells, but may also activate T suppressor cells. According to this hypothesis the ability of a crossreacting antigen or second carrier molecule to break tolerance would be a function of the balance between its ability to stimulate T helper cells and T suppressor cells.

Thus, in one experiment, simultaneous injection of HSA *and BSA* into a BSA-tolerant animal failed to terminate the state of tolerance.[4] Since we already know that HSA can break tolerance to BSA, it appears that the low dose of BSA included in the challenge inoculum was able to block the activity of HSA-induced T helper cells. This may have been the result of the activation of BSA-specific suppressor cells (see Fig. 8-11).

Nonspecific Stimulation

There is another type of mechanism available for bypassing T-cell tolerance. The T-helper-cell block could be overridden by a powerful, nonspecific stimulatory signal. Although this mechanism has not yet been shown to play a causal role in

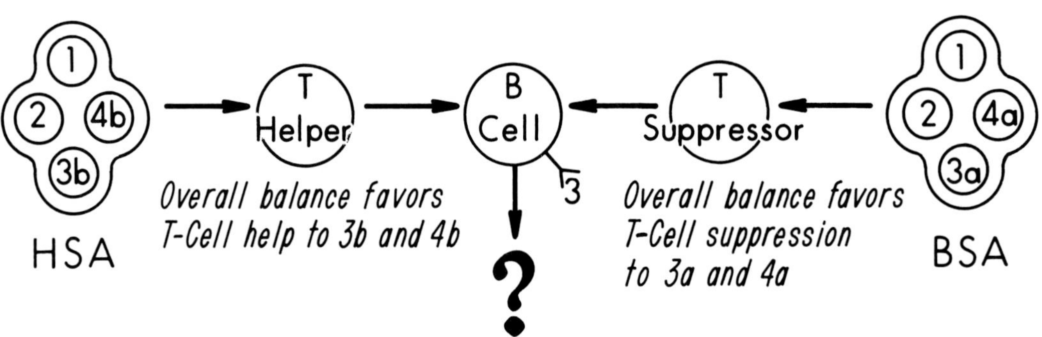

Fig. 8-11. The balance between T-cell help and T-cell suppression may determine whether or not an immune response is induced to a given determinant.

autoimmune disease, the production of autoantibodies has been induced experimentally by procedures designed to provide just such a stimulus. For example, the injection of allogeneic cells into mice can evoke antinuclear antibody production.[53] The allogeneic effect (see Chap. 5) provides a potent and nonspecific stimulation for antibody production, bypassing the necessity for antigen-specific T-cell help.

We would hardly pretend that naturally occurring autoimmune disease usually results from host exposure to allogeneic cells. However, other agents might be just as successful in providing a powerful nonspecific signal. One might speculate that a viral infection or any chronic infection or antigenic stimulation could lead to the production by activated lymphocytes of high levels of nonspecific stimulatory substances that could break tolerance to self-antigens and induce autoimmunity. Viral infections have been associated with several autoimmune diseases,[54] and although there are many other theories to explain this association (see below), this is one that must certainly be considered. Such a mechanism would undoubtedly be very nonspecific and one would expect to find antibodies directed against a variety of self-determinants. This is indeed the characteristic picture of many autoimmune diseases.

REMOVING THE T-CELL BLOCK

It is possible that the T suppressor cell does not serve merely as a second line of defense against autoimmunity, but may in many instances be primarily responsible for the maintenance of self-tolerance. Thus, the loss of suppressor cells might remove the major force mediating the state of unresponsiveness, freeing self-reacting clones to respond. It is not unreasonable to predict that self-reacting killer cells—if such exist—could also be released by the removal of suppressor cells, resulting in cell-mediated immunity against autoantigens as well as the production of autoantibodies. The role of cell-mediated immunity in autoimmunity has not been well defined.[55] We shall discuss the evidence for cell-mediated autoimmune processes later in this chapter when we examine the human autoimmune diseases. Also of importance in this regard is the section on Hashimoto's thyroiditis in Chapter 15.

The role of the T suppressor cell in autoimmune phenomena has been firmly established in several animal systems. Later in this chapter we will review the natural history of the New Zealand mice which develop autoimmunity concomitant with the loss of T suppressor cells. Similarly, Buffalo rats and Leghorn chickens develop spontaneous autoimmune thyroiditis which is accelerated by neonatal thymectomy. Presumably, thymus-derived cells are exerting a suppressive influence on antithyroid-reacting clones in these animals.

The loss of suppressor cells could also account for the high (60%) incidence of autoimmune phenomena in the elderly human population. Certain animal strains, notably the Strain A mice, have been observed to develop antinuclear antibodies as they age. This process can be prevented by the transfer of T cells from young animals.

THE DESTRUCTIVE POTENTIAL OF AUTOANTIBODIES

The demonstration of autoreactivity in diseases associated with tissue destruction does not, in and of itself, allow one to attribute the destruction to the presence of autoantibodies or autosensitized lymphocytes. Thus, autoantibodies are not always associated with clinically apparent tissue damage, as in the many elderly individuals in apparent good health who possess autoantibodies. It has often been suggested that autoreactivity may occur secondarily to prior tissue destruction by some nonimmune mechanism which may alter tissue antigens so that they become immunogenic. According to this view, autoimmune phenomena are merely sequelae to an underlying disease process. This is an important cautionary note to bear in mind in approaching diseases associated with autoimmune phenomena, and one to which we shall frequently refer.

Despite this qualification, autoreactive immune phenomena are clearly capable of producing tissue damage and it is not unlikely that they are responsible for the disease manifestations in many autoimmune diseases. Autoantibodies can do all the things that normal antibodies can do, and it is only the antigen against which they are directed that makes them unique. Thus, they can cause tissue destruction by (1) direct action aginst tissue antigens, and (2) the production of immune complex disease. The latter has been clearly demonstrated in some of the rheumatic autoimmune diseases (SLE, rheumatoid arthritis, etc.). The former has been more difficult to prove. However, there are a number of diseases in which the presence of autoantibodies appears to be related to direct tissue damage. Although we shall be discussing these diseases in subsequent chapters, a brief review of the role of autoantibodies in some of these diseases is worthwhile at this point:

1. *Autoimmune Hemolytic Disease* (see Chap. 14). Antibodies against erythrocyte antigens can mediate red-cell destruction via complement-mediated lysis, reticuloendothelial-system phagocytosis, and antibody-dependent cell-mediated cytotoxicity. The relative importance of each of these mechanisms is not known, and may vary from case to case.

2. *Immune Thrombocytopenic Purpura* (see Chap. 14). Antiplatelet antibodies may induce destruction of platelets by the same mechanisms as those mentioned above.

3. *Pemphigus* (see Chap. 15) Antibodies against the glycocalyx of the prickle cell layer in the skin may be responsible for disruption of the epidermis with resultant formation of bullae.

4. *Myasthenia Gravis* (see Chap. 12). Anti-acetylcholine-receptor antibodies may impair neuromuscular transmission.

5. *Graves' Disease* (see Chap. 15). Antibody against the thyroid-stimulating hormone (TSH) receptor may stimulate the thyroid as well as be responsible for the refractoriness of the organ to feedback suppression.

6. *Goodpasture's Syndrome* (see Chap. 15). Anti-basement-membrane antibody may contribute to both the pulmonary and renal lesions seen in this disease.

7. *Pernicious Anemia* (see Chap. 15) Anti-intrinsic-factor antibodies may prevent the absorption of vitamin B_{12} in the distal ileum. This may result either by blocking the binding of B_{12} to intrinsic factor or by blocking the binding of intrinsic factor to its intestinal receptor.

8. *Other tissue-destructive changes* associated with the presence of autoantibodies are seen in Hashimoto's thyroiditis, idiopathic Addison's disease, atrophic gastritis and others. Whether or not these antibodies contribute to organ destruction in these disorders is not known.

THE NEW ZEALAND MICE

The New Zealand black mice (NZB) and their NZB × NZW (white) F_1 hybrids (NZB/W) provide the outstanding animal models for human autoimmune disease.[56,57] Both of these animals pursue a relentless (although very different) clinical course, marked by characteristic immunologic and pathologic changes and terminating in premature death. Much of what we know about the possible pathogenetic mechanisms of autoimmunity has been derived from intensive study of these animals. In this section we will review the natural history and immunology of the New Zealand mice as a prelude to a discussion of human autoimmune disease.

NATURAL HISTORY OF THE NZB MOUSE

The disease process of the NZB mouse is highlighted by the development of an autoimmune hemolytic anemia and immune-complex renal disease. By three months of age a small percentage of these animals have antibodies against erythrocyte antigens detectable on the surface of their red cells. The figure reaches 100 per cent by the time the mice are 12 to 15 months of age. These autoantibodies can be demonstrated in the serum one to two months after they can first be detected on the red-cell surface. They can be of all classes, but IgG predominates.[58] Autoantibody titers generally increase with the age of the animal. Several months after the appearance of these autoantibodies, most animals will develop an autoimmune hemolytic anemia with marked reticulocytosis and spherocytosis. Many develop splenomegaly with extramedullary hematopoiesis and some develop hepatomegaly as well. The severity of the anemia worsens with age and is a frequent cause of death.

Fifty per cent of NZB mice have azotemia at the time of death. However, renal failure is not a frequent cause of mortality. Renal biopsy typically reveals a pathologically severe membranous glomerulonephritis, although only rarely are there accompanying signs of clinical deterioration. A small percentage of animals eventually go on to develop a severe proliferative glomerulonephritis.

About 50 per cent of NZB mice produce low titers of autoantibodies against DNA by the time they reach nine months of age. The production of antinuclear antibodies, of which anti-DNA antibodies are clearly representative, is one of the hallmarks of many animal and human autoimmune diseases, and can contribute significantly to overall morbidity and mortality. The NZB mouse provides an excellent illustration of the clinical importance of antinuclear antibodies. IgG and complement can be readily demonstrated in the renal lesions of these animals. DNA can also be detected in these lesions, and about 50 per cent of the kidney-bound IgG has specificity for nuclear antigens.[59] It is believed that circulating immune complexes of antibody and nuclear antigens deposit in the kidney and are responsible for much of the damage that is observed there. A small percentage of the IgG has specificity for antigens of the Gross leukemia virus, a hint at a possible viral etiology for NZB mouse disease (see below).[59]

A final aspect of the remarkable pathogenic process in these animals is a pronounced proliferation of lymphoid cells throughout the body. An increase in serum IgG levels can be noted even before the onset of autoimmune phenomena.[58] When the animals are between 3 and 11 months of age lymphoid hyperplasia is evident in the spleen, lymph nodes, thymus, lungs and liver,[60] and may eventually give way to a massive proliferation of plasma cells and reticulum cells. There may be pronounced splenomegaly and lymphadenopathy. Follicular aggregates of lymphoid cells may appear in the thymus. The thymus of the NZB mouse also displays a marked decrease in a number of epithelial cells.[61] About 20 per cent of NZB mice develop a frank malignancy, usually a thymoma, a pleomorphic lymphoma, or a reticulum-cell sarcoma.

NZB mice live for an average of about 15 to 18 months. The most common cause of death is hemolytic anemia, but death from renal failure or malignancy can occur.

NATURAL HISTORY OF THE NZB/W MOUSE

The clinical course of the NZB/W mouse is extremely severe, terminating in a rapidly progressive membranoproliferative glomerulonephritis, usually around one year of age. Some animals will produce antibodies against erythrocyte antigens and a few will develop a hemolytic anemia, but this is almost always of less clinical significance than the production of antinuclear antibodies. Antinuclear antibodies can first be detected by two months of age, and are present in all animals who live to be one year old. They are heterogeneous, and among their antigenic targets are single-stranded RNA and DNA, double-stranded RNA and DNA, nucleic acid-protein complexes, and nuclear protein. The anti-DNA antibodies are felt to be primarily responsible for the severe renal disease.[62] As with the NZB mouse, antibodies with specificity for both nuclear and viral antigens can be eluted from the renal lesions.[59]

Lymphoproliferation is also observed in these animals and thymic lesions have been noted.[61] A proliferation of lymphoid cells in the lacrimal and salivary glands may resemble Sjögren's syndrome (see below). Only 1 to 5 per cent of NZB/W mice develop a lymphoid malignancy (usually thymoma), but this low figure may be attributed to their short life span.

Immunologic Dysfunction of the New Zealand Mice

1. Early maturation of the immune system 1-week-old animals produce an adult-level antibody response to SRBCs and display an enhanced ability to reject sarcomas.
2. Enhanced humoral responsiveness until late in life
   a. Nonspecific increase in serum IgG levels
   b. Increased antibody responses to T-cell-dependent and T-cell-independent antigens
3. Diminished cellular reactivity with aging; 6-month-old animals demonstrate:
   a. Decreased reactivity to T-cell mitogens
   b. Decreased graft-versus-host reactivity
   c. Decreased ability to reject tumors
4. Loss of ability to be tolerized
   a. To foreign proteins and viral antigens
   b. To self-components: production of antinuclear and antierythrocyte Ab
5. Production of a thymocytotoxic antibody
6. Loss of thymosin-like activity in serum by 2 months of age
7. Lymphoid hyperplasia may develop into a frank malignancy.

IMMUNOLOGY AND PATHOGENESIS OF NEW ZEALAND MOUSE DISEASE

The production of antibodies against erythrocyte antigens and antinuclear antibodies is the most striking evidence that something is wrong with these animals' immune systems. In general, the immune dysfunction of the New Zealand mice can be viewed as one of B-cell hyperreactivity and depressed T-cell activity.[56]

The New Zealand mice show an early maturation of both the humoral and cellular limbs of the immune system. Thus one-week-old animals produce adult-level antibody responses to sheep erythrocytes, and their enhanced ability to reject virally induced sarcomas testifies to a prematurely competent cellular response.[63-65] However, their enhanced cellular reactivity is lost with aging. When these animals are about six months of age one can demonstrate a decreased responsiveness to T-cell mitogens and a diminished ability to partake in graft-versus-host reactions or to reject tumors.[66,67]

The humoral response remains hyperactive until late in the animal's life. There is an enhanced antibody response to T-cell-independent antigens (such as pneumococcal polysaccharide and synthetic nucleic acids) and to certain T-cell-dependent antigens (for example, sheep erythrocytes and various foreign proteins). These responses decline as the animals age.[68]

Final evidence of immune dysfunction is the rapid loss of tolerance to self and foreign proteins. The former is clearly evident in the production of autoantibodies. The latter can be demonstrated by administering deaggregated bovine gammaglobulin (BGG) to very young animals. Ordinarily, this regimen is tolerogenic, but the New Zealand mice are unable to be successfully tolerized.[69] Another example is the production of antibodies to Gross leukemia viral antigens. Like other mice, the New Zealand mice carry the Gross leukemia virus throughout life, but unlike other animals, they break tolerance and begin to produce antibodies against this agent.[70]

An explanation for these immunologic abnormalities has been suggested by the following experiments.[71] Neonatal thymectomy has been found to accelerate the autoimmune disease of the New Zealand mice, whereas thymectomy in 10-week-old mice has no effect on the course of the disease. This result indicates that a population of suppressor cells is present in the thymus of very young New Zealand mice, but disappears by the time the animals are 10 weeks old. Confirmation of this hypothesis has been obtained by demonstrating that the consequences of neonatal thymectomy can be prevented by transplanting 2-week-old thymuses into thymectomized hosts. Thymic cells from 1-month-old mice are also able to reduce the excess antibody responses of 10-month-old NZB mice. A loss of T suppressor cells could account for the humoral hyper-responsiveness and the loss of tolerance to self and foreign antigens. The rapid decline in cell-mediated immunity could be attributed to a subsequent loss of other T-cell subpopulations, for example, T killer cells.

We need finally to consider the possible etiology of the immune defects and severe disease of the NZB and NZB/W mice. Essentially three types of pathogenetic mechanisms have been proposed: genetic, immunologic and viral.

Genetic Factors

The definitive association of these immunologic and pathologic processes with the New Zealand mice clearly establishes a genetic basis for the disease. However, it has proved extremely difficult to define the precise mode of inheritance; backcross studies have not been very illuminating. Most observers feel that several genes are involved.

Immunologic Factors

It is very possible that a genetic abnormality predisposes to an immunologic defect. Two immune mechanisms have been suggested to explain the general decline in T-cell function:

All NZB mice produce a natural thymocytotoxic antibody (NTA) which is detectable by three months of age. Fifty per cent of NZB/W mice produce similar antibodies within three to six months.[72,73] Although occasionally present in other strains, NTA is only found in high titers in the New Zealand mice. NTA is an IgM that reacts optimally at 4°C. but is also reactive at 37°C. It appears to react only against T cells, and promotes their phagocytosis *in vitro*. The *in vivo* significance of NTA has not yet been established.

In Chapter 5 we explored the possibility that thymic hormones may be essential for maintaining normal T-cell function *in vivo*. Thymosinlike activity has been found to disappear from the serum of NZB and NZB/W mice by two months of age.[74] However, reports that exogenous thymosin restores certain T-cell functions of these animals *in vitro*[75,76] have been countered by claims that replacement with thymic extracts does not affect the natural history of these animals.[76a] Interestingly, thymosin is felt to be a product of the thymic epithelium which has been shown to be abnormal in the New Zealand mice.

Viral Factors

The presence of murine leukemia viral antigens and antibody directed against those antigens in the kidney eluates of NZB and NZB/W mice with glomerulonephritis has been offered as evidence of a viral etiology.[70,77] More detailed analysis has shown that the major envelope glycoprotein of the leukemia virus is the primary viral antigen deposited in the kidney.[78] C-type viral particles can be easily demonstrated by electron microscopy almost everywhere in these animals.[57] There are several reports that various manifestations of New Zealand mouse disease can be transmitted to healthy recipients with cell-free filtrates of NZB tissues and cells, but other investigators have failed to confirm this.[57,79-81]

It is important to emphasize that the presence of abnormal amounts of viral antigens and antibodies could well be secondary to a primary immune dysfunction. On the other hand, a virus might be responsible for the immunologic abnormalities in any of a number of ways (see earlier in this chapter). One interesting possibility has been raised by a report that thymocytes carrying a murine leukemia virus are cytotoxic for syngeneic tissues *in vitro*.[82]

Summary

In summary, the NZB and NZB/W mice pursue characteristic courses marked by profound immunologic and pathologic changes. The etiology of New Zealand mouse disease has not been firmly established, but genetic, immunologic and viral factors may all be important. Many of the features of New Zealand mouse disease closely mimic various human diseases. Most prominent among these are the rheumatic, or connective tissue diseases, and we shall look at these next.

SYSTEMIC LUPUS ERYTHEMATOSUS

The most distinctive feature of SLE is its ability to involve almost any tissue of the body to varying extents in different people. The protean manifestations and diverse presentation of the disease have necessitated the development of criteria for establishing a diagnosis of SLE. These classification criteria are listed below.[83] Even these criteria are often inadequate to differentiate SLE from other connective tissue disorders.

The A.R.A. Criteria for the Diagnosis of Systemic Lupus Erythematosus

A patient having any 4 of the following manifestations is said to have SLE:

1. Facial erythema (butterfly rash)
2. Discoid lupus (erythematous skin lesions with scaling and follicular plugging)
3. Raynaud's phenomenon
4. Alopecia
5. Photosensitivity
6. Oral or nasopharyngeal ulceration
7. Arthritis without deformity
8. Positive LE cell prep
9. Chronic false-positive STS
10. Proteinuria greater than 3.5 gm. per day
11. Cellular casts
12. Pleuritis or pericarditis
13. Psychosis or convulsions
14. Hemolytic anemia or leukopenia (WBC<4000) or thrombocytopenia (platelets <100,000)

SLE can present acutely as a rapidly progressing, systemic disease with fever, cutaneous manifestations, synovial effusions, polyarthritis and central nervous system disease, or it may pursue an indolent course marked by spontaneous remissions and exacerbations with the only clinical symptoms being malaise, myalgias and arthralgias. In one large study, 95 per cent of patients had musculoarticular symptoms, 81 per cent had cutaneous symptoms, 77 per cent had fever, 59 per cent had neuropsychiatric manifestations, 53 per cent had renal involvement, 48 per cent had pulmonary involvement, and 38 per cent had cardiac involvement at some time during the course of their illness.[84] Renal failure is the primary cause of death, but the complications of long-term steroid therapy also make a significant contribution to mortality of patients with long-standing disease.[85]

Three patterns of renal involvement are recognized histologically: focal glomerulonephritis, diffuse proliferative glomerulonephritis and membranous glomerulonephritis.[86] It is now believed that these patterns are not static within a given patient, but can progress one to the other. The renal disease occurs on an immune complex basis, with nuclear antigen-antibody complexes probably the major culprits (see below and also Chap. 7).

The cutaneous manifestations of SLE are often pronounced, but are not specific for the disease. Dermatologic findings include erythema (the typical butterfly rash), scaling, follicular plugging, telangiectasias and photosensitivity; the lesions may progress to scarring and atrophy.[87] Immune complexes can be detected at the dermal-epidermal junction. A detailed discussion of the immune complex etiology of the skin lesions of SLE can be found in Chapter 15.

There are few characteristic pathologic findings in SLE. One is present in the renal glomerulus, and involves basement-membrane thickening and the presence of hyaline thrombi and hematoxylin bodies in the renal capillaries. Hematoxylin bodies are free cell nuclei which have been coated with IgG and, as a result, swell to give a homogenous, ground-glass appearance. When they are phagocytosed by neutrophils, they give rise to the typical LE cell (Fig. 8-12). The LE cell is found most frequently in SLE but can also be demonstrated in other rheumatic and inflammatory diseases.

Other pathologic findings include a vasculitis of varying intensity and distribution, and periarteriolar fibrosis in the spleen, often felt to be characteristic of SLE. There have been reports that the thymus in some SLE patients is small and atrophic with marked cortical lymphocytic depletion, disorganization, cystic Hassall's corpuscles, and the formation of aggregates of epithelial cells.[88,89] These thymic abnormalities correspond to those of the New Zealand mice, but their significance remains unclear.

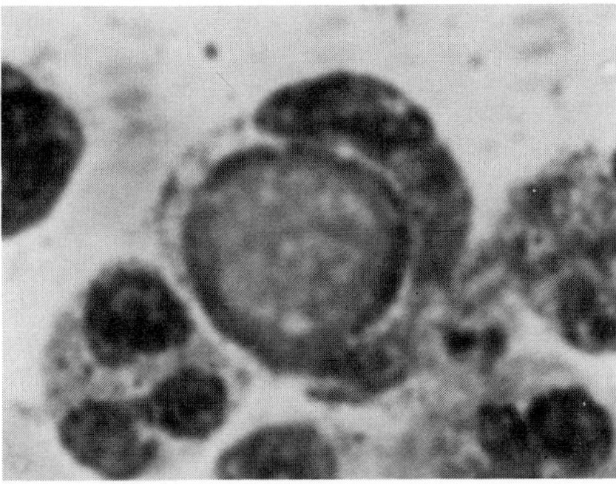

Fig. 8-12. An LE cell.

IMMUNOLOGY

Patients with SLE have numerous abnormalities of both the humoral and cellular limbs of the immune system. Abnormalities of the former have been much more carefully defined and are probably more significant in the overall disease process.

Patients with active SLE have a pronounced hypergammaglobulinemia consisting primarily of IgG and reflecting an increase in immunoglobulin synthesis per cell.[89a] Most notable, however, is the abundant production of a vast, heterogeneous array of autoantibodies. These are predominantly IgG, but IgM autoantibodies are present as well.[90] One can detect antibodies against erythrocyte antigens, antibodies to platelets and clotting factors which can lead to hemostatic abnormalities,[91] antibodies to lymphocytes (see below), antibodies responsible for a false-positive syphilis test, and antinuclear antibodies. Included in the last category are the antibodies responsible for the LE cell phenomenon (the nuclear antigen is a DNA-histone complex)[92] and antibodies to DNA, RNA and other nuclear antigens. Anticytoplasmic antibodies are also present. Patients may also have antibodies to double-stranded RNA, not a constituent of normal human cells.[93]

Antibody to DNA is most closely correlated with active disease and renal involvement.[94-96] Anti-DNA antibodies

Nuclear and Cytoplasmic Antigenic Targets of Autoantibody Production in SLE

Nuclear
DNA
DNA-histone
Nuclear RNA-protein
  a. Ribonuclease-insensitive component (Sm)
  b. Ribonuclease-digestible component (ENA)
Histone
Nucleolar antigen (precursor rRNA?)

Cytoplasmic
Ribosomes
Ro
Cytoplasmic RNA-protein (La)
Single-stranded RNA

Other
Double-stranded RNA
DNA-RNA hybrids

and DNA antigen have been eluted from the kidneys of patients with SLE nephritis, and it is believed that immune complexes of DNA–anti-DNA are responsible for the renal damage of SLE.[97] These complexes can fix complement. In general, patients with anti-DNA antibodies and depressed complement levels are most likely to have renal involvement.[94]

Decreased complement titers have been correlated with active disease.[8] Both the classical and the properdin complement pathways are activated and components of each can be found deposited along the glomerular basement membrane.[99,100] However, several studies have shown that the major reason for the decline in complement titers in patients with SLE is the decreased synthesis of complement components.[101,102] Complexes of DNA–anti-DNA and decreased complement levels are also found in the cerebrospinal fluid of patients with lupus meningitis.[103,104]

An antibody present in patients with SLE that has excited great interest is the antibody directed against double-stranded RNA. High titers of these antibodies are found only in patients with SLE, and approximately 40 to 50 per cent of patients with SLE have anti-double-stranded RNA antibody.[105,106] The antibody will react with synthetic and viral double-stranded RNA, but not with single-stranded RNA. The presence of anti-double-stranded RNA antibodies has been interpreted as evidence of a viral infection in patients with SLE.

A nuclear antigen which may prove to be of special clinical significance has only recently been described and has been termed extractable nuclear antigen (ENA).[107] ENA appears to be a complex of nuclear RNA and protein and may be a part of the chromosomal structure.[93,108] Patients who possess antibodies to the ribonuclease-insensitive component of ENA are virtually indistinguishable from other patients with SLE (about 50 per cent of patients with SLE have antibody to ENA).[109,110] However, patients with antibodies to the ribonuclease-sensitive component have been recognized as comprising a unique clinical syndrome now called *mixed connective tissue disease.*[110] These patients express features of SLE, progressive systemic sclerosis and polymyositis. The most common clinical symptoms include arthritis and/or arthralgias, swollen hands, Raynaud's phenomenon, abnormal esophageal motility, myositis and lymphadenopathy. About 80 per cent of patients with mixed connective tissue disease have hypergammaglobulinemia.

The identification of a group of patients with this particular constellation of findings has been reported to be of prognostic significance. In general, patients with mixed connective tissue disease have been described as responding favorably to corticosteroid therapy and having a very low incidence of nephritis.[110] Interestingly, these patients rarely possess antibodies to native DNA, and then it is only of a very low titer. It has therefore been suggested that antibodies to the ribonuclease-digestible portion of ENA may have a protective value for the host. The mechanism for such an effect is unknown, although one possibility that has been raised is that anti-ENA antibodies prevent the formation of DNA–anti-DNA complexes. Since ENA seems to be a part of the human chromosome, antibodies to ENA might conceivably block the antigenic sites on native DNA. Preliminary work has shown that injections of ENA into NZB/W mice significantly reduce the severity of their renal disease.[111]

The role of cell-mediated immunity in SLE has not been clearly established. Certain patients with SLE appear to have a pronounced depression in T-cell activity. These patients have a decreased percentage of peripheral blood lymphocytes bearing T-cell markers.[112,113] In addition, several observers have reported a diminished *in vitro* T-cell response to mitogens and antigens, as well as a decreased reactivity to skin test antigens.[114-118] The degree of T-cell depression has been correlated with the extent of disease activity. This evidence of depressed immune function may partially explain the increased susceptibility to infection of patients with SLE.[119]

Two immune mechanisms have been offered to explain the compromised T-cell function, and these are similar to the explanations offered for the New Zealand mice:

1. The serum from some patients with active disease has been shown to inhibit T-cell reactivity of autologous and normal heterologous lymphocytes.[115,120] Lymphocytotoxic IgG antibodies have been described, and these appear to be specific for T cells.[121-123] One additional study suggests that only a subpopulation of T cells may be susceptible.[124] It is still uncertain whether these antibodies are responsible for the inhibitory effects of SLE serum on T-cell function. It is also not known in what manner the lymphocytotoxic antibodies are destructive to T cells, although antibody-dependent cell-mediated cytotoxicity has been postulated.[124] The *in vivo* significance of these antibodies has recently been questioned since lymphocytotoxic activity does not correlate with the severity of SLE.[124a]

2. It has been suggested that a defect in thymosin production may be responsible for the diminished T-cell reactivity, although with considerably less evidence than for the NZB mouse. One *in vitro* study showed that the addition of thymosin could increase the percentage of sheep-erthrocyte-rosetting cells, but the significance of this finding remains obscure.[125]

PATHOGENESIS

Ideas similar to those that have been offered to explain the genesis of New Zealand mouse disease have been advanced to explain the etiology of SLE. We have already discussed the possible pathogenetic role of immune mechanisms and shall now focus on the genetic and viral factors.

Genetic Factors

A number of family studies have convincingly demonstrated a genetic element in SLE. The essential conclusions of these studies are as follows:

1. One to 2 per cent of the first-degree relatives of patients with SLE have the disease themselves.[126] This is considerably above the incidence of SLE in the general population. Several large family aggregates with SLE have been reported.[127]

2. Over 50 per cent of monozygotic twins, at least one of whom has SLE, have been found to be clinically concordant for SLE.[128] A similar high percentage has not been found for dizygotic twins.

3. There is an increased incidence of hypergammaglobulinemia and autoantibody production in otherwise healthy relatives of patients with SLE.[127,129]

Although little is known about the genetic basis for the inheritance of SLE, these studies are highly suggestive that some genetic factors are instrumental in this disease.

Viral Factors

Electron microscopic studies have revealed particles with a viral-like appearance in SLE tissues,but identical particles have been seen in other diseases, and may only represent a nonspecific product of tissue injury.[130] Electron microscopic studies have, in general, been inconclusive. Viral-core proteins have been detected in high concentrations in tissues of patients with SLE, and viral antigens are expressed on the surface of the lymphocytes of some patients with SLE.[131-133] The existence of antibodies to double-stranded RNA, an antigen found only in virally infected tissues, is further evidence for a viral presence in SLE. All of this data does not establish a viral etiology for SLE, but should provide a powerful stimulus for further investigation.

DRUG-INDUCED SLE

A large number of pharmacologic agents have been found that can induce a clinical picture very much like SLE.[134] These can be grouped into two broad categories:[135] (1) many drugs will occasionally elicit an allergic reaction which can lead to a full-blown SLE syndrome; (2) a smaller group of drugs induces antinuclear antibody production in a large percentage of patients taking the drugs for a long time, and an SLE syndrome in a smaller percentage of patients, presumably via a direct pharmacologic effect of the drugs themselves. We will focus on the latter class of drugs in the following discussion.

The most common offenders in this second group of drugs are hydralazine, isoniazid, procainamide, chlorpromazine and the hydantoins. The SLE-like syndrome that can result from (usually) chronic ingestion of these agents includes fever, arthritis, rash, polyserositis and the production of various autoantibodies. Renal disease is very rare, and this is the major distinction between the drug-induced syndrome and classical SLE.

Hydralazine-induced lupus has been the most carefully studied form of drug-induced lupus. Hydralazine can form complexes with nucleoprotein, and antibodies to the drug-nucleoprotein complex can be demonstrated.[136] There is, however, no evidence that hydralazine alters the antigenicity of the nuclear constituents.[137] More than 50 per cent of patients taking hydralazine for long periods of time develop antinuclear antibodies.[138] A clue to the predisposition of certain people to develop antinuclear antibodies while taking hydralazine has been obtained by studying the way in which these people metabolize the drug. Hydralazine is normally metabolized in the liver by an acetyltransferase. It has been shown that patients who are "slow acetylators," and in whom the drug has an increased half-life, are highly predisposed to develop antinuclear antibodies. All patients who go on to develop a lupus-like syndrome have been found to be slow acetylators.[138]

Isoniazid probably acts by a mechanism similar to hydralazine, but it is a less potent inducer of antinuclear antibodies. Patients receiving isoniazid do not develop anti-DNA antibodies, and this may be the explanation for the sparing of the kidneys in this and all forms of drug-induced lupus.

Procainamide also does not induce antibody to native DNA, but does induce autoantibodies to denatured DNA and nucleohistone.[139] Virtually all patients taking this drug develop antinuclear antibodies. Procainamide can be photochemically induced to complex to DNA, but whether such complexes form *in vivo* is unclear. Chlorpromazine can likewise be artificially linked to nucleic acids by ultraviolet light.[140]

Diphenylhydantoin and related anticonvulsants may elicit antinuclear antibody production by a different mechanism. Diphenylhydantoin increases membrane permeability and may be responsible for a leakage of soluble nuclear antigens out of cells.[135] It has also been hypothesized that diphenylhydantoin can bind to nuclear antigens and perhaps alter their antigenicity.

ANTINUCLEAR ANTIBODY FLUORESCENT PATTERNS

Autoantibodies directed against nuclear antigens were first described in patients with SLE and have since been demonstrated in the other rheumatic diseases. They may also be present as an uncommon finding in several unrelated diseases, and on rare occasions in perfectly healthy individuals.

The ability to detect antinuclear antibodies has become a useful clinical tool with the development of immunofluorescent techniques. It is now recognized that antibodies to particular nuclear antigens are associated with specific patterns of nuclear immunofluorescence. The technique is rapid and accurate, and is performed as follows: cultured animal cells (e.g., African green monkey kidney cells) are incubated with the patient's serum at 37°C. for 30 minutes. The cells are washed and then incubated with fluorescein-labelled anti-immunoglobulin antisera for another 30 minutes. The label will be detectable only in those areas of the cells where the patient's serum antinuclear antibodies have bound.

In SLE and all of the rheumatic diseases with the exception of rheumatoid arthritis, IgG antinuclear antibody titers are much greater than the titers of IgM antinuclear antibodies, and the most valuable information is obtained using anti-IgG fluorescein-labelled antisera.

With this technique, several patterns of nuclear staining have been described (Fig. 8-13):[141]

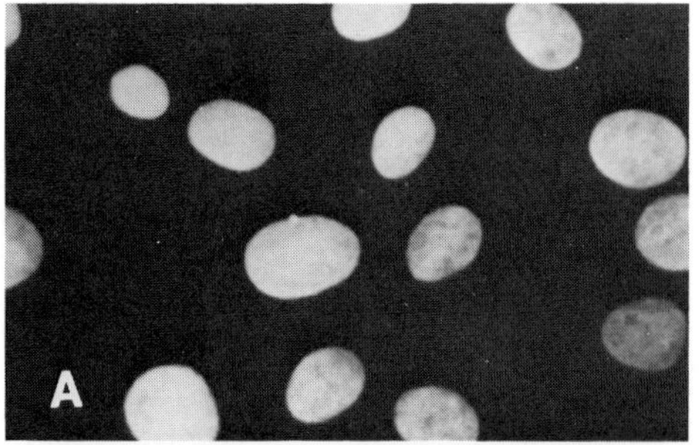

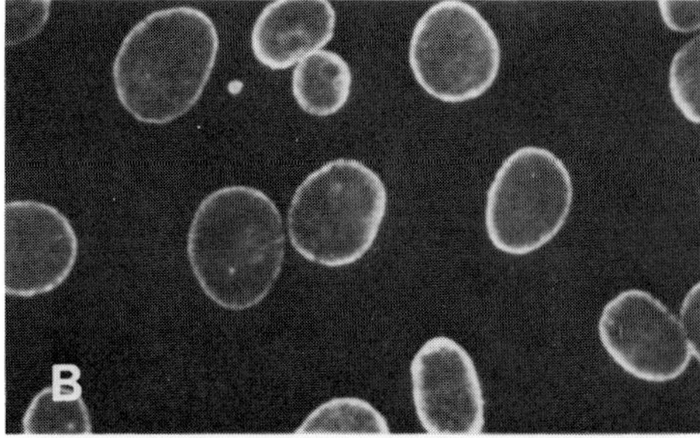

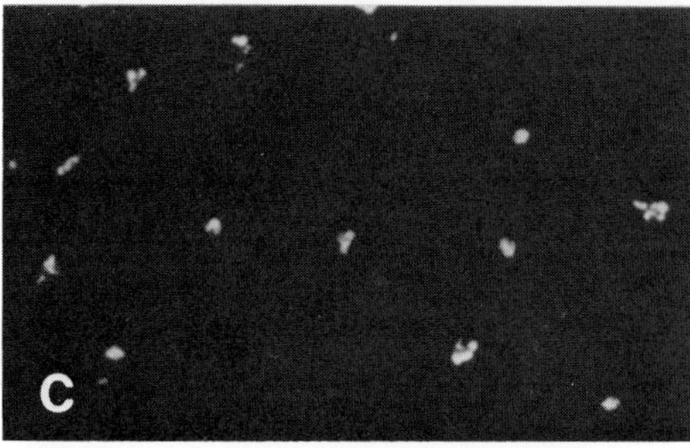

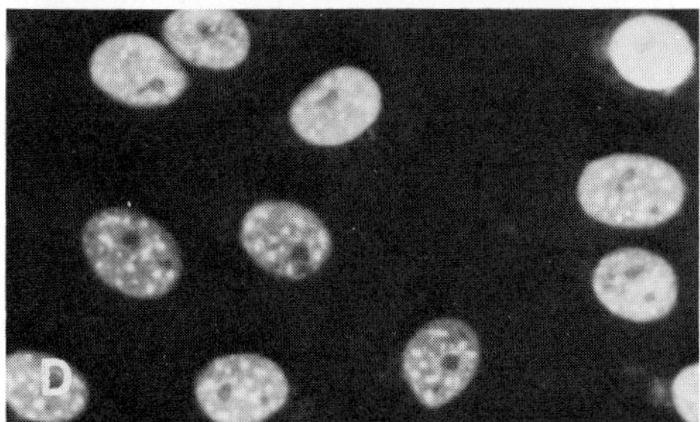

Fig. 8-13. Fluorescent antinuclear staining patterns: (*A*) homogeneous pattern; (*B*) peripheral pattern; (*C*) nucleolar pattern; (*D*) speckled pattern. (Parker, M.D., and Kerby, G. P.: Combined titre and fluorescent patterns of IgG antinuclear antibodies using cultured cell monolayers in evaluating connective tissue disorders. Ann. Rheum. Dis., *33*:465, 1974.)

1. *Homogeneous Pattern* (Fluorescence of the Entire Nucleus). This has been shown to be due to antibodies reacting with particulate nucleoprotein, the same antibodies responsible for the LE cell phenomenon.[142]

2. *Peripheral (Rim) Pattern* (Fluorescence of Just the Outer Edge of the Nucleus). It is associated with antibody to DNA and to soluble nucleoprotein.[143]

3. *Nucleolar Staining* (Fluorescence of Just the Nucleolus). This is most likely the result of reactivity with a precursor ribonucleoprotein.[144]

4. *Speckled Pattern* (an Irregular Salt and Pepper Appearance of the Entire Nucleus). This pattern can be produced by autoantibodies to at least two different antigenic targets. One is the Sm antigen, which is resistant to DNase, RNase and trypsin.[145] The second is the extractable ribonucleoprotein antigen that we have already discussed in association with mixed connective tissue disease.[146]

Patients with SLE can have very high titers of antinuclear antibodies and all patterns of nuclear staining can be seen, although the nucleolar pattern is very rare. The presence of a peripheral or a peripheral plus homogeneous pattern is seen almost exclusively in active SLE.[141] Since the peripheral pattern is associated with antibody to DNA, it is not surprising that it correlates very highly (85%) with the presence of nephritis. A solely homogeneous pattern with titers of greater than 1:640 is also seen virtually only in SLE. Regardless of the pattern of nuclear staining, the titers of antinuclear antibody correlate with the activity of the disease.

Patients with mixed connective tissue disease possess very high titers of antinuclear antibodies. The nuclear staining pattern is always speckled and can be removed with ribonuclease. The diagnosis of mixed connective tissue disease requires this RNase-digestible staining pattern and the typical clinical picture.

OTHER RHEUMATIC DISEASES

In the following paragraphs we shall be examining the immunologic features of the other rheumatic diseases with special emphasis on the patterns of antinuclear staining. It is important to note that with our increasing awareness of these diseases, the number of patients who both clinically and immunologically fall somewhere in between the classical descriptions below (the so-called overlap syndromes) is increasing. Thus, it is not unusual to find patients presenting with a clinical picture with features of several of these diseases. Evidence of autoimmunity is usually present but may not fall into one of the well-established patterns that we shall be describing. It may therefore be useful to consider the rheumatic diseases as lying along a spectrum of disease. Each disorder then represents a frequently encountered cluster of clinical and immunologic features. Such an interpretation could account for the existence of overlap syndromes as well as serve to focus our attention on understanding the pathogenesis of autoimmunity in general.

RHEUMATOID ARTHRITIS

Rheumatoid arthritis is extremely common, affecting as many as 3 per cent of adult females and 1 per cent of adult males. Specific criteria for making the diagnosis of rheumatoid arthritis have been established by the American Rheumatism Association.[147] Like SLE, the course of rheumatoid arthritis is variable, with frequent remissions and exacerbations. Often the disease is mild, affecting only a limited number of joints and causing little functional disability. The disease may even disappear entirely. However, the inflammatory process will often persist, eventually leading to joint destruction and deformity. The joints most often affected are the small joints of the hands (the proximal interphalangeal (PIP) and metacarpophalangeal (MCP) joints) and feet, the wrists and the knees. However, any articular surface can be affected. Involvement is usually bilaterally symmetrical, and can be recognized by the symptoms of pain, warmth, swelling and tenderness of the joint. Constitutional symptoms are usually associated with, and may precede, active joint disease. Fever is very common. Fifteen to 20 per cent of patients develop subcutaneous nodules over pressure points. In occasional patients, the disease is unusually aggressive and produces rapidly progressive joint destruction. This form of the disease is often referred to as "malignant rheumatoid arthritis," and is often associated with pleuritis, pericarditis, myocarditis, and all the evidence of an extensive vasculitis (digital gangrene, peripheral neuropathy, etc.).

Laboratory features often include a moderate anemia and a leukocytosis, although patients may present with leukopenia and splenomegaly (Felty's syndrome, see Chap. 14). Hypergammaglobulinemia is usually present. Among the abnormal immunoglobulins present are rheumatoid factor and various antinuclear antibodies. A complete discussion of the etiology and clinical importance of rheumatoid factor was presented in Chapter 7.

Fewer than 50 per cent of patients with rheumatoid arthritis possess antinuclear antibodies. The IgG antinuclear antibody titers are rarely high and do not exceed 1:160. The presence of IgG antinuclear antibodies does not appear to correlate with disease activity.[141] With rare exceptions, only homogeneous staining patterns with IgG are observed. Rheumatoid arthritis is the one rheumatic disease in which IgM antinuclear antibody titers often exceed IgG titers. The IgM staining pattern is frequently speckled.

PROGRESSIVE SYSTEMIC SCLEROSIS

Progressive systemic sclerosis (PSS) is a systemic disease of the connective tissue. The most obvious and most frequently encountered lesions are those of the skin (scleroderma). The patient's initial complaint is often that of Raynaud's phenomenon, or painless edema, tightening and thickening of the skin over the fingers. Visceral involvement most often affects the esophagus, but intestinal, pulmonary and myocardial fibrosis may also be seen. Renal disease is one of the most serious complications of PSS, and is often associated with an explosive malignant hypertension. Renal failure and malignant hypertension have been correlated with structural and functional changes in the circulation of the renal cortex.[148] Other manifestations of PSS include arthritis, myopathy and pathologic calcification of the soft tissues (calcinosis). Fever is common in patients with active disease, and anemia may accompany visceral involvement. Serologic findings include hypergammaglobulinemia in about 50 per cent of patients, and a positive rheumatoid factor and LE cell prep in some patients.

Cutaneous involvement is characterized by edema, inflammation and fibrosis. Skin biopsy reveals an increased density of collagen in the dermis, and this appears to be the result of increased collagen synthesis. Amino acid analysis has revealed no striking differences between PSS collagen fibrils and fibrils from normal individuals. Some investigators have suggested that abnormal aggregation of the collagen fibrils may be responsible for the skin lesions.[149]

An immunologic pathogenesis for PSS has been proposed on the evidence of a systemic vasculitis, the existence of an overlap syndrome with SLE (mixed connective tissue disease), the finding of immunoglobulin and complement in the kidneys of patients with PSS, and the presence of antinuclear antibodies. However, although immunoglobulin and complement can be found in diseased renal arterioles, the sites of IgG and C3 deposition do not appear to correlate well with sites of renal damage.[150,151]

Patients with PSS almost invariably have antinuclear antibodies, often in very high titers. Both nucleolar and speckled patterns have been described, the former being the more common. The presence of high titers of antinuclear antibodies giving a nucleolar pattern is seen almost exclusively in PSS.

POLYMYOSITIS

Polymyositis is an inflammatory disease of the muscles which, when accompanied by cutaneous manifestations, is referred to as *dermatomyositis*. Often a difficult diagnosis to make, five criteria have recently been recommended for defining these disease entities:[152] (1) symmetrical weakness of the proximal musculature progressing over weeks to months. This most often affects the limb-girdle muscles, the anterior neck flexors, and sometimes the respiratory muscles. (2) Muscle biopsy evidence of necrosis with an inflammatory infiltrate; (3) elevation in muscle enzymes, especially creatine phosphokinase, and often aldolase, lactate dehydrogenase, and the serum transaminases; (4) characteristic electromyographic findings; (5) for the diagnosis of dermatomyositis, the presence of characteristic cutaneous lesions. These include an erythematous dermatitis over the dorsum of the hands, as well as the knees, elbows, face and upper torso, and a purple-hued heliotrope rash on the upper eyelids. Atypical skin lesions such as sclerodermatous changes and atrophy may occasionally be seen.

The most frequent clinical complaints are due to muscular involvement, and can include weakness, dysphagia and dysphonia. In addition, patients often complain of Raynaud's phenomenon and a mild, often transitory, arthritis. Serologic findings include elevated muscle enzymes, frequently a positive rheumatoid factor, and hypergammaglobulinemia. Antinuclear antibodies are not always detectable and are never present in very high titers.[141] Positive LE cell preps are rare.

An immunologic basis for polymyositis has been suggested by the presence of chronic inflammatory cells in the muscular lesions. IgG, IgM and complement have been detected in the blood vessel walls of skeletal muscles in approximately 40 per cent of patients.[153] Antimyosin and anti-whole-muscle antibodies have been found in the sera of patients with polymyositis, but can also be found in other dystrophic and neurogenic disorders.[154] There have been several reports that lymphocytes from patients with active disease are toxic to autologous and fetal muscle preparations, suggesting a possible role for cell-mediated immunity in the tissue destruction of polymyositis.[155,156]

One puzzling aspect of this disorder is the high coincidence rate of malignancy. Although figures as high as 70 per cent have been quoted, the frequency of associated malignancy probably approaches 15 per cent.[152,157] Neoplasia develops most commonly in men over the age of fifty with dermatomyositis. Although this is an intriguing association, its implications in terms of the pathogenesis of dermatomyositis remain obscure. The etiology of polymyositis remains unknown. A viral mechanism has been suggested on the basis of reports of viral-like structures in the muscle cells of affected patients, but these claims are subject to the same objections as the reports of similar structures in SLE.[158]

SJÖGREN'S SYNDROME

Sjögren's syndrome is characterized by keratoconjunctivitis sicca and xerostomia (dry eyes and dry mouth) due to reduced secretion of the lacrimal and salivary glands (sicca complex). About 50 per cent of these patients have an associated connective tissue disease, most commonly rheumatoid arthritis. About 10 to 15 per cent of patients with rheumatoid arthritis have Sjögren's syndrome. Complications of diminished lacrimal and salivary gland secretions include ulceration of the cornea, difficulty with talking and chewing, ulcers of the tongue, lips and buccal membranes, and dental caries. Occasionally the dryness may extend to affect the nose, pharynx, larynx and the rest of the tracheobronchial tree. About half the patients have parotid gland enlargement that is often accompanied by fever.

Serologic findings can include anemia, leukopenia, hypergammaglobulinemia and a positive rheumatoid factor. Some patients present with splenomegaly, leukopenia and leg ulcers, as in Felty's syndrome, even without an accompanying arthritis. LE cells are often present, and about 50 per cent of patients have detectable antinuclear antibodies.[159] Antinuclear antibodies are more common in people with sicca complex plus rheumatoid arthritis than sicca complex alone. A homogeneous pattern is most common although low-titer nucleolar and speckled patterns can occur.[160] Antibodies to native DNA are not found. Many patients have antibodies to salivary duct antigens,[160] including about 10 to 20 per cent of patients with sicca complex alone and nearly two thirds of patients with sicca complex plus rheumatoid arthritis.[161] Antibodies to salivary duct antigens rarely appear in patients with rheumatoid arthritis alone.

Renal involvement is uncommon in Sjögren's syndrome, and this may be partially due to the absence of antibodies to native DNA. When renal disease does occur, it is the result of a direct infiltration of lymphocytes and plasma cells and not secondary to immune complex deposition. Glomerular disease does not occur; the most common renal lesion is renal tubular acidosis.[162]

The characteristic histologic lesion of the involved glands is an infiltrate of lymphocytes and plasma cells. There are reports that the majority of infiltrating cells are B cells, although some investigators have described the presence of both B and T cells.[163,164] In either case, the lymphoid infiltrates produce high amounts of immunoglobulin, including specific antibodies such as rheumatoid factor.[161] The disease process is usually benign and the cellular infiltrate is most often confined to the secretory glands per se. However, in some patients the lymphoid infiltrate extends beyond the glands to involve the lymph nodes, lung, kidney and bone marrow. These cells can form tumorlike aggregates to give the picture of *pseudolymphoma*. The diffuse lymph-node involvement of pseudolymphoma may mimic active lymphoma, but the infiltrating cells are histologically benign.[161,165] In some individuals the disease process eventually acquires the characteristics of a malignancy, most commonly lymphoma, reticulum cell sarcoma or Waldenström's macroglobulinemia.[161,165]

RHEUMATIC HEART DISEASE: AUTOIMMUNITY ASSOCIATED WITH CROSSREACTING ANTIGENS

Rheumatic heart disease most commonly affects the endocardium with valvular involvement, but can also affect the myocardium and pericardium. Fever and arthritis are the most frequent accompanying symptoms. The disease is initiated by infection with group A streptococci. The characteristic pathologic lesion is the granulomatous Aschoff body. Areas of chronic inflammatory infiltration and myocardial degeneration, although less specific for rheumatic heart disease, are also present.

An immunologic basis for this disease has been suspected for a long time, and an impressive array of supportive evidence has been accumulated.[166,167] The first significant finding was the detection of autoantibodies directed against the patients' own heart tissue in the serum of affected patients. These autoantibodies may be detected either before or after the appearance of clinical evidence of rheumatic fever. In some patients, the titer and frequency of positive tests for anti-heart antibodies correlate with the presence and severity of active disease.

Investigators were next able to demonstrate that group A streptococci possess antigens which crossreact with human heart tissue. Several different streptococcal antigens present in both the bacterial cell wall and cell membrane appear to crossreact with components of the human heart, including the myocardium and heart valves. Other human tissues also crossreact with streptococcal antigens, including cartilage, smooth muscle, skeletal muscle, and the renal glomerular basement membrane. Antibodies to the glomerular basement membrane may play a role in chronic poststreptococal glomerulonephritis.

Patients with rheumatic heart disease possess high titers of crossreactive antibodies in their sera. Thus, if the sera of these patients is first absorbed with group A streptococci, no reactivity against heart tissue remains.

Autopsy studies of rheumatic hearts have revealed the presence of local deposits of immunoglobulin and complement in the myocardium and heart valves. The distribution of these antibodies corresponds to the sites where the crossreacting antibodies can be shown to bind to heart tissue *in vitro*. This evidence is highly suggestive that circulating crossreacting antibodies bind to the hearts of affected patients *in vivo*.

Despite the weight of this accumulated data, it has still not been shown that these crossreacting antibodies are responsible for the cardiac lesions of rheumatic heart disease rather than representing simply a nonspecific response to cardiac injury. In fact, there is evidence that these antibodies are not toxic to heart tissue *in vitro* unless the tissue has been previously damaged by some other agent.[168] Anti-heart antibodies can also be demonstrated in many patients with streptococcal infections but without any evidence of cardiac disease. The pathogenic significance of the crossreacting antibodies in patients with rheumatic heart disease clearly needs further evaluation.

AUTOANTIBODIES ASSOCIATED WITH PRIOR TISSUE DAMAGE: POST-MYOCARDIAL INFARCTION SYNDROME (DRESSLER'S SYNDROME)

Following a myocardial infarction, approximately 3 per cent of patients exhibit a syndrome of clinical findings referred to as post-myocardial infarction syndrome, or Dressler's syndrome. This can develop anywhere from several days to several months after the initial insult, and includes fever and chest pain which may radiate to the neck, back and epigastrium. There is often an accompanying pericarditis and pleuritis with effusions, and not infrequently patients will complain of myalgias and arthralgias. Symptomatic relief is often obtained with corticosteroid therapy.

One fourth to one third of patients with post-myocardial infarction develop anti-heart antibodies.[169] These antibodies appear to be directed against multiple antigens but do not react with streptococcal antigens. Anti-heart antibodies are present in patients with the clinical syndrome described above but are also found in patients without any post-myocardial infarction symptomatology.[170] It is thus unlikely that anti-heart antibodies alone are responsible for the post-myocardial infarction syndrome. Most observers feel that these antibodies represent a harmless response to prior tissue injury, and are not instrumental in the pathogenesis of the post-myocardial infarction syndrome.

IMMUNOLOGIC STATUS OF THE FETUS

The immunologic status of the fetus presents one of the most fascinating problems in tolerance. Since the fetus inherits genes from both parents, the fetus should express cell-surface antigenic determinants of both the mother and the father. One of the oldest dilemmas in immunology is how the fetus, expressing paternal antigens, escapes immunologic rejection by the mother.

One of the earliest theories was that the uterus might be an immunologically privileged site, in some way exempt from interaction with the immune system. This view is no longer tenable since there have now been many demonstrations of immunologic reactivity occurring within the uterus.[171,172]

Investigation in this field next shifted to the trophoblast, the physiologic barrier between the mother and the fetus. The trophoblast is genetically identical to the fetus and its cells are in direct contact with maternal blood. Some observers have suggested that the trophoblast might be deficient in transplantation antigens, but this does not appear to be true.[173-175] An alternate possibility is that the trophoblast secretes a substance which coats its surface, thereby masking any surface-expressed transplantation antigens. A sialomucinlike substance has been described which may partly serve this function. However, it has been shown that this barrier is incomplete, and further, that maternal cellular elements may be able to cross into the fetal circulation.[176,177] Thus, the existence of a nonspecific masking substance by itself does not appear to account for fetal survival, although it may be a contributing factor.

The most rewarding studies have focused on the immunologic status of the mother. Several investigators have presented evidence indicating a generalized depression of the maternal immune system during pregnancy. These findings have included negative skin testing, diminished reactivity to mitogen stimulation *in vitro*, and delayed rejection of skin grafts.[174,178,179] However, a large percentage of pregnant women respond normally by these parameters.

Others have sought to determine whether the maternal serum might possess some substance (or substances) which could act as a general immune depressant. There have been two leading candidates:

1. *Glucocorticoids.* During pregnancy there is an increase in the maternal production of glucocorticoids, but this has not been shown to make a significant contribution to maternal immunosuppression.[180]

2. *Gestational Hormones.* One of the hallmarks of pregnancy is the production of placental hormones including human choriogonadotropin (HCG). There are several reports that HCG can act as a powerful immunosuppressant.[181,182] However, most of these studies have employed supraphysiologic doses of HCG or have made use of experimental animals whose immunocompetent cells may differ greatly from human cells in their response to this hormone. In one very careful study using human cells and human sera, physiologic levels of HCG were demonstrated to be ineffective in depressing lymphocyte function.[183] Only levels several times higher than those obtained in maternal serum during pregnancy were found to be suppressive. It has been suggested, however, that very high local concentrations of gestational hormones could be maintained at the fetal-maternal interface such that a serum measurement would not reflect this local accumulation.[184] Such a possibility has not been adequately tested.

Recent work has implicated another serum factor in permitting fetal survival, and this may turn out to be of great importance. When trophoblast cells are cultured *in vitro* with maternal cells, a potent cytotoxic reaction usually occurs. This finding indicates not only that the mother is sensitized against fetal antigens, but that she possesses antifetal cytotoxic cells. However, the cytotoxic effect of these maternal cells can be blocked by the addition of maternal serum to the *in vitro* culture medium. The nature of the blocking substance in the serum has not been well characterized, but may be IgG.[185,186] In most studies, this blocking factor appears to be specific for the paternal antigen. The importance of blocking antibodies and antigen-antibody complexes in other systems is discussed in Chapter 13.

REFERENCES

1. Owen, R. D.: Immunogenetic consequences of vascular anastomoses between bovine twins. Science, *102*:400, 1945.
2. Billingham, R. E., Brent, L., and Medawar, P. B.: Actively acquired tolerance of foreign cells. Nature, *172*:603, 1953.
3. Brent, L., and Gowland, G.: Cellular dose and age of host in the induction of tolerance. Nature, *192*:1265, 1961.
4. Weigle, W. O.: Immunological unresponsiveness. Adv. Immunol., *16*:61, 1973.
5. Felton, L. D.: The significance of antigen in animal tissues. J. Immunol., *61*:107, 1949.
6. Howard, J. G.: Cellular events in the induction and loss of tolerance to pneumococcal polysaccharides. Transplant. Rev., *8*:50, 1972.
7. Weigle, W. O.: Immunological unresponsiveness. *In* Najarian, J., and Simmons, R. L. (eds.): Transplantation. P. 174. Philadelphia, Lea & Febiger, 1972.
8. Mitchison, N. A.: Induction of immunological paralysis in two zones of dosage. Proc. R. Soc. Lond. [Biol.], *161*:275, 1964.
9. Weigle, W. O.: *In* Katz, D. H., and Benacerraf, B. (eds.): Immunological Tolerance. P. 57. New York, Academic Press, 1974.
10. Chiller, J. M., Habicht, G. S., and Weigle, W. O.: Cellular sites of immunologic unresponsiveness. Proc. Natl. Acad. Sci., U.S.A., *65*:551, 1970.
11. ———: Kinetic differences in unresponsiveness of thymus and bone marrow cells. Science, *171*:813, 1971.
12. Sanfilippo, F., and Scott, D. W.: Cellular events in tolerance. III. Carrier tolerance as a model for T cell unresponsiveness. J. Immunol., *113*:1661, 1974.
13. Boyden, S. V.: The effect of previous injections of tuberculoprotein in the development of tuberculin sensitivity following BCG vaccination in guinea pigs. Br. J. Exp. Pathol., *38*:611, 1957.
14. Borel, Y., Fauconnet, M., and Miescher, P. A.: Selective suppression of delayed hypersensitivity by the induction of immunologic tolerance. J. Exp. Med., *123*:585, 1966.
15. Parish, C. R.: Immune response to chemically modified flagellin. J. Exp. Med., *134*:1, 21, 1971.
16. Dresser, D. W.: Specific inhibition of antibody production. II. Paralysis induced in adult mice by small quantities of protein antigen. Immunology, *5*:378, 1962.
17. Golub, E. S., and Weigle, W. O.: Studies on the induction of immunologic unresponsiveness. III. Antigen form and mouse strain variation. J. Immunol., *102*:389, 1969.
18. Das, S., and Leskowitz, S.: The cellular basis for tolerance or immunity to bovine-gamma-globulin in mice. J. Immunol., *112*:107, 1974.
19. Blaese, R. M.: Macrophages and the development of immunocompetence. *In* Bellanti, J. A., and Dayton, D. H. (eds.): The Phagocytic Cell in Host Resistance. P. 309. New York, Raven Press, 1975.
20. Diener, E., Kraft, N., Lee, K. C., and Shiozowa, C.: Antigen recognition. IV. Discrimination by antigen-binding immunocompetent B cells between immunity and tolerance is determined by adherent cells. J. Exp. Med., *143*:805, 1976.
21. Howard, J. G.: Immunological tolerance and immunosuppression. *In* Porter, R. R. (ed.): Defense and Recognition. P. 103. Baltimore, University Park Press, 1973.
22. Felton, L. D., Kauffmann, E., Prescott, B., and Ottinger, B.: Studies on the mechanism of the immunological paralysis induced in mice by pneumococcal polysaccharide. J. Immunol., *74*:17, 1955.
23. Janeway, C. A., and Sela, M.: Synthetic antigens composed exclusively of L- or D-amino acids. Immunology, *13*:29; *14*:225, 1967.
24. Howard, J. G., Christie, G. H., Jacob, M. J., and Elson, J.: Studies on immunological paralysis. Clin. Exp. Immunol., *7*:583, 1970.
25. Burnet, F.: The Clonal Selection Theory of Acquired Immunity. Cambridge, Cambridge University Press, 1959.
26. Lederberg, J.: Genes and antibodies. Science, *129*:1649, 1959.
27. Nossal, G. J. V.: Principles of immunological tolerance and immunocyte receptor blockade. Adv. Cancer Res., *20*:93, 1974.
28. Vitetta, E. S., and Uhr, J. W.: Immunoglobulin-receptors revisited. Science, *189*:964, 1975.
29. Allison, A. C.: *In* Katz, D. H., and Benecerraf, B. (eds.): Immunological Tolerance: Mechanisms and Potential Therapeutic Applications. P. 25. New York, Academic Press, 1974.
30. Clagett, J. A., and Weigle, W. O.: Roles of T and B lymphocytes in the termination of unresponsiveness to autologous thyroglobulin in mice. J. Exp. Med., *139*:643, 1974.
31. Unanue, E. R.: Antigen-binding cells. I. Their identification and role in the immune response. J. Immunol., *107*:1168, 1971.
32. Humphrey, J. H., and Keller, H. U.: *In* Sterzl, J.,

and Riha, I. (eds.): Developmental Aspects of Antibody Formation. Vol. 2, p. 485. New York, Academic Press, 1970.

33. Davie, J. M., and Paul, W. E.: Antigen-binding receptors on lymphocytes. Cont. Top. Immunobiol., *3*:171, 1974.
34. Ivanyi, J., and Salerno, A.: Cellular mechanisms of escape from immunological tolerance. Immunology, *22*:247, 1972.

34a. Sjöberg, O.: Rapid breaking of tolerance against *Escherichia coli* lipopolysaccharide *in vivo* and *in vitro*. J. Exp. Med., *135*:850, 1972.

35. Howard, J. G., Christie, G. H., and Courtenay, B. M.: Studies on immunological paralysis. Proc. R. Soc. Lond. [Biol.], *180*:347, 1972.
36. Katz, D. H., and Bernacerraf, B.: Immunological Tolerance: Mechanisms and Potential Therapeutic Applications. P. 249. New York, Academic Press, 1974.
37. Greenberger, J. S., Aaronson, S. A., Rosenthal, D. S., and Moloney, W. C.: Low doses of DNP-D-GL, a potent hapten-specific tolerogen, are immunogenic *in vitro*. Nature, *257*:141, 1975.
38. Ault, K. A., Unanue, E. R., Katz, D. H., and Benacerraf, B.: Failure of lymphocytes to reexpress antigen receptors after brief interaction with a tolerogenic D-amino acid copolymer. Proc. Natl. Acad. Sci., U.S.A., *71*:3111, 1974.
39. Katz, D. H., Davie, J. M., Paul, W. E., and Benacerraf, B.: Carrier function in antihapten antibody responses. J. Exp. Med., *134*:201, 1971.
40. Diener, E., and Feldmann, M.: Mechanisms at the cellular level during induction of high zone tolerance *in vitro*. Cell. Immunol., *5*:130, 1972.
41. Feldmann, M., Howard, J. G., and Desaymard, C.: Role of antigen structure in the discrimination between tolerance and immunity by B cells. Transplant. Rev., *23*:78, 1975.
42. Cohen, I. R., Livnat, S., Livnat, D., Steiner, E., and Waksal, H.: Molecular events in the induction of autosensitization of initiator T lymphocytes. *In* Rosenthal, A. S. (ed).: Immune Recognition. P. 201. New York, Academic Press, 1975.
43. Sterzl, J.: Immunological tolerance as the result of terminal differentiation of immunologically competent cells. Nature, *209*:416, 1966.
44. Gershon, R. K.: T. cell control of antibody production. Contemp. Top. Immunobiol., *3*:1, 1974.
45. Whittingham, S., Irwin, J., Mackay, I. R., Marsh, S., and Cowling, D. C.: Autoantibodies in healthy subjects. Aust. Ann. Med., *18*:130, 1969.
46. Weigle, W. O.: Studies on the termination of acquired tolerance to serum protein antigens following injection of serologically related antigens. Immunology, *7*:239, 1964.
47. ———: The immune response of rabbits tolerant to bovine serum albumin to the injection of other heterologous serum albumins. J. Exp. Med., *114*:111, 1961.
48. Zabriskie, J. B.: Mimetic relationships between group A streptococci and mammalian tissues. Adv. Immunol., *7*:147, 1967.
49. Rowley, D., and Jenkin, C. R.: Antigenic cross-reaction between host and parasite as a possible cause of pathogenicity. Nature, *193*:151, 1962.
50. Isacson, P.: Myxoviruses and autoimmunity. Prog. Allergy, *10*:256, 1967.
51. Weigle, W. O.: Termination of acquired immunological tolerance to protein antigens following immunization with altered protein-antigens. J. Exp. Med., *116*:913, 1962.
52. Allison, A. C., Denman, A. M., and Barnes, R. D.: Cooperating and controlling functions of thymus-derived lymphocytes in relation to autoimmunity. Lancet, *2*:135, 1971.
53. Fialkow, P. J., Gilchrist, C., and Allison, A. C.: Autoimmunity in chronic graft versus host disease. Clin. Exp. Immunol., *13*:479, 1973.
54. Ziff, M.: Viruses and the connective tissue diseases. Ann. Intern. Med., *75*:951, 1971.
55. Stiller, C. R., Russell, A. S., and Dossetor, J. B.: Autoimmunity: present concepts. Ann. Intern. Med., *82*:405, 1975.
56. Talal, N., and Steinberg, A. D.: The pathogenesis of autoimmunity in New Zealand black mice. Curr. Top. Microbiol. Immunol., *64*:79, 1974.
57. Howe, J. B., and Simpson, L. O.: Autoimmune disease in NZB mice and their hybrids. *In* Davies, E. L. (ed.): Lupus Erythematosus. Chap. 4, suppl. 2, p. 124. Los Angeles, University of Southern California Press, 1974.
58. Warner, N. L., and Wistar, R.: Immunoglobulins in NZB/BL mice. I. Serum immunoglobulin levels and immunoglobulin class of erythrocyte autoantibodies. J. Exp. Med., *127*:169, 1968.
59. Dixon, F. J., Oldstone, M. B. A., and Tonietti, G.: Pathogenesis of immune complex glomerulonephritis of New Zealand mice. J. Exp. Med., *134*:65s, 1971.
60. East, J., deSousa, M. A. B., and Parrott, D. M. V.: Immunopathology of New Zealand black (NZB) mice. Transplantation, *3*:711, 1965.
61. deVries, M. J., and Hijmans, W.: Pathological changes of thymic epithelial cells and autoimmune disease in NZB, NZW and (NZB × NZW) F_1 mice. Immunology, *12*:179, 1967.
62. Lambert, P. H., and Dixon, F. J.: Pathogenesis of the glomerulonephritis of NZB/W mice. J. Exp. Med., *127*:507, 1968.
63. Siegel, B. V., and Morton, J. I.: Response of NZB mice to immunization with sheep erythrocytes. J. Reticuloendothel. Soc., *4*:439, 1967.
64. Evans, M. M., Williamson, W. G., and Irvine, W. J.: The appearance of immunological competence at an early age in New Zealand black mice. Clin. Exp. Immunol., *3*:375, 1968.
65. Gazda, A. F., Beitzel, W., and Talal, N.: The age-related responses of New Zealand mice to a murine sarcoma virus. Clin. Exp. Immunol., *8*:501, 1971.
66. Leventhal, B. G., and Talal, N.: Response of NZB and NZB/NZW spleen cells to mitogenic agents. J. Immunol., *104*:918, 1970.

67. Cantor, H., Asofsky, R., and Talal, N.: Synergy among lymphoid cells mediating the graft-versus-host response. J. Exp. Med., *131*:223, 1970.
68. Salomon, J. C., and Benveniste, J.: The immune response in NZB × NZW F_1 hybrid mice. Clin. Exp. Immunol., *4*:213, 1969.
69. Staples, P. J., and Talal, N.: Relative inability to induce tolerance in adult NZB and NZB/NZW F_1 mice. J. Exp. Med., *129*:123, 1969.
70. Mellors, R. C., *et al.*: Wildtype gross leukemia virus and the pathogenesis of the glomerulonephritis of New Zealand mice. J. Exp. Med., *133*:113, 1971.
71. Steinberg, A. D.: Pathogenesis of autoimmunity in New Zealand mice. V. Loss of thymic suppressor function. Arthritis Rheum., *17*:11, 1974.
72. Shirai, T., and Mellors, R. C.: Natural thymocytotoxic autoantibody and reactive antigen in New Zealand black and other mice. Proc. Natl. Acad. Sci., U.S.A., *68*:1412, 1971.
73. Goldblum, R., Pillarisetty, R., and Talal, N.: Independent appearance of anti-thymocyte and anti-RNA antibodies in NZB/NZW F_1 mice. Immunology, *28*:621, 1975.
74. Bach, J.-F., Dardenne, M., and Salomon, J.-C.: Studies on thymus products. IV. Absence of serum "thymic activity" in adult NZB and (NZB × NZW) F_1 mice. Clin. Exp. Immunol., *14*:247, 1973.
75. Dauphinee, M. J., Talal, N., Goldstein, A. L., and White, A.: Thymosin corrects the abnormal DNA synthetic response of NZB mouse thymocyte. Proc. Natl. Acad. Sci., U.S.A., *71*:2637, 1974.
76. Gershwin, M. E., *et al.*: Correction of T cell function by thymosin in New Zealand mice. J. Immunol., *113*:1068, 1974.
76a. Gershwin, M. E., Steinberg, A. D., Ahmed, A., and Derkay, C.: Study of thymic factors. Arthritis Rheum., *19*:862, 1976.
77. Mellors, R. C., Aoki, T., and Huckner, R. J.: Further implication of murine leukemia-like virus in the disorders of NZB mice. J. Exp. Med., *129*:1045, 1969.
78. Yoshiki, T., Mellors, R. C., Strand, M., and August, J. T.: The viral envelope glycoproteins of murine leukemia virus and the pathogenesis of immune complex glomerulonephritis of New Zealand mice. J. Exp. Med., *140*:1011, 1974.
79. Mellors, R. C., and Huang, C. Y.: Immunopathology of NZB/Bl mice. V. Viruslike (filtrable) agent separable from lymphoma cells and identifiable by electron microscopy. J. Exp. Med., *124*:1031, 1966.
80. ——:Immunopathology of NZB/Bl mice. VI. Virus separable from spleen and pathogenic for Swiss mice. J. Exp. Med., *126*:53, 1967.
81. Croker, B. P., *et al.*: Immunopathogenicity and oncogenicity of murine leukemia viruses. I. Induction of immunologic disease and lymphoma in (BALB/c × NZB) F_1 mice by Scripps leukemia virus. J. Exp. Med., *140*:1028, 1974.
82. Provitt, M. R., Hirsch, M. S., and Black, P. H.: Murine leukemia: a virus-induced autoimmune disease. Science, *182*:821, 1973.
83. Cohen, A. S., Reynolds, W. E., and Franklin, E. C.: Bull. Rheum. Dis., *21*:643, 1971.
84. Estes, D., and Christian, C. L.: The natural history of systemic lupus erythematosus by prospective analysis. Medicine, *50*:85, 1971.
85. Urowitz, M. B., *et al.*: The bimodal mortality pattern of systemic lupus erythematosus. Am. J. Med., *60*:221, 1976.
86. Decker, J. L., *et al.*: Systemic lupus erythematosus: contrasts and comparisons. Ann. Intern. Med., *82*:391, 1975.
87. Tuffenelli, D. L.: Lupus erythematosus. Arch. Dermatol., *106*:553, 1972.
88. Hare, W. S. C., and Mackay, I. R.: Thymic size in systemic lupus erythematosus. Arch. Intern. Med., *124*:60, 1969.
89. Goldstein, G., and Mackay, I.: The thymus in systemic lupus erythematosus; a quantitative histopathological analysis and comparison with stress involution. Br. Med. J., *2*:475, 1967.
89a. Jasin, H. E., and Ziff, M.: Immunoglobulin synthesis by peripheral blood cells in systemic lupus erythematosus. Arthritis Rheum., *18*:219, 1975.
90. Talal, N.: Antibodies to nucleic acids in human and murine lupus. J. Rheum., *2*:130, 1975.
91. Lee, S. L., and Miotti, A. B.: Disorders of hemostatic function in patients with systemic lupus erythematosus. Semin. Arthritis Rheum., *4*:241, 1975.
92. Holman, H., and Diecher, H. R.: The reaction of the lupus erythematosus cell factor with deoxyriboneucleoprotein of the cell nucleus. J. Clin. Invest., *38*:2059, 1959.
93. Reichlin, M., and Mattioli, M.: Antigens and antibodies characteristic of systemic lupus erythematosus. Bull. Rheum., Dis., *24*:756, 1974.
94. Schur, P. H., and Sandson, J.: Immunologic factors and clinical activity in systemic lupus erythematosus. N. Engl. J. Med., *278*:533, 1968.
95. Casals, S. P., Friou, G. J., and Myers, L. L.: Significance of antibody to DNA in systemic lupus erythematosus. Arthritis Rheum., *7*:379, 1964.
96. Rothfield, N. F., and Stollar, B. D.: The relation of immunoglobulin class, pattern of antinuclear antibody, and complement-fixing antibodies to DNA in sera from patients with systemic lupus erythematosus. J. Clin. Invest., *46*:1785, 1967.
97. Koffler, D., Schur, P. H., and Kunkel, H. G.: Immunological studies concerning the nephritis of systemic lupus erythematosus. J. Exp. Med., 126:607, 1967.
98. Williams, R. C., and Law, D. H.: Serum complement in connective tissue disorders. J. Lab. Clin. Med., *52*:273, 1958.
99. Morse, J. H., Muller-Eberhard, H. J., and Kunkel, H. G.: Antinuclear factors and serum

complement in systemic lupus erythematosus. Bull. N.Y. Acad. Med., *38*:641, 1962.

100. Rothfield, N. R., Ross, A., Minta, J. O., and Lepow, I. H.: Glomerular and dermal deposition of properdin in systemic lupus erythematosus. New Engl. J. Med., *287*:681, 1972.
101. Teisberg, P.: Complement system studies in systemic lupus erythematosus. Acta Med. Scand., *197*:131, 1975.
102. Sliwinski, A. J., and Zvaifler, N. J.: Decreased synthesis of the third component of complement in hypocomplementemic systemic lupus erythematosus. Clin. Exp. Immunol., *11*:21, 1972.
103. Phillips, P. E., and Christian, C. L.: Virus antibody studies in the connective tissue diseases. Arthritis Rheum., *14*:180, 1971.
104. Keeffe, E. B., *et al.*: Lupus meningitis: antibody to deoxyribonucleic acid and DNA-anti DNA complexes in cerebrospinal fluid. Ann. Intern. Med., *80*:58, 1974.
105. Davis, P., Cunnington, P., and Hughes, G. R. V.: Double stranded RNA antibodies in systemic lupus erythematosus. Ann. Rheum. Dis., *34*:239, 1975.
106. Schur, P. H., Stollar, B. D., Steinberg, A. D., and Talal, N.: Incidence of antibodies to double stranded RNA in systemic lupus erythematosus and related diseases. Arthritis Rheum., *14*:342, 1971.
107. Sharp, G., Irwin, W., Holman, H., and Tan, E.: A distinct rheumatic disease syndrome associated with antibody to a particular nuclear antigen and unusual responsiveness to corticosteroid therapy. Clin. Res., *17*:359, 1969.
108. Holman, H. R.: Partial purification and characterization of an extractable nuclear antigen which reacts with systemic lupus erythematosus sera. Ann. N.Y. Acad. Sci., *124*:800, 1965.
109. Farber, S. J., and Bole, G. G.: Antibodies to components of extractable nuclear antigen: clinical characteristics of patients. Arch. Intern. Med., *136*:425, 1976.
110. Sharp, G. C., Irwin, W. S., Tan, E. M., Gould, R. G., and Holman, H. R.: Mixed connective tissue disease—an apparently distinct rheumatic disease syndrome associated with a specific antibody to an extractable nuclear antigen. Am. J. Med., *52*:148, 1972.
111. Morris, A. D., *et al.*: Modification of NZB/NZW nephritis by extractable nuclear antigen. Program and Abstracts of the 35th Annual Meeting of the American Rheumatism Assoc. Section of the Arthritis Foundation. Abstract No. 32, New York, June, 1971.
112. Messiner, R. P., Lindström, F. D., and Williams, R. G.: Peripheral blood lymphocyte cell surface markers during the course of systemic lupus erythematosus. J. Clin. Invest., *52*:3046, 1973.
113. Scheinberg, M. A., and Cathcart, E. S.: B cell and T cell lymphopenia in systemic lupus erythematosus. Cell. Immunol., *12*:309, 1974.
114. Hahn, B. H., Bagby, M. K., and Osterland, C. K. Abnormalities of delayed hypersensitivity in systemic lupus erythematosus. Am. J. Med., *55*:25, 1973.
115. Horwitz, D. A., and Cousar, J. B.: A relationship between cellular immunity, humoral suppression of lymphocyte function and severity of systemic lupus erythematosus. Am. J. Med., *58*:829, 1975.
116. Rosenthal, C. J., and Franklin, E. C.: Depression of cellular-mediated immunity in systemic lupus erythematosus: relation to disease activity. Arthritis Rheum., *18*:207, 1975.
117. Lockshin, M. D., *et al.*: Cell-mediated immunity in rheumatic diseases. Arthritis Rheum., *18*:245, 1975.
118. Patty, J. G., *et al.*: Impaired cell-mediated immunity in systemic lupus erythematosus: a controlled study of 23 untreated patients. Am. J. Med., *59*:769, 1975.
119. Staples, P. J., Gerding, D. N., Decker, J. L., and Gordon, R. S.: Incidence of infection in systemic lupus erythematosus. Arthritis Rheum., *17*:1, 1974.
120. Williams, R. C., Jr., Lies, R. B., and Messner, R. P.: Inhibition of mixed leukocyte culture responses by serum and gamma-globulin fractions from certain patients with connective tissue disorders. Arthritis Rheum., *16*:597, 1973.
121. Thomas, D. B.: Antibodies specific for human T lymphocytes in cold agglutinin and lymphocytotoxic sera. Eur. J. Immunol., *3*:824, 1973.
122. Lies, R. B., Messner, R. P., and Williams, R. C., Jr.: Relative T-cell specificity of lymphocytotoxins from patients with systemic lupus erythematosus. Arthritis Rheum., *16*:369, 1973.
123. Weinet, P., and Kunkel, H. G.: Antibodies to a specific surface antigen of T cells in human sera inhibiting mixed leukocyte reactions. J. Exp. Med., *138*:1021, 1973.
124. Glinski, W., Gershwin, M. E., and Steinberg, A. D.: Fractionation of cells on a discontinuous ficoll gradient: study of subpopulations of human T cells using anti T-cell antibodies from patients with systemic lupus erythematosus. J. Clin. Invest., *57*:604, 1976.

124a. Zvaifler, N. J., and Bluestein, H. G.: Lymphocytotoxic antibody activity in cryoprecipitates from serum of patients with SLE. Arthritis Rheum., *19*:844, 1976.

125. Scheinberg, M. A., Cathcart, E. S., and Goldstein, A. L.: Thymosin-induced reduction of "null cells" in peripheral blood lymphocytes of patients with systemic lupus erythematosus. Lancet, *1*:424, 1975.
126. Block, S. R., and Christian, C. L.: The pathogenesis of systemic lupus erythematosus. Am. J. Med., *59*:453, 1975.
127. Leonhardt, E. T. G.: Family studies in systemic lupus erythematosus. Clin. Exp. Immunol., *2*:743, 1967.
128. Block, S. R., *et al.*: Studies of twins with systemic lupus erythematosus: a review of the

literature and presentation of 12 additional sets. Am. J. Med., *59*:533, 1975.

129. Siegel, M., *et al.*: A comparative family study of rheumatoid arthritis and systemic lupus erythematosus. N. Engl. J. Med., *273*:893, 1965.
130. Andres, G. A., Spiele, H., and McCluskey, R. T.: Virus-like structures in systemic lupus erythematosus. Prog. Clin. Immunol., *1*:23, 1972.
131. Strand, M., and August, J. T.: Type-C RNA virus gene expression in human tissue. J. Virol., *14*:1584, 1974.
132. Lewis, R. M., Tannenberg, W., Smith, C., and Schwartz, R. S.: C-type viruses in systemic lupus erythematosus. Nature, *252*:78, 1974.
133. Schwartz, R. S.: Viruses and systemic lupus erythematosus. N. Engl. J. Med., *293*:132, 1975.
134. Lee, S. L., and Chase, H. P.: Drug-induced systemic lupus erythematosus: a critical review. Semin. Arthritis Rheum., *5*:83, 1975.
135. Alarcon-Segovia, D., and Fishbein, E.: Patterns of antinuclear antibodies and lupus-activating drugs. J. Rheum., *2*:167, 1975.
136. Alarcon-Segovia, D., Fishbein, E., and Betancourt, V. M.: Antibodies to nucleoprotein and to hydrazide-altered soluble nucleoprotein in tuberculous patients receiving isoniazid. Clin. Exp. Immunol., *5*:429, 1969.
137. Tan, E. M.: Drug-induced autoimmune disease. Fed. Proc.., *33*:1894, 1974.
138. Perry, H. M., Tan, E. M., Carmody, S., and Sakamoto, A.: Relationship of acetyl transferase activity to antinuclear antibodies and toxic symptoms in hypertensive patients treated with hydralazine. J. Lab. Clin. Med., *76*:114, 1970.
139. Blomgren, S. E., Condemi, J. J.,and Vaughan, J. H.: Procainamide-induced lupus erythematosus: clinical and laboratory observations. Am. J. Med., *52*:338, 1972.
140. Kahn, G., and Davis, B. P.: *In vitro* studies on longwave ultra violet light-dependent reactions of the skin photosensitizer chlorpromazine with nucleic acids, purines, and pyrimidines. J. Invest. Derm., *55*:47, 1970.
141. Parker, M. D., and Kerby, G. P.: Combined titer and fluorescent pattern of IgG antinuclear antibodies using cultured cell monolayers in evaluating connective tissue diseases. Ann. Rheum. Dis., *33*:465, 1974.
142. Lachmann, P. J., and Kunkel, H. G.: Correlation of antinuclear antibodies and nuclear staining patterns. Lancet, *2*:436, 1961.
143. Tan, E. M.: Relationship of nuclear staining patterns with precipitating antibodies in systemic lupus erythematosus. J. Lab. Clin. Med., *70*:800, 1967.
144. Beck, J. S.: Autoantibodies to cell nuclei. Scott. Med. J., *8*:373, 1963.
145. Tan, E. M., and Kunkel, H. G.: Characteristics of a soluble nuclear antigen precipitating with sera of patients with systemic lupus erythematosus. J. Immunol., *96*:464, 1966.
146. Sharp, G. C., *et al.*: Mixed connective tissue disease. Am. J. Med., *52*:148, 1972.
147. Ropes, M. W., *et al.*: Proposed diagnostic criteria for rheumatoid arthritis. Bull. Rheum. Dis., *7*:121, 1956.
148. Cannon, P. J., *et al.*: The relationship of hypertension and renal failure in scleroderma to structural and functional abnormalities of the renal cortical circulation. Medicine, *53*:1, 1974.
149. Grio, M. G., Peserico, A., and Volpin, D.: Collagen and elastin in scleroderma. Connec. Tis. Res., *2*:309, 1974.
150. Gerber, M. A.: Immunohistochemical findings in the renal vascular lesions of progressive systemic sclerosis. Human Pathol., *6*:343, 1975.
151. Scott, D. G., and Rowell, N. R.: Immunohistological studies of the kidney in systemic lupus erythematosus and scleroderma using antisera to IgG, C3, fibrin, and human renal glomeruli. Ann. Rheum. Dis., *33*:473, 1974.
152. Bohan, A., and Peter, J. B.: Polymyositis and dermatomyositis. N. Engl. J. Med., *292*:344, 403, 1975.
153. Whitaker, J. N., and Engel, W. K.: Vascular deposits of immunoglobulin and complement in idiopathic inflammatory myopathy. N. Engl. J. Med., *286*:333, 1972.
154. Caspary, E. A., Gulbay, S. S., and Stern, G. M.: Circulating antibodies in polymyositis and other muscle-wasting disorders. Lancet, *2*:941, 1964.
155. Johnson, R. L., Fink, C. W., and Ziff, M.: Lymphotoxin formation by lymphocytes and muscle in polymyositis. J. Clin. Invest., *51*:2435, 1972.
156. Mastaglia, F. L., and Currie, S.: Immunological and ultra-structural observations on the role of lymphoid cells in the pathogenesis of polymyositis. Acta Neuropathol., *18*:1, 1971.
157. Williams, R. C.: Dermatomyositis and malignancy: a review of the literature. Ann. Intern. Med., *50*:1174, 1959.
158. Chou, S. M.: Myxovirus-like structures and accompanying nuclear changes in chronic polymyositis. Arch. Pathol., *86*:649, 1968.
159. Shearn, M. A.: Sjögren's Syndrome. Philadelphia, W. B. Saunders, 1971.
160. Whaley, K., *et al.*: Sjögren's syndrome. 2. Clinical associations and immunological phenomena. Quart. J. Med., *42*:513, 1973.
161. Cummings, N. A., *et al.*: Sjögren's syndrome—newer aspects of research, diagnosis, and therapy. Ann. Intern. Med., *75*:937, 1971.
162. ———: Recent clinical and experimental developments in Sjögren's syndrome. West. J. Med., *122*:50, 1975.
163. Talal, N., *et al.*: T and B lymphocytes in peripheral blood and tissue lesions in Sjögren's syndrome. J. Clin. Invest., *53*:180, 1974.
164. Chused, T. M., Hardin, J. A., Frank, M. A., and Green, I.: Identification of cells infiltrating the minor salivary glands in patients with Sjögren's syndrome. J. Immunol., *112*:641, 1974.
165. Anderson, L. G., and Talal, N.: The spectrum of benign tumor malignant lymphoproliferation in Sjögren's syndrome. Clin. Exp. Immunol., *10*:199, 1971.

166. Zabriskie, J. B.: The relationship of Streptococcal crossreactive antigens to rheumatic fever. Transplant. Proc., *1*:968, 1969.
167. Kaplin, M. H., and Frengley, J. D.: Autoimmunity to the heart in cardiac disease: current concepts of the relation of autoimmunity to rheumatic fever, postcardiotomy, and postinfarction syndromes and cardiomyopathies. Am. J. Cardiol., *24*:459, 1969.
168. Tagg, J. R., and McGiven, A. R.: Some possible autoimmune mechanisms in rheumatic carditis. Lancet *2*:686, 1972.
169. Ehrenfeld, E. N., Gery, I., and Davies, A. M.: Specific antibodies in heart disease. Lancet, *1*:1138, 1961.
170. Vander Geld, H.: Antiheart antibodies in the postpericardiotomy and the post myocardial infarction syndromes. Lancet, *2*:617, 1964.
171. Schlesinger, M.: Uterus of rodents as site for manifestation of transplantation immunity against transplantable tumors. J. Natl. Cancer Inst., *28*:927, 1962.
172. Beer, A. E., Billingham, R. E., and Hoerr, R. A.: Elicitation and expression of transplantation immunity in the uterus. Transplant. Proc., *3*:609, 1971.
173. Loke, Y. W., Joysey, V. C., and Borland, R.: HLA antigens on human trophoblast cells. Nature, *232*:403, 1971.
174. Ceppellini, R., *et al.*: Mixed leukocyte cultures and HLA antigens. 1. Reactivity of young fetuses, newborns and mothers at delivery. Transplant. Proc., *3*:58, 1971.
175. Currie, G. A.: Immunological studies of trophoblast *in vitro*. Obstet. Gynaecol., Br. Commonw., *74*:841, 1967.
176. Beer, A. E., and Billingham, R. E.: Immunobiology of mammalian reproduction. Adv. Immunol., *14*:1, 1971.
177. Billingham, R. E.: The transplantation biology of mammalian gestation. Am. J. Obstet. Gynecol., *111*:469, 1971.
178. Lichtenstein, M. R.: Tuberculin reaction in tuberculosis during pregnancy. Am. Rev. Tuber. Pul. Dis., *46*:89, 1942.
179. Andresen, R. H., and Monroe, C. W.: Experimental study of the behavior of adult human skin homografts during pregnancy: a preliminary report. Am. J. Obstet. Gynecol., *84*:1096, 1962.
180. Kasakura, S.: Is cortisol responsible for inhibition of mixed leukocyte culture reactions by pregnancy plasma? Nature, *246*:496, 1973.
181. ———: A factor in maternal plasma during pregnancy that suppresses the reactivity of mixed leukocyte cultures. J. Immunol., *107*:1296, 1971.
182. Han, T.: Inhibitory effect of human chorio gonadotropin on lymphocyte blastogenic response to mitogens, antigens and allogeneic cells. Clin. Exp. Immunol., *18*:529, 1974.
183. Schiff, R. I., Mercier, D., and Buckley, R. H.: Inability of gestational hormones to account for the inhibitory effects of pregnancy plasmas on lymphocyte responses *in vitro*. Cell. Immunol., *20*:69, 1975.
184. Adcock, E. W., III, *et al.*: Human chorionic gonadotropin: its possible role in maternal lymphocyte suppression. Science, *181*:845, 1973.
185. Taylor, P. V., and Hancock, K. W.: Antigenicity of trophoblast and possible antigen-masking effects during pregnancy. Immunology, *28*:973, 1975.
186. Pence, H., Petty, W. M., and Rocklin, R. E.: Suppression of maternal responsiveness to paternal antigens by maternal plasma. J. Immunol., *114*:525, 1975.

9 Immunogenetics and Transplantation

THE MAJOR HISTOCOMPATIBILITY COMPLEX

The epic work of Landsteiner on blood groups at the turn of the century established that the surface antigenicity of human cells determines whether a cell from one individual is viewed as foreign or not when introduced into the system of another individual. It was recognized quite early that the success of blood transfusions depended upon matching the donor blood to that of the recipient. Transfusions of blood against which the recipient possessed antibodies would often result in a serious transfusion reaction.

The availability of inbred animal strains opened for study the factors that are responsible for graft rejection. Tissue grafts between genetically identical individuals of a single strain (syngeneic) survived indefinitely, whereas grafts from one strain to another (allogeneic) were rejected. The ability of a graft to be accepted by a host is a measure of the "histocompatibility" of the donor and the recipient. Histocompatibility is a reflection of the similarity of surface antigens on donor and recipient cells. In humans, the major histocompatibility determinants are the ABO antigens. These were the antigens that Landsteiner and his successors discovered in their work on blood transfusions. We shall examine the ABO and other red-cell antigen systems in Chapter 14. More recently another very important system of cell-surface antigens detectable on many body tissues has been described. These antigens were first recognized as the targets of antisera produced against white blood cells in patients receiving multiple transfusions or in multiparous women.[1] These cell-surface determinants are called the *HLA antigens*.

HLA antigens are the gene products of part of a large genetic region on the sixth chromosome (Fig. 9-1).[2] The entire region, termed HL-1, is referred to as the major histocompatibility complex (MHC). The MHC codes for many different products, some of which appear to be related to various aspects of immune function. The HLA antigens were the first of these products to be discovered and defined. They are readily detected by specific antisera and are therefore often referred to as *serologically defined* (SD) *antigens*.[3] We will begin our discussion of the MHC with a look at the HLA antigens.

THE HLA ANTIGENS

The most recent work suggests that each person displays up to six different HLA antigens.[4] Three are the gene prod-

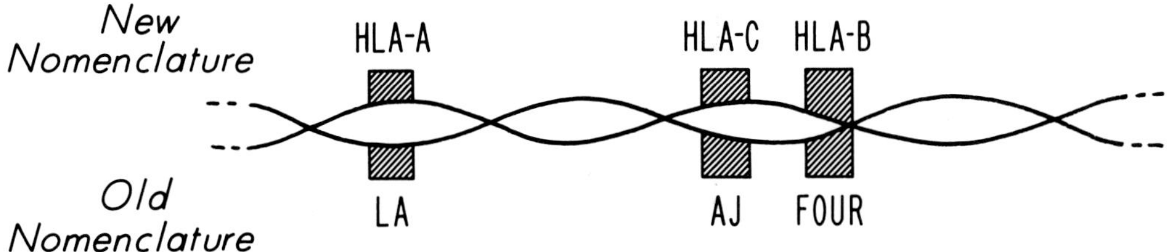

Fig. 9-1. Segment of the sixth chromosome containing the human MHC, illustrating the major SD loci.

ucts of the paternally inherited chromosome, and three are inherited from the mother. The MHC inherited from each parent contains three closely linked loci each of which codes for a specific HLA antigen. The three loci were initially given identifying abbreviations: LA (the first locus, or SD-1); FOUR (the second locus, or SD-2); and AJ (the third locus, or SD-3). There is still some question as to whether AJ truly represents a separate and distinct locus.

Recently a new and simpler nomenclature has been adopted for the HLA system.[5] The LA locus is now referred to as HLA-A, the FOUR locus as HLA-B, and the AJ locus as HLA-C. We shall use this newer nomenclature throughout the remainder of this chapter.

Each child inherits the ability to express two antigens from the A series (one from each parent), and likewise two from the B series and two from the C series. All genes that are inherited are expressed, and, therefore, the HLA genes are *codominant*. The set of antigens inherited from each parent is called a *haplotype*. Each child thus inherits two haplotypes. From simple Mendelian genetics we can see that any pair of siblings can fall into one of three groups: they can be identical at both haplotypes, share one identical haplotype, or share neither haplotype (see Fig. 9-2).

The importance of the HLA antigens to human transplantation has been the object of considerable research.[6] Early experiments using genotypic matching among siblings showed that those sibpairs that had inherited identical HLA genes exchanged skin grafts relatively successfully while those sibpairs lacking surface identity rapidly rejected each other's grafts.[7]

More precise examination of sibling graft rejection correlated skin graft survival patterns with each of the three haplotype groups of sibpairs.[8,9] Those that shared no HLA determinants rejected earliest, those sharing both haplotypes had the longest survival, and those expressing haploidentity exhibited intermediate survival (Fig. 9-3). Note that the HLA-identical sibpairs still rejected their grafts (no attempts at immunosuppression were made). This has been felt to be the result of minor or other antigenic differences not tested for by HLA typing.

Offspring inherit haplotypes and not, as a rule, separate loci. This is a reflection of the close genetic linkage between loci. For individual loci to be transmitted separately, a crossover event must occur between chromosomal chains such that one locus separates from its neighbor. The likelihood of such recombination is proportional to the distance between loci on the chromosome. The recombinant frequency between the A and the B loci is about 0.8 per cent and thus these two loci are quite close to each other on the chromosome.[10]

One of the most intriguing characteristics of the HLA system is a property termed *polymorphism*.[11] This term refers to the multiallelic nature of each of the HLA loci. At each of the three loci on

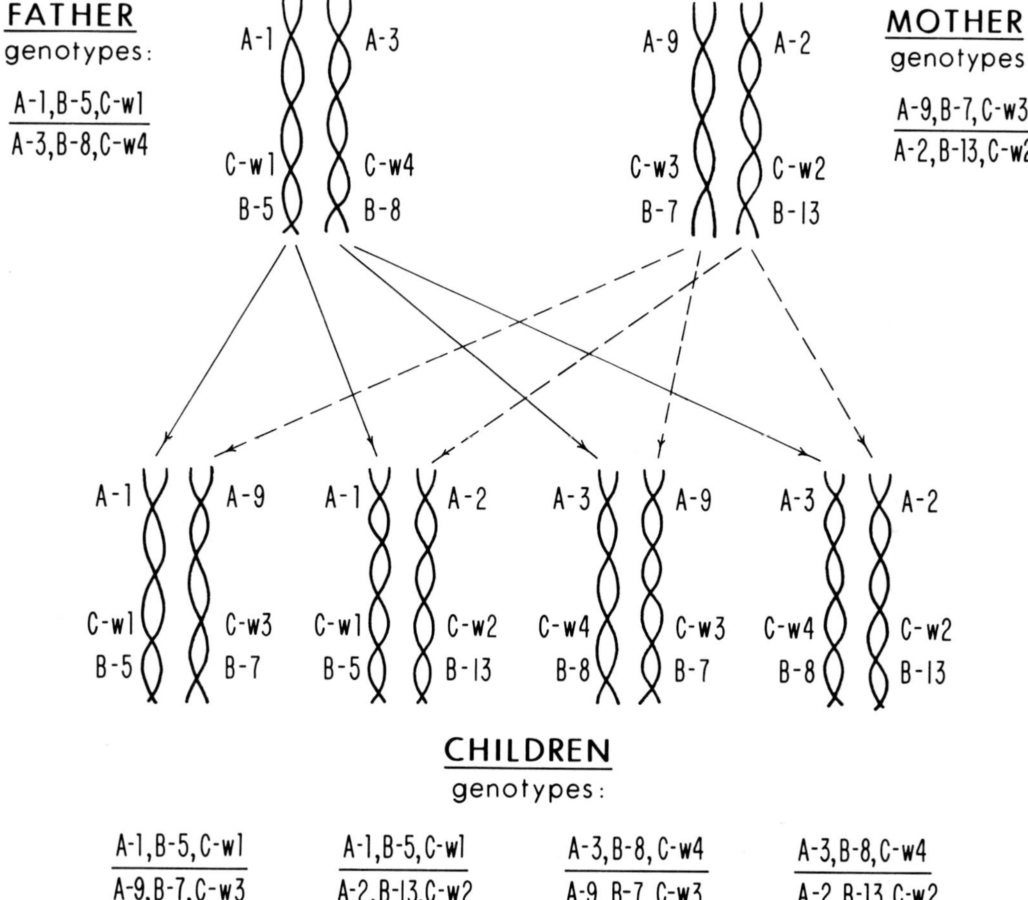

Fig. 9-2. Inheritance of HLA haplotypes. Each child receives one haplotype from each parent, resulting in four possible genotypes.

each copy of the sixth chromosome a given individual may have one of many alleles. Each allele is identified according to a different serologic specificity of its product—the HLA antigen. Since each person has two chromosomes, both with three loci each of which can possess any one of a large variety of alleles, the chances of finding HLA identity between two unrelated people is extraordinarily small. Table 9-1 shows a partial list of the different specificities that have been found for each locus. It is not known how many specificities or distinct HLA antigens there are.

If a calculation is made based upon each person having any two of the known A specificities, two of the known B specificities and two of the known C specificities, we find that there are about one million unique HLA genotypes. Population studies, however, have demonstrated that HLA antigens are distributed *nonrandomly* among populations.[12] Certain populations commonly express particular HLA specificities whereas other groups rarely express those same antigens. This is a reflection of the limited gene pool present in a defined population.

The restriction of HLA expression in specific populations has some interesting applications to anthropologic studies. The degree of inbreeding and isolation in particular groups as well as the migration

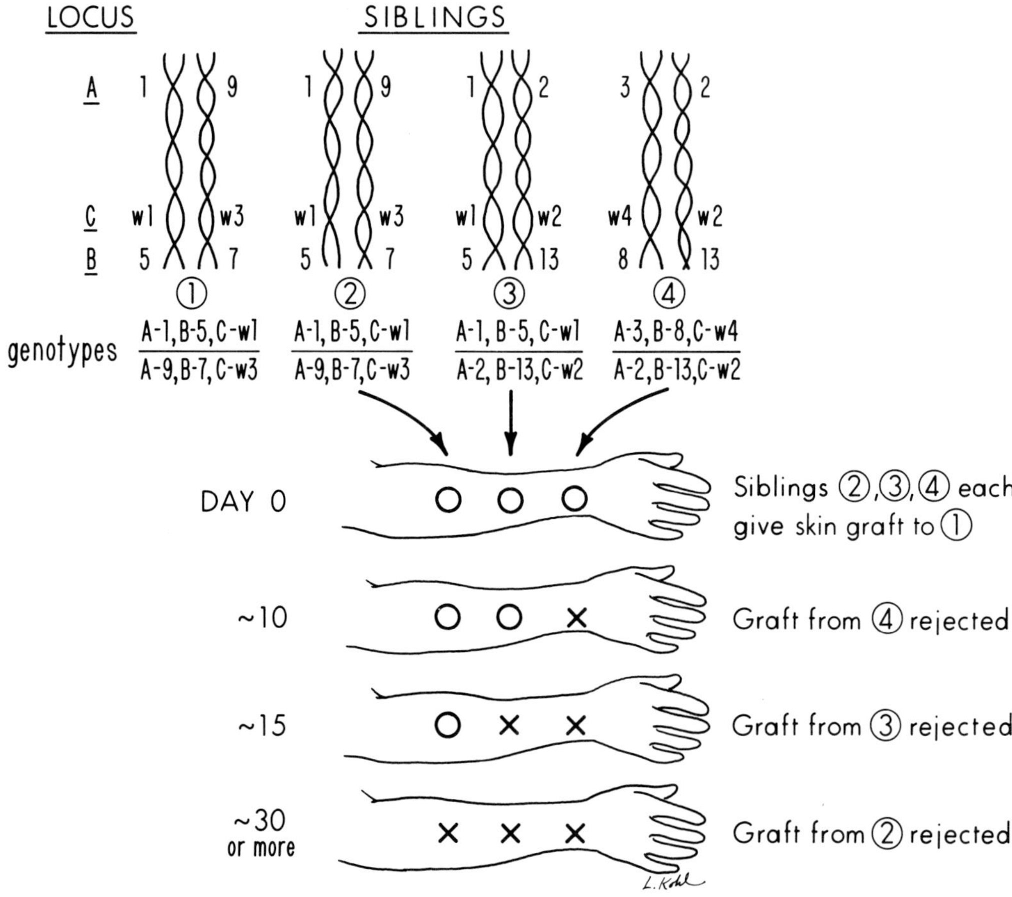

Fig. 9-3. Skin grafts among siblings. Each sib donates a skin graft to sib 1 on day 0. Sib 4 shares no genetic identity with sib 1 and his graft is rapidly rejected by day 10. Sib 3 is haploidentical to sib 1 and his graft remains viable until day 15. Sib 2 is HLA-identical to sib 1 and his graft survives the longest.

patterns of populations have been studied. For example, a striking similarity of HLA gene frequencies between Asian populations across the Bering Strait and Eskimos and some American Indians attests to the probable Asian origin of these groups.

The inheritance of certain specificities at one locus may sometimes show a high correlation with the inheritance of particular specificities at another locus.[13] This phenomenon is called *linkage disequilibrium*. One way to understand this concept is as follows: if the frequency of finding the first locus HLA antigen, α, in a given population is x, and the gene frequency of finding the second locus HLA antigen, β, in the same population is y, then the expected frequency of finding α and β together in any individual in that population is the product xy. The frequency xy would be observed only if α and β are *not* in linkage disequilibrium. Sometimes, however, the frequency of finding a given pair of HLA genes in a single haplotype is quite different than the expected value as derived above. An example is the observation in Caucasian populations that the frequency of finding the first locus gene A1 along with the second locus gene B8 is much higher than the product of their individual gene frequencies. Thus A1 and B8 are in linkage dis-

Table 9-1. The HLA Antigens

A Locus (Old Name LA)	*B Locus (Old Name FOUR)*	*C Locus (Old Name AJ)*	*D Locus (Old Name MLR-S)*
A1	B5	Cw1	Dw1
A2	B7	Cw2	Dw2
A3	B8	Cw3	Dw3
A9	B12	Cw4	Dw4
A10	B13	Cw5	Dw5
A11	B14		Dw6
A28	B18		
A29	B27		
Aw19	Bw15		
Aw23	Bw16		
Aw24	Bw17		
Aw25	Bw21		
Aw26	Bw22		
Aw30	Bw35		
Aw31	Bw37		
Aw32	Bw38		
Aw33	Bw39		
Aw34	Bw40		
Aw36	Bw41		
Aw43	Bw42		

equilibrium in these populations. Linkage disequilibrium is a puzzling phenomenon and its meaning is obscure. It has been suggested that certain locus combinations have a selective advantage and thus have been conserved throughout evolution. Just what the advantages might be is unknown.

We have said that each HLA antigen is defined serologically; a unique antiserum defines a unique antigen. However, the actual situation is more complex.[14] Antisera can be raised that react with more than one HLA antigen.[15] This finding has led to the notion that different sets of HLA antigens belong to different cross-reactive groups. Investigators have thus described the existence of different levels of antigenic specificity expressed by HLA antigens. *Subtypic determinants* (also referred to as private specificities) are determinants unique to one particular HLA gene product. *Supertypic determinants* (or public specificities) are determinants shared by more than one HLA antigen. One way to view this phenomenon is that a single HLA antigen contains both private and public specificities (Fig. 9-4).[16] These reside on the same molecule but represent distinct and separate parts of the HLA antigen. Thus many HLA antigens share structures giving rise to public specificity and each antigen also has a unique aspect to its structure reflected in the private specificity. It is interesting that the antigens sharing public specificity are all found within the same locus, suggesting that the HLA alleles de-

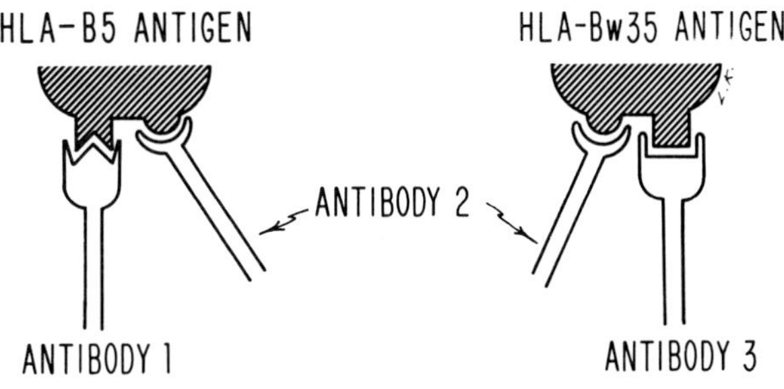

Fig. 9-4. Shematic of one possible relationship between subtypic and supertypic determinants. The supertypic determinant is present on both HLA antigens, while each antigen also bears unique subtypic determinants.

rived from mutation at the three separate SD loci. Thus, within the group from each locus, mutations gave rise to the private specificities while retaining determinants common to the series. It is important, however, to bear in mind that the exact molecular basis of crossreactivity in the HLA system is not yet known.

This conceptualization of the relationship between private and public specificities is only one of several possible models. Several experiments in mice support the idea that the different specificities may be part of the same molecule as shown in Figure 9-4.[17] However, there is some recent evidence, again from the mouse, that public and private specificities need not be part of one molecule.[18] This finding does not support the model depicted above.

Each HLA antigen consists of two components that are noncovalently bound to each other.[19] The larger part is a glycoprotein with a molecular weight of about 30,000 to 40,000. This component contains all of the antigenic specificity of the HLA gene product. The smaller component is a polypeptide with a molecular weight of about 11,000, called β_2 microglobulin.[20] This component is identical for all HLA antigens. There is extensive amino acid sequence homology between β_2 microglobulin and the constant region of the IgG heavy chain.[21] This finding has led to speculation that β_2 microglobulin acts like the heavy chain region of IgG responsible for binding to cell surfaces. However, there is no evidence that it serves as the link between the HLA antigen and the cell membrane. Although the HLA antigens are linked to β_2 microglobulin on the cell surface, most of the β_2 microglobulin found on the cell is not associated with HLA gene products.[22] β_2 Microglobulin is produced by many cells and its structure has been highly conserved throughout the evolution of different species, suggesting a basic and important functional role.

Most if not all cells in the body express HLA antigens, but there are marked differences in the amount of antigen present on the surface of different cell types.[23] White blood cells, especially lymphocytes, are the cells most richly endowed with HLA antigens. Platelets have a considerable amount while red cells have very little. HLA antigens are also found in order of descending density, on spleen, lung, liver, kidney and heart tissue; practically none is found in fat or brain tissue. In addition, different HLA antigens may be expressed to varying extents on the surfaces of different cells.

The experiments exchanging skin grafts among siblings led early investigators to conclude that the HLA antigens might be the sole determinants of tissue acceptance and rejection. HLA compatibility between two siblings was a very reliable indicator of the probable success of a graft. However, HLA matching between unrelated individuals proved to be of far less value in predicting graft acceptance.[23a] This observation was interpreted to mean that yet another genetic locus closely linked to the HLA loci was the real determinant of tissue rejection. Thus it was postulated that HLA identity between siblings correlates highly with graft acceptance only because it can serve as a general marker of the identity of the whole chromosome (assuming no crossover has taken place). The failure of HLA identity to predict with equal certainty the success of grafts between unrelated individuals was felt to be the result of a dissociation between the inheritance of HLA loci and the postulated locus.[24] In other words, although they may be matched for HLA identity, unrelated individuals are likely to be allogeneic at many other loci on the same chromosome.

Much work has gone into defining the nature of this hypothetical locus. Two *in vitro* tests have been employed extensively; the mixed lymphocyte reaction

(MLR) and the cell-mediated lymphocytolysis assay (CML). Both of these tests have been used in attempts to explore the interactions between lymphocytes and target cells, and specifically to determine which antigens are responsible for triggering immunologic recognition and destruction of foreign cells.

IN VITRO STUDIES OF LYMPHOCYTE–TARGET-CELL INTERACTIONS

The Mixed Lymphocyte Reaction and Graft Rejection

We can monitor the recognition of foreign cells by using the mixed lymphocyte reaction (see Chap. 4, especially Fig. 4-5). The mixing of allogeneic cells results in blastogenic changes in the responding lymphocytes with proliferation and DNA synthesis. Lymphocytes are usually employed as the stimulatory cells but epithelial cells can also be used. When an allogeneic cell stimulates a population of lymphocytes, up to several per cent of the lymphocytes respond. Most evidence points to the T cell as the responding lymphocyte. Studies attempting to determine whether the HLA antigens on the stimulatory cells provide the stimulus for T-cell activation have shown that most combinations of lymphocytes from HLA-identical, unrelated individuals will produce a positive MLR.[25] More definitive observations have shown that 1 per cent of HLA-identical siblings will stimulate each other's lymphocytes in this reaction.[26] The converse has also been observed in which siblings without HLA identity do not stimulate in an MLR.[27] All of this data suggests the existence of a separate antigenic locus responsible for the MLR. It has been named the *mixed lymphocyte reaction stimulating locus* (MLR-S) and recently renamed HLA-D.[28] Thus, expression of an MLR-S product that is not identical to the MLR-S product of the responder lymphocytes allows a cell to act as a stimulator in the MLR. The MLR-S locus is closely linked to the HLA-B and HLA-C loci (Fig. 9-5) and this may explain why HLA identity at HLA-B between sibs is better correlated with the ability to transfer grafts than is HLA-A locus identity. The observation that 1 per cent of histoidentical sibling pairs demonstrates a positive MLR is due to the 1 per cent recombinant frequency between the SD and the MLR-S loci (Fig. 9-6).[29] Similarly the fact that most pairs of unrelated HLA-identical people will stimulate in an MLR reflects their having inherited different MLR-S genes. That 10 per cent of these pairs do not stimulate each other is a consequence of linkage disequilibrium between the SD loci and the MLR-S.[30]

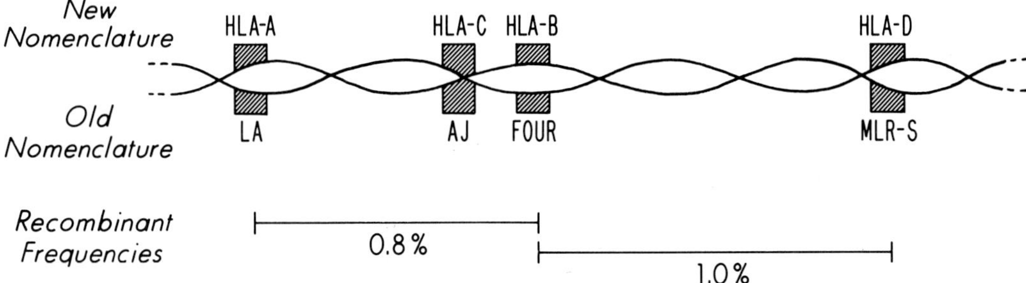

Fig. 9-5. The human MHC including all four major loci and their relative distances from each other. The distance between the loci is reflected in the recombinant frequencies. The higher the frequency of recombination between two loci, the further they are from each other.

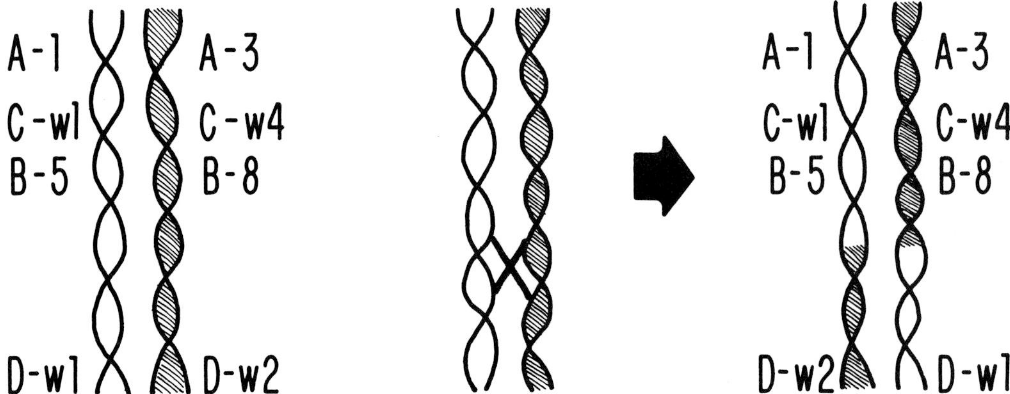

Fig. 9-6. Example of a DNA crossover event leading to recombination between the SD and LD loci.

Lymphocytes that are stimulated by a specific MLR-S gene product represent a clonally restricted set of cells.[31] This means that these lymphocytes probably have surface receptors for specific MLR-S antigens; hence the T cells that recognize and proliferate in response to one MLR-S specificity are different than the T cells responding to another MLR-S. The antigenic specificity of the MLR-S was originally defined by the proliferative response of lymphocytes; hence these antigens have been called "lymphocyte defined" or LD determinants.[32] Recently, however, it has become possible to raise antisera against specific MLR-S determinants, thus making the designation LD somewhat of a historical one.[33] According to the new nomenclature the LD or MLR-S locus (or loci) is designated HLA-D. Because the literature remains filled with references to "LD" antigens, we will continue to employ the term although we will include it in quotes in order to emphasize that "LD" should not be taken as a literal description.

The range of cells that express "LD" determinants seems to be restricted. The "LD" determinants are found primarily on lymphocytes and may also be present on macrophages, epidermal cells and spermatocytes. Recently it has been reported that the B lymphocyte is the major carrier of these surface determinants.[34] At least some T cells (in the mouse) which express the SD antigens do not appear to possess the "LD" antigens and are not capable of stimulating an MLR.[35]

If the "LD" antigens determine the ability to stimulate T cells then we can ask whether "LD" identity between donor and recipient is the critical factor in transplant acceptance. That this might be true was at first supported by the occasional reports of successful "LD"-identical but HLA-incompatible bone marrow transplants.[35] Such cases, however, seem to be exceptional.

When skin grafts have been studied, the role of the "LD" antigens becomes even less clear. There is no quantitative relationship between the extent of MLR stimulation and graft survival.[36,37] Unrelated individuals who are both HLA- and "LD"-identical reject each other's grafts more quickly than do related individuals with both SD and "LD" identity.[13] These and other findings, reminiscent of the earlier discussion of the inadequacy of HLA differences in explaining graft rejection, suggest that there is still another locus that may ultimately determine the fate of a transplant.[28]

Cell-Mediated Lymphocytolysis and Graft Rejection

The failure of the "LD" locus to fully explain graft rejection encouraged the development and utilization of a second *in vitro* assay that might be more closely related to the events of tissue rejection *in vivo*. CML measures the activity of killer lymphocytes in the presence of foreign cells. Lymphocytes are mixed with target cells that have been labelled with radioactive chromium (Cr^{51}). After an appropriate incubation time, the number of target cells that have been destroyed can be estimated by measuring the amount of free chromium that has been released.

With this system it has been shown in animals that whereas antigenic differences which produce an MLR can induce the *proliferation* of T cells, those differences alone may not be sufficient to produce *killer* lymphocytes. In other words, the production of an MLR need not be associated with the active killing of target cells. If one assumes that target-cell destruction *in vitro* is closely analogous to the events of tissue rejection *in vivo*, it is therefore not surprising that the HLA-D locus (by extrapolation to man) fails to account completely for tissue rejection. One can then draw either of two conclusions:

1. There is yet another MHC-linked locus that is actually responsible for graft rejection and the generation of killer cells *in vitro*.
2. Instead of continuing to look for a single locus that determines graft rejection, one could postulate that it is rather particular arrays or patterns of surface antigens that provide the stimulus for immunologic destruction of foreign cells. The search for a single genetic locus that is responsible for the acceptance or rejection of a tissue graft may therefore be continually frustrated by the presence of several different loci that directly or indirectly contribute to graft rejection. The precise loci which are involved may even differ from one donor-host relationship to another.

At present it is impossible to say which of these two theories will turn out to be correct.

The CML assay may indeed prove to be the most reliable marker for transplant success. In one study, the failure of renal transplants was closely correlated with the presence of a positive CML against the donor cells.[38] Conversely, the absence of CML augured well for transplant success. A preliminary report of work in animal systems has claimed a perfect correlation between the presence of a positive CML and the failure of skin grafts.[39]

The finding that a positive MLR need not be associated with a positive CML has had some important implications for our understanding of the mechanisms of recognition and destruction of foreign cells. These may bear directly upon our appreciation of the events surrounding transplant rejection. Because the great majority of this work has been pursued in animal systems, we have reserved a detailed discussion of it for the end of this chapter (see the section entitled *In-Vitro* Studies of the T-Cell Response to Foreign Cells).

RENAL TRANSPLANTATION

Renal transplantation is no longer an uncommon procedure and many centers throughout the world perform numerous transplantations each year. The current figures on graft survival vary widely from institution to institution.[40,41] The success of a transplant is as much an immunologic question as a surgical one, and several steps are now taken routinely to insure an optimum immunologic setting for the transplant:

1. All centers HLA type donors and recipients. Among siblings, HLA identity gives reasonably good assurance for the success of a transplant. Among HLA-identical unrelated individuals the probability of success is considerably less, but in many series is significantly greater than the chances of success between unmatched pairs.
2. Immunosuppressive drugs are used

in all transplant recipients, whatever their HLA identity or nonidentity.[42] Azathioprine and steroids are the agents most commonly used, and many institutions add antilymphocyte serum (ALS) to the immunosuppressive regimen.

3. Other *in vitro* tests may soon be employed to further guarantee immunologic compatibility between donor and host. MLR measurements in unrelated individuals have been found to give an overall probability of graft survival but offer little in the way of prognosis for individual cases.[43] More promising is the CML assay, which, as we have just discussed, may correlate very closely with the eventual outcome of a graft.[38]

IMMUNOLOGIC MECHANISMS OF TRANSPLANT REJECTION

Transplant rejection can occur in at least three different ways. Each has its characteristic clinical and pathologic features, and has been correlated with specific immune effector mechanisms.

Hyperacute Rejection

Hyperacute rejection is the most rapid and fatal of the possible pathways of graft rejection.[44] It occurs within minutes to hours after a kidney is implanted. Examination of the transplant during hyperacute rejection reveals an active destructive process in the vasculature of the new kidney, consisting of a granulocytic inflammatory infiltrate and blockage of the small vessels with thrombi of platelets and fibrin. The kidney is rapidly depleted of its own blood supply and ischemic cortical necrosis ensues, with death of the transplant complete within a few days. Such a kidney must be removed from the patient.[45]

Hyperacute rejection is most likely to occur in recipients who have been presensitized to antigens present on the donor tissue. These people possess circulating antidonor antibodies which are rapidly precipitated within the transplant.[46] Hyperacute rejection is therefore a *humoral* rather than a cell-mediated immune process. Supporting this view is the observation that IgG and the third component of complement are deposited in the glomerular and peritubular capillary walls whereas the presence of lymphocytes in the inflammatory infiltrate is rare.

People may become sensitized to cellular antigens of other individuals through previous exposure derived from pregnancy, blood transfusions or infectious agents that antigenically crossreact with donor antigens.[47,48] Transplantation antigens are not very potent humoral immunogens and multiple exposures may have to take place before antibodies will be generated.

There are several techniques available for detecting the presence of pre-existing antidonor antibodies in a potential transplant recipient.[49] There is a very high probability of hyperacute rejection if a recipient can be shown to possess antidonor antibodies, and screening donor-recipient pairs for these antibodies has greatly reduced the incidence of hyperacute rejection.[50] It does not seem clinically important which donor antigen is the target of the humoral rejection.

The antibodies responsible for hyperacute rejection are capable of activating the complement pathway once they have combined with donor antigen. The target antigen (or antigens) may be expressed on the surface of the donor endothelial cells so that the circulating antibodies attach to the vessel walls, or donor tissue may shed the target antigen into the circulation where antigen-antibody complexes are formed that precipitate in the walls of the small vessels of the graft. A combination of these two processes may occur. Activation of the complement pathway releases powerful neutrophil chemotactic factors and neutrophils rapidly accumulate at the site of complement fixation.

The neutrophils degranulate, releasing lysosomal digestive enzymes. This process leads to destruction of the endothelium which in turn provokes platelet aggregation and release, resulting in the initiation of coagulation. In this way the characteristic histologic picture of hyperacute rejection is produced (Fig. 9-7).

The role of preformed antibodies, complement and neutrophils in hyperacute rejection has been demonstrated experimentally.[51] Hyperacute rejection can be produced by injecting preformed antidonor antibodies into an animal who has received a renal transplant. Rejection can be prevented by depleting the animal of either complement or neutrophils.

The best method for preventing hyperacute rejection (which cannot be treated with immunosuppression) is to carefully screen for the presence of preformed antidonor antibodies. However, there are certain instances of hyperacute rejection in which the histologic picture is one of fibrin deposits and coagulation in the transplant vessels producing infarction and necrosis without the accompaniment of any significant inflammation.[52] The role of preformed antibodies in these cases is unclear. This type of reaction resembles a Schwarzmann-type reaction classically described as a diffuse intravascular coagulation initiated by bacterial endotoxemia. The true pathogenesis of this phenomenon is not known and its relationship to immune mechanisms is uncertain. This sort of rejection has been diagnosed by the clinical picture of a severe coagulopathy and may be treatable with anticoagulation.

The two other forms of transplant rejection are believed to take place in hosts that have not been previously sensitized against donor antigens.

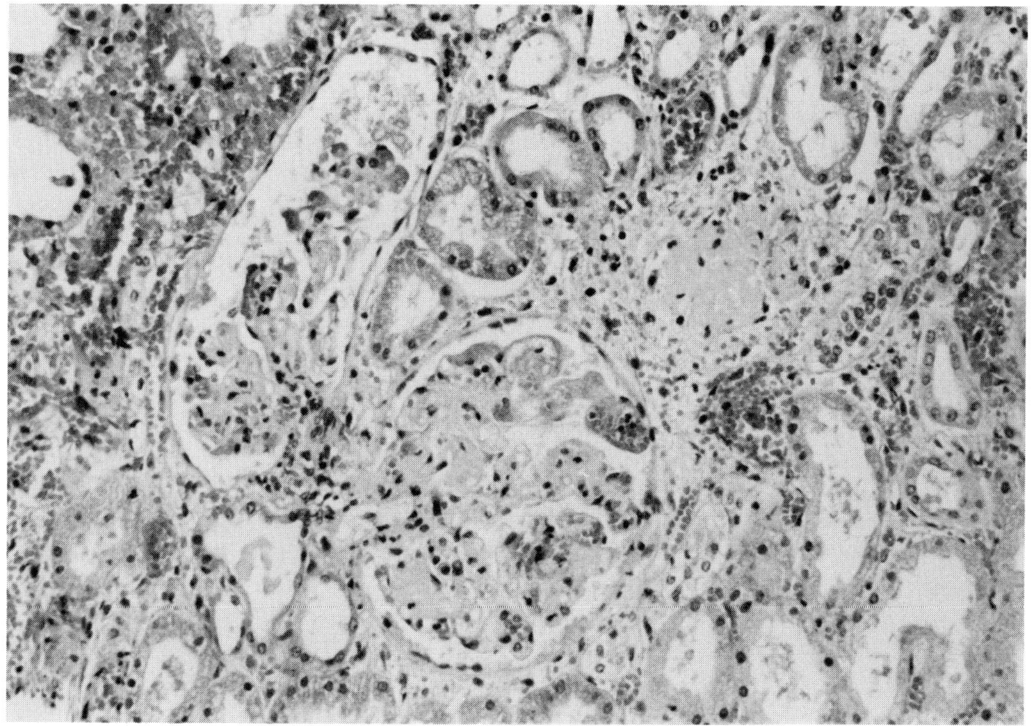

Fig. 9-7. The kidney in hyperacute rejection.

Acute Rejection

Acute rejection usually occurs within the first few weeks after transplantation but in some instances may take a long as several months. The first immunologic event is the sensitization of the host. There are several possible routes of sensitization.

1. Antigen may be leaked from the graft into the renal vein and distributed throughout the host. In experimental systems an antigen leak has been observed within ten minutes of implantation.[53] The transplant acts as a depot for the continuous systemic infusion of immunogen. This is a form of *central* sensitization since the antigen must make its way to the lymphoid organs where sensitization occurs.

2. Some investigators have proposed that donor passenger lymphocytes, carried over in the transplant organ, are the major stimuli to the host's immune system.[54] We have already described how lymphocytes may express certain MHC surface antigens that may not be carried by other cells. Some of these antigens may be crucial in stimulating graft rejection. In some experiments where the passenger lymphocytes were deliberately destroyed, improved kidney-graft survival was seen, although rejection still occurred.[55]

3. The principal mode of sensitization probably results from the blood-borne passage of *host* lymphocytes through the transplant.[56] These lymphocytes become sensitized to the foreign antigens, leave the graft in the venous blood, and make their way either to splenic or peripheral lymphoid tissue where they can recruit effector T cells (see Chap. 1). Thus these circulating recruiter T cells establish a pattern of *peripheral* sensitization and must return to the lymphoid organs before the actual cytotoxic cells are generated.

Whatever the mode of sensitization, the process occurs quickly, usually within the first few hours postimplant. Once sensitization has been accomplished, the normal circulatory pattern of the host lymphocytes is disrupted and the directed migration of lymphocytes to the graft begins.[57] The migration and accumulation of lymphocytes in the graft is the hallmark of acute rejection. Once in the graft, the lymphocytes are intensely active and display the characteristic pattern of antigenic stimulation, undergoing blast transformation and proliferating rapidly. Most of these accumulated lymphocytes are believed to be the expanding clones that are specific for the foreign antigens.[58]

Lymphocytes are not the only cells attracted to the graft. Monocytes comprise up to 30 per cent of the infiltrating cells.[59] These cells are probably attracted to the transplant by lymphocyte-derived chemotactic factors. Once at the site of rejection they are most likely transformed into active macrophages and subserve the many functions that are necessary for a complete immune response. Sensitized T cells may also elaborate a lymphokine called *macrophage arming factor* (MAF) that can stimulate direct macrophage cytotoxicity against the graft.[60]

All of these infiltrating and proliferating cells crowd the renal cortex. Their cytotoxic activities cause injury primarily to the capillary endothelial cells with the subsequent dissolution of the basement membrane. Focal necrosis of the cells of the proximal convoluted tubule is also seen. As the destruction progresses, necrosis of the small arteries ensues, leading to thrombosis and ischemic death of the kidney (Fig. 9-8).

Thus the major effector mechanism in acute rejection is a cell-mediated immune reaction. This type of mechanism is most susceptible to immunosuppressive therapy. Episodes of acute rejection can often be controlled with the immunosuppressive regimens discussed earlier as well as with local x-irradiation.

At the same time that the destructive

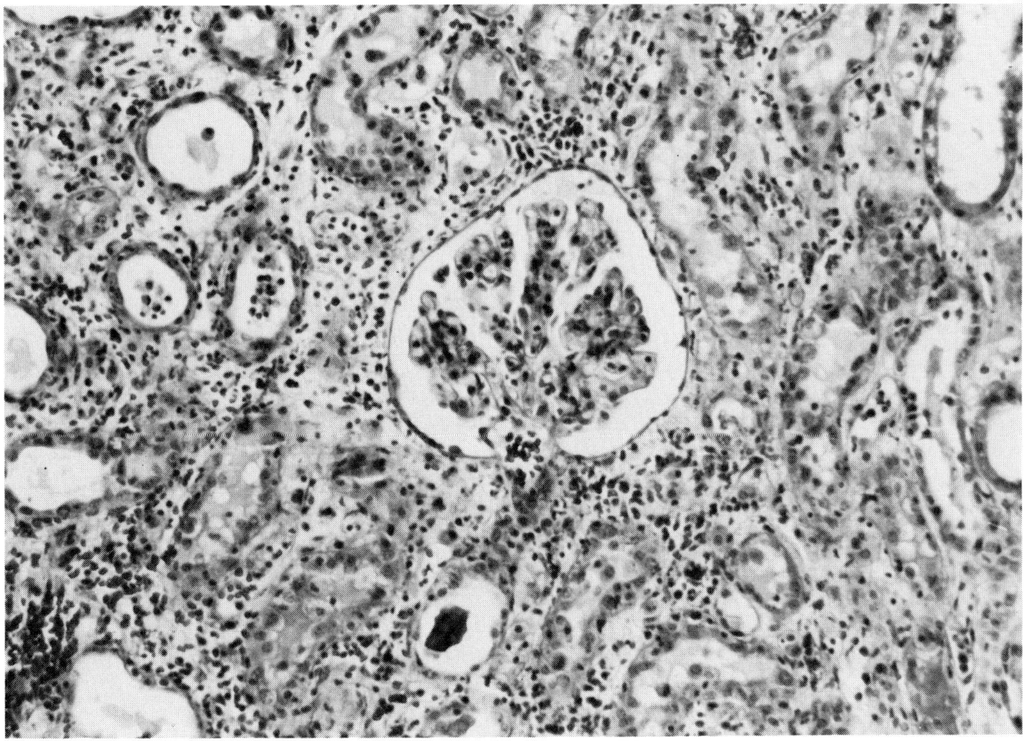

Fig. 9-8. The kidney in acute rejection.

cellular response is evolving, a humoral response is produced.[57] The importance of these antidonor antibodies is not known. Antibodies can be detected in many patients who have received transplants, and recently a correlation between the presence of cytotoxic antibodies and poor graft function has been made.[59] Often the antibody seems to be sequestered in the transplant and cannot be detected free in the circulation.[61] Although thrombosis and platelet aggregation do occur in acute rejection, there is little evidence that this results from a hyperacute type of mechanism. Antibody-dependent cell-mediated cytotoxicity activity has been detected in sera from patients with renal allografts and may play a role in the destruction of donor cells (see Chap. 6).[62]

There is evidence that blocking antibodies or immune enhancement may be important mechanisms in the acceptance of a kidney graft. Among successful renal-transplant recipients, two groups have been defined on the basis of their immunologic status.[63] In one group the host lymphocytes do not attack the donor cells in *in vitro* tests, suggesting true unresponsiveness. In the other successful transplant group, host lymphocytes are cytotoxic to donor cells but this cytotoxicity is blocked by the recipient's serum. This blocking activity resides in the IgG serum fraction. Interestingly, blocking activity has been reported to be lost after about three years of successful transplant function. Accompanying this is a loss of host-versus-donor cytotoxicity.[64] Because of these findings, experimenters have sought to determine whether immune enhancement can be used by the clinician to augment transplant survival. Animal experiments designed to induce immune enhancement by the injection of donor cells in adjuvants prior to transplant have produced encouraging results.[65] In mice the use of antilymphocyte serum with donor-cell injections seems to select for the production of blocking antibodies. The application of this technique to human transplantation awaits further research.

The acute rejection of a renal transplant is a setting in which a full range of immune mechanisms is expressed. The outcome of the graft is the final product of many interesting forces:

1. The directly cytotoxic immune responses, including:
   a. Killer T cells
   b. Cytotoxic macrophages
   c. Antibody-induced cell destruction mediated via humoral mechanisms such as complement.
   d. Antibody-dependent cell-mediated cytotoxicity
2. Mechanisms inhibiting these effector pathways, including:
   a. The development of tolerance to the graft
   b. The effect of blocking antibodies
   c. The effect of immunosuppressive therapy

Chronic Rejection

The third type of rejection poses a frequent and long-term threat to the ultimate outcome of the graft. Chronic rejection is characterized by the proliferation of vessel walls most commonly involving the interlobular arcuate arteries (Fig. 9-9).[66] These lesions may evolve over months to years. The cause of these changes is obscure. Some investigators say that they represent the long-term residuum of acute rejection episodes with chronic scarring following an initial insult. Others maintain that an immune phenomenon is involved that is primarily humoral in nature. There are varying reports of subendothelial deposition of immunoglobulin in the vessel walls in certain cases of chronic rejection. When such

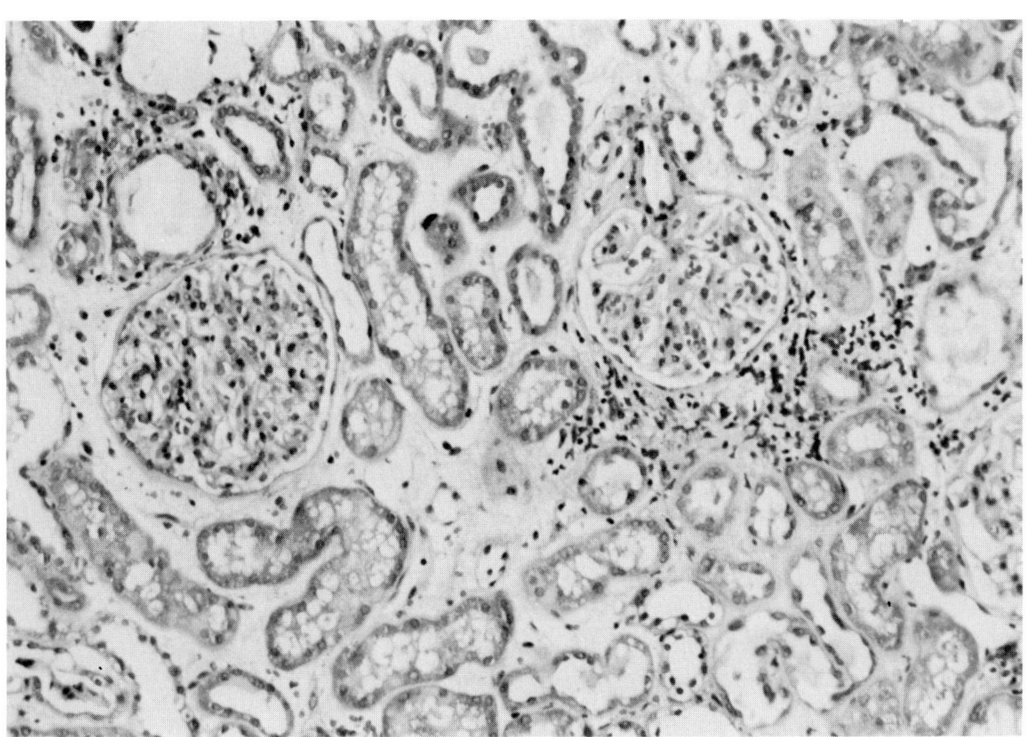

Fig. 9-9. The kidney in chronic rejection.

Table 9-2. Mechanisms of Renal Transplant Rejection

Type of Rejection	*Time Course*	*Immune Mechanisms*	*Histology*
Hyperacute	Minutes to hours	Humoral via preformed antibodies; IgG and C3 deposit in vessel walls	Granulocytic infiltrate; small vessel thrombosis
Acute	1 to several weeks	Cell-mediated immunity; may also see serum blocking factors	Lymphocytic infiltrate; destruction of endothelial cells; arteriolar necrosis
Chronic	Months to years	Unknown; may be a low-level humoral response—possible to detect IgM in vessel walls	Proliferation of vessel walls

deposits are seen they usually consist of IgM.[67] This is in contrast to acute rejections where immunofluorescence often reveals IgG or both IgG and IgM deposition.[68] Production of IgM without IgG in an immune response may sometimes reflect the lower intensity of that response. Such a long-term low-level immune response may lead to the slowly progressive changes of chronic rejection.

GENETICS OF IMMUNE RESPONSIVENESS

We cannot close our discussion of immunogenetics without discussing a phenomenon already alluded to several times in this text. The abilty to mount an immune response against a given antigen is inherited as an autosomal dominant trait and is called *immune responsiveness*.[69] The genes responsible are termed immune response (Ir) genes and are part of the MHC.[70] Thus far their existence in several animal species including the mouse,[71] guinea pig[72] and rat[73] has been well documented. However, there is at present only suggestive evidence that these genes exist in man.[74] In the next several paragraphs we will be discussing immune responsiveness in these animal systems.

The discovery of Ir genes has introduced an entirely new concept into the field of immunology. Their existence implies the evolution of a complex set of genetic controls that determine the immunogenicity of an antigen in a given host. These genes have been implicated in the control of responsiveness to a variety of antigens, including synthetic linear and branched copolymers, alloantigens and more conventional antigens.[75] An Ir gene determines both the humoral and cell-mediated immune responsiveness to the appropriate antigen.[70]

Ir genes have been shown to have either of two effects on the immune response, depending upon the antigen and particular animal strain under study:[76]

The presence of an Ir gene can wholly determine an animal's *ability* to respond to a given antigen. Such an animal is called a "responder." The absence of the gene is associated with the total inability to respond; such an animal is termed a "nonresponder." Thus, in certain circumstances, Ir genes can determine the difference between a complete response and no response.

Ir genes can control the *level* of response to an antigen. The presence of an Ir gene can convey a high level of responsiveness to an antigen, and its absence can be associated with a low level of response. Such animals are called high and low responders respectively.

The most complete genetic analysis of

the Ir system has been carried out in the mouse where the largest number of genetically characterized strains has been studied. Genetic mapping in the mouse has localized the Ir genes to the I region of the MHC (see p. 228, The MHC of the Mouse).[77] When a large number of different genetic strains of mice were tested for responsiveness to a battery of over twenty different antigens, no two strains were found to give identical reaction patterns.[78] These mice all possess different MHC haplotypes. This finding strongly suggests that the different Ir genes controlling the responsiveness to particular antigens are distinct from each other.

Much recent work has been directed toward understanding the specificity of antigen responsiveness controlled by an individual Ir gene.[78] The humoral response to three similar linear copolymers was found to consist of antibody that crossreacted very strongly with all of the three substances. Thus antibody molecules do not strongly distinguish one molecule from the other. Nevertheless, different Ir genes appear to control the responsiveness to each of these antigens. Thus Ir-gene-controlled responsiveness can be very discriminating in terms of antigen specificity.

Although the Ir gene can be a remarkably specific regulator of responsiveness, no one knows how many Ir genes there are. The repertoire of antigen responsiveness that is controlled by these genes is still undefined. Most investigators, however, believe that the scope of antigen-specific responses controlled by the Ir genes does not approach the tremendous array of antibody specificities.[78]

Recently experiments have raised the possibility that the immune response to a particular antigen may be controlled by two Ir genes. This work has indicated that an animal must possess the appropriate gene at each of two loci in order to mount an effective response.[79,80]

Over the past several years, experiments in the mouse and other animals have begun to elucidate the function of the Ir genes. The following observations have led to the view that Ir genes primarily determine the reactivity of *T cells* to particular antigens:

1. Ir genes are absolutely required for the development of cell-mediated immunity against the appropriate antigen.[70]

2. The Ir genes govern the response to the carrier moiety of a hapten-carrier complex.[81] In guinea pigs, one strain (strain 2) is a responder to low doses of BSA and a nonresponder to low doses of guinea pig albumin (GPA). Strain 2 animals will not produce an anti-DNP antibody response to DNP-GPA but will produce an anti-DNP antibody when given DNP-BSA. Therefore, a nonresponder cannot produce carrier-specific helper function when the molecule against which the animal cannot respond is used as a carrier.

This point is further emphasized by the observation that non-responder animals are perfectly capable of mounting a response against the antigen if it is presented as a hapten coupled to an immunogenic carrier.[82] In other words, if an antigen to which an animal cannot respond is itself presented on an immunogenic carrier, the antibody response is identical to that seen if the antigen is given to a responder animal. For example, animals who are nonresponders to a particular molecule called GAT, nevertheless can mount a normal anti-GAT response if challenged with GAT coupled to methylated BSA (Fig. 9-10). Thus the B-cell function in a nonresponder appears to be intact, while T helper function is deficient. It has been observed that there are equal numbers of specific antigen-binding B cells in responder and nonresponder strains, and, further, that a nonresponder can produce a response if T-derived helper function is provided by a nonspecific stimulus such as the allogeneic effect (see Chap. 5).[83,84]

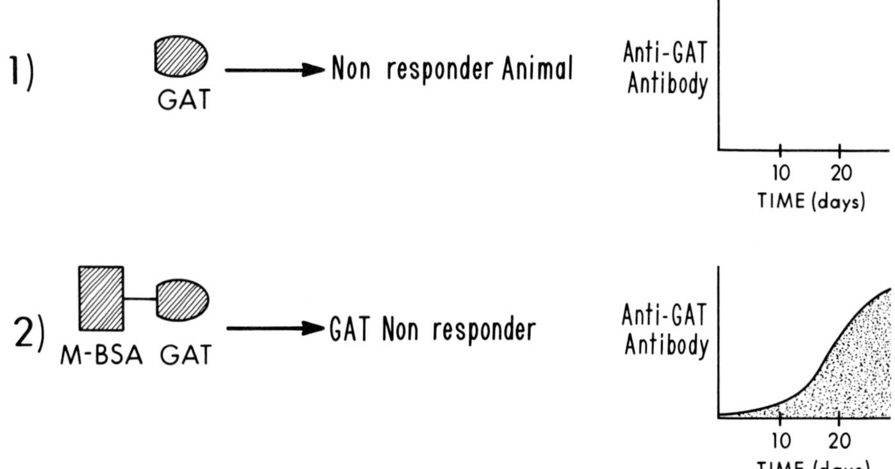

Fig. 9-10. GAT alone will not stimulate anti-GAT antibody production in a nonresponder animal. However, if GAT is coupled to a carrier that is capable of stimulating an immune response in that animal, anti-GAT antibody will be produced. Thus, GAT conjugated to M-BSA will elicit an anti-GAT response in the same animal, indicating that anti-GAT B cells are present in the nonresponder.

3. Certain nonresponders can mount an IgM response against a specific antigen but are unable to produce IgG or a secondary response, both of which are heavily T-dependent (see Chap. 5).[85] All antigens which have thus far been found to be involved in Ir-gene-controlled responsiveness have been T-cell-dependent antigens.

4. The differences between a nonresponder and a responder can be abolished in certain animals by neonatal thymectomy of the responders (Fig. 9-11).[86]

5. Finally, the macrophage does not seem to be the target of Ir-gene control. Some experiments have shown that macrophages from nonresponders are perfectly capable of reconstituting the immune response to the appropriate antigen when added to macrophage-depleted cultures of lymphocytes from responder animals.[87]

These observations suggest that nonresponsiveness is primarily a T-cell phenomenon. Both B cells and macrophages from nonresponders appear to be immunologically capable of responding to the appropriate antigen. This lack of responsiveness by the T cells could conceivably arise as the result of one of two mechanisms: the T cells could be unreactive to the antigen, or the specific antigen could selectively stimulate the production of T suppressor cells in the nonresponders.[88]

In mouse systems both of these mechanisms may be operative.[89] Thus certain strains of nonresponder mice clearly develop T suppressor cells when stimulated by the appropriate antigen.[90] Other nonresponder strains do not produce specific suppressor cells but merely fail to react to the particular antigens.

It has been proposed that there may be genes that code for the ability of suppressor cells to be stimulated by particular antigens as well as the set of genes that determine the ability to produce helper functions in response to specific antigens.[90] According to this idea, genetically controlled responsiveness may either result from the lack of genes coding for specific helper function or the presence of

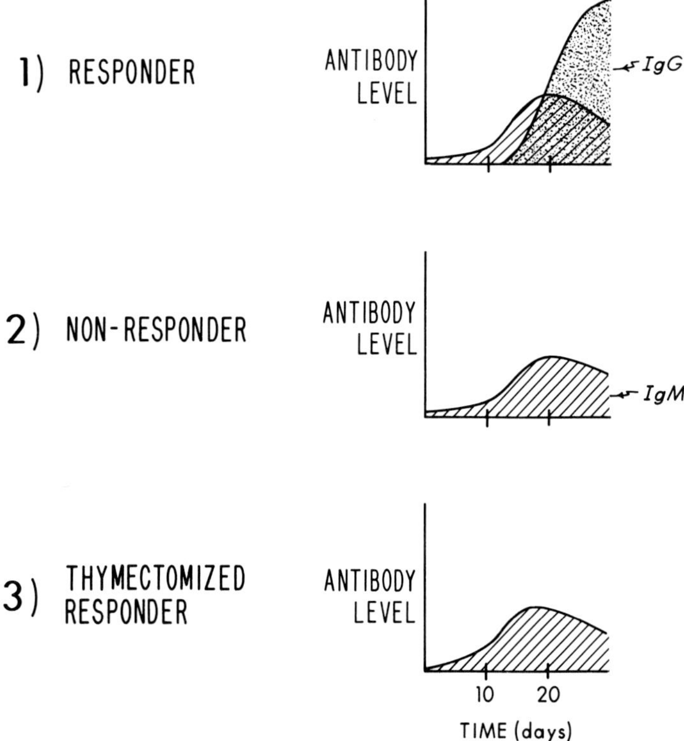

Fig. 9-11. (1) A responder animal produces a normal IgG and IgM response. (2) A nonresponder may produce only IgM. (3) If a responder is thymectomized, his antibody response may now resemble that of a nonresponder.

genes coding for specific suppressor function. These ideas remain hypothetical at present.

The products of the Ir genes have not yet been defined. It has been proposed by several investigators that they are cell-surface molecules that are intimately associated with the cell-surface receptors for antigen, and in some way modify the cell's response to antigen-receptor binding.[91] Too little is known at present to support any particular model of the action of these genes and their products.

There is only suggestive evidence that Ir genes may exist in man. Several investigators have reported a linkage between HLA haplotype and immune responsiveness to the ragweed antigen E.[92] Recently, the postulated Ir gene for this antigen has been mapped outside of the SD loci and close to the MLR-S.[93] This is similar to the location of the Ir genes in mice (see the section on the MHC of the mouse at the end of this chapter). The response to several other types of antigens have also recently been linked to MHC haplotypes in man.[74]

CELLULAR INTERACTIONS

There is still another way in which the MHC influences immune responsiveness. Recently, in animal systems, a region of the MHC that includes the I region has been shown to be important in the interactions of the various immunocompetent cells.

Effective interaction of T helper cells with B cells requires that both share identical I-region genes.[94] Thus a T cell will only be able to serve as a T helper cell if it is syngeneic to the B cell at the appropriate I-region loci.

Similarly, certain interactions between lymphocytes and macrophages, critical for a normal immune response, may require I-region identity.[95] This particular requirement appears to hold only for secondary responses.

Why genetic identity at these particular loci is required in order for cells to interact is not yet understood. Recent observations have provided some intriguing information as to the role of the I region in immunologic communication. We discussed the existence of several soluble helper and suppressor factors in Chapter 5. These newly discovered molecules can act as intercellular messengers carrying either antigen-specific or nonspecific information between immunocompetent cells. Several of these factors appear to bear I-region-coded antigens, that is, they serologically crossreact with antigens coded for by certain I-region loci (the Ia antigens). These findings suggest a further link between the I-region genes and their ability to determine suppression or help. Thus, if the I-region gene products determine the activity of the intercellular messengers, then one gene product may be received as a suppressive message while another may convey a helper signal.

THE MHC AND DISEASE

The discovery that susceptibility to certain cancers in mice was associated with major histocompatibility haplotypes led to the investigation of whether human disease states might also be associated with the MHC.[96] Many studies have since been carried out to answer this question, most of them looking at possible associations between various diseases and HLA antigens because of the availability of antisera against these antigens.

Several diseases have been found to have statistically significant correlations with particular HLA genotypes (see Table 9-3).[97] HLA B27 has a very high association with ankylosing spondylitis. Thus, about 90 per cent of patients with ankylosing spondylitis have this allele compared to less than 8 per cent of the normal population. The B27 antigen is also seen in much higher than expected frequency in patients with Reiter's disease, acute anterior uveitis, and reactive arthritis following infection with Yersinia and Salmonella species. HLA-B8 is highly correlated with celiac disease, myasthenia gravis and idiopathic Addison's disease. HLA-B13 is associated with psoriasis vulgaris and HLA-A3 has been strongly correlated with idiopathic hemochromatosis.[97a] Other correlations have been made but are less impressive.[98]

Table 9-3. HLA and Disease: Some Associations

Disease	*HLA Locus*	*Relative Risk*
Ankylosing spondylitis	B27	120
Reiter's disease	B27	40
Acute anterior uveitis	B27	30
Psoriasis vulgaris	B13 Bw17	4 4
Dermatitis herpetiformis	B8	4
Celiac disease	B8 Dw3	10 Very high
Idiopathic hemochromatosis	A3	Very high
Myasthenia gravis	B8	4-5

It is interesting to note that virtually all of the correlations involve alleles of the HLA-B locus. Since this locus is much closer than the A locus to the MLR-S locus, it has been suggested that the latter region may be the crucial one in terms of disease associations. In other words, the HLA correlations may actually be reflecting the tight linkage of the HLA-B loci to specific "LD" alleles. Only recently has it been possible to type "LD" alleles, employing batteries of mixed lymphocyte reactions.[99] Matching these alleles with disease states has produced some encouraging results. For example, the MLR-S allele Dw3 is highly associated with celiac disease. Dw2 may be associated with multiple sclerosis, although this finding has yet to be confirmed.[100]

Similar findings of a high "LD" association have been reported with several organ-specific endocrine diseases.[101] Juvenile-onset diabetes, idiopathic Addison's disease and Grave's disease all show a high correlation with HLA-Dw3. Other HLA haplotypes have been associated with an increased risk of developing juvenile diabetes mellitus, including both HLA-B8 and HLA-B15. Interestingly, in some healthy individuals carrying these two HLA alleles, diminished insulin responsiveness to an intravenous glucose tolerance test has been reported.[101] This finding hints at a particular relationship between these alleles and islet-cell function.

It should be added that MLR-S typing does not always provide a better MHC-disease marker than the HLA-B locus; ankylosing spondylitis is better correlated with the HLA allele than with any tested MLR-S type.

Several mechanisms have been proposed to explain MHC associations with disease.[102] One possibility is that an Ir gene product may be etiologically related to certain diseases, perhaps by permitting an immune response to an antigen or antigens which otherwise cause no problem for the host. For example, HLA-B8 may be linked with an Ir gene determining immune responsiveness to gluten. Any person carrying this Ir gene product would be hypersensitive to gluten and would present with the clinical picture of celiac disease. In the HLA-Dw3-positive individuals we may really be seeing the linkage of that locus with an immune response gene (or genes) controlling responsiveness to a self-antigen expressed on the target organs. Thus it has been shown that HLA-Dw3-positive individuals with Addison's disease often possess antiadrenal antibodies. Similarly, both Grave's disease and diabetes mellitus (especially the juvenile-onset form) have been associated with autoimmune phenomena. Although the pathogenetic relationships between these observations and the respective diseases are unknown, their possible association with a "forbidden" Ir gene is intriguing.

Other possible mechanisms for MHC-disease associations include molecular mimicry. According to this hypothesis, certain MHC antigens may bear a structural similarity to certain infectious agents. An immune response to these agents would result in cross-reactivity against the cell-surface antigen. This has been offered as an explanation for the association of HLA-B27 with post-Yersinia arthritis but has not been verified.

Because the human MHC contains genes that code for components of both the classical and properdin complement pathways, specific alleles may be associated with either defective or overactive complement production, both of which might lead to pathologic states. Finally, linkage disequilibrium between the MHC and other loci on the sixth chromosome *outside* the MHC has been offered as an explanation for the association in certain families of HLA types with spinal anomalies such as spina bifida and asymmetric facet joints.[13]

HLA genotypes may also affect the course of human disease in more indirect ways. For example, HLA-A2 has been associated with a more favorable prognosis in patients with leukemia.[103] It has been suggested that since about 50 per cent of blood donors are A2-positive, these individuals would not produce antibodies against this common transfusion antigen, thereby allowing HLA-A2-positive leukemics to benefit more fully from random blood transfusion than HLA-A2-negative leukemics.

THE MHC OF THE MOUSE

A great amount of experimental work in transplantation and immunogenetics has been performed with mice. One of the advantages of this system has been the availability of carefully characterized genetic strains. Much of our understanding of immunogenetics derives from work with murine systems, and it is therefore useful to take a brief look at the mouse MHC (see reference 104 for an excellent and detailed discussion of this material).

The mouse MHC is a tightly linked genetic region found on chromosome 17 (Fig. 9-12). It is referred to as the H-2 gene complex. A map of this region as it is currently understood is shown below. The K region and the D region code for major serologically determined histocompatibility antigens analogous to HLA-A, HLA-B and HLA-C. The marker loci are called H2K and H2D respectively. The S region contains genes that control the levels of a particular serum beta globulin. It may also control levels of complement components. The I region is divided into three subregions and contains genes that code for a variety of immune-related functions. These include:

1. *Ir genes*. These genes control the level of the immune response against various antigens.

2. *Lad Genes*. These apparently code for surface antigens that lead to stimulation in an MLR. These genes also seem to code for antigens that stimulate the graft-versus-host reaction; it is possible that the assays for graft-versus-host reactivity and mixed lymphocyte reactivity may at least partly measure similar phenomena (see Chap. 5).

3. *Histocompatibility Genes*. This locus, designated H-2I, codes for an antigen that is capable of stimulating skin-graft rejection in the face of antigen identity between the H-2K and H-2D loci.

4. *T-B, T-T and T-Macrophage Interaction Genes*. The genes governing the requirement for genetic identity between cells for immune interactions are contained in this region.

It is not known whether all of these functions reflect the activity of separate genes. Furthermore, the precise characteristics of the gene products of the I region have still not been defined. The I-region genes are defined by purely functional means such as graft rejection, MLR and immune responsiveness. Several gene products of this region have recently been defined serologically. The resultant antibodies react against cell-surface antigens which have been called Ia antigens. It is not known whether these newly detected Ia antigens are the gene products of the functional loci (Ir, Lad, etc.) described above.

There is some recent evidence to suggest that some of the Ia antigens may represent the Lad gene products. Some Ia antigens may also represent Ir gene products, although certain disparities between the two exist. Ia antigens have been mapped in all three subregions of the I region while all of the Ir genes that have been mapped are in the Ir-IA or Ir-IB subregions. Ia antigens are also primarily expressed on B cells, consistent with their being Lad gene products, whereas one would expect Ir gene products to be present on the T cell as well.

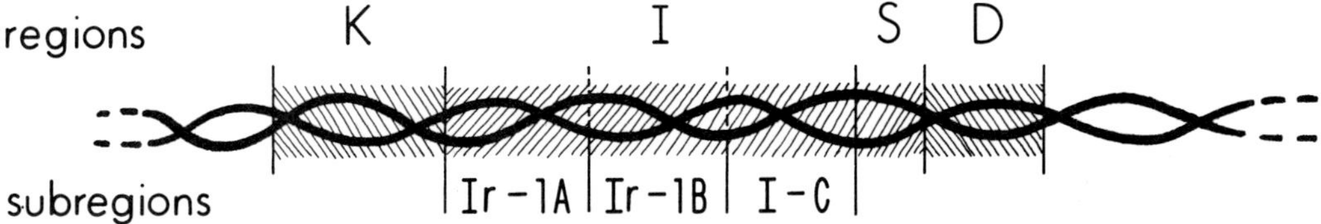

Fig. 9-12. H-2 region of chromosome 17 of the mouse, containing the mouse MHC (see text for details).

We must emphasize that the definition of the I-region antigens is still in its infancy. At present, few definite conclusions have been reached. Our approach has been to summarize the state of the art as currently perceived by most investigators in the field. Figure 9-13 shows a tentative placement of immune functions within the H-2 complex.

IN VITRO STUDIES OF THE T-CELL RESPONSE TO FOREIGN CELLS

There are two major aspects of the response of T lymphocytes to allogeneic cells. These are: (1) recognition and proliferation; and (2) production of specific cytotoxic effector cells. Each of these functions can be monitored by an *in vitro* test. Recognition and proliferation are measured in a "one-way MLR." Cytotoxicity is measured by the cell-mediated lymphocytolysis (CML) assay.

Over the past few years, a number of investigators have carried out experiments that have examined the genetic details of the T-cell response to allogeneic cells. Out of this work has emerged an exciting and complex picture of cell-cell interactions. Most of this work has been done in mouse systems and we will be referring to this animal in the following discussion.

The mixed lymphocyte reaction occurs because T cells recognize particular alloantigens which are coded for by the I region of the H-2 complex.[105] In the MHC of humans the specific genes coding for the antigens that stimulate an MLR are called MLR-S. In the murine MHC these genes are called Lad. It is not known how

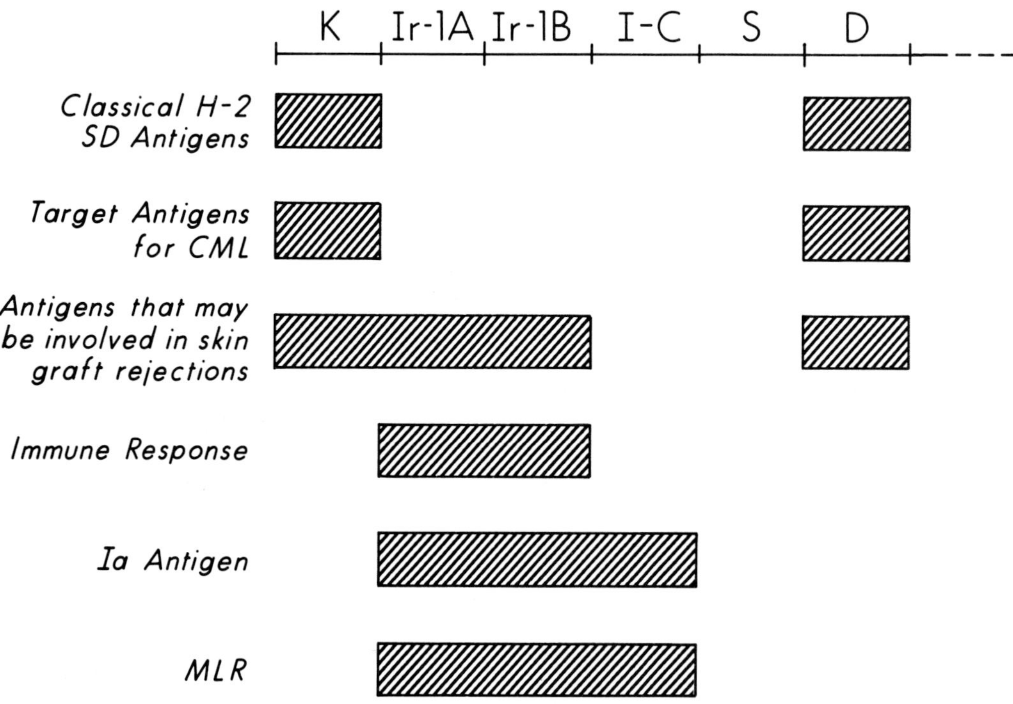

Fig. 9-13. Location of various functions and antigens on the mouse MHC. (Adapted from Sheffler, D. C., and David, C. S.: The H-2 major histocompatibility complex and the I immune response region: genetic variation, function and organization. Adv. Immunol., *20*:125, 1975.)

many genes code for Lad surface antigens nor has the exact location of the genes within the I region been established.

In the normal reaction between two allogeneic cell lines, the appearance of cytotoxic T lymphocytes (CTL) accompanies the mixed lymphocyte proliferative response. However, when lymphocytes from mice that were genetically identical at all loci except certain parts of the I region were mixed, an excellent proliferative response occurred without the generation of CTL.[106] This experiment showed that the MLR does not necessarily lead to the production of CTL, and that the MLR-S antigens by themselves do not stimulate killer-cell production.

This result led to a search to find the locus that codes for those surface antigens that do stimulate the production of CTL. Most experiments have pointed to the SD antigens of the D and K regions as the stimuli to killer-cell development.[107] In other words, if a cell is to stimulate the production of specific killer T cells it must be allogeneic to the responding cells at the D or K loci. Killer cells so stimulated are directed against the stimulating alloantigens and not against alloantigens in other regions of the MHC.[108] This observation implies that the foreignness of a particular antigen is not in itself sufficient to generate specific killer cells. Instead, only certain alloantigens can stimulate these effector T cells.

Questions have been raised as to whether the target antigens for CML are truly K or D SD antigens or are other antigens coded for by loci that are closely linked to the K and D regions. Although there is some evidence to support the latter view,[109] at present the bulk of experimental work appears to support the SD antigens as the CML target.

Although an MLR can take place without the production of cytotoxic T cells, it has been questioned whether a positive MLR is required for killer-cell induction. In certain studies, a positive MLR appeared to be requisite for a positive CML test.[110] However, other systems have shown that SD-region differences that give only minimal MLR will nevertheless lead to anti-SD-antigen killer cells.[111] At present it is therefore not known whether an MLR is required to produce killer cells. There is some evidence that SD differences alone may be capable of stimulating killer-cell production.[112] However, the level of killer-cell production seems to be less than if an accompanying "LD"-stimulated MLR is seen.

Recently some of the intricacics of the relationship between the MLR and CML have begun to be elucidated. One of the most important observations is that the T cells which can recognize the I-region MLR-S antigens and proliferate in the MLR may represent a subpopulation of lymphocytes antigenically distinct from either killer cells or precursors of killer cells (see Chap. 5).[113] It is presently believed that the killer cells and the proliferating cells interact with each other in order to produce a maximally effective cytotoxic reaction. One model for their interaction considers the T cell that proliferates in the MLR to be an amplifier cell. This is the T_2 cell referred to in Chapter 5. The prekiller cell, or T_1 lymphocyte, is induced to become a cytotoxic cell by SD or SD-related differences. The cytotoxicity of the anti-SD killer cell is augmented by the "LD"-stimulated amplifier T cell. According to this model, "LD"-stimulated T_2 cells act synergistically with the SD-stimulated T_1 cell to produce maximal killing. The killing however is only directed against the SD antigens that induced T_1-cell activation.

This scheme is illustrated by a set of experiments using animals that are allogeneic at restricted MHC loci.[114] These experiments can be outlined as follows (Fig. 9-14):

1. The target cell is allogeneic at the "LD" locus but syngeneic at the SD loci.

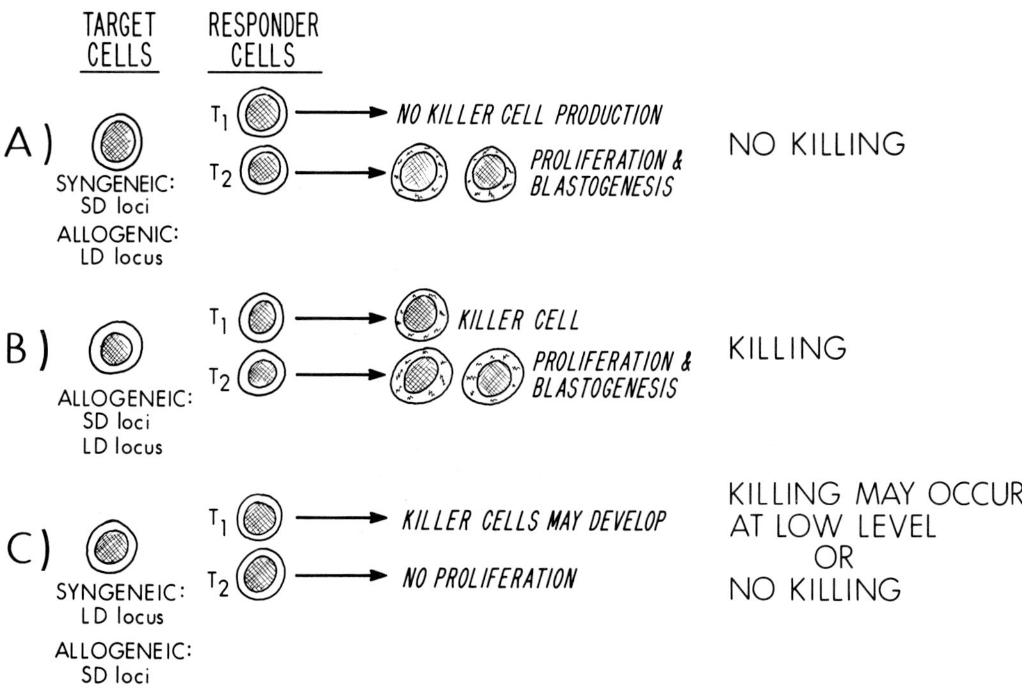

Fig. 9-14. Cell-stimulation experiments illustrate the relationship between specific MHC loci and foreign T-cell responsiveness (see text for details).

This stimulates the proliferation and blastogenesis of the T_2 helper cells but does not lead to any killer-cell activity against the target (Fig. 9-14A).

2. The target is allogeneic at both the "LD" and the SD loci. This stimulates both the T_1 and the T_2 subclasses leading to proliferation as well as the destruction of the targets by stimulated T_1 killer cells. If these stimulated T_1 killers are removed and added to a new target-cell population, they will destroy only those new targets that have identical SD antigens as the original target. The stimulated T_1 cells will kill such second targets even if they are "LD"-identical to the killers. This implies that the "LD" antigens are not the targets of killer-cell activity (Fig. 9-14B).

3. The target is allogeneic at an SD locus but syngeneic at the "LD" locus. In this situation less proliferation is seen and the T_2 helper cells are not stimulated. Some killing is observed by the SD-stimulated T_1 cells but this is at a lower level than would be seen if the enhancing effect of stimulating T_2 helper cells were present (Fig. 9-14C).

We must still ask how all of these findings relate to graft rejection. Unfortunately, it is not yet understood exactly what the precise antigenic parameters may be that determine the graft-host relationship. In one report, a non-SD I-region difference alone was responsible for the rejection of skin grafts.[115] In summary, present knowledge has not yet reached the point where one can make a definite statement as to the functional genetic definition of histocompatibility.

It will be important to determine whether the various experimental results obtained in the mouse are applicable to man. Much of the work done in the animal systems was possible because of the use of genetically controlled strains. This is clearly impossible with man. However, some evidence suggests that the results from these experiments with mice may be reliably extrapolated to man. Experiments with human cells appear to support the "LD"-SD dichotomy discussed above.[116,117] Thus, "LD" antigens stimulate an MLR while SD-related antigens are the targets for CML. It is interesting that these experiments have revealed a marked difference in the relevance of the first (A) as opposed to the second (B) major HLA locus in providing the targets for cytotoxic lymphocytes. Cells that are allegeneic at the B locus provide excellent killer-cell targets while A-locus differences stimulate only weak or sometimes no cytotoxicity.[118] Recent experiments have suggested that CML may be directed against a non-SD determinant closely linked to the HLA SD loci.[119] Unfortunately little is known about different T-cell subpopulations in man and a clear-cut distinction between amplifier and killer cells has not been made in the human "LD"-SD system. However, the fact that so much of the work in mice appears to be applicable to humans is encouraging.

REFERENCES

1. Van Rood, J. J., Eernisse, J. G. and Van Leeuwen, A.: Leukocyte antibodies in sera from pregant women. Nature, *181*:1735, 1958.
2. Van Someren, H. *et al.*: Human antigen and enzyme markers in man/Chinese hamster somatic cell hybrids. Proc. Natl. Acad. Sci. U.S.A., *71*:962, 1974.
3. Terasaki, P. I.: HL-A histocompatibility determinants. D. M., Dec., 1971.
4. Thorsby, E., Sandberg, L., Lindholm, A., and Kissmeyer-Nielsen, F.: The HLA system: evidence of a third sub-locus. Scand. J. Haematol., *7*:195, 1970.
5. ——: WHO-IUIS terminology committee nomenclature for factors of the HLA system. Eur. J. Immunol., *3*:889, 1975.
6. Van Rood, J. J.: The (relative) importance of HLA matching in kidney transplantation. Prog. Immunol., *1*:1027, 1971.
7. Van Rood, J. J., *et al.*: Leukocyte groups and their relation to homotransplantation. Ann. N.Y. Acad. Sci., *129*:467, 1966.
8. Amos, D. B., *et al.*: Skin donor selection by leukocyte typing. Lancet, *1*:300, 1966.
9. Amos, D. B., Seigler, H. F., Southworth, J., and Ward, F. E.: Skin graft rejection between subjects genotyped for HLA. Transplant. Proc., *1*:342, 1969.
10. Svejgaard, A., *et al.*: The recombination fraction of the HLA system. Tiss. Antigens, *1*:81, 1971.
11. Dausset, J.: Polymorphism of the HLA system. Transplant. Proc., *3*:1139, 1971.
12. Svejgaard, A., Hauge, M., Kissmeyer-Nielsen, F., and Thorsby, E.: HLA haplotype frequencies in Denmark and Norway. Tiss. Antigens, *1*:184, 1971.
13. Amos, D. B., and Ward, F. E.: Immunogenetics of the HLA system. Physiol. Rev., *55*:206, 1975.
14. Thorsby, E., and Kissmeyer-Nielsen, F.: New HL-A alleles. Vox Sang., *18*:134, 1970.
15. Eguro, S., Dorf, M., and Amos, D. B.: Cross reactions of HLA antibodies. VI. Dissection of a complex serum. Tiss. Antigens, *3*:195, 1973.
16. Mittal, K., and Terasaki, P.: Serological cross-reactivity in the HLA system. Tiss. Antigens, *4*:146, 1974.
17. Hauptfeld, V., and Klein, J.: Molecular relationship between private and public H-2 antigens as determined by antigen redistribution method. J. Exp. Med., *142*:288, 1975.
18. Lemonnier, F., Neuport-Sautes, C., Kourilsky, F. M., and Demant, P.: Relationships between private and public H-2 specificities on the cell surface. Immunogenetics, *2*:517, 1975.
19. Cresswell, P., Turner, M., and Strominger, J.: Papain-solubilized HL-A antigens from cultured human lymphocytes contain two peptide fragments. Proc. Natl. Acad. Sci. U.S.A., *70*:1603, 1973.
20. Peterson, P., Rask, L., and Lindblan, J.: Highly purified papain-solubilized HLA antigens contain β-2-microglobulin. Proc. Natl. Acad. Sci. U.S.A., *71*:35, 1974.
21. Peterson, P., Cunningham, B., Berggard, I., and Edelman, G.: Beta-2-microglobulin-A free immunoglobulin domain Proc. Natl. Acad. Sci. U.S.A., *69*:1697, 1972.
22. Solheim, B., and Thorsby, E.: Beta-2-microglobulin. Part of the HLA molecule in the cell membrane. Tiss. Antigens, *4*:83, 1974.
23. Beral, M., Hors, J., and Dausset, J.: A study of HLA antigens in human organs. Transplantation, *9*:185, 1970.

23a. Bach, F. H., and van Rood, J. J.: The major histocompatibility complex—genetics and biology. N. Engl. J. Med., *295*:927, 1976.

24. van Hooff, V. P., Schippers, H. M. A., Hendricks, G. F. J., and van Rood, J. J.: Influence of possible HL-A haploidentity on renal-graft survival in eurotransplant. Lancet, *1*:1130, 1974.
25. Koch, C., Fredericks, E., Eijsvoogel, V., and Van Rood, J. J.: MLC and skin graft data in unrelated HLA identical individuals. Lancet, *2*:1334, 1971.
26. Thorsby, E.: The human major histocompatibility system. Transplant. Rev., *18*:51, 1974.
27. Yunis, E. J., Plate, J. M., Ward, F. E., Seigler, H.

F., and Amos, D. B.: Anomalous MLR responsiveness among siblings. Transplant. Proc., *3*:118, 1971.

28. Yunis, E. J., and Amos, D. B.: Three closely linked genetic systems relevant to transplantation. Proc. Natl. Acad. Sci. U.S.A., *69*:3031, 1971.
29. Dupont, B., Staub-Nielsen, L, and Svejgaard, A.: Relative importance of FOUR and LA loci in determining MLR. Lancet, *2*:1336, 1971.
30. Hirschberg, H., and Thorsby, E.: Histocompatibility antigens causing stimulation in mixed lymphocyte culture interactions. Transplantation, *16*:451, 1973.
31. Zoschke, D. C., and Bach, F. H.: Specificity of allogeneic cell recognition by human lymphocytes *in vitro*. Science, *172*:1350, 1971.
32. Widmer, M., Alter, B., Bach, F., Bach, M., and Bailey, D.: Lymphocyte reactivity to serologically undetected components of the MHC. Nature [New Biol.], *242*:239, 1973.
33. Van Rood, J. J., Van Leeuwen, A., Parlevliet, J., Termijtelen, A., and Keuning, J. J.: LD typing by serology. *In* Kissmeyer-Nielsen, F. (ed.): Histocompatibility Testing. Copenhagen, Munksgaard, 1975.
34. Simpson, E.: Stimulation of MLC and cytotoxic response: evidence that T cells express SD but not LD antigens whereas B cells express both. Eur. J. Immunol., *5*:456, 1975.
35. Gatti, R. A., Meuwissen, H. J., Terasaki, P I., and Good, R. A.: Recombination within the HLA locus. Tiss. Antigens, *1*:239, 1971.
36. Seigler, H. F., Ward, F. E., and Amos, D. B., Phaup, M. B., and Stickel, D. L.: The immunogenicity of human HLA haplotypes as measured by skin graft survival times and mixed leukocyte reactions. J. Exp. Med., *133*:411, 1971.
37. Seigler, H. F., Ward, F. E., Amos, D. B., and Stickel, D. L.: Comparisons of mixed leukocyte reactions with skin graft survival in families genotyped for HLA. Transplant. Proc., *3*:115, 1971.
38. Stiller, C. R., *et al.*: Anti-donor immune responses in prediction of transplant rejection. N. Engl. J. Med., *294*:978, 1976.
39. Klein, J., and Hauptfeld, V.: Ia antigens: their serology, molecular relationships, and their role in allograft reactions. Transplant. Rev., *30*:83, 1976.
40. Starzl, T., *et al.*: Renal homotransplantation: Part I. Curr. Probl. Surg., April, 1974.
41. Van Rood, J. J., *et al.*: Graft survival in unrelated donor-recipient pairs matched for MLC and HLA. Transplant. Proc., *5*:409, 1973.
42. Starzl, T., *et al.*: Renal homotransplantation: Part II. Curr. Probl. Surg., May, 1974.
43. Hamburger, J., Crosnier, J., Descamps, B., and Rowinska, D.: The value of present methods used for the selection of organ donors. Transplant. Proc., *3*:260, 1971.
44. Boehmig, H., *et al.*: Hyperacute rejection of renal homografts: with particular reference to coagulation changes, humoral antibody and formed blood elements. Transplant. Proc., *3*:1105, 1971.
45. Williams, G., *et al.*: Studies in hyperacute and chronic renal homograft rejections in man. Surgery, *62*:204, 1967.
46. Kissmeyer-Nielsen, F., Olsen, S., Petersen, V., and Fjeldborg, O.: Hyperacute rejection of kidney allografts associated with preexisting humoral antibodies against donor cells. Lancet, *2*:662, 1966.
47. Patel, R., and Terasaki, P.: Significance of positive crossmatched test in kidney transplantation. N. Engl. J. Med., *280*:735, 1969.
48. Hirata, A., and Terasaki, P.: Cross-reactions between streptococcal M proteins and human transplantation antigens. Science, *168*:1095, 1970.
49. Revillard, J., and Betuel, N.: Circulating antibodies in allograft recipients. Adv. Nephrol., *5*:257, 1975.
50. Pierce, J., and Lee, H.: The kidney cell crossmatch in retransplantation. Surgery, *76*:101, 1974.
51. Clark, D., Fober, J., Good, R., and Varco, R.: Humoral factors in canine renal allograft rejection. Lancet, *1*:8, 1968.
52. Starzl, T., *et al.*: Schwartzmann reaction after human renal homotransplantation. N. Engl. J. Med., *278*:642, 1968.
53. Najarian, J., *et al.*: Mechanism of antigen release from canine kidney homotransplants. Ann. N.Y. Acad. Sci., *129*:76, 1966.
54. Elkins, W., and Guttmann, R.: Pathogenesis of a local graft versus host reaction: immunogenicity of circulating host lymphocytes. Science, *159*:1250, 1968.
55. Guttmann, R., and Lindquist, R.: Renal transplantation in the inbred rat. Transplantation, *8*:490, 1969.
56. Strober, S., and Gowans, J.: The role of lymphocytes in the sensitization of rats to renal homografts. J. Exp. Med., *122*:347, 1965.
57. Pedersen, N., and Morris, B.: The role of the lymphatic system in the rejection of homografts. J. Exp. Med., *131*:936, 1970.
58. Strom, T., Tilney, N., Carpenter, C., and Busch, G.: Identity and cytotoxic capacity of cells infiltrating renal allografts. N. Engl. J. Med., *292*:1257, 1975.
59. Hamburger, J.: Recent advances in the understanding of rejection. Adv. Nephrol., *5*:101, 1975.
60. Dimitriu, A., Dy, M., Thomson, N., and Hamburger, J.: Macrophage cytotoxicity in the mouse immune response against a skin graft. J. Immunol., *114*:195, 1974.
61. Milgrom, F., Litvak, B. I., Kano, K., and Witebsky, E.: Humoral antibodies in renal homografts. J.A.M.A., *198*:226, 1966.
62. Stiller, C., *et al.*: Lymphocyte dependent antibody and renal graft rejection. Lancet, *1*:953, 1975.
63. Garovoy, M., *et al.*: Antibody modulation of cellular reactivity post renal transplantation. Transplant. Proc., *5*:129, 1973.

64. Quadracci, L., *et al.*: Homograft survival and serum-blocking factors. Transplant. Proc., *5*:649, 1973.
65. Monaco, A., Lugois, A., Wood, M., and Clark, A.: Active enhancement of tissue allografts with ALS and bone marrow. Adv. Nephrol., *5*:135, 1975.
66. Callard, P., *et al.*: The arterial lesions in the course of renal allograft rejection phenomena. Adv. Nephrol., *5*:333, 1975.
67. Andres, G. A., *et al.*: Human renal transplants III. Immunopathologic studies. Lab. Invest., *22*:588, 1970.
68. Busch, G., *et al.*: Human renal allografts. Medicine, *50*:29, 1971.
69. McDevitt, H. O., and Benacerraf, B.: Genetic control of specific immune responses. Adv. Immunol., *11*:31, 1969.
70. Benacerraf, B., and McDevitt, H.: Histocompatibility-linked immune response genes. Science, *175*:273, 1972.
71. McDevitt, H., and Chinitz, A.: Genetic control of the antibody response: relationship between immune response and H-2 type. Science, *163*:207, 1969.
72. Ellman, L., Green, I., Master, W., and Benacerraf, B.: Linkage between the poly-L-lysine gene and the locus controlling the major histocompatibility antigens in strain 2 guinea pigs. Proc. Natl. Acad. Sci. U.S.A., *66*:322, 1970.
73. Gunther, E., Rude, E., and Stark, O.: Antibody response in rats to the synthetic polypeptide (T,G)-A-L genetically linked to the major histocompatibility system. Eur. J. Immunol., *2*:151, 1972.
74. Buckley, C. E., *et al.*: HLA linked human immune response genes. Proc. Natl. Acad. Sci. U.S.A., *70*:2157, 1973.
75. Green, I.: Genetic control of immune responses. Immunogenetics, *1*:4, 1974.
76. Merryman, C., and Maurer, P.: Genetic control of immune response to glutamic acid, alanine, tyrosine, co-polymers in mice. J. Immunol., *108*:135, 1972.
77. McDevitt, H., *et al.*: Genetic control of the immune response. J. Exp. Med., *135*:1259, 1972.
78. Benacerraf, B., and Katz, D.: The histocompatibility-linked immune response genes. Adv. Cancer Res., *21*:121, 1975.
79. Schwartz, R. H., Dorf, M. E., Benacerraf, G., and Paul, W. E.: The requirement for two complementing Ir-GL Φ immune response genes in the T-lymphocyte proliferative response to poly (glu^{53} Lys^{36} Phe^{11}). J. Exp. Med., *143*:892, 1976.
80. Dorf, M. E., Maurer, P. H., Merryman, C. F., and Benacerraf, B.: Inclusion group systems and Cis-trans effects in responses controlled by the two complementing Ir-G1 genes. J. Exp. Med., *143*:889, 1976.
81. Green, I., and Benacerraf, B.: Genetic control of immune responsiveness to limiting doses of proteins and hapten protein conjugates in guinea pigs. J. Immunol., *107*:374, 1971.
82. Kapp, J., Pierce, C., and Benacerraf, B.: Genetic control of immune responses *in vitro*. J. Exp. Med., *138*:1107, 1973.
83. Dunham, E., Unanue, E., and Benacerraf, B.: Antigen binding and capping by lymphocytes of genetic nonresponder mice. J. Exp. Med., *136*:403, 1972.
84. Ordal, J., and Grumet, C.: Genetic control of the immune response. J. Exp. Med., *136*:1195, 1972.
85. Grumet, C.: Genetic control of the immune response. J. Exp. Med., *135*:110, 1972.
86. Mitchell, G., Grumet, C., and McDevitt, H.: Genetic control of the immune response. J. Exp. Med., *135*:126, 1971.
87. Kapp, J., Pierce, C., and Benacerraf, B.: Genetic control of immune responses *in vitro*. J. Exp. Med., *138*:1121, 1973.
88. Gershon, R., Maurer, P., and Merryman, C.: A cellular basis for genetically controlled immunological unresponsiveness in mice: tolerance induction in T cells. Proc. Natl. Acad. Sci. U.S.A., *70*:250, 1972.
89. Benacerraf, B., *et al.*: The stimulation of specific suppressor T cells in genetic nonresponder mice by linear random copolymers of L-amino acids. Transplant. Rev., *26*:21, 1975.
90. Kapp, J., Pierce, C., and Benacerraf, B.: Genetic control of immune responses *in vitro*. J. Exp. Med., *140*:172, 1974.
91. Katz, D., and Benacerraf, B.: The function and interrelationship of T-cell receptors, Ir genes and other histocompatibility gene products. Transplant. Rev., *22*:175, 1975.
92. Levine, B., Sternber, R., and Fotino, M.: Ragweed hayfever: genetic control and linkage to HLA haplotypes. Science, *178*:1201, 1972.
93. Blumenthal, M., *et al.*: Genetic mapping of Ir locus in man: linkage to a second locus of HLA. Science, *184*:1201, 1974.
94. Katz, D., *et al.*: Cell interaction between histoincompatible T and B lymphocytes. J. Exp. Med., *141*:263, 1975.
95. Rosenthal, A. S., and Shevach, E. M.: Function of macrophages in antigen recognition by guinea pig T lymphocytes. J. Exp. Med., *138*:1194, 1973.
96. McDevitt, H., and Landy, M. (eds.): Genetic Control of Immune Responses: Relationship to Disease Susceptibility. New York, Academic Press, 1972.
97. Terasaki, P., and Mickey, M.: HLA haplotypes of 32 diseases. Transplant. Rev., *22*:105, 1975.
97a. Simon, M., Bourel, M., Fauchet, R. and Genetet, B.: Association of HLA-A3 and HLA-B14 antigens with idiopathic hemochromatosis. Gut, *17*:332, 1976.
98. Svejgaard, A., *et al.*: HLA and disease associations—a survey. Transplant. Rev., *22*:3, 1975.
99. Van Rood, J. J., Van Hooff, J., and Keuning, J.: Disease predisposition, immune responsiveness and the fine structure of the HLA supergene. Transplant. Rev., *22*:75, 1975.

100. Jerslid, C., *et al.*: Histocompatibility determinants in multiple sclerosis. Transplant. Rev., *22*:148, 1975.
101. Thomsen, M., *et al.*: MLC typing in juvenile diabetes mellitus and idiopathic Addison's disease. Transplant. Rev., *22*:125, 1975.
102. Dausset, J., and Hors, J.: Some contributions of the HLA complex to the genetics of human disease. Transplant. Rev., *22*:44, 1975.
103. Rogentine, G., Trapani, R., Yankee, R., and Henderson, E.: HLA antigens and acute lymphocytic leukemia: the nature of the HLA-2 association. Tiss. Antigens, *3*:470, 1973.
104. Shreffler, D. C., and David, C. S.: The H-2 major histocompatibility complex and the I immune response region: genetic variation, function, and organization. Adv. Immunol., *20*:125, 1975.
105. Meo, T., Vives, J., Miggiano, V., and Shreffler, D.: A major role for the Ir-1 region of the mouse H-2 complex in the MLR. Transplant. Proc., *5*:377, 1973.
106. Schendel, D., and Bach, F.: Genetic control of cell mediated lymphocytolysis in the mouse. J. Exp. Med., *140*:1534, 1974.
107. Nabholz, M., *et al.*: Cell-mediated lysis *in vitro*: Genetic control of killer cell production and target specificities in the mouse. Eur. J. Immunol., *4*:378, 1974.
108. Sorensen, S., and Hawkes, S.: The genetic basis for CML in mice. Transplant. Proc., *5*:1361, 1973.
109. Edidin, M., and Henney, C.: The effect of capping H-2 antigens on the susceptibility of target cells to humoral and T cell-mediated lysis. Nature [New Biol.], *246*:47, 1973.
110. Alter, B., *et al.*: Cell mediated lympholysis. J. Exp. Med., *137*:1303, 1973.
111. Schendel, D., Alter, B., and Bach, F.: The involvement of LD and SD region differences in MLC and CML: a three cell experiment. Transplant. Proc., *5*:1651, 1973.
112. Demant, P.: H-2 gene complex and its role in alloimmune reactions. Transplant. Rev., *15*:164, 1973.
113. Cantor, H., and Boyse, E.: Functional subclasses of T lymphocytes bearing different Ly antigens. J. Exp. Med., *141*:1390, 1975.
114. Bach, F., *et al.*: *In* Rosenthal, A., (ed.): The Immune Response P. 173. New York, Academic Press, 1975.
115. Klein, J., Hauptfeld, M., and Hauptfeld, V.: Evidence for a 3rd Ir-associated histocompatibility region in the H-2 complex of the mouse. Immunogenetics, *1*:45, 1974.
116. Eijsvoogel, V., *et al.*: Lymphocyte activation and destruction *in vitro* in relation to MLC and HL-A. Transplant. Proc., *5*:1301, 1973.
117. Bonnard, G., *et al.*: SD versus LD antigens as targets for lymphocyte-mediated cytotoxicity. Transplant. Proc., *5*:1679, 1973.
118. Eijsvoogel, V., *et al.*: The specificity and activation mechanism of CML in man. Transplant. Proc., *5*:1675, 1973.
119. Sondel, P., and Bach, F.: Recognitive specificity of human cytotoxic T lymphocytes. J. Exp. Med., *142*:1339, 1975.

10 The Immunodeficiency Diseases

The immunodeficiency diseases include a wide spectrum of disorders characterized by the inability of affected individuals to perform normal immunologic functions. Because of the emormous complexity of the immune system, there are many loci at which dysfunction may lead to clinically overt immunodeficiency. The precise clinical manifestations will vary, depending upon the particular aspect of the immune system affected and the extent of the compromise.

An immunodeficiency disease can be a primary defect of the immune system, part of a more generalized systemic defect or secondary to a disease involving other tissues. It can be inherited, congenital or acquired, and may present as a stable defect, as a progressive loss of immunocompetence or as a reversible deficiency. In this chapter, we shall focus on the primary immunodeficiency diseases.

There are three major types of primary defects that can lead to immunodeficiency:

1. Some immunodeficiency states result from the *failure of one or more of the essential elements of the immune system to develop properly*. Examples are the failure to develop a fully competent thymus or the absence of precursor cells which would ordinarily differentiate into a population of immunocompetent cells.

2. *Metabolic defects* can compromise the ability of immunocompetent cells to perform their normal functions. Specific metabolic defects have recently been described in certain immunodeficiency diseases.

3. Most of the primary immunodeficiency diseases appear to result from the absence of particular immune functions associated with *the failure to develop specific functionally competent cell populations*. These are not necessarily gross anatomical developmental defects, as those mentioned in paragraph 1 above, but rather failures of specific cellular differentiation. Because so many of the immunodeficiency diseases appear to fall into this category, we will first examine what is currently known about the normal course of differentiation of immunocompetent cells. It is hoped that a clear understanding of this process will eventually enable the characterization of specific immunodeficiency disorders on the basis of particular lesions along the various pathways of differentiation.

THE DIFFERENTIATION OF IMMUNOCOMPETENT CELLS

A knowledge of the normal pathways of differentiation of the various immunocompetent cell lines would afford a much greater understanding of the immune system than we now possess. Although a considerable amount of experimental work has been directed toward understanding lymphocyte differentiation, the entire field is evolving so rapidly that any attempt to describe a sequence of differentiation is bound to be promptly outdated. One further difficulty in presenting an accurate picture of immune development in man comes from the fact that most experiments have employed animal systems and it is far from clear how much of this information can be extrapolated to humans.

The hematopoietic elements of the body are believed to arise from a pluripotential stem cell.[1] Erythrocytes and granulocytes as well as immunocompetent lymphocytes are felt to derive from this primordial cell.[2] The next step may be the appearance of "differentiated" stem cells committed to producing cells of one particular line, i.e., erythroid, myeloid or lymphoid. Somewhere after this point, lymphoid precursors become committed to one of two pathways: those which are destined to become T cells migrate to the thymus; those which will become B cells do not.[3] (See Fig. 1-17.)

The B Cell

Stem-cell differentiation gives rise to a population of precursor B cells which can be found in the marrow and spleen but not in the lymph nodes (Fig. 10-1).[4] These cells cannot actively secrete antibody in response to antigen, nor do they appear capable of expressing immunoglobulin on their surface.[5] The ability to express surface immunoglobulin is acquired next.[6] Only fully mature B cells can synthesize immunoglobulin, express it on their surfaces, and differentiate into cells capable of secreting antibody in response to antigenic stimulation. The mature small B lymphocyte is itself only a precursor for the blast cells, plasma-blasts and plasma cells that appear upon antigenic stimulation. A deficient humoral immune system can result from the failure of these terminal stages of differentiation despite the presence of normal-appearing small B lymphocytes.

Deficient T helper function can also compromise the humoral response. Production of IgA, IgG and IgE appears to require T helper function. IgM production is less dependent upon T-cell help.[7] It is still uncertain whether IgG-, IgM-, IgA- and IgE-producing cells represent different B-cell lines or whether they are separately differentiated states of the same cell line (Fig. 10-2; see Chap. 6).[8,9]

B cells carry other surface markers such as the Fc and complement receptors. Little is known about the relative order of appearance of these markers. Work in mice suggests that B cells acquire the capacity to express surface immunoglobulin before the C3 receptor is acquired.[10] Some evidence suggests that surface-immunoglobulin-bearing B cells appear in humans

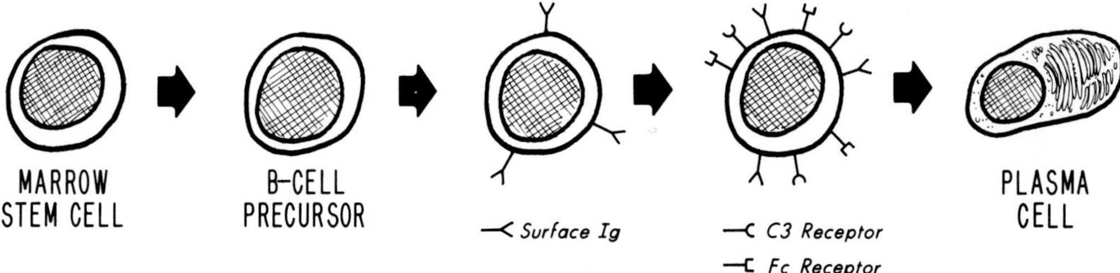

Fig. 10-1. Scheme of B-cell differentiation. The postulated pluripotential stem cell is believed to give rise to a precursor B cell which eventually develops the typical surface markers of a mature B cell. The final differentiative step to an antibody-producing plasma cell is driven by antigenic stimulation (or other forms of stimulation).

Fig. 10-2. Two proposed schemes for the generation of B-cell class diversity. (1) B cells develop sequentially in the order IgM→ IgG→ IgA. (2) There may be distinct B-cell precursors for each of the major immunoglobulin classes.

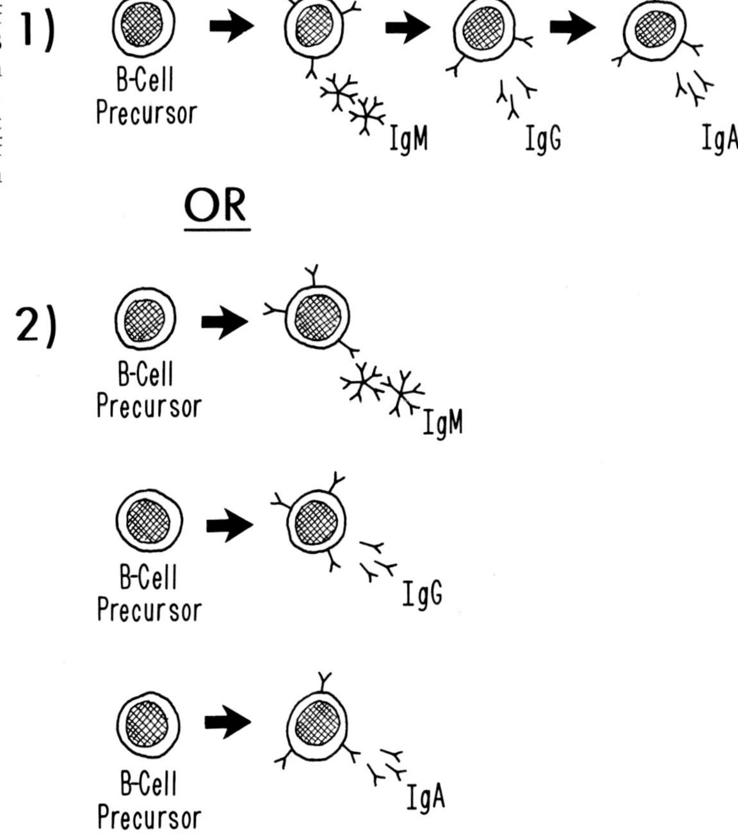

before Fc- or C3-receptor-bearing cells can be detected.[11]

The development of the secretory IgA system has certain unique features. There is a high percentage of B cells and plasma cells committed to IgA synthesis in the lamina propria of the intestine and in gut-associated lymphoid tissue.[12] Many of these cells have been reported to bear IgA surface molecules.[13] In mice there is a subpopulation of lymphocytes in the mesenteric lymph nodes which specifically homes to gut-associated lymphoid tissue and gives rise to IgA-secreting plasma cells.[14] It is likely that the specific homing of lymphocytic precursor cells to the gut is a necessary event in the development of the *local* secretory immunoglobulin system. Whether precursors already committed to IgA production home to the region or whether there is a local inductive mechanism which stimulates uncommitted cells to become IgA producers is not known (Fig. 10-3).[15] In order to develop a normal secretory IgA system, not only must the IgA-producing lymphocytic line be fully competent but the epithelial cells must be capable of producing secretory component. The production of secretory component in humans is detectable at birth whereas IgA itself may not appear in significant amounts until several weeks postpartum.[16]

The T Cell

The most commonly held view concerning the development of mature T cells postulates the existence of precursor lymphoid cells which mature into im-

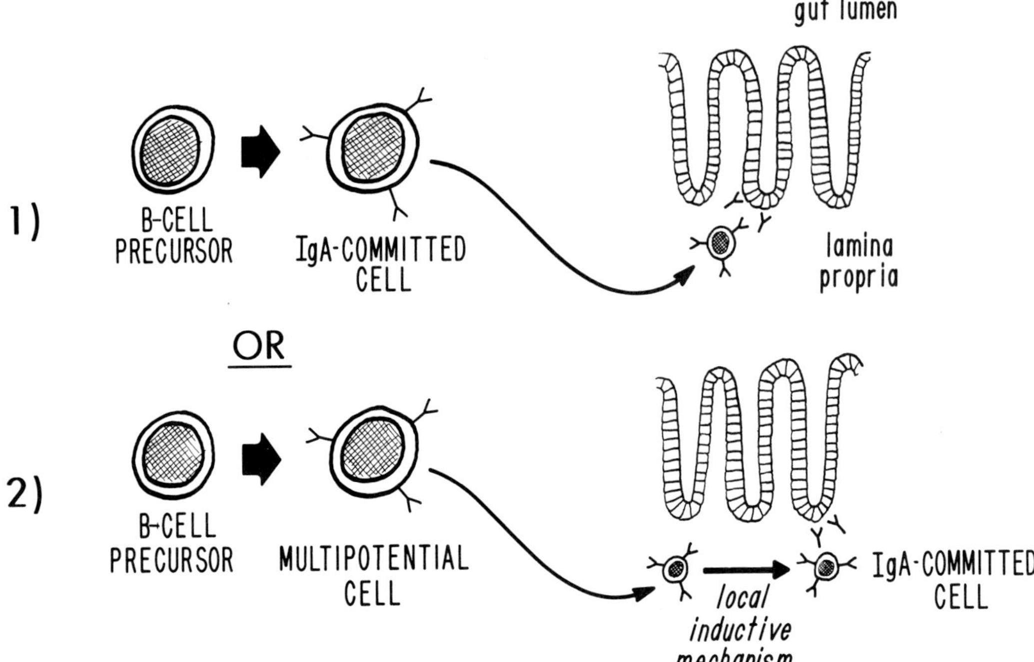

Fig. 10-3. Two proposed schemes for the development of gut-associated IgA-committed B cells. (1) IgA-committed B cells specifically home to gut tissue. (2) Uncommitted B cells circulate through gut tissue where they are induced to become IgA-committed cells.

munocompetent T cells under the influence of the thymus. The details of this process are not well understood. The mouse system has been most amenable to attempts at delineating a pathway of maturation within the thymus. Experimental evidence in the mouse suggests that two sequential steps may be involved (Fig. 10-4).[17,18] These studies propose that there is an early "prethymic" cell which

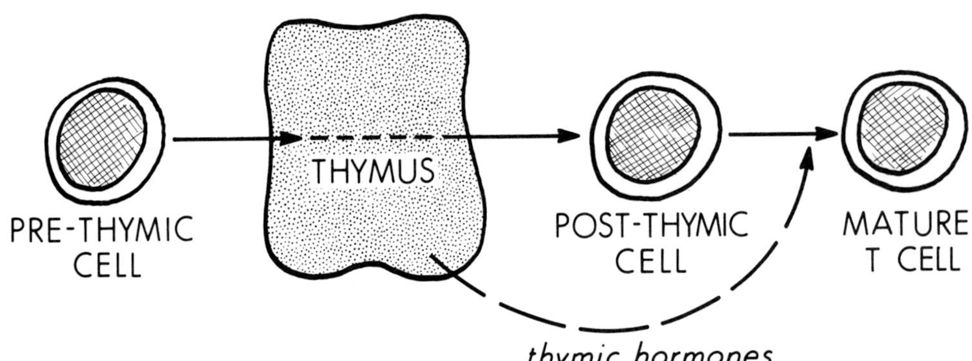

Fig. 10-4. Proposed T-cell development illustrating two possible stages of maturation. Prethymic cells must pass through the thymus where they mature into post-thymic cells. Post-thymic cells can leave the thymus and further develop into mature T cells under the influence of thymic humoral factors.

must migrate to an intact thymus gland where it differentiates into a "post-thymic" cell. This latter cell can then further differentiate into an immunocompetent T cell under the influence of thymic hormones (see Chap. 5).[19-21] The existence of prethymic and post-thymic cells is still somewhat controversial.

There have been very few studies of the fetal development of T cells in man. One study documented the time course for the development of different T-cell functions in the various fetal tissues.[22] PHA-responsive cells were first detected within the thymus at about ten weeks of gestation and were later found in the spleen and peripheral blood. Responsiveness to alloantigens (as measured in the mixed lymphocyte reaction) appeared to be acquired by the fetus earlier than mitogen responsiveness since mixed lymphocyte reactivity could be detected in the fetal liver lymphoid cells at about five to seven weeks. However, MLR-responsive cells were not detected in the thymus until about twelve weeks.

In the *post*natal human, thymic precursors are believed to be present in the bone marrow.[23] There appears to be a distinct population of bone marrow cells in man that is capable of responding to alloantigens but does not form spontaneous rosettes and does not respond to PHA.[24]

Several investigators have reported the effectiveness of thymic extracts in inducing the differentiation of human bone marrow cells *in vitro*.[25] Incubation of marrow cells with thymic extracts can induce the appearance of T-cell surface-antigen markers as well as a slight increase in the number of cells forming spontaneous sheep erythrocyte rosettes.[26]

At present it is difficult to organize the available information concerning the maturation and differentiation of human T cells into a single scheme. Certain points should be kept in mind when considering possible defects in T-cell development:

1. The thymus undoubtedly plays a crucial role in the normal maturation of T cells. The requirements for intrathymic development and the role of thymic humoral factors remain uncertain. Data from animal models suggests that both may be important.
2. T-cell functions and physical characteristics (such as rosette formation) may mature in a particular time sequence. Thus, alloantigen responsiveness may precede mitogen responsiveness and so on. However, one must be cautious in interpreting reports of sequential development. It is important to know whether the reported observations reflect the sequential development of separate T-cell subpopulations or the sequential acquisition of different functions by a single lymphocyte population.

THE CLINICAL PRESENTATION OF THE IMMUNODEFICIENT PATIENT

As we explore the various immunodeficiency states, it will become apparent that recurrent infection is the hallmark of the immunodeficient patient, reflecting the tremendous importance of the immune system in dealing with microorganisms. There is an increase in the incidence of infection in almost all of the immunodeficiency diseases. The nature of the immune deficit determines, in part, the spectrum of infections that may be encountered. Thus, primary T-cell deficits with diminished cell-mediated immunity permit an unusual amount of intracellular infections (see Chap. 11). These may be caused by viruses, fungi and certain bacteria such as tuberculosis. B-cell deficits allow infections by organisms that are largely disposed of by opsonization, that is, by encapsulated bacteria such as the pneumococcus, staphylococcus, etc. This distinction between T-cell and B-cell-dependent infections is not exact and is certainly less compelling than much of the literature

Table 10-1. **The Immunodeficiency Diseases**

Disease	*Cell-Mediated Immunity (CMI)*	*Humoral Immunity*
DiGeorge's syndrome	Failure of the thymus to develop; diminished CMI	Normal serum Ig levels; decreased antibody responses
Nezelof's syndrome	Thymic dyplasia; diminished CMI	Normal or increased serum Ig; decreased antibody responses; often a dysgamma-globulinemia
X-linked agammaglob-ulinemia	Normal, except decreased *in vitro* mitogenesis	Decreased serum Ig; decreased antibody responses
IgA deficiency	Normal	Decreased IgA levels
Hyper-IgM syndrome	Normal	Normal or increased IgM; decreased IgA and IgG
Hyper-IgE syndrome	Decreased	Increased immediate hyper-sensitivity; decreased responses of other antibody classes
Severe combined immuno-deficiency	Decreased	Decreased antibody responses
Nucleoside phosphorylase deficiency	Decreased	Normal
Common variable hypogam-maglobulinemia	Variable	Decreased serum Ig levels; most have Ig+ cells but lack plasma cells.
Wiskott-Aldrich syndrome	Decreased CMI to antigens; normal response to mitogens	Increased IgE, decreased IgM levels; increased Ig catabolism; decreased response to antigens, normal to mitogens
Ataxia-telangiectasia	Decreased	Decreased IgA and IgE levels; impaired response to antigens

might lead one to believe, but it does roughly reflect the variation in specific immune mechanisms normally employed against different infectious agents. The many manifestations of each particular immunodeficiency disease will be discussed separately below (see Table 10-1).

DISORDERS WITH PREDOMINANT ABNORMALITIES OF CELL-MEDIATED IMMUNITY

Immunodeficiency diseases are often divided into T-cell disorders, B-cell disorders and mixed disorders. This division is merely a reflection of the major phenotypic expression of the individual disease. Because T- and B-cell functions are so deeply intertwined, a deficiency in T-cell function almost invariably results in abnormal B-cell reactivity. There is one noted exception that we would like to mention here. Recently, a patient has been described whose B-cell function appears entirely normal in the face of compromised cellular immunity.[27] This patient can mount perfectly adequate antigen-specific antibody responses, but cannot mount T-cell responses. It is possible that this patient's defect is one of failure to differentiate T-cell effector functions while maintaining the ability to perform helper functions.

Several well-defined syndromes appear to affect primarily the T-cell lineage. In these disorders, which include DiGeorge's and Nezelof's syndromes, humoral immunity is typically depressed as well, and may reflect the absence of T-cell cooperative functions.

DiGEORGE'S SYNDROME

DiGeorge's syndrome, or congenital thymic hypoplasia, is at present the only immunodeficiency syndrome with a well-defined developmental etiology.[28]

Clinical Presentation

DiGeorge's syndrome presents in the neonate with hypocalcemic tetany due to severe hypoparathyroidism. Associated malformations include tracheal, esophageal and cardiovascular anomalies (notably a right-sided aortic arch) and a characteristic facies with hypotelorism, bowed mouth and notched pinnae.[28] Compromised immune function is evident in the great susceptibility of these infants to infections. Extensive mucocutaneous candidiasis is often present and is refractory to normal antimycotic therapy. Most infections are usually fungal or viral in nature, although gram-negative bacterial infections are also seen. These children may also become infected with *Pneumocystis carinii*, a type of protozoan, leading to severe pneumonitis and respiratory failure. Since the organism is ordinarily nonpathogenic in man, *P. carinii* infection is virtually diagnostic of immunologic compromise due to primary immunodeficiency or immunodeficiency associated with systemic diseases such as autoimmune diseases and lymphoreticular malignancies. If untreated, children with DiGeorge's syndrome die in infancy from overwhelming infection.

Pathophysiology and Immunology

The underlying pathologic abnormality of DiGeorge's syndrome is the dysmorphogenesis of the embryonic third and fourth pharyngeal pouches.[29] Failure of the development of the thymus and the parathyroid glands is responsible for the major clinical findings. The cause of this developmental anomaly is unknown. The developmental defect may range from a complete absence of the thymus (thymic aplasia) to varying degrees of thymic hypoplasia.[30,31]

Thymic insufficiency is responsible for all of the immunologic abnormalities in these children. Lymph node biopsy characteristically reveals marked diminu-

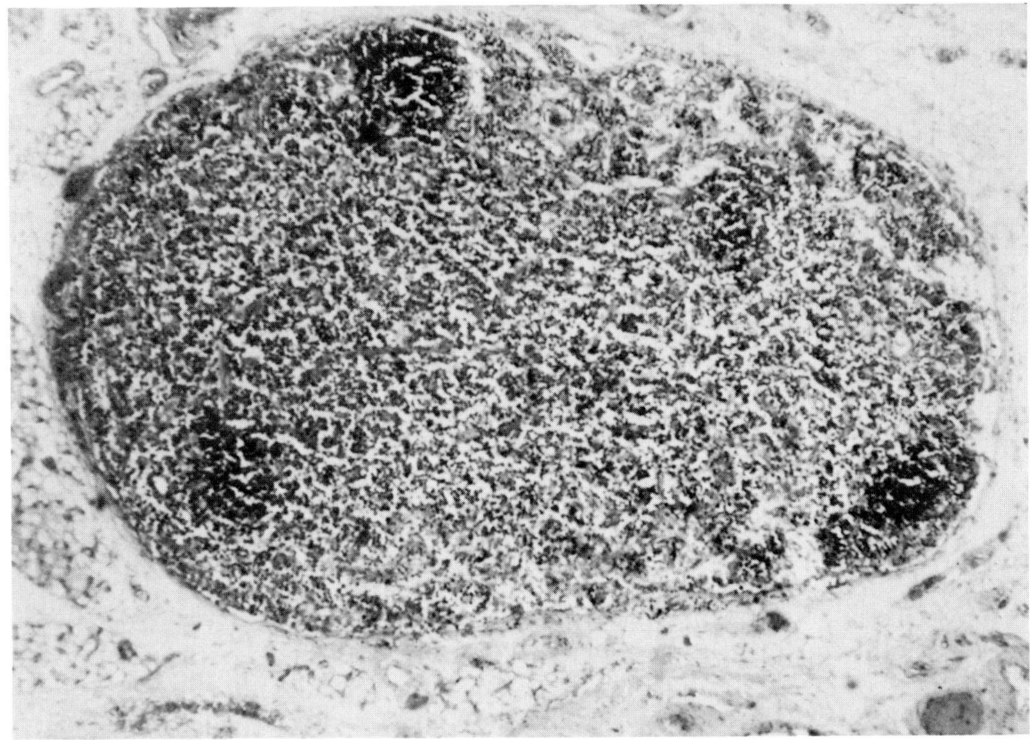

Fig. 10-5. Lymph node from a patient with DiGeorge's Syndrome. Follicles are present, but the paracortical region is only sparsely populated with lymphocytes. (Courtesy Dr. R. H. Buckley.)

tion of the number of lymphocytes in the paracortical (T-cell) regions (Fig. 10-5).[32] The level of peripheral blood lymphocytes is usually normal, although some of these children do eventually develop lymphopenia, perhaps as a result of chronic infection.[33] Surface characterization of the peripheral lymphocytes reveals an abnormally high percentage of cells bearing surface immunoglobulin and very low numbers of cells forming spontaneous sheep erythrocyte rosettes.[33]

The ability to carry out T-cell-related immune functions is markedly impaired although it varies from patient to patient. This can be demonstrated by the diminished ability of these patients to reject allografts and to mount delayed hypersensitivity reactions to skin test antigens.[33] T-cell *in vitro* reactivity, such as mitogen responsiveness, is also compromised.[34] T helper function may also be affected. Thus, although serum immunoglobulin levels are often normal, the capacity to mount humoral responses to specific antigens can be depressed.[35]

The thymic defect in these patients appears primarily to manifest itself as an inability to induce the differentiation of a normal population of precursor T lymphocytes. Patients may have up to 10 to 20 per cent of the normal amount of thymic tissue and still be functionally deficient in cases of partial DiGeorge's syndrome.[33] Recent studies suggest that precursor cell from patients with DiGeorge's syndrome can be induced to express certain T-cell markers when cultured with normal human thymic extracts.[36]

Therapy

The most promising innovation in the treatment of DiGeorge's syndrome is the transplantation of human allogeneic fetal thymuses.[37] Successful transplants result in a reversal of the immunodeficient state and the development of mature and functioning T cells. These T lymphocytes appear to be of *host* origin.[38] Because the donor thymus is fetal it is generally believed that lymphocytes carried in the graft cannot mount a graft-versus-host (GvH) reaction against the recipient.[39] Furthermore, since the patient's own immune system is likely to be incapable of distinguishing self from nonself constituents, the graft is not rejected. With subsequent T-cell maturation, tolerance to the graft is probably achieved since the transplanted thymus would be effectively viewed as "self" by the newly emergent immune system.

NEZELOF'S SYNDROME

This is a syndrome of thymic dysplasia often associated with near normal or even elevated levels of circulating immunoglobulins.[40] Neutropenia is a frequent accompaniment. This syndrome affects young children from about six months of age, presenting with failure to thrive, recurrent infections (predominantly viral and fungal) and chronic diarrhea. The course as well as the age of onset are somewhat variable. The syndrome appears to be inherited as either an autosomal recessive or X-linked recessive trait.[41]

The thymus in Nezelof's syndrome is hypoplastic and embryonal in character, with an absence of Hassall's corpuscles and no corticomedullary differentiation. There is an associated lymphopenia and a deficiency of well-differentiated T cells. T-cell dysfunction is evident in a decreased *in vitro* responsiveness to mitogens and a failure to exhibit cutaneous delayed hypersensitivity. However, these patients' cells often retain the ability to proliferate in an MLR. Thus, it has been suggested that the ability to react against allogeneic cells is acquired earlier in T-cell differentiation than mitogen responsiveness and that MLR reactivity is "less thymic-dependent" than other T-cell functions.

B-cell function is also impaired. Despite normal levels of circulating immunoglobulins in about 50 per cent of patients, these children are unable to mount specific antibody responses to an antigenic challenge. Most patients have plasma cells in their lymph nodes, but the lymph node architecture is abnormal, lacking follicles and germinal centers. Fifty per cent of patients present with some sort of dysgammaglobulinemia, usually a deficiency of IgA alone or a deficiency of both IgA and IgG. These classes of immunoglobulin are highly susceptible to a loss of T helper function.

The variable age of onset of symptoms (anywhere from infancy to several years of age) and the reports of a progressive loss of immunologic function, including declining immunoglobulin levels, raise the possibility that this is a degenerative process.[41,42] Many severely affected children show evidence of a healthier immune system earlier in their lives, e.g., by the presence of specific isoagglutinins and negative Shick tests.[41]

DISORDERS WITH PREDOMINANT ABNORMALITIES OF HUMORAL IMMUNITY

X-LINKED AGAMMAGLOBULINEMIA

X-linked agammaglobulinemia, described by Bruton, was the first immunodeficiency disease to be recognized.[43] Young males present with recurrent infections including pneumonia, otitis, sinusitis and meningitis beginning at about six months of age. Unlike the children with DiGeorge's syndrome,

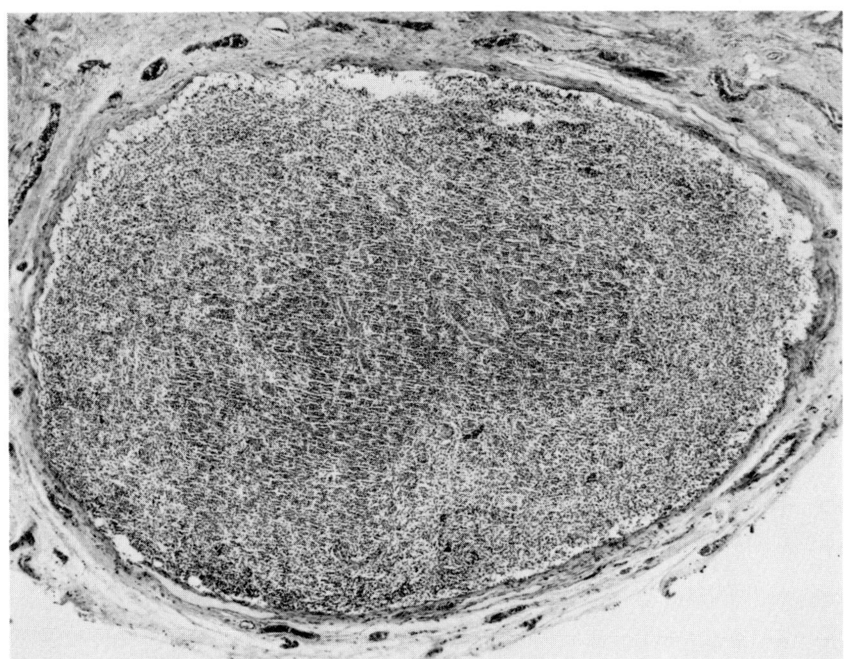

Fig. 10-6. Lymph node from a patient with X-linked agammaglobulinemia. Note the lack of follicles, germinal centers and plasma cells. Compare this node to the one shown in Figure 1-18. (Courtesy Dr. R. H. Buckley)

these patients primarily suffer from bacterial infections, especially with encapsulated pneumococci and streptococci.[44] They are less likely to be susceptible to viral and fungal infections. One apparent exception is an increased susceptibility to hepatitis virus. These patients have also been reported to display prolonged shedding of polio virus after vaccination. Other complications include rheumatoid arthritis, seen in up to 50 per cent of patients, dermatomyositis, and an increased incidence of lymphoreticular malignancies.[45-48]

Immunologic Features

The primary immunologic finding is one of very low levels of circulating immunoglobulin of all classes.[49] These children are rarely completely agammaglobulinemic, as the name of the disease would otherwise indicate. The peripheral lymphoid tissue is hypoplastic and the lymph nodes lack cortical follicles, germinal centers and plasma cells (Fig. 10-6). Peripheral blood lymphocyte levels are usually normal as one might expect, since the majority of circulating lymphocytes in healthy individuals are T cells.

The patients have deficient humoral immunity and are unable to opsonize bacteria for eventual phagocytosis and clearance from the body. The passive transfer of maternal immunoglobulin during fetal life affords protection against these pathogens lasting for the first six months of life. Humoral unresponsiveness against both T-cell-dependent and T-cell-independent antigens is strong evidence for a primary B-cell defect. In most patients there is an absence of surface immunoglobulin-bearing cells, although occasional patients have been reported with normal or only reduced levels of immunoglobulin-bearing lymphocytes.[50,51] Patients may nevertheless have normal numbers of cells bearing complement receptors.[52] These patients' cells cannot be stimulated to produce immunoglobulin when cultured *in vitro*.[53]

The cellular immune system seems to be generally competent at handling viral, fungal, parasitic and intracellular infections. The thymus develops normally and thymic-dependent areas of peripheral lymphoid tissue are well populated. Spontaneous rosette formation, allograft rejection and the development of cutaneous hypersensitivity are all normal. The only evidence of T-cell impairment is in the *in vitro* response to mitogens. PHA responsiveness has been reported to be selectively diminished while responsiveness to Con A and PWM is normal.[52] It has been hypothesized that PHA may activate a more mature population of T cells than Con A.[54]

Treatment

Patients with X-linked agammaglobulinemia are treated with periodic injections of gammaglobulin.[55] This has been shown to work well in reducing the incidence of infections. Sinopulmonary infections, however, will often persist since secretory IgA cannot be replaced by parenteral injections of immunoglobulin.

IgA DEFICIENCY

Selective IgA deficiency is the most common of all the immunodeficiency disorders, affecting up to one in every 500 people.[56] There is a strong familial tendency, and the deficiency appears to be inherited. The mode of inheritance is not known; autosomal recessive and autosomal dominant with variable penetrance are considered the most likely modes of transmission. Patients with IgA deficiency have an almost complete absence of both serum and secretory IgA.[57]

Clinical Features

Many people with selective IgA deficiency appear to be asymptomatic. However, there is increasing evidence that the deficiency is frequently associated with a definite symptom complex. These symptoms can be considered in four separate categories.[58]

1. Most common are symptoms referrable to the mucosal surfaces. Eighty per cent of symptomatic patients report recurrent sinopulmonary infections. Gastrointestinal manifestations can include gluten-sensitive enteropathy, ulcerative colitis, pernicious anemia and intestinal disaccharidase deficiency. Malabsorption is a relatively frequent problem and is often caused by chronic infection with Giardia.

2. Some atopic disease is present in about 50 per cent of symptomatic patients.

3. Individuals with selective IgA deficiency have an increased incidence of autoimmune phenomena and autoimmune disease. These include autoimmune hemolytic anemia, Addison's disease, SLE, rheumatoid arthritis, and others. Various autoantibodies can be demonstrated, including anti-IgA (50% of patients), anti-IgM (35% of patients) and anti-collagen (35% of patients). These autoantibodies may exist in the absence of any overt clinical manifestations.[59]

4. These individuals have a high incidence of malignancies compared to normal controls,[60] including malignancies of the lung, gastrointestinal tract and lymphoreticular system.

Immunologic and Related Features

The only obvious immunologic deficiency in these patients is the lack of IgA. The importance of *serum* IgA is not understood, and the consequences of its deficiency—if any—cannot yet be appreciated. On the other hand, *secretory* IgA has a well-defined role as the major class of immunoglobulin present in the body's secretions: (1) secretory IgA contributes to the neutralization of infectious agents at their portal of entry.[61] (2) In addition, IgA has been postulated to limit the absorption of noninfectious antigens from the outside, including those introduced by breathing and those carried in by food.[62]

Absence of the protective effects of IgA against the invasion of microorganisms undoubtedly plays a role in the frequently encountered sinopulmonary infections in some of these patients. Many patients with selective IgA deficiency escape these infections, and it has been suggested that these people are protected by a compensatory increase in the level of other immunoglobulin classes in their secretions.[63]

The precise mechanisms by which these people become atopic and are susceptible to autoimmune disease and malignancies are not known, but a hypothesis based upon the possible consequences of IgA deficiency has been offered. Secretory IgA may ordinarily prevent many antigens from entering the body in significant amounts.[62] With a deficiency in secretory IgA, the body could become flooded with both commonly and uncommonly encountered antigens. The presence of abnormal antifood antibodies in these patients may be a reflection of this abnormal antigen load.[64] Antigen flooding could account for:

1. *Atopy.* Antigens normally excluded by IgA could react with IgE bound to mast cells and produce immediate hypersensitivity reactions.

2. *Autoimmune Disease.* The increased influx of antigens could increase the possibility of the systemic immune system encountering antigens which crossreact with self-determinants, thus eliciting autoantibody production. In addition, IgA has been postulated normally to prevent reabsorption of certain self-antigens, such as those present on mucosal surfaces, that are continually being shed into the body's secretions.[62] Several patients with IgA deficiency have been found to have a spruelike syndrome associated with the presence of anti-epithelial-cell antibodies.[65]

3. *Malignancy.* Chronic irritation or inflammation resulting from a high antigenic load could be responsible for the high incidence of pulmonary and gastrointestinal cancers. Alternatively, the inability to prevent local microbial invasions at these sites could lead to neoplasia if tumor-causing agents were to gain entry to the body. Chronic antigenic stimulation has also been suggested as a possible causal mechanism in some lymphoproliferative diseases (see Chaps. 12 and 13).

Pathogenesis

We shall consider three possible explanations of how selective IgA deficiency may develop (this is not an exhaustive list of possibilities; see Fig. 10-7).

1. IgA deficiency could result from a lack of precursors of IgA-secreting cells. Despite the current controversy over the precise nature of the immunoglobulin receptors on B cells (see Chap. 3), many investigators feel that IgA-secreting cells express IgA molecules on their surfaces. They report that patients with selective IgA deficiency have normal numbers of IgA-bearing cells in their circulation.[66] Thus it has been hypothesized that these IgA-committed B cells are incapable of differentiating into IgA-producing plasma cells. Other reports, however, indicate that the cells of at least some IgA-deficient patients can be stimulated by mitogens *in vitro* to produce IgA.[53]

2. IgA production has a strict requirement for T-cell helper function, and is perhaps the most dependent of all the immunoglobulin classes on T helper activity (see Chap. 6).[67] There are several reports of thymic dysplasia in man being associated with a selective IgA deficiency.[68] However, in almost all patients with selective IgA deficiency there is no evidence of a T-cell functional abnormality although a diminished percentage of spontaneous rosette-forming cells has been reported.[57] It remains possible that the lack of T helper function for IgA production may be a subtle and selective de-

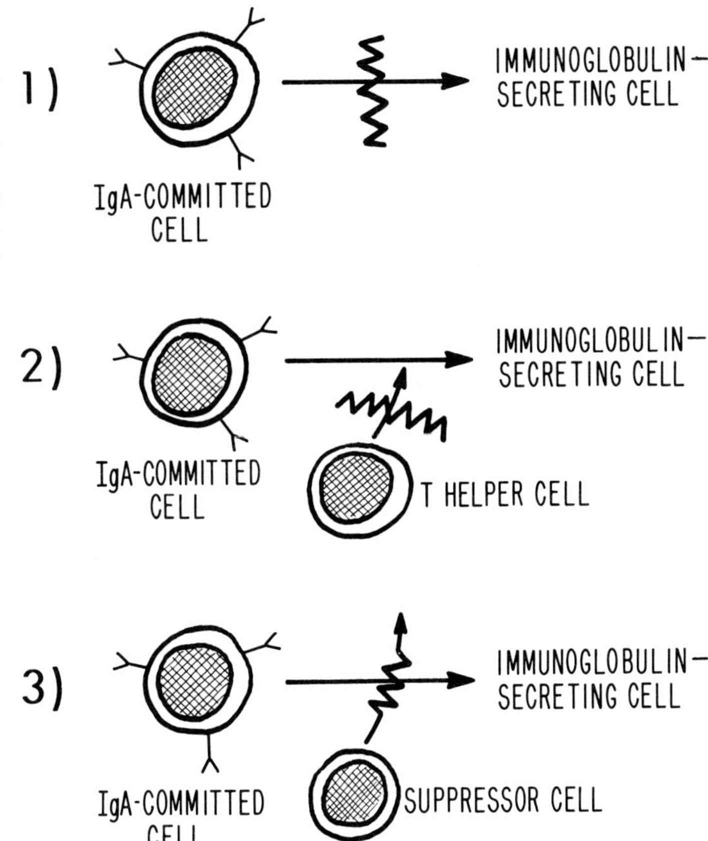

Fig. 10-7. Three possible mechanisms for selective IgA deficiency. (1) Intrinsic failure of the IgA-committed B cell to become an IgA-producing cell. (2) Absence of IgA-specific T helper cells. (3) Specific suppression of IgA production, possibly by class-specific suppressor cells.

fect not reflected in normal assays of T-cell function.

3. IgA production in these individuals may be under the regulation of an immunologic suppressor mechanism. One attractive possibility would be the existence of a population of overactive IgA-specific suppressor cells. Another possible suppressive mechanism is suggested by the observation that over 50 per cent of IgA-deficient individuals have detectable anti-IgA antibodies in their serum.[69] These are usually IgG and are directed against class-specific heavy-chain determinants. Most of these people have no history of exposure to exogenous IgA. The cell-surface IgA may be the target for these autoantibodies. In some animal systems anti-alpha-chain antibodies have been found to prevent the secretion of IgA, possibly by binding to lymphocytes bearing surface IgA.[70] This inhibition may be analogous to the phenomenon of allotype suppression discussed in Chapter 6. Whether such an inhibitory mechanism is operative in patients with IgA deficiency remains to be established. The presence of anti-IgA antibodies may have additional significance in that these patients can develop anaphylactic reactions if given blood or plasma transfusions that contain IgA.[59,71]

Recently, a patient with an interesting variant of selective IgA deficiency has been described.[72] This patient does not produce any detectable secretory component and thus lacks secretory IgA despite normal serum levels.[73] Also of interest is the finding that his jejunal lymphocytes do not produce IgA. The investigators suggest that secretory component may provide a homing signal to precursors of

IgA-producing lymphocytes for migration to the mucosal surfaces. Without the production of secretory component, these cells would not migrate to the gastrointestinal mucosa, and little or no IgA-producing potential would be found there.

HYPER-IgM SYNDROME

This syndrome is believed to have an X-linked mode of inheritance, but recent descriptions of occurrences in females place this in some doubt. Affected children suffer from infections similar to those encountered in X-linked agammaglobulinemia with a marked susceptibility to pyogenic bacteria. Infections most commonly involve the respiratory tract. In contrast to patients with X-linked agammaglobulinemia, these patients often present with generalized lymphadenopathy, enlarged tonsils and adenoids, and splenomegaly.[74,75]

The diagnosis is established in the laboratory. Immunoelectrophoresis reveals a marked diminution of IgA and IgG with normal or, even more commonly, elevated levels of IgM. The IgM does not form a sharp monoclonal spike but is rather a broad, polyclonal band. The lymph nodes may appear normal, but many patients have diminished numbers of follicular plasma cells. There are normal numbers of circulating lymphocytes with stainable surface immunoglobulin. Despite the high levels of IgM, attempts to immunize patients against specific antigens have often met with failure. However, most patients appear to be capable of producing at least some antigen-specific IgM as evidenced by the existence of blood-group isoagglutinins (see Chap. 14).

Pathophysiology

The coincidence of low levels of IgG with high titers of IgM suggests that these patients may have lost the usual negative feedback that IgG may exert upon 19S IgM production (Fig. 10-8A; see Chap. 6). An intrinsic defect in the B-cell population may prevent the switch from IgM to IgG, resulting in excess IgM production. Support for this hypothesis is derived from observations that the administration of exogenous IgG to these patients can lower their levels of IgM.[76] A second possibility is that these people lack appropriate T helper function (Fig. 10-8B). IgG, we recall, is heavily dependent upon T helper function, IgM much less so. A deficiency in T helper function could result in an immune system which is capable only of responding to T-independent antigens. This may explain why only certain antigens elicit a response from affected individuals. Thymic abnormalities have been documented in several of these patients.[77]

HYPER-IgE SYNDROME

These young patients are plagued with recurrent pyogenic (especially staphylococcal) infections with the formation of cutaneous, pulmonary and joint abscesses. Chronic dermatitis and growth retardation are also seen. An IgE aberration was first suggested by the observation of exaggerated immediate hypersensitivity reactions. The high level of IgE in these patients is polyclonal and is associated with an eosinophilia. Immediate hypersensitivity can be elicited by many different antigens. The other immunoglobulin classes circulate in normal levels.[78]

IgE levels may normally be rigorously controlled by T suppressor cells (see Chap. 6), and a deficiency of suppressor cells may contribute to the pathogenesis of this syndrome. This view is supported by other evidence of T-cell dysfunction in these patients. There is poor delayed hypersensitivity reactivity; these children cannot be sensitized to produce a cell-mediated response against the common

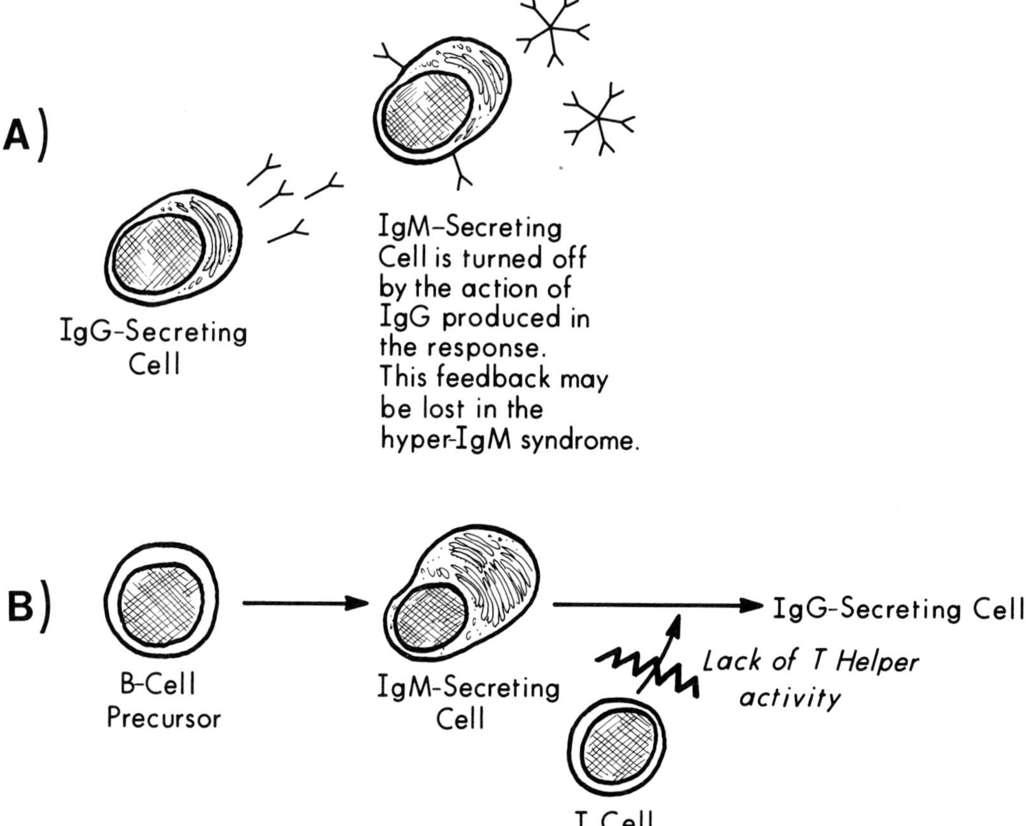

Fig. 10-8. Two theoretical schemes to explain the hyper-IgM syndrome. (A) Lack of IgG feedback. (B) Lack of T helper activity.

skin test antigen, DNCB (dinitrochlorobenzene). Although blastogenesis by PHA stimulation is normal, their lymphocytes do not respond to antigenic stimuli *in vivo*. These patients also have marked deficiencies in their ability to mount humoral responses against antigenic challenges. They do, however, have normal blood-type isoagglutinins, reminiscent of those patients with the hyper-IgM syndrome. The abnormal *in vivo* antibody responsiveness in these patients may be indicative of defective T helper function. The many indications of T-cell dysfunction in these patients enhance the possibility that a deficiency of T suppression of IgE responses may be at fault.

DISORDERS WITH COMBINED DEFECTS OF CELL-MEDIATED AND HUMORAL IMMUNITY

IMMUNODEFICIENCY WITH HEMATOPOIETIC HYPOPLASIA

Children born with this rare disease are both lymphocytopenic and granulocytopenic, and suffer from a severe immunodeficiency of both the humoral and cellular limbs of the immune system. They succumb to overwhelming infections within the first several weeks of life. The pathogenesis is obscure, but may be a failure of differentiation beyond the pluripotential stem cell.[79]

Table 10-2. Clinical Manifestations and Immunopathology of the Immunodeficiency Diseases

Disease	*Clinical Presentation*	*Immunopathologic Findings*
DiGeorge's syndrome	Hypocalcemic tetany, infections (especially candidiasis, viral, bacterial and *P. carinii*), and tracheal, esophageal and cardiovascular anomalies	Thymic hypoplasia; absence of T cells in lymph nodes
Nezelof's syndrome	Failure to thrive, recurrent infections (especially fungal and viral) and diarrhea	Hypoplastic and embryonal thymus; lymphopenia; abnormal lymph node architecture (no follicles or germinal centers)
X-linked agammaglobulinemia	Recurrent infections beginning at about 6 months of age, mostly bacterial, and rheumatoid arthritis	Hypoplastic lymphoid tissue without germinal centers, follicles or plasma cells
IgA deficiency	Sinopulmonary infections gastrointestinal disorders including malabsorption, atopy and autoimmune disease	——
Hyper-IgM syndrome	Infection—mostly bacterial	Lymphadenopathy
Hyper-IgE syndrome	Recurrent pyogenic infections, often with abscess formation, and growth retardation and dermatitis	——
Severe combined immunodeficiency	Failure to thrive, overwhelming infections, diarrhea with malabsorption	Marked lymphoid hypoplasia
Without ADA deficiency	As above	Small and embryonic thymus
With ADA deficiency	As above plus bony abnormalities	Small but *not* embryonic thymus
Nucleoside phosphorylase deficiency	Recurrent infections	——
Common variable hypogammaglobulinemia	Recurrent infections and gastrointestinal disorders including malabsorption	——
Wiskott-Aldrich syndrome	Eczema, thrombocytopenia and recurrent infections	——
Ataxia-telangiectasia	Progressive ataxia, oculocutaneous telangiectasia, sinopulmonary infections, skin changes and endocrine abnormalities	Cerebellar cortical atrophy; bizarre cellular changes throughout the body; hypoplastic and embryonal thymus; lymphoid hypoplasia

SEVERE COMBINED IMMUNODEFICIENCY (SCID)

Severe combined immunodeficiency is a rare disease which affects both the humoral and cellular limbs of the immune system. It is one of the most severe of all of the immunodeficiency states. Inheritance can be autosomal recessive or X-linked recessive although sporadic cases have also been reported. The autosomal recessive form has been called Swiss-type combined immunodeficiency.[80] Recently it has become possible to divide severe combined immunodeficiency into two types: (1) severe combined immunodeficiency without any known specific biochemical defect; and (2) severe combined immunodeficiency with a deficiency in the enzyme adenosine deaminase (ADA).

In both of these forms, the patients present before six months of age with failure to thrive.[81] These infants get severe infections, notably mucocutaneous candidiasis. Other infections are caused by viruses, fungi and opportunistic pathogens such as *Pneumocystis carinii*. Chronic pneumonia as well as diarrhea with malabsorption (often on an infectious basis) are common. These children often die at a very young age.

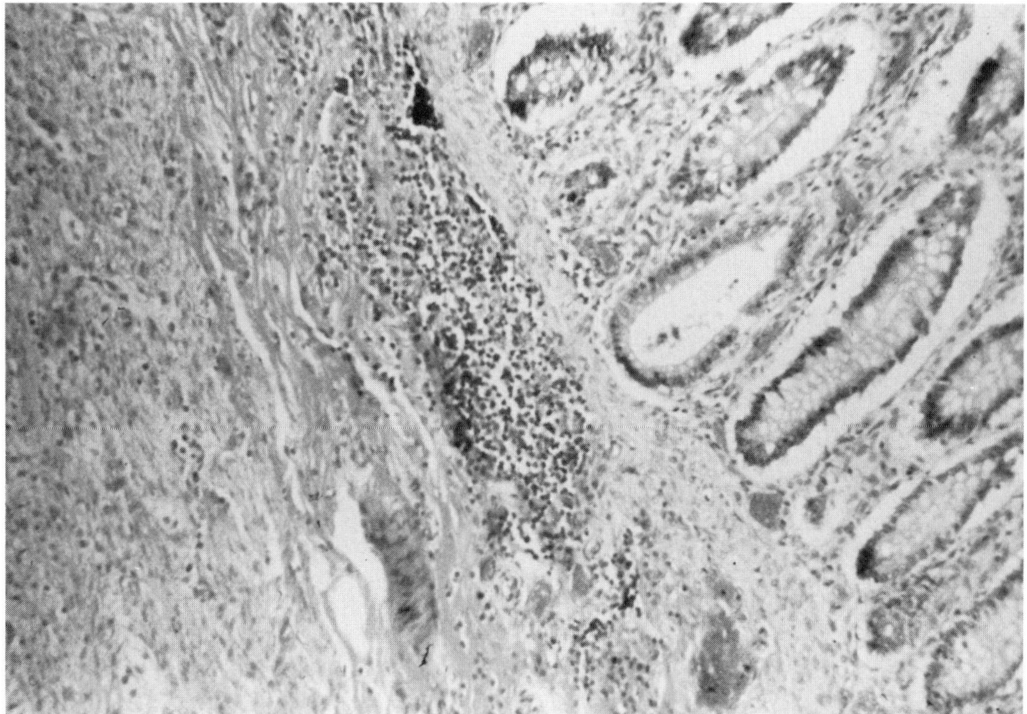

Fig. 10-9. Hypoplastic lymphoid tissue (Appendix) from a patient with severe combined immunodeficiency. (Courtesy Dr. R. H. Buckley.)

Severe Combined Immunodeficiency Without ADA Deficiency

These patients are markedly lymphopenic and both the B- and T-cell areas of the peripheral lymphoid tissue are depleted of lymphocytes (Fig. 10-9). Their immunologic function is depressed by all measurable parameters. They are anergic and cannot be sensitized to cutaneously applied antigens. Their lymphocytes will not respond to antigens, allogeneic cells or mitogens *in vitro*. These patients are panhypogammaglobulinemic and do not make specific antibodies.[82] Their thymuses are small and embryonic, lacking evidence of cortico-medullary differentiation or Hassall's corpuscles (Fig. 10-10).[83]

Investigators have attributed certain aspects of this global immunodeficiency to the grossly abnormal thymus. Unlike DiGeorge's syndrome, however, these patients' cells do not respond *in vitro* to thymic extracts, indicating that the primary defect may instead lie with an unresponsive precursor-cell population.[26] Thus, fetal thymic transplantations have only rarely been helpful. Further support for a primary precursor-cell defect is derived from the several reports of the successful use of bone marrow transplants in these patients.[84]

Recent work suggests that a thymic defect may be causally involved in at least one aspect of the disease, despite the treatment failures cited above. It was first proposed in mouse systems that T-cell precursors pass through two stages of differentiation, one where they must physically interact with the thymic epithelium, and a later stage where further maturation can occur with exposure to thymic extracts (see earlier).[17,18] Extending this work to humans, a recent report has demonstrated that incubation of the

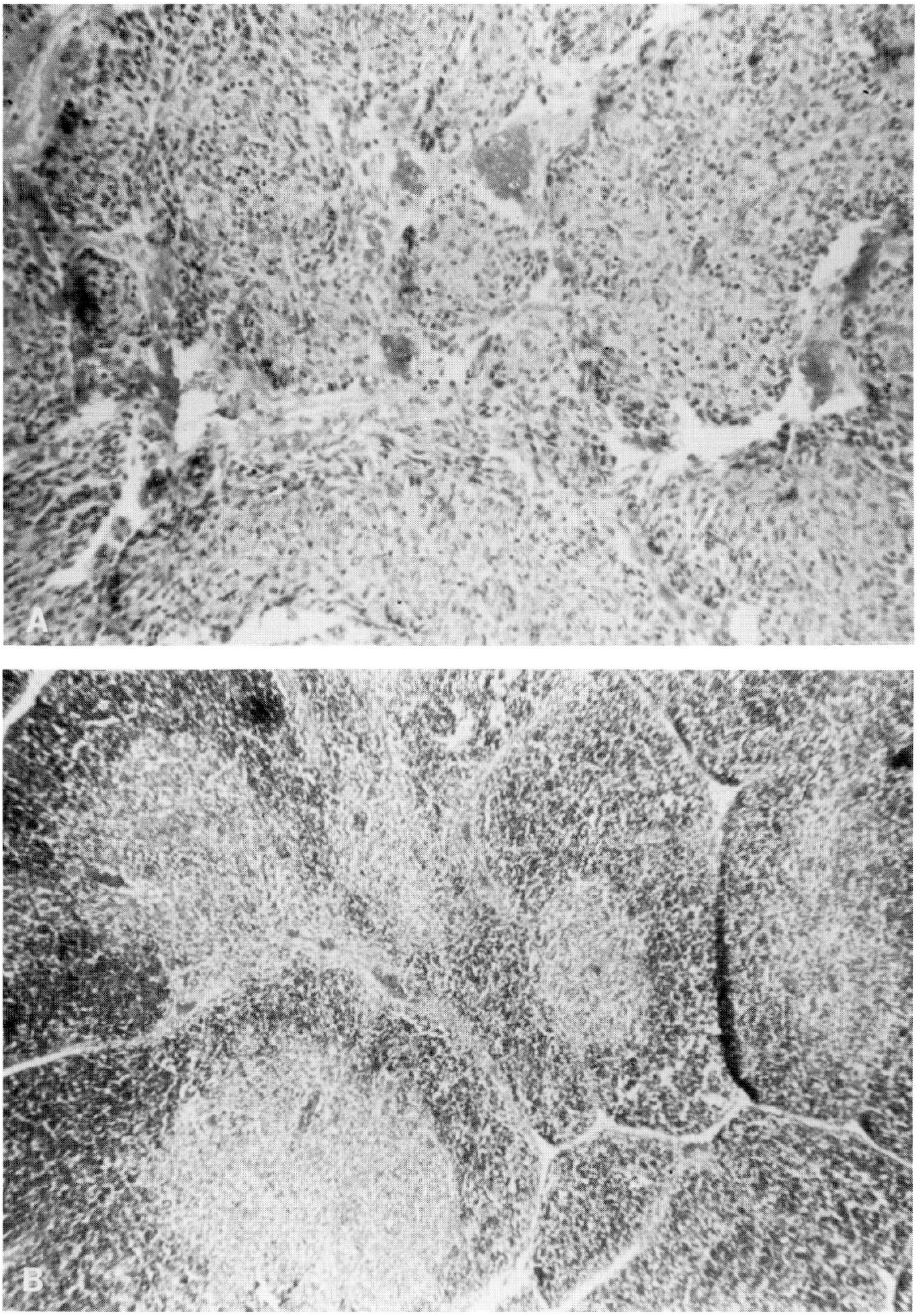

Fig. 10-10. (A) Hypoplastic, embryonic thymus from a patient with severe combined immunodeficiency. (B) Normal thymus is shown for comparison. (Courtesy Dr. R. H. Buckley.)

lymphocytes of patients with SCID with a thymic extract failed to produce any response. However, direct incubation of those lymphocytes with normal thymic tissue could induce T-cell differentiation; cells capable of forming spontaneous sheep erythrocyte rosettes could be demonstrated, as could humoral responses to T-cell-dependent antigens.[83] This work indicates that a thymic defect in inducing early stages of T-cell differentiation may be involved in the pathogenesis of severe combined immunodeficiency.

Severe Combined Immunodeficiency with ADA Deficiency

An apparent breakthrough in identifying specific defects that may lead to immunodeficiency was achieved when two patients with severe combined immunodeficiency were demonstrated to lack the enzyme adenosine deaminase (ADA).[85] The clinical features of the syndrome are essentially as stated above. In all forms of severe combined immunodeficiency, radiographic analysis often reveals the absence of adenoidal and thymic shadows as well as evidence of pneumonia. In ADA-deficient patients there is also a high frequency of associated bony abnormalities on x-ray including cupping and flaring of anterior rib ends.[86]

Immunologic Features

Most patients with ADA deficiency present with laboratory evidence of severe combined immunodeficiency with an absence of all aspects of immune function.[87] However, some patients have been described with less severe aberrations of their immune system although totally deficient in the enzyme. These patients have not been followed long enough to know whether they eventually will develop complete immunodeficiency.

Patients have small and involuted thymuses but the epithelium is well differentiated and Hassall's corpuscles are present, a sign of thymic maturity.[88] There is significant lymphopenia reflected in a marked deficiency of lymphocytes in the peripheral blood, lymph nodes and spleen, and there are few if any Peyer's patches. Those lymphocytes that are present are generally found to be without demonstrable immunologic competence and carry few B- or T-cell markers. The cells are incapable of responding to antigenic or mitogenic stimuli. In the most severely affected patients there is little or no detectable circulating immunoglobulin.

Pathophysiology

ADA catalyzes the conversion of adenosine to inosine and therefore can contribute to the regulation of intracellular adenosine levels.[89] ADA exists in several tissue-specific isoenzymatic forms, but no case of ADA deficiency has yet been reported with a selective deficiency of only one or several of these isoenzymes.[90] ADA deficiency is inherited as an autosomal recessive trait and can be diagnosed by measuring the level of the enzyme in the patient's red blood cells.[91] Parents of affected children are heterozygotes and have one half the normal level of ADA. Nevertheless, they are clinically normal.[92]

It has not been proven that ADA deficiency is responsible for the severe immunodeficiency in patients lacking the enzyme. Many thousands of apparently healthy people have been screened for ADA deficiency, and thus far only one young boy from the Kalahari Desert has been found to lack the enzyme.[93] Although he has not been carefully studied, he appears to be fully immunocompetent. The reason for the dissociation between his enzyme deficiency and his immune status is unknown.

There are two ways in which a deficiency of ADA could theoretically com-

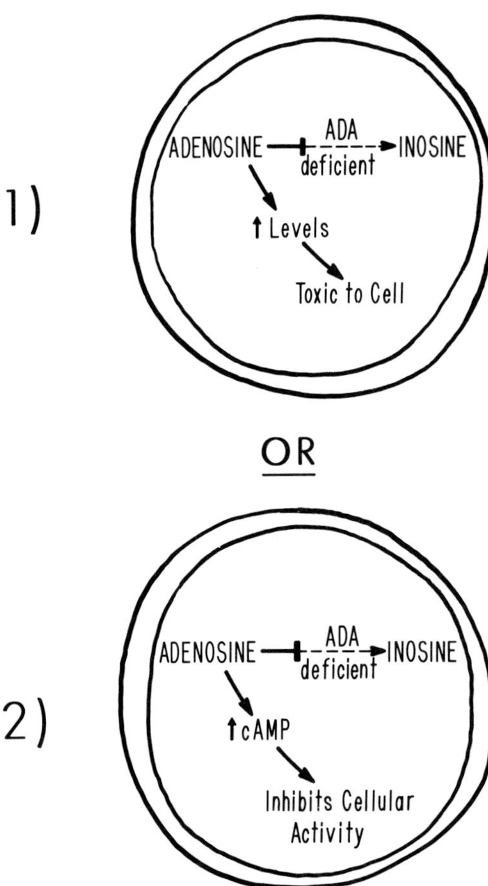

Fig. 10-11. Proposed mechanisms of lymphocyte depression in ADA deficiency. (1) Increased adenosine levels are toxic to the cell. (2) Increased intracellular cAMP inhibits lymphocyte function.

promise immunologic function (Fig. 10-11):

1. ADA deficiency might lead to high intracellular levels of adenosine. It has been suggested that high levels of adenosine can be toxic to the cell by inhibiting pyrimidine synthesis and thereby leading to pyrimidine starvation.[94] This hypothesis has garnered the most support at present.

2. Figure 10-12 illustrates the adenosine cycle. It is conceivable that a buildup of adenosine could lead to an increase in the intracellular levels of cyclic AMP,[95,96] a molecule shown to be able to inhibit many aspects of lymphocyte function (see Chap. 4). The conversion of adenosine to cyclic AMP in the presence of adenosine accumulation is compatible with the established kinetics of at least some of the enzymes involved.[97]

If ADA deficiency is responsible for the severe immunologic compromise in these patients, we must wonder why this deficiency so strongly and selectively affects the immune system. No answer is available at present.

Treatment

Treatment of this disease has been difficult. In an attempt to assess whether thymic transplantation would be of value, patients' cells have been treated *in vitro* with thymic extracts in a manner similar to that used with success in DiGeorge's syndrome. Such treatment is without effect in patients with SCID. The patients' precursor cells appear to be unable to respond to the thymic stimulus.

Histocompatible bone marrow transplants have been attempted with occasional successes in reconstituting the immune system,[98] and in one instance transplantation of fetal liver was of benefit.[99] It is not known whether success depends on the establishment of a viable donor lymphocyte line which can perform the required immunologic functions, or whether one is merely providing donor cells with sufficient ADA to detoxify and reduce adenosine levels. Since adenosine is permeable across cell membranes, reduction in one cellular compartment could conceivably affect adenosine levels elsewhere. In support of this latter view, a recent report indicates that transfusions of normal red cells possessing high levels of ADA may correct the immunologic defects.[100]

NUCLEOSIDE PHOSPHORYLASE DEFICIENCY

Following the excitement of the description of ADA deficiency in severe combined immunodeficiency, many pa-

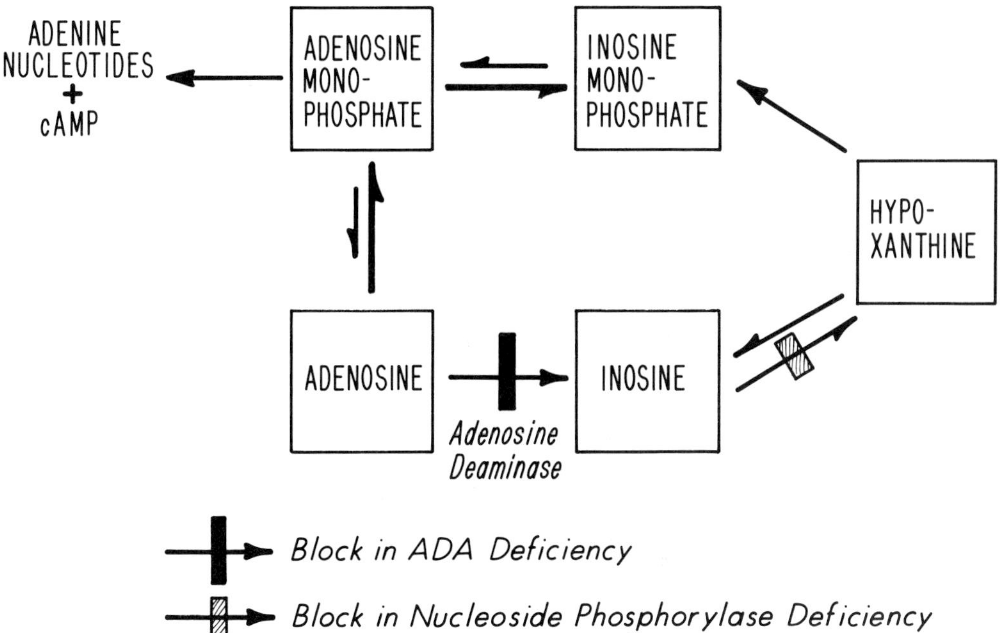

Fig. 10-12. Metabolism of adenosine illustrating the adenosine-inosine cycle and the site of specific blocks in ADA deficiency and nucleoside phosphorylase deficiency.

tients with various immunodeficiencies have been screened for other types of enzymatic defects in purine metabolism. One such defect appears to have been found in a young girl whose red cells lack any nucleoside phosphorylase activity,[101] and this defect has since been found in other immunodeficient individuals.

The girl's clinical course has been marked by recurrent infections (otitis media and pneumonia) and diarrhea. She also has had a persistent anemia. Her immunologic status is severely compromised. She has a marked lymphopenia with a decreased percentage of spontaneous rosette-forming cells. Poor T-cell function is evident in the inability of her cells to respond to PHA or to allogeneic cells, and in her failure to exhibit positive skin tests. B-cell function appears to be intact. Serum immunoglobulin levels are normal and her cells mount adequate antibody responses against both T-independent (pneumococcal polysaccharide) and T-dependent (keyhole-limpet hemocyanin) antigens. The last finding is especially intriguing since it indicates that her T helper function may be normal despite the apparent loss of T effector functions. The same selective T-cell deficiency has been noted in the other patients studied with this disease.

Pathophysiology

Both of the parents of this child (who are cousins) have only half the normal activity of nucleoside phosphorylase and are probably heterozygotes, suggesting that the defect is inherited as an autosomal recessive trait. Nucleoside phosphorylase converts inosine to hypoxanthine, the step following the reaction requiring ADA activity in the catabolism of adenosine (Fig. 10-12). Nucleoside phosphorylase deficiency may therefore produce cellular biochemical abnormalities similar to ADA deficiency, but this possibility has not yet been studied. Red-cell transfusions appear to improve the patient's success in handling infections, a finding similar to that in patients with ADA deficiency.

COMMON VARIABLE HYPOGAMMAGLOBULINEMIA

The term common variable hypogammaglobulinemia (CVH) actually encompasses a spectrum of disorders presenting with varying degrees of hypogammaglobulinemia and with a variable age of onset.[102] Within this general syndrome patients are also seen with varying degrees of demonstrably deficient T-cell function.[103,104] As with all the clinically significant immunodeficiency diseases, infections are the most common and serious problem. Patients frequently have gastrointestinal disorders, including malabsorption, and an increased incidence of malignancy has been observed.[104a]

Clinically, these patients resemble those with X-linked agammaglobulinemia. However, unlike patients with X-linked agammaglobulinemia, most of these people have circulating B cells bearing surface immunoglobulin.[105] Twenty-five per cent of patients have normal amounts of surface immunoglobulin-bearing cells, 50 per cent have a slightly diminished immunoglobulin-bearing cell population, and another 25 per cent have a significantly decreased number of immunoglobulin-positive cells. Most patients have well-developed lymphoid tissue with normally populated B- and T-cell areas. The majority of patients possess mature B cells but lack plasma cells, suggesting that a block in the differentiation of B cells to plasma cells is instrumental in the pathogenesis of this disorder. Only those patients with a greatly decreased level of immunoglobulin-bearing cells appear to lack mature B cells.

Of those patients with normal or near normal numbers of immunoglobulin-bearing cells, two groups can be identified by *in vitro* assays of humoral function.[105] Upon exposure to mitogenic factors the cells of one group of patients synthesize immunoglobulin but are unable to secrete it.[106] Another subset of patients has lymphocytes that will neither synthesize nor secrete immunoglobulin when stimulated.

Recent work has implicated an overactivity of T suppressor cells as the pathogenetic mechanism in many of these patients.[107] The peripheral blood lymphocytes of patients with CVH respond with only minimal immunoglobulin secretion to pokeweed mitogen (PWM) stimulation. The addition of purified T cells from affected patients to PWM-stimulated cultures of normal cells suppresses normal immunoglobulin secretion as much as 100 per cent (Fig. 10-13).[107]

Treatment of these patients could theoretically be accomplished by decreasing the number or activity of their T suppressor cells. It is therefore almost paradoxical that this immunodeficiency syndrome may eventually be treated by immunosuppressive therapy, with agents such as steroids, antilymphocyte serum or x-irradiation.

WISKOTT-ALDRICH SYNDROME

Clinical Features

This syndrome is inherited as an X-linked recessive trait and remains one of the most puzzling immunodeficiency diseases from an immunologic standpoint.[108] Patients present early in life with the clinical triad of eczema, thrombocytopenia with a bleeding diathesis and recurrent infections due to a variety of organisms. Bloody diarrhea, recurrent otitis, pneumonia and skin abscesses are all common. The eczema is not present at birth but develops at a young age. Thrombocytopenia is associated with increased numbers of marrow megakaryocytes, suggesting a peripheral depletion of platelets, possibly due to an intrinsic defect in the platelets.[109] Other hematologic abnormalities can include anemia, which

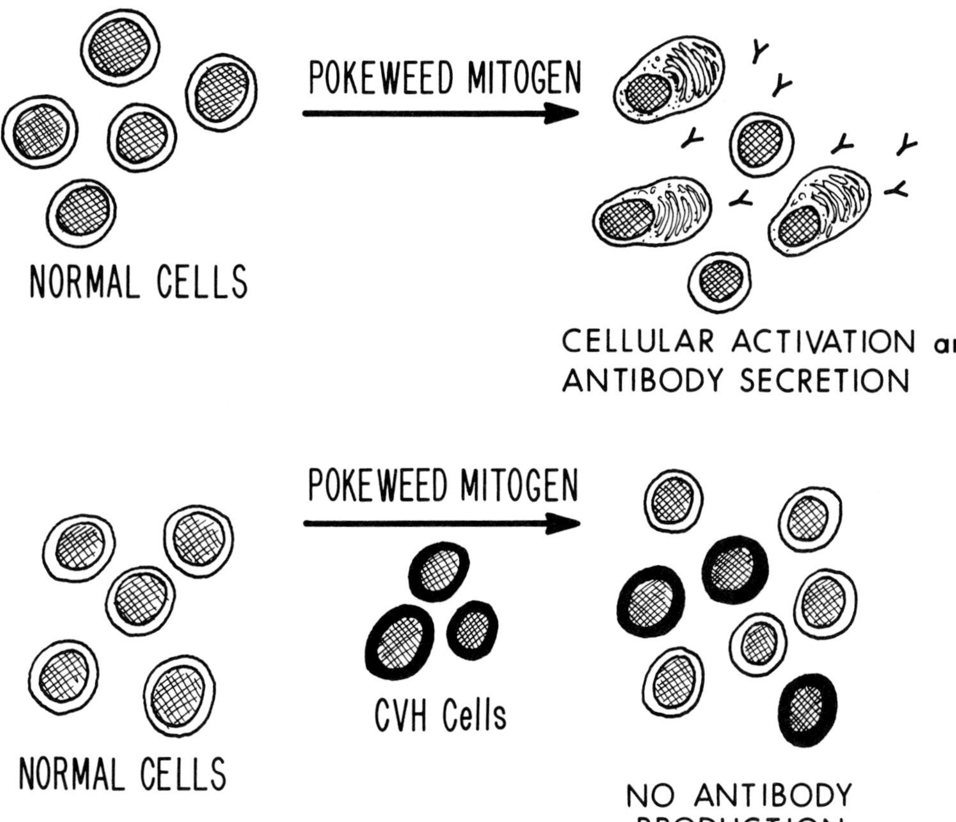

Fig. 10-13. The presence of suppressor T cells in common variable hypogammaglobulinemia prevents the stimulation of immunoglobulin production by pokeweed mitogen.

in some patients is autoimmune in nature, neutropenia and eosinophilia. Affected children often die young as a result of infection or occasionally as victims of lymphoreticular malignancies, which occur in about 10 per cent of these children.[110] Death from cerebral hemorrhage is also not uncommon.

Immunology and Pathophysiology

There is a wide spectrum of immunologic abnormalities in these patients.[111] Anergy to skin testing and prolonged allograft rejection suggest a T-cell dysfunction. Patients have normal numbers of cells that react with anti-T-cell antisera although they exhibit a decreased percentage of spontaneous rosette-forming cells.[112] *In vitro* studies reveal that lymphocytes from affected patients may exhibit normal activation by optimum concentrations of mitogens but diminished responsiveness to specific antigens.[113-115]

Studies of the humoral limb of the immune system have shown that although these patients have normal total serum immunoglobulin levels, the class distribution is decidedly abnormal.[111] IgE is markedly elevated, IgA and IgD may also be elevated, IgG is normal, and IgM is decreased. The metabolism of immunoglobulin molecules is also unusual.[116] There is a marked increase in the catabolism of immunoglobulins (as well as of albumin), and, in order to keep up with this increased destruction, the synthetic rate of IgE is elevated by 300 per cent and that of IgA by about 500 per cent. IgM synthesis is not increased, and hence the serum level of IgM is low.

Wiskott-Aldrich patients have normal numbers of immunoglobulin-bearing B cells as well as normal numbers of cells with Fc and complement receptors.[111,117] However, they are unable to mount optimal antibody responses against specific antigens.[111] Most patients are deficient in natural isoagglutinins and do not raise antibodies in response to specific immunization.[118] This B-cell dysfunction mirrors the T-cell findings in that the B cells will respond to nonspecific mitogenic stimulation but not to antigenic stimulation *in vitro*.

The peculiarity of the observations regarding T- and B-cell function in these patients has led to the proposal that the defect in the Wiskott-Aldrich syndrome resides in the afferent limb of the immune system. Thus, it has been suggested that antigens are either not recognized by the patient's immune system or else are abnormally processed and/or presented to the immunocompetent cells.[118,119] The first possibility has not been vigorously pursued, but the second has aroused considerable interest and has turned people's attention to the macrophage-monocyte.

As we discussed in Chapter 5, it is believed that an antigen must first interact with the macrophage population before it can induce an immune response. An intrinsic macrophage defect does not appear to be present in patients with the Wiskott-Aldrich syndrome since macrophages from affected patients can participate normally in antigen-induced lymphocyte transformation using lymphocytes from healthy individuals.[120] On the other hand, it has been reported that some patients with this syndrome may have a subnormal number of monocytes bearing Fc receptors.[115] Perhaps of even greater interest is a recent report that lymphocytes from affected patients spontaneously secrete a factor that inhibits the activity of both normal macrophages and macrophages from Wiskott-Aldrich patients.[121]

The lymphoreticular system, of which the macrophage is a prominent member, appears to be in a state of high activity in this illness. This is evident in the increased catabolism and synthesis of immunoglobulin that has been described. Further evidence comes from numerous reports of transient monoclonal gammopathies in affected children.[122] The high incidence of lymphoreticular neoplasms may also result from relatively uncontrolled activity of the lymphoreticular system.

Treatment

Therapy, as with all of the immunodeficiency diseases, has been difficult. The use of transfer factor obtained from the leukocytes of normal donors has been most encouraging.[123] Fifty per cent of patients show clinical improvement on transfer factor therapy.[124] Clinical improvement has been correlated with improvement in immune function both *in vivo* (conversion from cutaneous anergy to positive skin reactivity) and *in vitro* (MIF production upon antigenic challenge). However, *in vitro* attempts at stimulating lymphocyte proliferation with specific antigens have remained unsuccessful. Transfer factor therapy has been reported to induce a clearing of the eczematous skin disease, and, rarely, to reduce the bleeding tendency in association with an increase in the peripheral platelet count.

ATAXIA-TELANGIECTASIA

Clinical Features

Ataxia-telangiectasia is a progressive disease that is inherited as an autosomal recessive trait.[125,126] Early manifestations include truncal ataxia that progresses to involve the extremities, and oculocutaneous telangiectasias that may appear at any time from the patient's birth to several years of age. By the time the patients reach three years of age an increased incidence of sinopulmonary infections becomes obvious, involving a variety of organisms. Other abnormalities include insulin resistance, ovarian and testicular dysgenesis, hepatic abnormalities and pigmentary changes. These patients often show progeric (early aging) changes, including gray hair and atrophy of the skin. Most patients succumb at a young age to the effects of chronic infection, most commonly to pulmonary insufficiency. They also exhibit an increased incidence of lymphoreticular malignancies. There appears to be a mild variant of the disease which is compatible with survival into the fifth decade.

Pathology

Pathologic findings that accompany ataxia-telangiectasia include cerebellar cortical atrophy and degeneration with loss of Purkinje's cells, and extensive pulmonary changes compatible with chronic lung infection. Pathologic abnormalities have been reported in virtually every organ of the body and include nucleomegalic aneuploidy and bizarre cytoplasmic changes. Some investigators feel that these findings resemble viral lesions. The organs of the immune system are also histologically abnormal. The thymus is small and embryonal in character. One third of patients are lymphopenic, and an examination of the lymph nodes reveals few lymphocytes in both T- and B-cell areas.

Immunology[127]

Seventy per cent of patients with ataxia-telangiectasia have low levels of serum IgA and diminished secretory IgA levels, accounting for their frequent sinopulmonary infections. Some patients have anti-IgA antibodies. Serum levels of 7S IgG and 19S IgM are usually in the normal range. About 80 per cent of patients have a small (7 to 8S) serum IgM component. IgE levels are almost always diminished or absent. In one study 60 per cent of healthy relatives also had an IgE deficiency. The ability to produce specific antibodies in response to an antigenic challenge is variable; the IgA response is most uniformly impaired. The response to viral antigens seems to be more severely compromised than the response to bacterial antigens. These patients consistently display subnormal antiviral antibody titers despite normal quantitative IgG and IgM serum levels.

Cellular immune deficiencies are even more commonly encountered. Cellular immunity becomes increasingly impaired with the passage of time as measured by *in vitro* assays of mitogenic and antigenic activation. *In vivo* evidence of cellular immune abnormalities includes delayed graft rejection and the inability to mount cutaneous delayed hypersensitivity reactions.

Pathogenesis

Several ideas have been suggested concerning the possible etiology of this disease:

1. Some investigators believe that the widespread cellular degeneration can be attributed to progressive destruction by a slow virus. This would certainly account for many of the microscopic findings described above. However, no viral particles have been seen in any of the lesions.

2. Others have proposed that a generalized autoimmune destruction is responsible for the disease. There is little evidence to support this view.

3. A third explanation attributes the pathogenesis of the disease to a basic systemic developmental defect, involving either a defect in endodermal maturation or in the interaction of endodermal and mesenchymal elements. Consistent with this view is the presence of structural abnormalities of the liver, thymus, blood vessels and endocrine organs. A maturational arrest is strongly suggested by the

presence of an embryonal thymus and the recent finding of high levels of alpha-fetoprotein, a fetal antigen, in the serum of all of these patients.[128] This model fails only to explain the progressive nature of the disease.

COMPLEMENT DEFICIENCIES

See Table 10-3 for a list of the complement deficiencies[129] and their manifestations.

C1q

C1q deficiency has been found in association with certain immunodeficiency diseases, notably hypogammaglobulinemia[130] and severe combined immunodeficiency disease.[131] The reasons for this association are unclear, but some investigators have now demonstrated that patients with hypogammaglobulinemia have an increased rate of metabolism of C1q.[132] C1q has been described to interact reversibly with IgG under normal circumstances, and this may serve to limit the destruction or clearance of C1q. Such protection would be lost in hypogammaglobulinemia, and low levels of C1q could result.

C1r

The few patients with C1r deficiency who have been identified have suffered from recurrent infections, cutaneous and systemic manifestations resembling systemic lupus erythematosus, and glomerulonephritis.[133,134]

C1s

C1s deficiency has been documented in one patient with systemic lupus erythematosus.

C2

One of the more common complement deficiencies, C2 deficiency has now been described in several families. Some individuals with a complete absence of C2 appear to be perfectly healthy. Others show a marked susceptibility to systemic lupus and other autoimmune diseases.[135]

C3

Several types of C3 deficiencies have been described, all associated with an increased incidence of infection. Patients exhibit a decreased ability to opsonize bacteria and to generate complement-derived chemotactic factors. One patient with C3 deficiency has been shown to be unable to synthesize C3.[136] The affected patient was apparently homozygous for the defective gene because his parents each had half the normal C3 levels and were presumably heterozygotes. Two variants associated with increased catabolism of C3 have also been de-

Table 10-3. The Complement Deficiencies

Complement Defect	*Manifestations*
Deficiencies	
C1q	Associated with hypogammaglobulinemia and severe combined immunodeficiency
C1r	Recurrent infections, glomerulonephritis, lupus-like syndrome
C1s	Seen in one patient with SLE
C2	Increased incidence of SLE and other autoimmune disorders
C3	Increased infections
C4	Lupus-like syndrome
C5	Lupus-like syndrome, recurrent infections
C6	No disease
C7	Seen in one patient with scleroderma
C8	Seen in one patient with disseminated *N. gonorrhoeae* infection
C1 esterase inhibitor	Hereditary angioneurotic edema
Other	
C5 dysfunction	Dermatitis, diarrhea, recurrent infections, failure to thrive

scribed.[137] Type 1 appears to be due to a lack of C3b inactivator (KAF), the enzyme which degrades C3b to C3c and C3d and also contributes to the inactivation of factor D of the properdin pathway (see Appendix A). This patient was continually activating the properdin pathway, leading to consumption of C3 by the alternate C3 convertase. The serum of the patient with type 2 hypercatabolism was shown to contain a protein capable of catabolizing C3 without involving the properdin pathway.

C4, C5

Both of these deficiencies have been associated with a lupus-like syndrome. Patients with complete C5 deficiency can present with recurrent infections associated with markedly deficient chemotaxis (due to failure to generate C5b).

C6

The one individual described with C6 deficiency appears to be perfectly healthy.[138] This patient lacks the components for a complete lytic complement sequence. His normal state of health attests to the possibility that complement lysis may be relatively unimportant in host defense.

C7

The one patient described with C7 deficiency has scleroderma.

C8

One patient has been reported with an isolated deficiency of C8 and a history of prolonged disseminated infection with *Neisseria gonorrhoeae*. Her serum lacked bactericidal activity against the gonococcus and the addition of purified C8 restored serum lytic activity.[139]

C5 Dysfunction

Lenier's syndrome of children is characterized by dermatitis, diarrhea, recurrent infections and failure to thrive. This syndrome has recently been associated in one patient with dysfunction of C5. The levels of all complement components including C5 were normal, as was the patient's ability to opsonize bacteria. However, the patient could not opsonize yeast. This defect could be corrected by the addition of normal C5.[140] The role of C5 in opsonization is not understood, and we cannot explain why this patient had this very specific defect.

C1 Esterase Inhibitor[141,142]

C1 esterase inhibitor plays an important part in the regulation of the complement system as well as in the control of other inflammatory systems (including the kinin and coagulation systems). Hereditary angioneurotic edema is inherited as an autosomal dominant trait and is due to the defective synthesis of C1 esterase inhibitor. It is the most common genetic defect of the complement system. Most patients do not have a complete absence of the inhibitor but possess about 20 per cent of the normal level. Fifteen per cent of patients have normal levels and are presumably making a nonfunctional protein.

These patients experience episodic attacks of nonpainful, nonpruritic edema lasting for two to four days, affecting mainly the limbs, trunk and neck. The great danger during these attacks is airway obstruction due to involvement of the tissues of the upper airways. Patients also have attacks of severe abdominal pain due to swelling of the walls of the gastrointestinal tract. These attacks may be totally unrelated to the bouts of peripheral swelling.

It is presumed that these often severe episodes are due to the deficiency of the C1 esterase inhibitor leading to uncontrolled activation of the complement cascade and a subsequent inflammatory response. The stimulus for the attacks has not been defined. During an attack, C4 and C2 are depleted. Between attacks the levels may rise but C4 is almost always subnormal.

THE EVALUATION OF IMMUNODEFICIENCY IN THE PATIENT WITH RECURRENT INFECTIONS

As we have emphasized, the hallmark of the immunodeficient patient is the presence of infections which are usually persistent, recurrent and may be resistant to conventional antibiotic therapy. Often the infections are caused by opportunistic organisms that are nonpathogenic in the healthy individual. However, we must emphasize that *the presence of recurrent infection does not necessarily imply the presence of an immunodeficiency disease*. Anatomical defects may lead to chronic respiratory or renal infection, and nonimmunologic diseases such as cystic fibrosis and others may also be responsible for chronic infection.

The clinical setting in which one finds recurrent infections can be important in guiding one's thinking toward possible immunodeficiency states. Thus, initial presentation in the adult makes severe combined immunodeficiency, reticular dysgenesis, X-linked agammaglobulinemia, etc., distinctly unlikely. The coexistence of hypocalcemia and infections in infancy suggests DiGeorge's syndrome. Neurologic abnormalities may indicate ataxia-telangiectasia, and thrombocytopenia and eczema are suggestive of the Wiskott-Aldrich syndrome. The family history may be helpful since many of the immunodeficiency diseases we discussed have definite patterns of inheritance.

We mentioned earlier in this chapter that the type of infection may suggest defects in specific aspects of immune func-

Evaluation of the Immunodeficient Patient

History of Recurrent Infections

↓

Evaluate Clinical Setting

1. Age of patient
2. Associated abnormalities
3. Any underlying diseases
4. Family history
5. Types of infections

↓

Search for Lymphoid Tissue

1. Physical exam
2. X-ray

↓

Routine Blood Studies

1. Lymphopenia
2. Granulocytopenia

Evaluate Humoral Immunity	*Evaluate Cellular Immunity*
1. *In vivo* tests	1. *In vivo* tests
a. Serum Ig levels	a. Standard battery of skin tests
b. Blood group isoagglutinins	b. Skin tests with new antigens (e.g., DNCB)
c. Antiviral antibody titers	2. Surface markers—number of SRBC rosette-forming cells
d. Response to new antigens (e.g., KLH)	3. *In vitro* tests
2. Surface markers—number of Ig + cells	a. Blast transformation to mitogens
3. *In vitro* tests	b. Blast transformation in the MLR
a. Pokeweed stimulation	
b. Specific antigen stimulation	

4. Other tests
   a. Lymphokine production: measures both B- and T-cell function
   b. Evaluation of macrophage function
      1. Chemotaxis
      2. Phagocytosis

tion. Thus, for example, recurrent infections with encapsulated bacteria suggest a humoral defect. However, the nature of the infection should serve as no more than a general guideline to the patient's immune status. Thus, patients with humoral defects can have viral infections, and patients with cell-mediated defects can suffer from bacterial infections. Infection with *Pneumocystis carinii* is strong evidence of immune dysfunction. Infection with this organism has been felt by some to be seen primarily in patients with depressed cellular immunity, but a careful review of the literature shows that pneumocystis infections can be seen just as often in patients with decreased humoral immunity.[143]

Physical examination of the patient with a suspected immunodeficiency disease generally yields little information. Many of the positive findings relate to the infections themselves. However, a search for lymphoid tissue is useful. Lymph node enlargement can be seen in the hyper-IgM syndrome whereas lymphoid tissue is absent in many other immunodeficiency diseases. X-ray examination can be useful in documenting the presence or absence of adenoidal and thymic shadows.

Once an immunodeficiency is suspected, the work-up of the patient can proceed with varying degrees of sophistication. Certain crude measures of host defense function are first evaluated. Routine blood studies can be a valuable adjunct to understanding chronic infection. Thus, a severely granulocytopenic patient will likely present with recurrent infections that are difficult to treat. Likewise, defects in granulocyte function can lead to a similar clinical presentation. Differential blood counts can also reveal the presence or absence of lymphocytopenia.

The first approach to evaluating the humoral limb of the immune system is a measurement of serum immunoglobulin levels, best done by single radioimmunodiffusion (see Appendix C) to quantitate the level of each immunoglobulin class. Normal levels of each class have been defined for each age group and these measurements can pinpoint a dysgammaglobulinemia and establish the presence of panhypogammaglobulinemia. Secretory IgA levels can be measured in saliva or other secretions.

Preliminary measurement of cell-mediated immunity is best carried out by the use of skin tests. A battery of several common skin test antigens can be used which include candida, mumps, tetanus toxoid, streptokinase-streptodornase, PPD and others. Tests are read after 24 to 72 hours and are generally considered to be positive if induration of more than 10 mm. is present. Occasionally, patients will present with chronic infection by one particular organism (i.e., chronic mucocutaneous candidiasis; see Chap. 11). In these instances, skin test reactivity to antigens of the responsible organism may be informative. For example, many patients with chronic mucocutaneous candidiasis exhibit normal skin test reactions to a variety of antigens but are unresponsive to candida. Another test of cell-mediated immune function is the ability to reject a skin allograft. Only rarely are patients totally unable to reject allogeneic tissue, and diminished cell-mediated immunity is usually reflected in *delayed* rejection.

A higher level of sensitivity for detecting immune dysfunction can be achieved. Even in the face of normal immunoglobulin levels, humoral competence is best measured by the presence of specific antibodies. These can be detected by measuring naturally occurring, blood-group isoagglutinins or antibody titers against viruses.

A considerable amount of information can be garnered if the patient has previously received a specific vaccination. The use of a vaccine employing a live or attenuated organism may lead to the death of the severely immunocompromised host by overwhelming infection. Therefore the ability of a patient to cope with live vaccination attests to some level of immunocompetence. The use of a live vaccination, needless to say, is not a recommended test of immunocompetency in patients suspected of being immunodeficient. Once it is known that a patient has received a specific immunization, antibody titers can be measured. Furthermore, the patient can be rechallenged with the immunizing antigen and the level of the secondary response can be evaluated.

The ability of the patient to mount a primary antibody response can be evaluated *in vivo* by injecting new antigens such as keyhole-limpet hemocyanin. Likewise, the ability to sensitize the patient against a new skin test antigen can be used to evaluate that aspect of cell-mediated immunity. Dinitrochlorobenzene (DNCB) is the most commonly employed sensitizing antigen.

The majority of further tests involve *in vitro* investigation. The patient's lymphocytes can be examined for:

1. *Surface Markers* (see Chap. 3). Surface characterization can indicate, in a very gross way, whether there are normal numbers of mature B and T cells. These studies do not necessarily correlate with functional competence. Thus, the presence of normal surface marker distribution may be seen in the presence of a marked functional deficiency. There is an absence of lymphocytes with stainable surface immunoglobulin in X-linked agammaglobulinemia whereas there are often normal numbers of immunoglobulin-bearing B cells in common variable hypogammaglobulinemia. In Chapter 3 we mentioned that the "activated" spontaneous sheep red-cell rosette numbers may correlate with T-cell function in immunodeficiency states.

2. *In Vitro Functional Tests:*

Immunoglobulin Secretion. The ability to synthesize immunoglobulin can be assayed by stimulating the patient's lymphocytes, usually with pokeweed mitogen, and measuring the amount of immunoglobulin that is produced. This procedure can be used both to assay the intracellular synthesis of immunoglobulin as well as the ability of the stimulated cells to secrete immunoglobulin.

Lymphocyte Transformation. This is most frequently measured by stimulating lymphocytes with either mitogens or specific antigens, incubating the cells for several days, and measuring the amount of DNA, RNA or protein synthesis. DNA synthesis is most commonly measured and is quantitated by the amount of incorporation of ^{3}H-thymidine into DNA. Blast transformation upon exposure to specific antigens is generally considered a measure of T-cell activation. An important *in vitro* proliferative test is the MLR (described in Chap. 4).

Production of Lymphokines. In practice the only lymphokine commonly measured is MIF/MAF. Lymphocytes can be stimulated *in vitro* by mitogens, and the supernatants of the cultures are then assayed for the presence of MIF/MAF. Most often, investigators measure the ability of the supernatant to prevent guinea pig macrophages from migrating out of a capillary tube. In general, if migration is inhibited by greater than 20 per cent over the amount of migration seen without the addition of lymphocyte supernatant, the lymphocytes are felt to be producing normal amounts of MIF/MAF. There is presently some debate over how well MIF/MAF production reflects T-cell as opposed to B-cell activity.

This brief discussion has outlined the general ways in which lymphocyte function can be measured both *in vivo* and *in vitro*. However, it is important to emphasize that many of these tests, from delayed hypersensitivity skin reactivity to *in vitro* antigen transformation, require normal macrophage function in order to give positive results. For this reason, additional tests that one may wish to carry out in the patient with a suspected immunodeficiency involve direct measurement of monocyte-macrophage activity.

Some of these tests measure the ability of these cells to respond to chemotactic agents and their abilty to perform phagocytosis.

REFERENCES

1. Nowell, P. L., *et al.*: Evidence for the existence of multi-potential lympho-hematopoietic stem cells in the adult rat. J. Cell. Phys., *75*:151, 1970.
2. Edwards, G. E., Miller, R. G., and Phillips, R. A.: Differentiation of rosette-forming cells from myeloid stem cells. J. Immunol., *105*:719, 1970.
3. Good, R. A., *et al.*: The immunological deficiency diseases of man. Birth Defects, *4*:17, 1968.
4. Lafluer, L., Underdown, B. J., Miller, R. G., and Phillips, R. A.: Differentiation of lymphocytes: characteristics of early precursors of B lymphocytes. Ser. Haematol., *5*(2):50, 1972.
5. Melchers, F., Von Boehmer, H., and Phillips, R. A.: B lymphocyte subpopulations in the mouse. Transplant. Rev., *25*:26, 1975.
6. Strober, S.: Immune function, cell surface characteristics and maturation of B cell subpopulations. Transplant., Rev., *24*:84, 1975.
7. Janossy, G., and Greaves, M.: Functional analysis of murine and human B lymphocyte subsets. Transplant. Rev., *24*:177, 1975.
8. Cooper, M. D., Lawton, A. R., and Kincade, P. W.: A two stage model for development of antibody producing cells. Clin. Exp. Immunol., *11*:143, 1972.
9. Cooper, M. D., and Lawton, A. R.: Development of T and B cells and their functional interaction. Birth Defects, *11*:3, 1975.
10. Gelfand, M. C., Elfenbein, G. J., Frank, M. M., and Paul, W. E.: Ontogeny of B lymphocytes. J. Exp. Med., *139*:1125, 1974.
11. Jondal, M., Wigzell, H., and Aiuti, F.: Human lymphocyte subpopulations. Transplant. Rev., *16*:163, 1973.
12. Tomasi, T. B., and Grey, H. M.: Structure and function of immunoglobulin A. Prog. Allergy, *16*:81, 1972.
13. McWilliams, M., Lamm, M. E., and Phillips-Quagliata, J. M.: Surface and intracellular markers of mouse mesenteric and peripheral lymph node and Peyer's patch cells. J. Immunol., *113*:1326, 1974.
14. McWilliams, M., Phillips-Quagliata, J. M., and Lamm, M. E.: Characteristics of mesenteric lymph node cells homing to gut associated lymphoid tissue in syngeneic mice. J. Immunol., *115*:54, 1975.
15. Lamm, M. E.: Cellular aspects of IgA. Adv. Immunol., *22*:223, 1976.
16. South, M. A., *et al.*: The IgA system. J. Exp. Med., *123*:615, 1966.
17. Stutman, O., Yunis, E., and Good, R. A.: Studies on thymus function. J. Exp. Med., *132*:583, 1970.
18. ———: Studies on thymus function. J. Exp. Med., *132*:601, 1970.
19. Osaba, D.: The effects of thymus and other lymphoid organs enclosed in millipore diffusion chambers on neonatally thymectomized mice. J. Exp. Med., *122*:633, 1965.
20. Globerson, A., Umiel, T., and Friedman, D.: Activation of immune competence by thymus factors. Ann. N.Y. Acad. Sc., *249*:248, 1975.
21. Ceglowski, W. S., and LaBadie, G. U.: Influence of thymus extracts on the maturation of the immune response in neonatal mice. Ann. N.Y. Acad. Sci., *249*:343, 1975.
22. Stites, D. P., Carr, M. C., and Fudenberg, H. H.: Ontogeny of cellular immunity in man. Birth Defects, *11*:489, 1975.
23. Geha, R. S., *et al.*: Discontinuous density gradient analysis of human bone marrow. Clin. Immunol. Immunopathol., *2*:404, 1974.
24. Osaba, D.: Precursors of thymus lymphocytes. Ser. Haematol., *7*:446, 1974.
25. Touraine, J. L., *et al.*: Differentiation of human bone marrow cells to T lymphocytes by *in vitro* incubation with thymic extracts. Clin. Exp. Immunol., *17*:151, 1974.
26. Touraine, J. L., Touraine, F., Incefy, G. S., and Good, R. A.: Effect of thymic factors on the differentiation of human marrow cells into T lymphocytes *in vitro* in normals and in patients with immunodeficiencies. Ann. N.Y. Acad. Sci., *249*:335, 1975.
27. Ballow, M., and Good, R. A.: Report of a patient with T-cell deficiency and normal B-cell function. Cell Immunol., *19*:219, 1975.
28. DiGeorge, A. M.: Congenital absence of the thymus and its immunologic consequences: concurrence with congenital hypoparathyroidism. Birth Defects, *4*:116, 1968.
29. Gilmour, J. R.: Some developmental abnormalities of the thymus and parathyroids. J. Pathol., *52*:213, 1971.
30. Good, R. A., and Wortis, H. H.: Immune deficiency disease: thymic aplasia. Prog. Immunol., *1*:1271, 1971.
31. Lischner, H. W.: DiGeorge's syndrome(s). J. Pediatr., *81*:1042, 1972.
32. Good, R. A.: Studies on the immunodeficiencies in man. Am. J. Pathol., *69*:484, 1972.
33. Lischner, H. W., and Huff, D. S.: T-cell deficiency in DiGeorge's syndrome. Birth Defects, *11*:16, 1975.
34. Kretschner, N., Say, B., Brown, D., and Rosen, F. S.: Congenital aplasia of the thymus gland. N. Engl. J. Med., *279*:1295, 1968.
35. Lischner, H. W., and DiGeorge, A. M.: Role of the thymus in humoral immunity. Lancet, *2*:1044, 1969.
36. Touraine, J. L., *et al.*: Immunodeficiency diseases. 1. T-lymphocyte precursors and T-lymphocyte differentiation in partial DiGeorge syndrome. Clin. Exp. Immunol., *21*:39, 1975.
37. Cleveland, W. W., *et al.*: Fetal thymic transplant in a case of DiGeorge's Syndrome. Lancet, *2*:1211, 1968.

38. Cleveland, W. W.: Immunologic reconstitution in the DiGeorge syndrome by fetal thymic transplant. Birth Defects, *11*:352, 1975.
39. Biggar, W. D., *et al.*: Fetal thymus transplantation. Birth Defects, *11*:361, 1971.
40. Fulganiti, V. A., *et al.*: Dissociation of delayed-hypersensitivity and antibody-synthesizing capacities in man. Lancet, *2*:5, 1966.
41. Lawlor, G. J., *et al.*: The syndrome of cellular immunodeficiency with immunoglobulins. J. Pediatr., *84*:183, 1974.
42. Hitzig, W. H., Landolt, R., Muller, G., and Bodmer, P.: Heterogeneity of phenotypic expression in a family with Swiss-type agammaglobulinemia. Observations on the acquisition of agammaglobulinemia. J. Pediatr., *78*:968, 1971.
43. Bruton, O. C.: Agammaglobulinemia. Pediatrics., *9*:722, 1952.
44. Good, R. A., Kelly, W. D., Rotstein, J., and Varco, R. L.: Immunological deficiency diseases. Prog. Allergy, *6*:187, 1962.
45. Janeway, C. A., Gitlin, D., Craig, J. M., and Grice, D. S.: Collagen diseases in patients with congenital agammaglobulinemia. Trans. Assoc. Am. Physicians, *69*:93, 1956.
46. Good, R. A., Rotstein, J., and Mazzitella, W. F.: The simultaneous occurrence of rheumatoid arthritis and agammaglobulinemia. J. Lab. Clin. Med., *49*:343, 1957.
47. Cook, C. D., Rosen, F. S., and Banke, B. Q.: Dermatomyositis and focal scleroderma. Pediatr. Clin. North Am., *10*:979, 1963.
48. Page, A. R., Hansen, A. E., and Good, R. A.: Occurrence of leukemia and lymphoma in patients with agammaglobulinemia. Blood, *21*:197, 1963.
49. Good, R. A., *et al.*: The immunologic deficiency diseases of man. Birth Defects, *4*:17, 1968.
50. Gajl-Peczalska, K., Lim, S. D., and Good, R. A.: B lymphocytes in primary and secondary deficiencies of humoral immunity. Birth Defects, *11*:33, 1975.
51. Siegal, F. P., Pernis, B., and Kunkel, H. G.: Lymphocytes in human immunodeficiency states: a study of membrane associated immunoglobulin. Eur. J. Immunol., *1*:482, 1971.
52. Schiff, R. I., Buckley, R. H., Gilbertsen, R. B., and Metzgar, R. S.: Membrane receptors and *in vitro* responsiveness of lymphocytes in human immunodeficiency. J. Immunol., *112*:376, 1974.
53. Wu, L. Y. F., and Lawton, A. R.: Evaluation of human D lymphocyte differentiation using pokeweed mitogen stimulation. Clin. Res., *20*:798, 1972.
54. Stobo, J. D., and Paul, W. E.: Functional heterogeneity of murine lymphoid cells. J. Immunol., *110*:362, 1973.
55. Hitzig, W. H., and Muntener, U.: Conventional immunoglobulin therapy. Birth Defects, *11*:339, 1975.
56. Johansson, S. G. O., Hogman, C. F., and Killander, J.: Quantitative immunoglobulin determination. Acta Pathol. Microbiol. Scand., *174*:519, 1968.
57. Buckley, R. H.: Clinical and immunologic features of selective IgA deficiency: Birth Defects, *11*:134, 1975.
58. Horowitz, S., and Hong, R.: Selective IgA deficiency—some perspectives. Birth Defects, *11*:129, 1975.
59. Wells, J. V., Michaeli, D., and Fudenberg, H. H.: Autoimmunity in selective IgA deficiency. Birth Defects, *11*:144, 1975.
60. Gatti, R. A., and Good, R. A.: Occurrence of malignancy in immunodeficiency diseases. Cancer, *28*:89, 1971.
61. Tomasi, T. B., and Grey, H. M.: Structure and function of IgA. Prog. Allergy, *16*:81, 1972.
62. Walker, W. A., Isselbacher, K. J., and Block, K. J.: Intestinal uptake of macromolecules: effect of oral immunization. Science, *177*:608, 1972.
63. Stobo, J. D., and Tomasi, T. B.: A low molecular weight immunoglobulin antigenically related to 19S IgM. J. Clin. Immunol., *46*:1329, 1967.
64. Buckley, R. H., and Dees, S. C.: The correlation of milk precipitins with IgA deficiency. N. Engl. J. Med., *281*:465, 1969.
65. Ammann, A. J., and Hong, R.: Unique antibody to basement membrane in patients with selective IgA deficiency and celiac disease. Lancet, *1*:1264, 1971.
66. Lawton, A. R., Royal, S. A., Self, S., and Cooper, M. D.: IgA determinants on B-lymphocytes in patients with deficiency of circulating IgA. J. Lab. Clin. Med., *80*:26, 1972.
67. Mitchell, G. F., Mishell, R. I., and Herzenberg, L. A.: Studies on the influence of T cells in antibody production. Prog. Immunol., *1*:324, 1971.
68. Schlegel, R. J., *et al.*: Severe candidiasis associated with thymic dysplasia, IgA deficiency and plasma anti-lymphocyte effects. Pediatrics, *45*:926, 1970.
69. Ammann, A. J., and Hong, R.: Selective IgA deficiency: report of 30 cases and a review of the literature. Medicine, *50*:223, 1971.
70. Murgita, R. A., Mattioli, C. A., and Tomasi, T. B.: Production of a runting syndrome and selective IgA deficiency in mice by the administration of anti-heavy chain antisera. J. Exp. Med., *138*:209, 1973.
71. Schmidt, A. P., Taswell, H. F., and Gleich, G. J.: Anaphylactic transfusion reactions associated with anti-IgA antibodies. N. Engl. J. Med., *280*:188, 1969.
72. Strober, W., *et al.*: Secretory component deficiency: a disorder of the IgA immune system. N. Engl. J. Med., *294*:351, 1976.
73. Hanson, L. A.: Aspects of the absence of the IgA system. Birth Defects, *4*:292, 1968.
74. Rosen, F. S., *et al.*: Recurrent bacterial infections and dysgammaglobulinemia. Pediatrics, *28*:182, 1961.
75. Stiehm, E. R., and Fudenberg, H. H.: Clinical and immunologic features of dysgammaglobulinemia type I. Am. J. Med., *40*:805, 1966.
76. Davis, S. D.: Antibody deficiency diseases. *In*

Stiehm, E. R., and Fulginiti, V. A. (eds.): Immunologic Disorders in Infants and Children. P. 184. Philadelphia, W. B. Saunders, 1973.

77. Hong, R., Schubert, W. K., Perrin, E. V., and West, C. D.: Antibody deficiency syndrome associated with beta-2 macroglobulinemia. J. Pediatr., *61*:831, 1962.
78. Buckley, R. H., Wray, B. B., and Belmaker, E. Z.: Extreme hyper IgE and undue susceptibility to infection. Pediatrics, *49*:59, 1972.
79. deVaal, O. M., and Seynhaeve, V.: Reticular dysgenia. Lancet, *2*:1123, 1959.
80. Hitzig, W. H.: The Swiss-type of agammaglobulinemia. Birth Defects, *4*:82, 1968.
81. Cohen, F.: *In* Meuwissen, H. J., Pollara, B., Pickering, R. J., and Porter, I. H. (eds.): Combined Immunodeficiency and Adenosine Deaminase Deficiency. P. 245. New York, Academic Press, 1973.
82. Gelfand, E. W., Biggar, W. D., and Orange, R. P.: Immune deficiency: evaluation, diagnosis and treatment. Pediatr. Clin. North Am., *21*:745, 1974.
83. Pyke, K. W., Dosch, H. M., Ipp, M. M., and Gelfand, E. W.: Demonstration of an intrathymic defect in a case of severe combined immunodeficiency. N. Engl. J. Med., *293*:424, 1975.
84. Duke, K. A., van der Waay, D., and van Bekkun, D. W.: The use of stem-cell grafts in combined immunodeficiency. Birth Defects, *11*:391, 1975.
85. Giblett, E. R., *et al.*: Adenosine deaminase deficiency in two patients with severely impaired cellular immunity. Lancet, *2*:1067, 1972.
86. Wolpar, J. J., and Cross, V. F.: *In* Meuwissen, H. J., Pollara, B., Pickering, R. J., and Porter, I. H. (eds.): Combined Immunodeficiency and Adenosine Deaminase Deficiency. P. 255. New York, Academic Press, 1973.
87. Wara, D. W., and Ammann, A. J.: *In* Meuwissen, H. J., Pollara, B., Pickering, R. J., and Porter, I. H. (eds.): Combined Immunodeficiency and Adenosine Deaminase Deficiency. P. 247. New York, Academic Press, 1973.
88. Huber, J., and Kersey, J.: *In* Meuwissen, H. J., Pollara, B., Pickering, R. J., and Porter, I. H. (eds.): Combined Immunodeficiency and Adenosine Deaminase Deficiency. P. 279. New York, Academic Press, 1973.
89. Green, H.: *In* Meuwissen, H. J., Pollara, B., Pickering, R. J., and Porter, I. H. (eds.): Combined Immunodeficiency and Adenosine Deaminase Deficiency. P. 141. New York, Academic Press, 1973.
90. Hirschorn, R., *et al.*: Evidence for control of several different tissue-specific isozymes of adenosine deaminase by a single genetic locus. Nature [New Biol.], *246*:200, 1973.
91. Moore, E. C., and Meuwissen, H. J.: *In* Meuwissen, H. J., Pollara, B., Pickering, R. J., and Porter, I. H. (eds.): Combined Immunodeficiency and Adenosine Deaminase Deficiency. P. 219. New York, Academic Press, 1973.
92. Meuwissen, H. J., Pickering, R. J., and Pollara, B.: Adenosine deaminase deficiency in combined immunodeficiency. Birth Defects, *11*:117, 1975.
93. Jenkins, T.: Red blood cell adenosine deaminase deficiency in a "healthy" Kung individual. Lancet, *2*:736, 1973.
94. Green, H., and Chan, T. S.: Pyrimidine starvation induced by adenosine in fibroblasts and lymphoid cells. Role of adenosine deaminase. Science, *182*:836, 1973.
95. Blume, A. J., Dalton, C., and Sheppard, H.: Adenosine-mediated elevation of cyclic 3:5-AMP concentrations in cultured mouse neuroblastoma cells. Proc. Natl. Acad. Sci., U.S.A., *70*:3099, 1973.
96. Wolberg, G., *et al.*: Adenosine inhibition of lymphocyte-mediated cytolysis: a possible role of cyclic AMP. Science, *187*:957, 1975.
97. Snyder, F. F., and Henderson, J. F.: Pathways of deoxyadenosine and adenosine metabolism. J. Biol. Chem., *248*:5899, 1973.
98. Buckley, R. H.: Reconstitution: grafting of bone marrow and thymus. Prog. Immunol., *1*:1061, 1971.
99. Keightley, R. G., Lawton, A. R., Wu, L. Y. F., and Cooper, M. D.: In Meuwissin, H. J., Pollara, B., Pickering, R. J., and Porter, I. H.(eds.): Combined Immunodeficiency and Adenosine Deaminase Deficiency. P. 213. New York, Academic Press, 1973.
100. Red cells put lymphocytes to work. Med. World News, *16*(2):37, 1975.
101. Giblett, E. R., *et al.*: Nucleoside phosphorylase deficiency in a child with severely defective T-cell immunity and normal B-cell immunity. Lancet, *2*:1010, 1975.
102. Douglas, S. D., and Goldberg, L. S., and Fudenberg, H. H.: Clinical serological and leukocyte function studies on patients with idiopathic "acquired" agammaglobulinemia and their families. Am. J. Med., *48*:48, 1970.
103. Wilson, W. R., Hermans, P. E., and Ritts, R. E.: Idiopathic late-onset immunoglobulin deficiency with functional T-cell deficiency. Arch. Intern. Med., *136*:343, 1976.
104. Gajl-Peczalska, K., Park, B. H., Biggar, W. D., and Good, R. A.: B and T lymphocytes in primary immunodeficiency diseases in man. J. Clin. Inv., *52*:919, 1973.

104a. Hermans, P. E., Diaz-Buxo, J. A., and Stobo, J. D.: Idiopathic late-onset immunoglobulin deficiency. Am. J. Med., *61*:221, 1976.

105. Geha, R. S., Schneeberger, E., Merler, E., and Rosen, F. S.: Heterogeneity of "acquired" or common variable agammaglobulinemia. N. Engl. J. Med., *291*:1, 1974.
106. Choi, Y. S., Biggar, W. D., and Good, R. A.: Biosynthesis and secretion of immunoglobulin by peripheral blood lymphocytes in severe hypogammaglobulinemia. Lancet, *1*:1149, 1972.
107. Waldmann, T. A., *et al.*: Role of suppressor T cells in the pathogenesis of common variable hypogammaglobulinemia. Lancet, *2*:609, 1974.

108. Cooper, M. D., *et al.*: Immunologic defects in patients with Wiskott Aldrich syndrome. Birth Defects, *4*:378, 1968.
109. Grottum, K. A., *et al.*: The Wiskott Aldrich syndrome: qualitative platelet defects and short platelet survival. Br. J. Haematol., *17*:373, 1969.
110. Ten Bensel, R. W., Stadler, E. M., and Krivit, W.: The development of malignancy in the course of the Aldrich syndrome. J. Pediatr., *68*:761, 1966.
111. Blaese, R. M., Strober, W., and Waldmann, T. A.: Immunodeficiency in the Wiskott Aldrich syndrome. Birth Defects, *11*:250, 1975.
112. Wybran, J., Carr, M. C., and Fudenberg, H. H.: The human rosette-forming cell as a marker of a population of thymus-derived cells. J. Clin. Invest., *51*:2537, 1972.
113. Sherwood, G., and Blaese, R. M.: PHA induced cytotoxic effector lymphocyte function in patients with the Wiskott Aldrich syndrome. Clin. Exp. Immunol., *13*:515, 1973.
114. Oppenheim, J. J., Blaese, R. M., and Waldmann, T. A.: Defective lymphocyte transformation and delayed hypersensitivity in the Wiskott Aldrich syndrome. J. Immunol., *104*:835, 1970.
115. Spitler, L. E., *et al.*: The Wiskott Aldrich syndrome. Immunologic studies in nine patients and selected family members. Cell. Immunol., *19*:201, 1975.
116. Blaese, K. M., Strober, W., Levy, A. L., and Waldmann, T. A.: Hypercatabolism of IgG, IgA, and IgM and albumin in Wiskott Aldrich syndrome. J. Clin. Invest., *50*:2331, 1971.
117. Preud'homme, J. L., Griscelli, C., and Seligiman, M.: Immunoglobulin on the surface of lymphocytes in 50 patients with primary immunodeficiency diseases. Clin. Immunol. Immunopathol., *1*:241, 1973.
118. Blaese, R. M., Strober, W. S., Brown, R. S., and Waldmann, T. A.: The Wiskott Aldrich syndrome. Lancet, *1*:1056, 1968.
119. Cooper, M. D., *et al.*: Wiskott Aldrich syndrome: an immunologic deficiency disease involving the afferent limb of immunity. Am. J. Med., *44*:499, 1968.
120. Blaese, R. M., Oppenheim, J. J., Seeger, R. C., and Waldmann, T. A.: Lymphocyte-macrophage interaction in antigen induced *in vitro* lymphocyte transformation in patients with the Wiskott Aldrich syndrome and other diseases with anergy. Cell. Immunol., *4*:228, 1972.
121. Altman, L. C., Snyderman, R., and Blaese, R. M.: Abnormalities of chemotactic lymphokine synthesis in mononuclear leukocyte chemotaxis in Wiskott Aldrich syndrome. J. Clin. Invest., *54*:486, 1974.
122. Bruce, R. M., and Blaese, R. M.: Monoclonal gammopathy in the Wiskott Aldrich syndrome. J. Pediatr., *85*:204, 1974.
123. Levin, A. S., Spitler, L. E., Fudenberg, H. H.: Transfer factor. I. Methods of treatment. Birth Defects, *11*:445, 1975.
124. Spitler, L. E., Levin, A. S., and Fudenberg, H. H.: Transfer factor. II. Results of treatment. Birth Defects, *11*:449, 1975.
125. Boder, E.: Ataxia-telangiectasia: some historic clinical and pathologic observations. Birth Defects, *11*:255, 1975.
126. McFarlin, D. E., Strober, W., and Waldmann, T. A.: Ataxia-telangiectasia. Medicine, *51*:281, 1972.
127. Biggar, W. D., and Good, R. A.: Immunodeficiency in ataxia-telangiectasia. Birth Defects, *11*:271, 1975.
128. Waldmann, T. A., and McIntire, K. R.: Serum alpha fetoprotein levels in patients with ataxia-telangiectasia. Lancet, *2*:1112, 1972.
129. Day, N. K., and Good, R. A.: Deficiencies of the complement system in man. Birth Defects, *11*:306, 1975.
130. Kohler, P. F., and Müller-Eberhard, H. J.: Complement-immunoglobulin relation: deficiency of C1q associated with impaired IgG synthesis. Science, *163*:474, 1969.
131. Gewurz, H., *et al.*: Decreased C1q protein concentration and agglutinating activity in agammaglobulinemic syndromes. Clin. Exp. Immunol., *3*:437, 1968.
132. Kohler, P. F., and Müller-Eberhard, H. J.: Metabolism of human C1q. J. Clin. Invest., *51*:868, 1972.
133. Moncado, B., Day, N. K. B., Good, R. A., and Windhorst, D. B.: Lupus erythematosus-like syndrome with a familial defect of complement. N. Engl. J. Med., *286*:689, 1972.
134. Pickering, R. J., *et al.*: Deficiency of C1r in human serum. J. Exp. Med., *131*:803, 1970.
135. Agnello, V., *et al.*: Hereditary C2 deficiency in SLE and acquired complement abnormalities in an unusual SLE-related syndrome. Birth Defects, *11*:312, 1975.
136. Alper, C. A., *et al.*: Homozygous deficiency of C3 in a patient with repeated infections. Lancet, *2*:1179, 1972.
137. Alper, C. A., and Rosen, F. S.: Increased susceptibility to infection in patients with defects affecting C3. Birth Defects, *11*:301, 1975.
138. Frank, M. M., *et al.*: Hereditary C6 deficiency in man. Birth Defects, *11*:318, 1975.
139. Petersen, B. H., Graham, J. M., and Brooks, G. F.: Human deficiency of the 8th component of complement. J. Clin. Invest., *57*:283, 1976.
140. Miller, M. E., and Nilsson, U. R.: A familial deficiency of the phagocytosis-enhancing activity of serum related to a dysfunction of the 5th component of complement (C5). N. Engl. J. Med., *282*:354, 1970.
141. Frank, M. M., Gelfand, J. A., and Atkinson, J. P.: Hereditary angioedema: the clinical syndrome and its management. Ann. Intern. Med., *84*:580, 1976.
142. Donaldson, V. H., and Evans, R. R.: A biochemical abnormality in hereditary angioneurotic edema. Am. J. Med., *35*:37, 1963.
143. Burke, B. A., and Good, R. A.: Pneumocystis carinii infection. Medicine, *52*:23, 1973.

11 The Immunology of Infectious Disease

VIRAL IMMUNOLOGY

The interaction between a virus and the immune system can be of enormous consequence to the well-being and often the survival of the host. In this section, we shall explore five important aspects of this interaction: (1) the nature of the immune response to viral infections; (2) the immunology of persistent viral infections; (3) the role of the immune system in the pathogenesis of virally induced lesions; (4) the effect of viruses upon the immune system; and (5) immunoprophylaxis.

THE IMMUNE RESPONSE TO VIRAL INFECTIONS

Viral Antigens

A viral infection introduces a variety of new antigens into the body. Antigens present on the surface of the virus can incite an immune response; these antigens are most often structural components. Multiplication of the virus within the host can provide additional immunogens, including structural subunits, partially assembled capsids and viral products such as replicative enzymes.

Many viruses also produce alterations in the membranes of infected cells. These surface alterations can sometimes present as new surface antigens.[1] New cell-surface antigens often appear very early after infection, and are frequently detectable before any progeny viral particles have been produced. Some of these antigens are the result of the insertion of newly synthesized virally coded proteins into the cell membrane. Others are due to the production of new host-coded molecules induced by the presence of the virus. Furthermore, in some experimental systems, viral infection can lead to modification in the normal surface antigenicity of host cells. The effects of viruses on host cell membranes are extremely important, since the altered cells can become targets for the host immune system. Infections with certain viruses, such as the picornaviruses (which include the polio and Coxsackie viruses), do not lead to the appearance of new cell-surface antigens (Table 11-1).

The Life Cycle of a Virus

In order to understand both when and where a virus is susceptible to an immune attack, we must first examine the life cycle of a virus. The polio virus provides a fairly typical example.[2]

The polio virus, like most viruses, enters the body across the mucosal surface

Table 11-1. Types of Viruses Causing Antigenic Changes on Surfaces of Virus-Infected Cells

*Changes Reported In**	*Changes Not Reported In*
Adenovirus	Picornaviruses
Type 12	Polio
Arenavirus	ECHO
Lymphocytic choriomeningitis	Coxsackie
Herpesviruses	Reoviruses
Herpes simplex virus	Parvoviruses
Varicella-zoster	
Cytomegalovirus	
Epstein-Barr virus	
Orthomyxovirus	
Influenza, type A	
Paramyxoviruses	
Mumps	
Measles	
Respiratory syncytial virus	
Poxviruses	
Vaccinia	
Cowpox	
Rhabdovirus	
Rabies	

*This is only a partial list.

of either the respiratory or gastrointestinal tract. The free virus in the secretions can infect the cells lining the portal of entry and thus gain access to the local draining lymph nodes, including the tonsils, cervical nodes, Peyer's patches and mesenteric nodes. Here the virus can infect more cells and replicate, while at the same time inducing an immune response. Replicated viral particles are released into the lymph, and a minor viremia develops allowing dissemination of the virus.[3] At this point, the virus circulates freely and will infect susceptible tissues. Most viruses infect only certain tissues. The polio virus preferentially invades the liver and lymphoid tissue. Replication of the polio virus in these targets results in the release of a large number of progeny viruses, and a second, major viremia ensues. The polio virus disseminates throughout the body in high concentration and can now infect the central nervous system. Despite the viremia present in most infections with polio virus, only a minority of cases culminate in the clinical disease of poliomyelitis.

This general pattern of infection and dissemination is seen in almost all human viral infections, although there are notable exceptions.[4] Rhinovirus infections appear to be limited to the respiratory mucosa and wart viruses to the skin, so that these exceptional viruses may not possess a viremic phase. Certain viruses are inoculated directly into the bloodstream (including the arthropod-borne viruses and serum hepatitis virus) and do not pass through a stage of local replication at the mucosal surfaces.

One investigator has postulated two modes of viral transmission from cell to cell (Fig. 11-1). The extracellular spread of free virus is called type I viral transmission, and is the major mode of spread for most viruses. Some viruses can infect neighboring cells across intercytoplasmic bridges, and thus do not have to leave the intracellular environment in order to disseminate. This is referred to as type II viral transmission and has been demonstrated for herpes simplex virus, varicella zoster, measles, vaccinia and cytomegalovirus.[5,6] It is important to note that most viruses capable of type II transmission can also spread via a type I mechanism.

Antibody can directly affect a virus only when the virus is in the extracellular environment. Thus, antibody can interfere with type I spread while those viruses capable of type II transmission can evade the effects of antiviral antibody.

The Humoral Response

The Importance of Secretory and Serum Antibody in Viral Infections

The humoral response to viral infection can be divided into two phases: (1) the generation of secretory IgA, and (2) the production of circulating immunoglobulins of all classes. This division emphasizes the independence of locally pro-

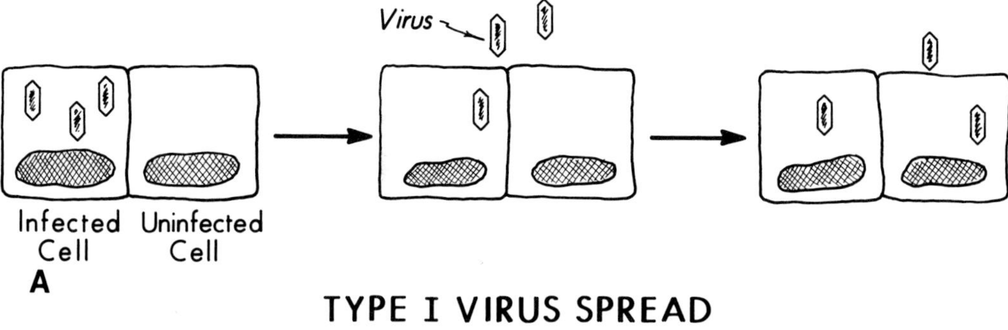

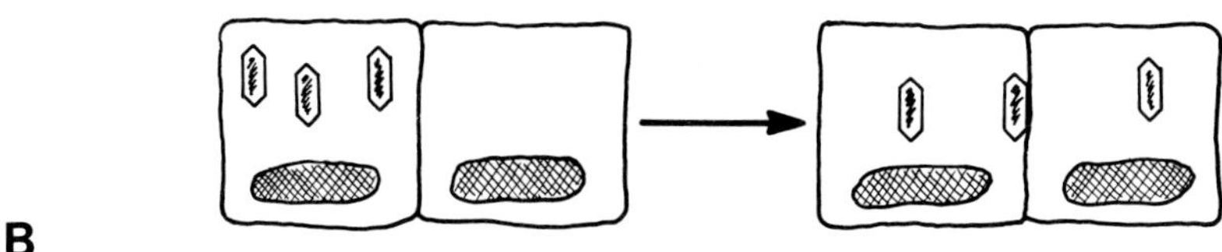

Fig. 11-1. Modes of viral spread. (A) Type I spread: the virus is released from an infected cell into the extracellular space from where it infects neighboring cells. (B) Type II spread: the virus passes from cell to cell via intercytoplasmic bridges without passing through the extracellular space.

duced secretory IgA from systemic antibody production. Furthermore, secretory IgA that is made in one location does not necessarily correlate with the production of secretory IgA in other regions of the respiratory or gastrointestinal tract. Thus, if virus is introduced into the distal colon, secretory IgA will appear in colonic excretions but not in other mucosal regions such as the nasopharynx.[7]

At the beginning of a primary infection, no preformed antibody is present at the mucosal surfaces to prevent a local infection, and mucosal antibody therefore can serve only to *prevent reinfection* by a previously encountered virus. Secretory IgA is the body's most important mechanism for preventing reinfection, and the level of antiviral secretory IgA at the appropriate portal of entry correlates quantitatively with resistance to reinfection.[8]

Secretory IgA production against the polio virus can usually be detected within approximately one week of inoculation. With certain viruses, secretory IgA levels can persist locally for several months.[9]

Although serum antibody may not contribute greatly to preventing reinfection, it does help to limit the extracellular spread of virus once it has gained access to the circulation. Serum antibody can prevent central nervous system disease due to polio virus dissemination even though local gastrointestinal infection has occurred. The consequence of the absence of serum antibody protection is illustrated by the high rate of polio virus dissemination and poliomyelitis in hypogammaglobulinemic children given live polio vaccine.[10]

Viral Neutralization

Antibody directed against certain antigens on the virus itself can destroy viral infectivity. This process is called *viral neutralization*, and the target antigens are called neutralization antigens. Attachment of antibody to the surface of free virus can prevent viral adsorption to the target cell surface, penetration into the cell, and proper uncoating of the virus once inside the cell (Fig. 11-2).[11] However, antibody binding does not always cause neutralization, and in certain situations antibody-coated virus particles can still be infectious.[12] Whether or not antiviral antibody actually neutralizes the virus depends upon the affinity of the antibody for the viral antigens, the site of attachment to the virus, and the ability of the antibody to fix complement.[13]

Low-affinity antibodies are commonly seen early in an antiviral response. They are capable of neutralizing a virus but tend to dissociate, allowing reactivation of the virus. Later in the response, high-affinity antibody is produced and is more effective at maintaining viral neutralization.

The mechanism by which antibodies can neutralize viruses is not completely understood. Perhaps the simplest and most widely accepted hypothesis is that antibody inhibits viral functions by sterically interfering with the viral surface. There is little definitive evidence that the neutralization of human viruses occurs via the covering up of specific viral "critical sites."

There are other ways in which direct antibody-mediated viral neutralization may occur. In some situations, antibody has been shown to induce conformational changes in the virus which are associated with neutralization.[14] Antibody-induced viral aggregation has also been proposed as a mechanism for neutralization.[15]

The binding of complement to antibody-coated viruses can promote viral neutralization.[16] In some cases, viral antibodies are dependent upon complement fixation for neutralization. Studies employing the sequential addition of complement components to antibody-virus complexes have helped to clarify the role of each component in viral neutral-

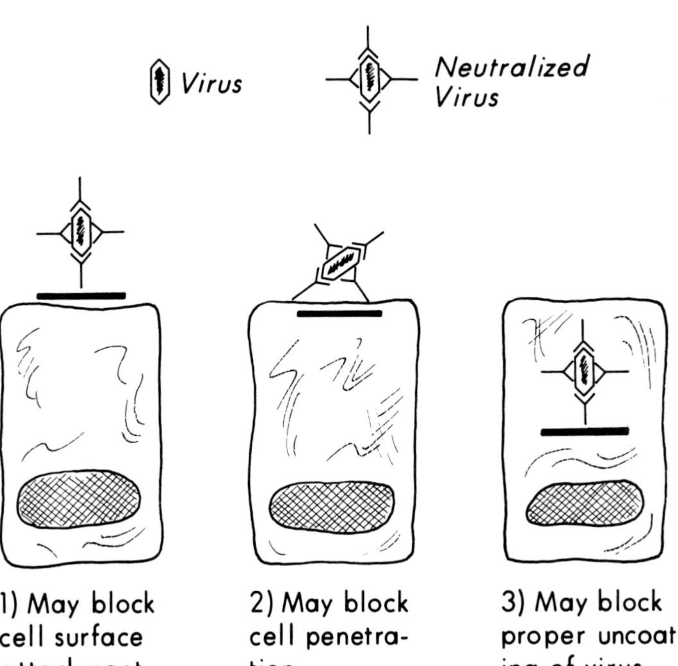

Fig. 11-2. Sites of action in antibody-mediated viral neutralization. (1) Prevention of cell-surface attachment. (2) Prevention of cell-surface penetration. (3) Prevention of uncoating.

ization.[17] Fixation of C1 alone does not lead to neutralization, but sequential addition of C4, C2 and C3 results in progressively greater and greater neutralization. The mechanism of neutralization by the early components of complement is not known, but they do not appear to destroy the virus and probably act by mechanisms similar to antibody-mediated neutralization.

The addition of the late complement components (C5 to C9) can further enhance neutralization, perhaps by inducing viral lysis.[18] Only some viruses have been shown to be susceptible to complement-mediated lysis.[19]

Neutralization is not the only mechanism by which antibody can nullify the infectivity of a virus. Antibody binding will also enhance the clearance of viral particles much as it does with any antigen. These two mechanisms, neutralization and opsonization, make the humoral response a powerful weapon against viral infection.

Antibody Directed Against Infected Cells

The appearance of new cell-surface antigens on infected cells can also induce a humoral response which may contribute to elimination of the infection. This response is directed against the infected cells themselves, and may involve two basic mechanisms. (1) Antibody-dependent *complement*-mediated cell lysis has been demonstrated *in vitro*.[20] (2) Antibody-dependent *cell*-mediated cytotoxicity can destroy virally altered host cells *in vitro*.[21] The relevance of each of these mechanisms *in vivo* remains to be confirmed.

The Cellular Response to Viruses

Whereas antiviral antibody can prevent viral dissemination and reinfection, the cellular limb of the immune system is considered to be responsible for the actual termination of an ongoing infection.

The T Cell

It has long been felt that the T lymphocyte is primarily responsible for host defense against a virus, whether as a T helper cell for the humoral response, as an activator of macrophages, or as a direct cytotoxic effector cell.[22] The idea that the T cell is the most important and formidable viral antagonist has been based largely upon extrapolation from studies of patients with various immunodeficiency syndromes.[23] Thus, patients with X-linked agammaglobulinemia who have intact T-cell function generally handle viral infections well, despite the lack of a competent humoral system. On the other hand, patients with T-cell deficiencies such as severe combined immunodeficiency and DiGeorge's syndrome often suffer from severe viral infections. We must caution, however, that although such evidence strongly implicates the T cell as a major factor in the defense against viral infection, there is little direct documentation *in vivo* in normal humans to support this conclusion.

The T lymphocyte appears to perform two major antiviral effector functions:[24]

Cytotoxicity. Whereas the activity of antibody is directed mostly against the viral particles themselves, T-cell effector function is primarily directed against the infected cells. The killing of virally infected cells by sensitized T cells may be of great importance since it provides a way for the immune system to abort an infection when the virus is sequestered within the host's cells. The T killer cell can destroy a cell bearing virally induced new surface antigens before the progeny viruses are assembled, and thus can quickly bring the infection to an end. However, lysis of infected cells by T killer cells is not always to the host's advantage. Thus, if T cells lyse the host's cells later in the infection, progeny viruses, which may now be fully mature, can be released and disseminated throughout the body.

Recent advances in immunogenetics

are beginning to alter our present picture of T-cell cytotoxicity against virally infected cells. A variety of animal experiments have shown that T cells can only lyse infected cells if the target cells are syngeneic to the killer lymphocytes.[24a] In the mouse, the requirement for genetic identity has been localized to the H2-K or H2-D regions (see Chap. 9). One interpretation of this work is that the killer cell responds against a complex of H-2 and viral antigens on the cell surface.[24b]

Release of Lymphokines. Among the many soluble substances released by sensitized lymphocytes are factors that recruit and activate host macrophages. Mechanisms may exist whereby macrophages can be specifically armed to respond to viral antigens to which the lymphocytes have been sensitized (see Chap. 6). Macrophage activity may be especially important in the ingestion and disposal of cell debris and the destruction of viral particles released from infected host cells that have been lysed by T lymphocytes.

The Macrophage

Macrophages ingest viruses at their portal of entry and within the local lymph nodes. If a virus is injected directly into the bloodstream, as are the arthropod-borne viruses, it is cleared by phagocytic cells lining the liver sinuses.[25] Once a virus has gained entrance to the host, macrophage ingestion helps to prevent the infection of target organs such as the liver and central nervous system.[26]

The role of the macrophage as a barrier to viral infection is illustrated by the susceptibility of newborn animals to viral inocula which are harmless to adult animals.[27] For example, injection of herpes simplex into neonates can cause a widespread and fatal infection, whereas adult animals of the same strain are comparatively resistant. The neonatal susceptibility to viral infection appears to be due to the immaturity of the macrophage population. Transfer of mature macrophages, but not lymphocytes, can convey resistance to the virus in these young animals.[28] One might speculate that macrophage immaturity is the reason for the relatively high frequency of disseminated, severe infections with rubella and cytomegalovirus in human fetuses.

Experimental work has shown that the macrophage has two possible relationships to a particular virus (Fig. 11-3). If the macrophage is *nonpermissive*, it will not support the replication of that virus. Macrophages have been found to be nonpermissive for several viruses including herpes simplex and Coxsackie.[29] If the macrophage is *permissive* for a virus, it will support viral replication. The consequences of a permissive relationship have been illustrated in animal systems.[30] One study showed that mice of one strain were susceptible to severe hepatitis by a viral inoculum that was *avirulent* to a second strain.[31] It was found that susceptibility was determined by a single dominant gene which controlled macrophage permissiveness toward the particular virus. The resistant strain lacked the dominant allele and would not support the multiplication of the virus.

Interferon

Interferon is a substance elaborated by many different types of cells when they are infected with certain viruses. Although its production is stimulated by the presence of a virus, interferon is coded for by the host genome. Interferon is a protein and requires host-cell macromolecular synthesis for its production. Interferon functions by derepressing a host gene which codes for a substance called *viral-inhibitory protein* (VIP) which in turn prevents the intracellular replication of viruses. This appears to be accomplished by the suppression of the translation of viral mRNA.[32,33] Interferon is released from the cell in which it is made and will afford protection to other host cells with which it comes in contact.

The relative importance of interferon in

1) NON-PERMISSIVE MACROPHAGE

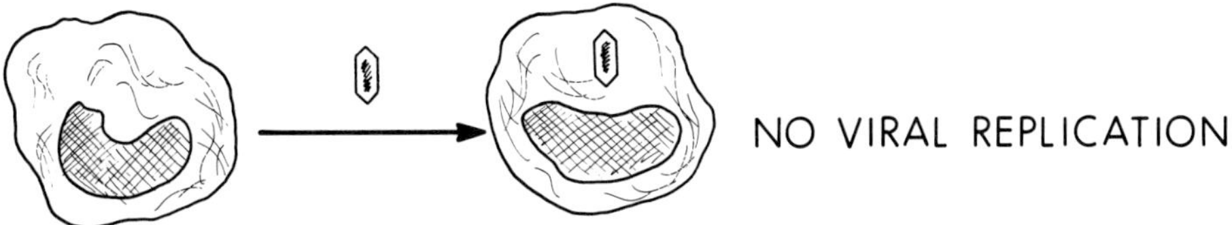

2) PERMISSIVE MACROPHAGE

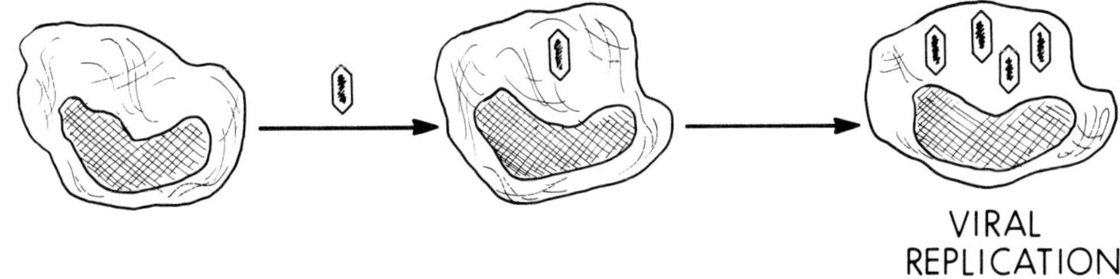

Fig. 11-3. (1) Viral infection of nonpermissive macrophages does not allow viral replication. (2) Viral infection of permissive macrophages allows infections to continue.

defense against viral infections has not been ascertained. During a primary infection, interferon can often be detected before specific antibody titers rise, and in some experimental systems the control of certain primary viral infections may be better correlated with the production of interferon than with the production of antiviral antibodies.[34]

The story of interferon is a fascinating and important chapter in molecular virology. However, a complete discussion of interferon is more appropriate for a text in virology than for one in immunology. Nevertheless, there are some recent experiments which have focused on its immunologic aspects. We will briefly review this area of interferon research while cautioning that it is but one small part of the study of interferon and one whose significance is still untested.

Lymphocytes are one cell type that can produce interferon, and they can release it as a lymphokine. Mitogens and both viral and nonviral antigens can stimulate interferon production by lymphocytes.[35-37] Sensitized lymphocytes do not have to be infected with whole virus in order to produce interferon, but need only recognize and respond to a particular sensitizing antigen. This is in contrast to interferon production by nonlymphoid cells. The production of interferon by lymphocytes may therefore be of great significance, since certain intact viruses rapidly shut down the synthetic machinery of infected cells, thereby preventing interferon synthesis in those cells.[38]

It has been reported that the interferon produced by lymphocytes in response to an antigenic challenge differs from standard nonlymphoid interferon in its biological, physical and serologic characteristics.[39,40] Whether lymphocyte-derived ("immune") interferon is more or less potent *in vivo* than interferon produced by other cell types has not been established.

The T lymphocyte appears to be the major producer of immune interferon.[41] Further examination has shown that a particular subpopulation of mature T cells is required for interferon production.[42] These cells are capable of immunologic memory; i.e., a second antigenic challenge has been demonstrated to induce a higher level of interferon production than the original sensitization.[43] Recently, B cells have also been found to be capable of producing interferon.[44] It is not clear whether the macrophage can also make interferon or whether it simply enhances interferon production by lymphocytes.[45]

Summary

The ability of the immune system to prevent, contain and terminate a viral infection involves all aspects of the immune response:

Antibody is important in (Fig. 11-4):

1. Preventing reinfection at portals of entry, primarily via secretory IgA
2. Inhibiting the dissemination of viral infections by neutralizing free virus that appears at various times in the infectious cycle of certain viruses
3. Enhancing the clearance of virus by the reticulo-endothelial system
4. Possibly aborting intracellular infections by lysing infected and antigenically altered cells either via a complement-mediated mechanism or ADCC

T-cell immunity is important in (Fig. 11-5):

1. Lysing antigenically altered infected cells
2. Producing immune interferon (Nonimmune infected cells also produce interferon.)
3. Providing helper function for the production of antiviral antibodies
4. Recruiting, activating and arming macrophages

Macrophages are important in:

1. Ingesting and destroying viruses and thus serving as a nonspecific primary barrier against the infection of parenchymal tissue
2. Clearing viral and cellular debris
3. Possibly aiding in the specific destruction of virally altered infected cells

The relative importance of each of these mechanisms can only be understood in terms of the biology of each individual virus. For example, certain enteroviruses do not induce antigenic changes in the surfaces of infected cells.[46] Thus T-cell cytolysis is unlikely to be a factor in these infections. On the other hand, these viruses disseminate by type I spread, and thus antiviral antibody is critically important in preventing the dissemination of these agents.

Viruses that can infect neighboring cells across cytoplasmic bridges (type II spread) may be protected from the effects of antibody. In these infections, T-cell immunity against the altered infected cells may be particularly important. However, T-cell lysis may fail to contain the infection, since by the time new surface antigens are first expressed, making lysis possible, progeny viruses may have already infected neighboring cells across the cytoplasmic bridges.[47,48] Thus, any immunologic response to infected cells bearing virally induced surface antigens might always remain one step behind the spread of the virus. This phenomenon has been reported in experimental infections with herpes simplex virus. In order to abort an infection with this virus, the host may have to rely on nonspecific effector functions. Although these have not been entirely defined, both macrophages and interferon are likely candidates. Macrophages seem to be able to destroy the intercellular bridges by a nonspecific toxic effect, and interferon may render the neighboring cells resistant to viral replication.[47] We must emphasize that it is still uncertain whether these conclusions can be extended beyond experimental herpes simplex virus infections.

THE IMMUNOLOGY OF PERSISTENT VIRAL INFECTIONS

Over the last few years it has become increasingly apparent that a number of viral infections do not merely represent acute episodes. Certain viral infections will persist, often for the entire lifetime of

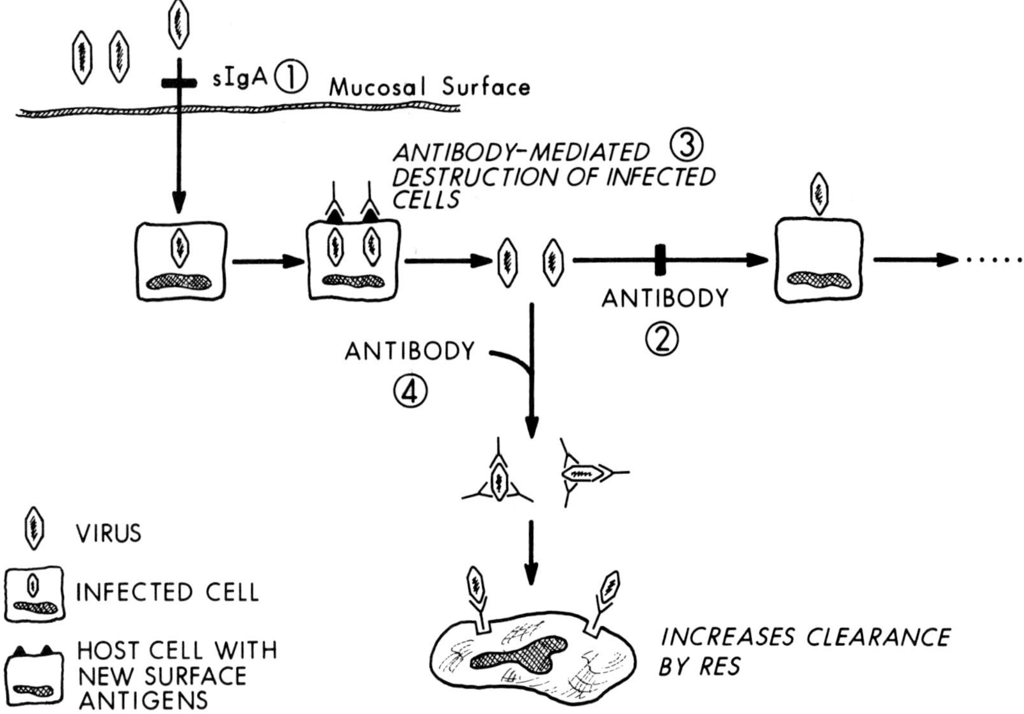

Fig. 11-4. Sites of antibody action in viral infection. (1) Secretory IgA can prevent infection across mucosal surfaces. (2) Antiviral antibody can prevent the spread of the virus and abort the infection. (3) Antibody directed against new cell-surface antigens can lead to cell lysis (either via complement or ADCC). (4) Viral clearance by the RES may be enhanced by the production of viral-antibody complexes.

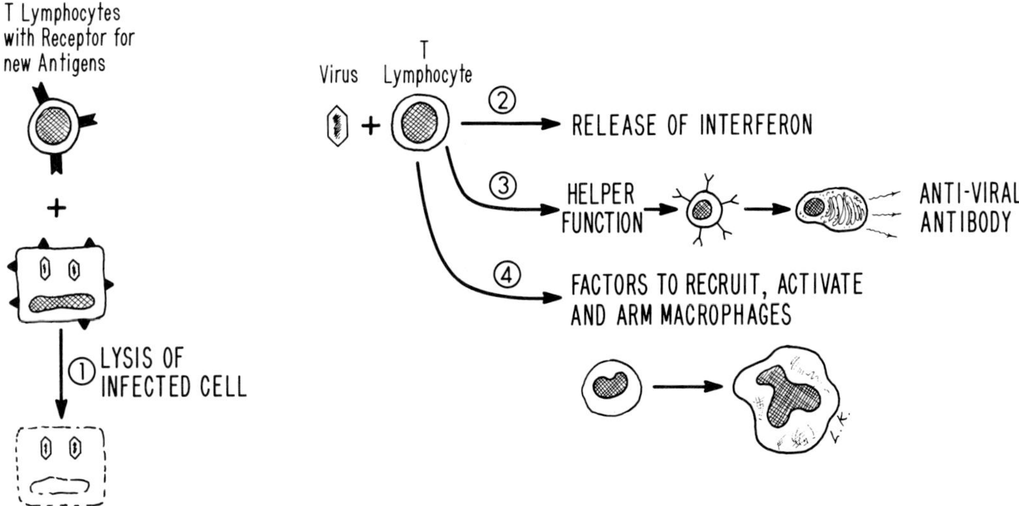

Fig. 11-5. Sites of T-cell action in viral infections. (1) Killer T cells can destroy virally infected cells that express new surface antigens. T cells recognizing the virus can (2) release interferon, (3) serve as helper cells for the production of antiviral antibody, and (4) release lymphokines to recruit and activate macrophages.

the host, and may or may not cause clinically evidence disease. Persistent viral infections have been described in both animals and man. Among the human diseases which have either been traced to or are being tentatively considered in terms of a persistent viral infection are subacute sclerosing panencephalitis (SSPE), herpes zoster, herpes simplex, kuru, Creutzfeldt-Jacob syndrome, and others. Among the viruses which may persist without causing any marked pathology are the hepatitis virus, cytomegalovirus and adenovirus.

Why does the immune system fail to eliminate certain viral agents? Many hypotheses have been advanced but no definitive answer is available at present. The human disease SSPE has been the focus of much experimental work attempting to elucidate the immunologic basis of viral persistence. We will therefore use SSPE as a model example for illustrating current ideas about the immunology of persistent infections.

Subacute Sclerosing Panencephalitis

SSPE is a rare, degenerative and fatal disease of the central nervous system that typically presents around ten years of age.[49] It is now believed to result from a persistent infection with the measles virus.[50] Measles antigen is found in cellular inclusions within the brain, and coculture of the brain cells of an affected patient with animal cells has resulted in the recovery of fully infectious virus.[51,52]

Why do most children who contract measles infections have an acute illness while a very few develop a persistent infection culminating in SSPE? A simple genetic predisposition to SSPE probably does not exist since there is one report of SSPE occurring in only one of a pair of identical twins, both of whom had had an acute measles infection at four years of age.[53] The age at which the primary measles infection occurs may play a role in the ultimate susceptibility to SSPE. Thus, over 50 per cent of patients with SSPE have had a clinically apparent measles infection before two years of age.[54]

Several explanations have been offered to account for the ability of the measles virus to persist in certain hosts.

1. Select individuals may be unresponsive to the measles virus.[55] In a high proportion of cases of SSPE, the patients' primary exposure to the virus occurred at a very young age when the immune system may be relatively immature and incapable of a maximal antiviral response. Consistent with this finding is a report that patients with SSPE have diminished cell-mediated immunity against the measles virus.[56] However, this report stands in opposition to others which have demonstrated intact cell-mediated immunity against the virus,[57] including the ability to kill measles-infected cells *in vitro*.[58] In addition, patients with SSPE have high levels of anti-measles antibody in their serum and in the cerebrospinal fluid,[59] and the presence of these antibodies is now often used to confirm the diagnosis of SSPE. Frequently, patients will possess a relatively homogeneous (oligoclonal) IgG spike in the cerebrospinal fluid that has specificity for the measles virus.[60] (In animals, oligoclonal antibody responses can be evoked by hyperimmunizing with a given antigen.[61]) Thus, most evidence indicates that the host immune system can respond against the measles virus and infected cells.

2. The SSPE virus may be an altered form of the measles virus, and might therefore be able to escape an anti-measles immune response.[62] Differences between the SSPE virus and the wild-type measles virus have been noted,[63] including variations in biological activity and susceptibility to measles-neutralizing antibody. However, the immune system in SSPE patients appears to be capable of destroying SSPE-virus-infected cells and reacting against the SSPE virus itself.[64,65]

3. Cells infected with the SSPE virus may not express antigenic targets which

are immunogenic for the host immune system, thus permitting the virus to persist intracellularly. There is little evidence *in vivo* to support this idea although measles-infected cells have been observed *in vitro* to go through periods in which very little antigen is expressed on their surfaces.[66] Cell-surface antigenicity may also be reduced by a process termed *antigenic modulation.*[67] In the presence of antibody against the measles virus, infected cells in culture have been shown to lose their surface antigenicity although they continue to produce infectious virus. Measles antigens continue to be detected in the cytoplasm. It is not known whether antigenic modulation is due simply to the masking of antigenic determinants by the antibody or to the actual loss of surface molecules, nor is it known whether antigenic modulation has any importance *in vivo*.

4. Patients with SSPE have been demonstrated to have blocking factors in their serum. These factors, which may be antigen-antibody complexes, can prevent sensitized lymphocytes from patients with SSPE from killing measles-infected cells *in vitro*.[68]

Although any of these hypotheses could theoretically explain viral persistence, they do not explain why, at some point, clinical deterioration sets in leading invariably to the death of the patient. Conceivably, the host may eventually acquire the capacity to destroy the infected cells, and the massive tissue destruction may therefore be more a result of an immunologically mediated process than a direct consequence of viral infection. This view, however, is purely speculative. In the section entitled The Immunopathogenesis of Viral Lesions, we shall review the role of the immune system in contributing to the pathology of viral infections.

Reactivation of Latent Viral Infections

Immunosuppression may be responsible, at least in part, for the reactivation and dissemination of certain latent persistent viral infections. This appears to be true for herpes zoster. The active disease is generally seen in settings of immunosuppression such as in patients with malignancies or those on immunosuppressive therapy.

It has been suggested that in some instances the immune system may maintain a persistent viral infection in a latent phase. About 20 per cent of people who are infected with herpes simplex virus have recurrent episodes of cutaneous viral lesions associated with the presence of active virus. During the latent periods the virus resides in sensory nerve ganglia.[69] The mouse also harbors herpes simplex virus in its ganglion cells, and there is evidence that antiviral antibody may interact with the surface of herpes-infected cells and maintain the dormancy of the virus.[70] However, there has been no demonstrable correlation betwen immune depression and detectable activity of the virus in man.[71]

THE IMMUNOPATHOGENESIS OF VIRAL LESIONS

A number of viruses can invade host cells and replicate while causing little or no damage to the infected cells. These viruses might persist indefinitely and in relative harmony with the host but for the intervention of the immune system. The immune response against these otherwise harmless viruses may be entirely responsible for the pathology of these infections. The two major ways in which the immune response against viral antigens can cause tissue damage are immune complex deposition[72] and the destruction of antigenically altered host cells.

The devastating potential for host destruction of the immune response to a viral infection has been convincingly demonstrated in mice infected with lymphocytic choriomeningitis (LCM) virus (Fig. 11-6).[73] When adult mice are injected intracerebrally with the LCM

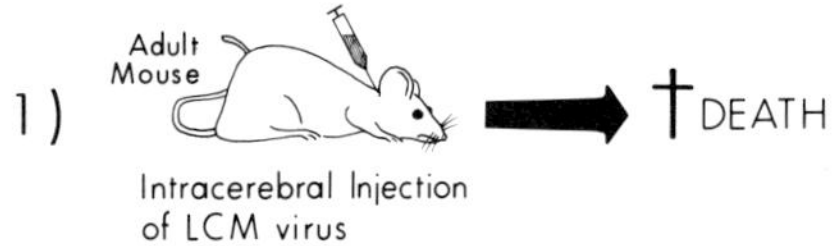

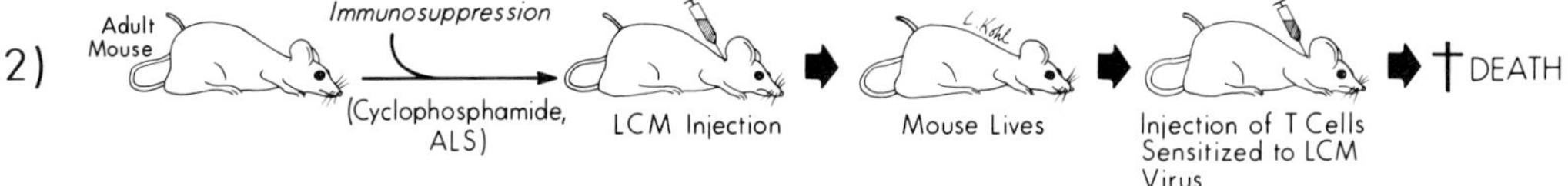

Fig. 11-6. Infection with LCM virus in the mouse. (1) An adult mouse infected intracerebrally with LCM virus dies within one week. (2) If that mouse is first immunosuppressed, the virus is relatively harmless. The reintroduction of sensitized lymphocytes leads to rapid death of the host.

virus, they develop an acute local infection that leads to death within one week. If the animals are first immunosuppressed with, for example, antilymphocyte serum or cyclophosphamide, no disease results although a persistent infection is established.[74,75] If these immunosuppressed and chronically infected animals are then given T cells sensitized to the LCM virus, a fatal central nervous system disease rapidly develops.[76] The cytotoxic T cells, in attempting to rid the host of a harmless viral infection, succeed only in destroying the infected brain cells and, in the process, destroying the host as well.

In humans, the hepatitis B virus provides an excellent example of a relatively benign virus provoking a destructive immune response. The clinical spectrum of this illness ranges from an inapparent infection to rare cases of acute, fatal, total destruction of the liver. The majority of patients develop an acute, self-limiting infection with a varying degree of hepatic damage. These infections may last from weeks to months, and eventually most patients recover as the virus is eliminated from the body. However, in approximately 15 per cent of these patients, the virus is not eliminated and a persistent infection results. Many of these patients maintain a mild to minimal hepatitis referred to as *chronic persistent hepatitis*. A lesser percentage of all patients with hepatitis develop the more destructive *chronic active hepatitis*.

The hepatitis B virus (HBV) is a double-stranded DNA virus. The DNA is contained within a protein inner core which, in turn, is surrounded by a complex coat. The surface of the core contains the antigen referred to as "hepatitis B core antigen" or "HBc-antigen."[77] The viral coat contains a protein antigen designated "HBs-antigen" also called Australia antigen or HAA) which can exist in any one of several serologic subtypes (Fig. 11-7).[78] HBc-antigen can be found in the nucleus of infected hepatocytes, and HBs-antigen can be detected in the cytoplasm and on the surface of infected cells.[79] The HBs-antigen is produced in great quantities and can be detected in the serum of in-

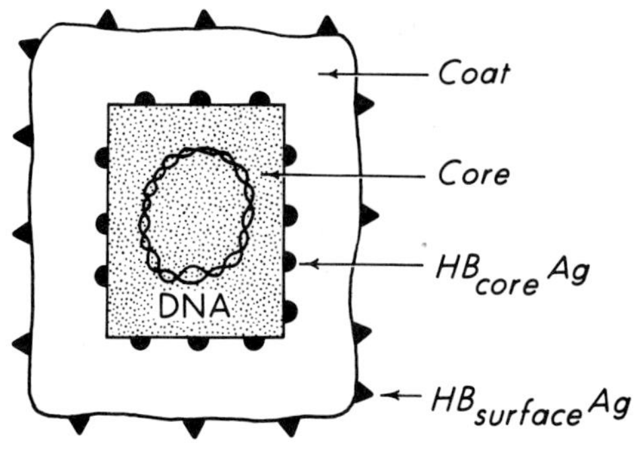

Fig. 11-7. Schematic rendering of the hepatitis B virus showing the localization of the HBs- and HBc-antigens.

fected patients.[80] One can measure antibody production against both antigens, the antibodies against the core antigen usually being detectable earlier in the infection than anti-HBs-antigen antibodies.[18] A third antigen "e", still poorly localized, seems to be closely related to infectivity.

The clinical manifestations of hepatitis B infections can be considered under two broad categories: systemic disease and liver involvement. Systemic involvement is not uncommon, and up to 25 per cent of patients experience an acute serum sickness type of illness as a prodrome several weeks before the onset of clinical hepatitis.[82] Symptoms are referable to involvement of the joints, skin, arterioles and renal glomeruli. The underlying cause of these systemic manifestations is an immune complex disease. Circulating complexes of antibody and HBs-antigen can be detected[83] and are able to fix complement.[84] In patients who develop a severe vasculitis, HBs-antigen, immunoglobulin and C3 can be detected in the walls of damaged blood vessels.[85] Thus, in this group of patients, there is evidence that the immune system may contribute to the pathologic involvement and destruction of tissues throughout the body.

Hepatic destruction in HBV infections does not appear to be caused by the virus which appears to exist in relative equilibrium with the host hepatocytes. Rather, parenchymal damage may be caused by the immune response to antigenically altered infected liver cells and/or the virus itself.

The two major HBV-associated antigens, HBs and HBc, are both targets of immune reactivity, but it is still controversial as to which is implicated in hepatic destruction. Some suggest that the HBs antigen is primarily involved since it appears to be more intimately associated with the hepatocyte cell surface where it would be an accessible target for the immune system.[86] On the other hand, the anti-HBc-antigen antibody response is often more closely correlated with the onset of clinical hepatitis; the anti-HBs-antigen antibody titers may not rise until after clinical evidence of active hepatic destruction has subsided (Fig. 11-8).[87] One further possibility is that *auto*reactivity against the host hepatocyte is stimulated in patients infected with HBV,[88] but there is little data pertaining to this point.

The relative importance of antibody-mediated liver destruction and cell-mediated destruction is presently unclear,[89] and it is entirely possible that both are involved. One aspect of antibody-dependent tissue damage that has recently been receiving attention is the observation that immune complexes and complement are deposited in the liver.[90] However, the histologic picture of the hepatic lesions is most consistent with a

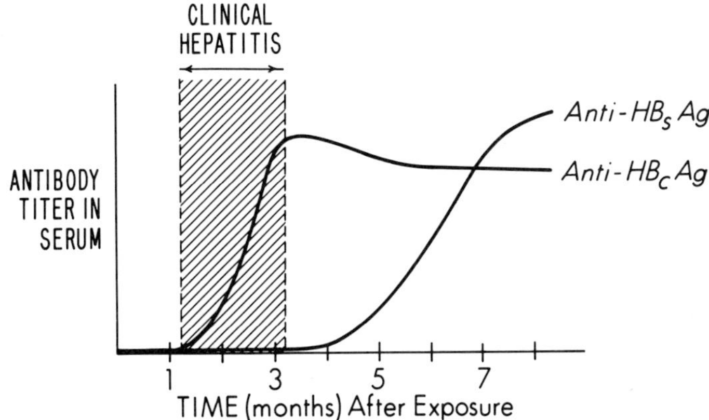

Fig. 11-8. Time course of antibody production during an infection with hepatitis B. Note that the production of anti-HBc is more closely correlated with the time course of clinical illness than is production of anti-HBs antibody. (Adapted from Hoofnagle, J. H., Gerety, R. J., and Barker, L. F.: Antibody to hepatitis B core antigen. Am. J. Med. Sci., *270*:179, 1975.)

cell-mediated response[87] and there is some evidence that depressed cell-mediated immunity may diminish hepatic destruction.[91,92] In one experiment, the passive transfer of lymphocytes from patients who had recovered from HBV infections to chronic HBV carriers resulted in a transient increase in the level of hepatic destruction in the recipients.[93]

Investigators have attempted to correlate the *in vitro* lymphocyte response to the HBs-antigen with the clinical course of affected patients. The results have led to a speculative model that attempts to relate the level of cell-mediated immunity to the outcome of the HBV infection.[94-96] Such a model is based upon the following observations: (1) asymptomatic carriers usually do not give evidence of cell-mediated immunity against the HBs-antigen. (2) Patients with chronic persistent hepatitis show little or no cell-mediated immunity against the HBs-antigen. (3) Patients with chronic active hepatitis often exhibit HBs-antigen sensitization. (4) Almost all patients with acute and self-limited infections exhibit cell-mediated immunity against the HBs-antigen. The results from one study suggest that the lymphocytes of this last group of patients show a consistently higher level of response than do the lymphocytes from patients with chronic active hepatitis.

The interpretation of this data is based on the hypothesis that lymphocyte reactivity against the HBs-antigen may also be directed against HBV-infected hepatocytes. It is proposed that patients whose lymphocytes are very active against the infected cells will abort the infection after an acute phase of hepatic destruction. At the other end of the spectrum are those asymptomatic individuals who mount no detectable response against the infected cells and continue to harbor the virus without clinical difficulty. Chronic active hepatitis seems to fall between these two groups and may represent a situation in which the immune response is weak enough to permit a persistent infection but potent enough to destroy a large number of infected cells. The data on chronic persistent hepatitis is not adequate to allow us to place it within this scheme.

In summary, although it is likely that the tissue destruction and the extrahepatic manifestations of HBV infections are due to the damaging effects of the immune response, the details of this process are still poorly understood.

THE EFFECT OF VIRUSES ON THE IMMUNE SYSTEM

Thus far we have looked at the effect that the immune system has upon the virus and upon the host. A viral infection can in turn have a marked effect upon the immune system.[97,98]

Viral-Induced Lymphopenia

Many viral infections are associated with lymphopenia at some point during the illness. Although the degree of lymphocyte depletion can be severe, the lymphopenia is usually transient. The T-cell "activated" rosette numbers in particular are depressed, and this finding may correlate with some of the T-cell functional defects observed during viral illnesses.[99]

There are two possible explanations for the lymphopenia associated with viral infections:

1. *Lymphocyte Destruction.* This could result from direct viral infection of the lymphocytes.[22] A second possible mechanism for viral-induced lymphocyte destruction has been suggested by the detection of antilymphocyte autoantibodies in a number of patients with a viral-associated lymphopenia.[100] These antibodies are toxic to the patients' lymphocytes *in vitro* in the presence of complement, but their importance *in vivo* remains to be determined.

2. *Lymphocyte Diversion.* Alternatively, the lymphocytes of a virus-infected lymphopenic patient may not be subjected to increased destruction, but rather may be diverted from their normal circulatory routes by the presence of the virus, thereby producing only an apparent depletion of cells. Suggestive evidence can be found in some animal systems but is lacking in man.[101] Changes in the lymphocyte surface induced by the virus have been postulated as the cause of this phenomenon.[102]

Viral Effects on Humoral Immunity

In general, viral infections have not been found to have significant effects on the humoral response in man. In animals, the ability to mount a specific antibody response is often depressed during a viral infection. In one experiment employing the measles virus, the source of the humoral hyporesponsiveness appeared to be depressed T-cell helper function and not a direct depression of hapten-specific B cells.[103]

Infection with certain viruses induces a generalized increase in serum immunoglobulin levels in both animals and man. In man, the best-studied example is the hypergammaglobulinemia accompanying infectious mononucleosis.[104]

Viral Effects on Cell-Mediated Immunity

The frequent transient depression of cell-mediated immunity accompanying viral infections was first recognized with the observation of the loss of tuberculin sensitivity during the acute stage of measles infections.[105] A number of *in vitro* indices of abnormal cell-mediated immunity correlate with the frequent loss of skin test delayed hypersensitivity. Thus, along with cutaneous anergy,[106] one often finds diminished *in vitro* responsiveness of T cells to mitogens, allogeneic cells and antigens.[107] Lymphopenia alone probably cannot fully account for the depressed T-cell function, and the precise mechanisms for the cellular hyporeactivity during viral infections are not known. Two interesting possibilities have been offered:

1. Macrophages infected with polio virus cannot cooperate adequately with lymphocytes in the response to T-cell mitogens.[108] Macrophage dysfunction could compromise T-cell function *in vivo*, but there is no evidence for this in man.

2. There is evidence that certain viruses can stimulate suppressor-cell activity.[109] Also of interest is the observation that interferon can suppress both humoral and cell-mediated responses *in vitro*.[110-114] Whether these findings are applicable to the *in vivo* immunosuppression of virally infected patients remains to be determined.

Viral Infections and Autoimmunity

A number of viral infections are associated with the transient production of autoantibodies. The ways in which a virus could potentially induce autoreactivity have been discussed in Chapter 8.

IMMUNOPROPHYLAXIS[115,116]

Jenner's use of a cowpox vaccine to immunize individuals against smallpox was perhaps the very first experiment in clinical immunology. Vaccines have been successfully used for smallpox, yellow fever, polio, measles, rubella, mumps, rabies and influenza. Most successful vaccines employ live attenuated viral strains. These include the vaccines against all the diseases mentioned above with the exception of rabies and influenza. Inactivated viruses are used for these two. At present, the possibility of using viral antigens alone as a potentially important alternative to live vaccines is being studied.[117]

The life cycle of the virus in question becomes an important consideration in developing a vaccine. Two basic patterns of infectivity are recognized as being important determinants of vaccination protocols: (1) some viruses replicate at the portal of entry and cause *local disease*. These are primarily respiratory- and gastrointestinal-associated infections, and include viruses such as the respiratory parainfluenza virus, rhinovirus and respiratory syncytial virus. (2) Other viral infections are characterized by a viremia with dissemination to one or several target organs where the primary disease occurs. Examples of this second type of virus are the measles virus and polio virus.

To prevent local infections, a vaccine must stimulate local antiviral immunity. Several studies have shown that local application of a vaccine to the site of natural viral infection can induce local protection, while systemic vaccination may fail to provide local immunity. In addition, live vaccines appear to be superior in affording site-specific immunity compared to inactivated viruses or viral antigens.[118,119]

Viruses that cause disease via dissemination to target organs can be effectively dealt with by vaccines which induce systemic immunity. The stimulation of circulating humoral immunity appears to be sufficient to prevent many disseminated viral diseases. This has been shown, for example, with inactivated polio virus vaccines. However, this particular vaccine will not stimulate local secretory immunity and thus will not prevent the virus from infecting the gastrointestinal tract and will not eradicate the virus from the community. The administration of live, attenuated polio virus can induce both systemic and local immunity and will therefore protect against both disease and infection.

Most live attenuated vaccines will convey long-term immunity to the host. Inactivated vaccines are generally less successful in this regard. For example, inactivated measles vaccine will stimulate anti-measles immunity and appreciable titers of anti-measles antibody. However, after several years, these antibodies are no longer detectable and the host is again susceptible to viral infection. Measles infection in these individuals can be very severe, even though the host immune system can mount a secondary anamnestic response to the measles virus.

THE IMMUNOLOGY OF BACTERIAL INFECTIONS

There are two general types of bacterial infections, those in which the infecting organisms primarily remain outside the host cells (extracellular infections) and those in which the invading bacteria spend much of their time within the cells (intracellular infections). The immune system is important in fighting both types, but the relative importance of the various limbs of the immune and inflammatory systems is very different for the two classes of bacterial infections.

EXTRACELLULAR BACTERIAL INFECTIONS

The Anti-bacterial Effect of Antibody

The humoral limb of the immune system is critical in the defense against extracellular bacterial infections, which include most of the commonly encountered organisms such as the staphylococcus, streptococcus, pneumococcus, *E. coli*, and so on. Thus, patients with X-linked agammaglobulinemia, who can have severely compromised humoral immunity with intact cell-mediated immunity, are highly susceptible to bacterial infections, especially by encapsulated organisms. The passive transfer of immunoglobulin to these patients restores much of their antibacterial immune competence.

There are three major ways in which antibody helps to eliminate extracellular bacterial infections (Fig. 11-9):

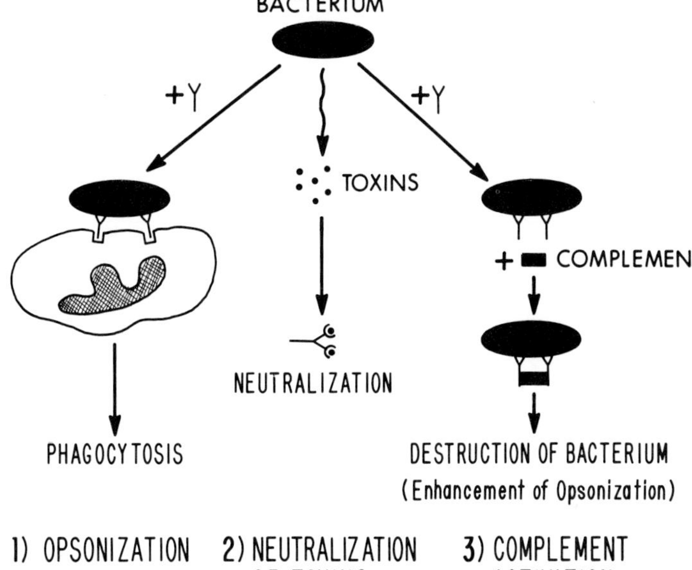

Fig. 11-9. Role of antibody in bacterial infections. (1) Opsonization. (2) Neutralization of toxins. (3) Complement activation can lead to bacteriolysis and/or enhancement of opsonization.

Opsonization. Complexes of IgG and bacteria adhere to the Fc receptors on phagocytic cells and are readily ingested. Phagocytosis without prior opsonization is much less efficient.

Neutralization of Toxins. Many bacterial pathogens cause severe damage to the host by the release of toxic substances into the host milieu. Well-known examples include the tetanus and diphtheria toxins. These toxins can further encourage infection by creating areas of tissue necrosis which are favorable to bacterial growth. Antibodies against bacterial toxins can effectively neutralize their toxic potential and thus prevent host tissue destruction and help to contain the infection.

Complement Activation. Antibody can fix complement to the surface of bacteria. There is evidence that the presence of C3 on the bacterial surface may be important for the efficient opsonization of many bacteria.[120] Fixation of the terminal complement components may lead to the lysis of the bacteria of several species.[121] For example, complement may attack the outer lipoprotein wall of *E. coli*,[122] allowing serum lysozyme to destroy the inner mucopeptide which may in turn give complement access to the cell membrane itself. Complement activation also leads to the release of complement-derived chemotactic factors which attract phagocytes to the site of reaction where they can ingest the infectious agents.

A number of bacteria and bacterial products, notably the polysaccharide endotoxins, can activate complement via the properdin pathway without the intervention of antibody.[123] The properdin pathway may provide an important first line of defense against bacterial infection.

Defective Granulocyte Function in Pyogenic Infections

It should be apparent from the brief review above that much of the antibacterial effect of antibody is dependent upon the presence of a population of competent phagocytic cells. The phagocytosis of opsonized bacterial cells is an essential defense mechanism against extracellular bacterial infections, and the circulating granulocytes are especially important in this regard. There are several syndromes of defective intrinsic granulocyte function associated with recurrent pyogenic infections:

Lazy Leukocyte Syndrome. Several patients have been described in whom the only demonstrable cellular defect is the failure of their leukocytes to respond to normal chemotactic stimuli. Thus, these patients fail to accumulate phagocytes at sites of infection, and at least one patient has been described who presented with recurrent infections. This disorder has been termed the *lazy leukocyte syndrome*.[124]

Chronic Granulomatous Disease (CGD) is a sex-linked or autosomal recessive disorder in which the patient's phagocytes display normal chemotaxis and phagocytosis but are unable to kill certain types of bacteria once they have been ingested. These patients frequently present with severe bacterial infections within the first year of life. The syndrome gets its name from the typical histologic picture of granulomas surrounding leukocytes which have ingested bacteria but have been unable to kill them. There are probably several intracellular bactericidal pathways, and the precise biochemical defect in CGD is not known. It has been proposed that the phagocytes of these patients are unable to generate sufficient bactericidal hydrogen peroxide (H_2O_2), a theory suggested by the finding that bacteria such as lactobacilli which cannot degrade their own H_2O_2 are killed normally following phagocytosis, presumably by the local accumulation of their own H_2O_2.[125] However, it is not unlikely that CGD is simply the end result of a variety of different functional metabolic defects, all giving rise to the identical clinical syndrome.

Myeloperoxidase Deficiency.[126] Several patients have been described who lack neutrophil and monocyte myeloperoxidase, an enzyme with intracellular bactericidal activity. Most of these patients do not have recurrent infections, suggesting that other bactericidal pathways can compensate for this deficiency.

The Chédiak-Higashi Syndrome is a rare, autosomal recessive disorder characterized by oculocutaneous albinism, a greatly increased susceptibility to pyogenic bacterial infections, and the presence of large peroxidase-positive granules in many of the cells of the body.[127] These patients usually die in infancy or childhood, most often from overwhelming infections. The large granules are found in the granulocytic cells, and also in Schwann cells, neurons, vascular endothelium, kidney, fibroblasts and melanocytes. The underlying defect appears to be a generalized abnormality of certain membrane-bound intracellular organelles found within these various cell types. Thus, the abnormal melanosomes in the body's melanocytes are responsible for the oculocutaneous albinism. The large granules in the leukocytes do not interfere with phagocytosis or intracellular metabolism, but do compromise the ability of the cells to kill intracellular bacteria. This is probably the result of a poorly coordinated delivery of bactericidal enzymes from these granules into the phagolysosomes. These cells also display a significantly depressed response to normal chemotactic stimuli.[128,129]

INTRACELLULAR BACTERIAL INFECTIONS

Much more is known—although perhaps less is understood—about the role of the immune system in combating intracellular bacterial infections. Commonly encountered intracellular pathogens include mycobacteria, pasteurella, brucella, *Listeria* and others. Humoral immunity is not of great importance in opposing these infections, and the cellular limb of the immune system, including the T cell and the macrophage, is primarily responsible for host defense.

Acute Infections

Listeria monocytogenes is a small, gram-positive organism that lives as a facultative intracellular parasite. Studies of listeria infection in the mouse have provided important information concerning the role of cell-mediated immunity in acute intracellular bacterial infections. When listeria is injected into a mouse, inflammatory cells rapidly accumulate at the site of injection. The nonspecific infiltrate is dominated first by neutrophils and then by monocytes. The bacteria are rapidly ingested by the mononuclear cells, but continue to multiply within these cells. On their own, the phagocytic macrophages are very inefficient at killing the ingested organisms.[130] The host's ability to eliminate the infection rests with the ability of the T-cell population to "activate" these cells, i.e., turn them into avid phagocytes with potent bactericidal capabilities (Fig. 11-10). T cells are sensitized to listeria antigens about three days after injection of the organism and secrete the lymphokine MAF. MAF provides a nonspecific stimulant which activates the macrophage population against many antigens, not just listeria. Following activation, the macrophages can kill the listeria and the infection is terminated acutely.

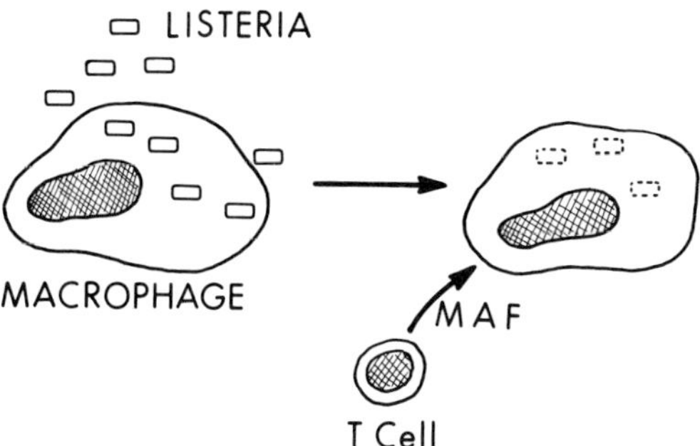

Fig. 11-10. Immune reactivity in listeria infections. Listeria will multiply within macrophages unless the phagocytic cells are activated by sensitized T cells. Activated macrophages kill the ingested organisms with great efficiency.

Chronic Infections

Tuberculosis

Tuberculosis results from infection with the bacterium *Myobacterium tuberculosis*. Although tuberculosis is a relatively common disease, asymptomatic infection with the myobacterium is even more common. In developed countries, the incidence and mortality of mycobacterial infections have declined markedly over the last several decades due to improved living conditions, widescale vaccination programs (notably in Europe) and the introduction of chemotherapy.

The primary infection usually is the result of inhalation of the organism followed by rapid seeding of the lungs. Once the infection is established, the bacteria multiply and spread, first via the lymphatics and then hematogenously, so that dissemination occurs quickly. The primary infection is usually not clinically apparent. Within a few weeks of infection, the host has mounted an immune response against the organism and the infection is contained. Occasionally the infection cannot be controlled by the host, particularly in infants whose immature defense systems make them especially susceptible to a devastating, widespread and progressive disease.

It is important to note that in the healthy individual a successful response is said only to *contain* the infection. This is because most evidence indicates that *primary infections are not completely aborted.* The bacteria are probably never totally eliminated from the body; instead, a prolonged phase of latency without any noticeable clinical effects begins. The latent infection may persist asymptomatically throughout the remainder of a person's life. However, under certain conditions, the disease may reactivate (see below).

The natural history of the disease that we have outlined thus far reflects a complex relationship between the mycobacterium and the host defense mechanisms. Granulocytes and macrophages nonspecifically accumulate at the site of the initial infection (usually the lungs). The mycobacteria are quickly ingested by these phagocytes and begin to replicate. Infected macrophages look different than their normal counterparts and have been termed *epithelioid cells*. The infected macrophages are inefficient at killing the organisms and the bacteria multiply and spread to other macrophages. The inefficiency of bacteriolysis is probably due both to the poor lytic capacity of the unactivated macrophages and the high intrinsic resistance of the mycobacteria to normal lytic mechanisms. The typical pathologic lesion is the *granuloma*, the result of an intense inflammatory response, and containing many epithelioid cells (Fig. 11-11). Granulomas occur wherever the disseminating mycobacteria establish an infectious focus.

By three to four weeks following infection, the host immune system has become optimally sensitized to the mycobacteria. Antimycobacterial antibodies can be detected but there is no evidence that these play any role in the defense against the organism. The sensitized T cells are primarily responsible for acquired immunity to the infection. Thus sensitized animals will resist infection by a second challenge of mycobacteria, and this resistance can be transferred to unsensitized animals only with sensitized T cells.[131]

Sensitized T cells are instrumental in containing the primary infection. In some animal studies, the course of infection has been divided into three phases (Fig. 11-12):[132]

1. *The Nonimmune Phase.* The

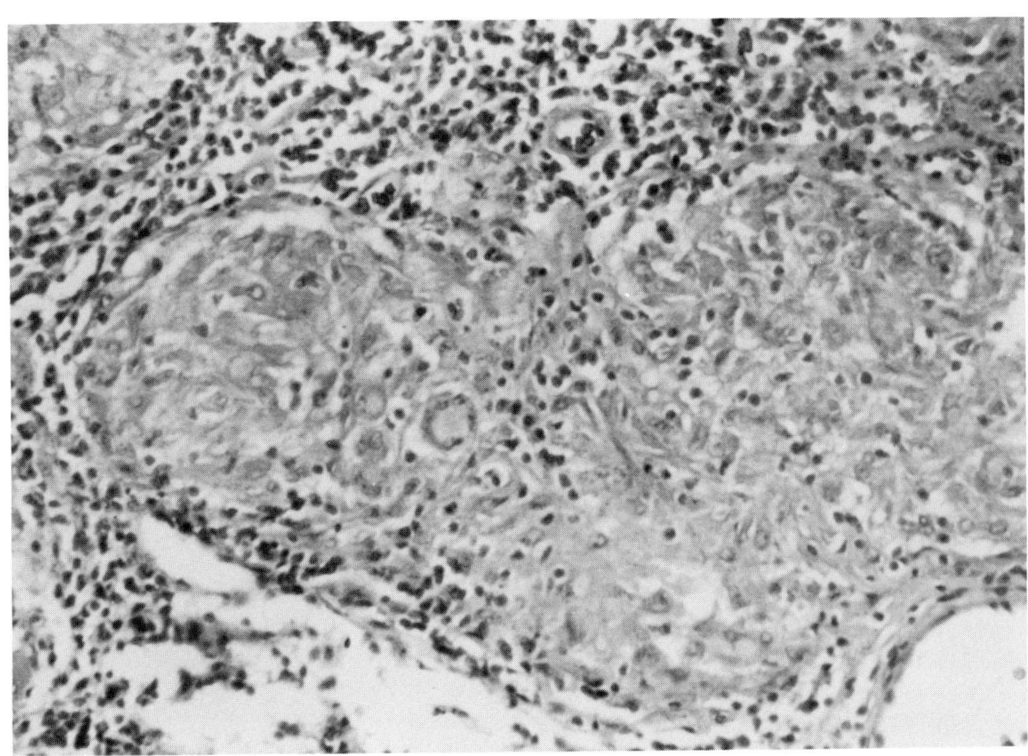

Fig. 11-11. A granuloma containing epithelioid cells and multinucleated giant cells.

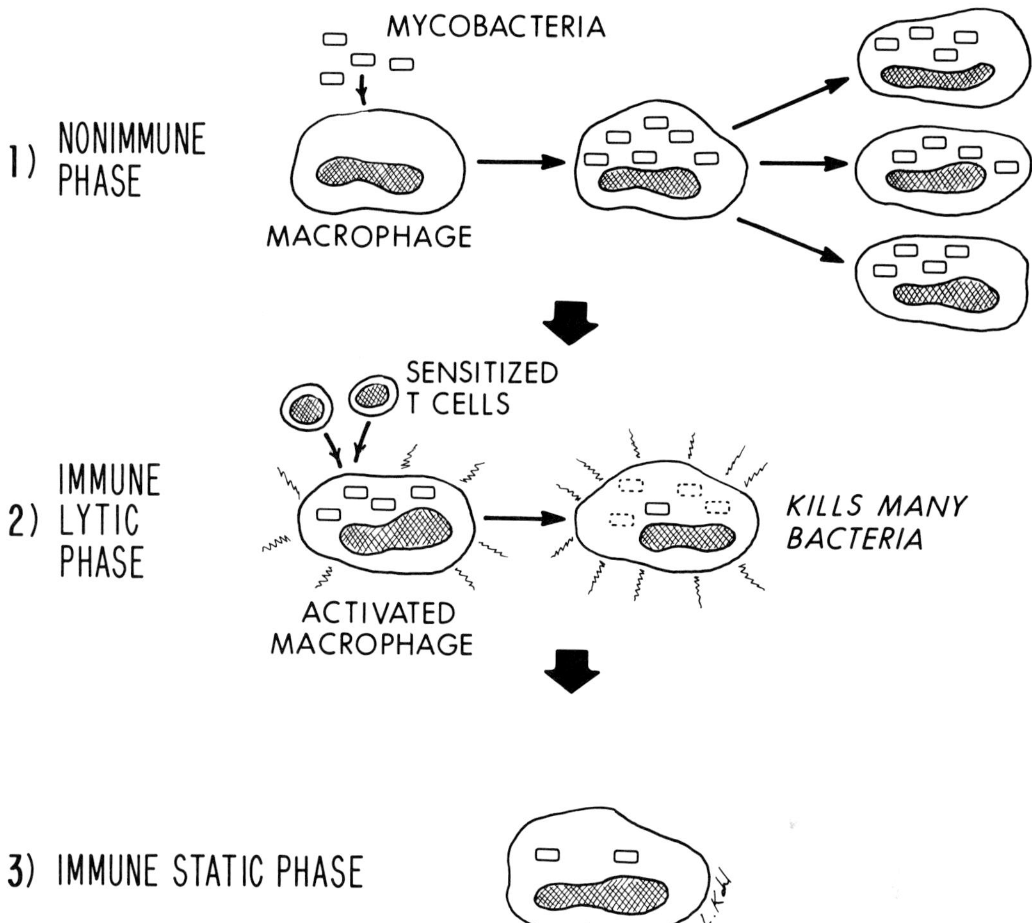

Fig. 11-12. Postulated scheme of three phases of mycobacterial infection. (1) Nonimmune phase; mycobacteria enter and multiply within macrophages and spread to other macrophages. (2) Immune lytic phase: the activation of infected macrophages by sensitized T cells leads to the killing of many of the bacteria. (3) Immune static phase: a steady state is established in which a low number of bacteria remain alive in the sensitized host for an indefinite period of time.

mycobacteria rapidly multiply within macrophages and spread to other macrophages.

2. *The Immune Lytic Phase.* The macrophages are activated by sensitized T cells and acquire a greatly enhanced lytic potential. During this phase many of the mycobacteria are killed by the activated phagocytes. As in the response to listeria, the macrophages are activated nonspecifically by T-cell-derived factors, but there is also evidence suggestive of a specific component to the acquired macrophage resistance to mycobacteria.[133-135] The importance of this latter process remains to be determined.

3. *The Immune Static Phase.* A steady state is finally reached in which a relatively constant number of organisms remain viable within infected macrophages. This state corresponds to the latent phase described above. The macrophages appear to be bacteriostatic, preventing the growth of the bacteria without being able to abort the infection. We do not know why the infection cannot be eliminated;

in other intracellular infections, for example, *Bordetella pertussis*, this third, bacteriostatic, phase is comparatively short and is followed by a second lytic phase which destroys the infection.[136]

Active tuberculosis represents the reactivation of primary endogenous foci of infection. The mycobacteria appear to survive best in areas of high oxygen tension such as the apices of the lungs, the bones and the kidneys, and reactivation commonly occurs in these loci. It has long been believed that reactivation occurs in the setting of a weakened immune system, for example, due to advancing age, steroid therapy, debilitating disease, and so on.[137] Active tuberculosis can, in turn, depress the immune system further. A majority of untreated patients with active tuberculosis cannot be sensitized to the skin test antigen DNCB, reflecting a depression in cell-mediated immunity.[138] It has been estimated that up to 1 per cent of patients with active tuberculosis are totally anergic by all measurable criteria, and no delayed hypersensitivity can be elicited.[139]

The Tuberculin Skin Test. T-cell sensitization to mycobacteria is most commonly demonstrated by the ability to elicit a cutaneous delayed hypersensitivity reaction to mycobacterial antigens. Several different preparations of skin test antigens have been developed; the two most widely used are old tuberculin (OT) and purified protein derivative (PPD). Once a person has been infected with *Mycobacterium tuberculosis*, that individual will display a positive skin reaction to these antigens. This cutaneous reactivity is long-lasting, often for the lifetime of the individual, and is probably the result of the persistence of immunologic memory and the continued presence of the organism in the host.[140] Tuberculin testing is an excellent measure of whether or not a person has ever been exposed to a mycobacterial infection.

Does delayed hypersensitivity to tuberculoprotein, as measured by positive cutaneous reactivity, necessarily indicate immunity to infection? Despite the frequent coincidence of these two findings, the answer is no.[134] Several findings have led to the realization that tuberculin skin test reactivity and acquired immunity may represent sensitization to separate antigenic determinants:

1. Animals can be desensitized to tuberculin so that they become negative to the skin test and yet retain their immunity.[141]
2. Certain antigens can be given which will convey tuberculin delayed hypersensitivity without conferring immunity to infection in people never previously exposed to mycobacteria.[142,143]
3. Antigens of the mycobacteria can be used to induce specific acquired immunity to tuberculosis without producing evidence of tuberculin delayed hypersensitivity.[144]

Thus, although tuberculin reactivity and immunity most commonly go hand in hand, they do not necessarily do so, and a positive skin test should be used only as evidence of infection with *Mycobacterium tuberculosis* or other related mycobacteria and not as an absolute assurance of immunity.

There is a second limitation to the tuberculin skin test. Since patients with active tuberculosis often have depressed cellular immunity, the tuberculin skin test can be falsely negative. False negative skin tests are seen most commonly in severe infections. As the patient is treated with chemotherapeutic agents, T-cell responsiveness will return and tuberculin reactivity will become positive again. False negative tuberculin tests may also occur in various states of immune suppression such as lymphoreticular malignancies, steroid therapy and viral infections. Thus, a negative tuberculin skin test does not rule out the presence of active tuberculosis.

Immunoprophylaxis. A live vaccine of an attenuated mycobacterial strain has been widely used to prevent mycobacterial infection and tuberculosis. This strain is called Bacillus Calmette-Guerin, or BCG,[145] and has been remarkably effective in conveying immunity to *Mycobacterium tuberculosis*. Recipients of the vaccine almost always display positive skin reactivity to tuberculin antigens. Unlike *Mycobacterium tuberculosis* this organism is eventually eliminated from the body and the skin reactivity may be lost with time. Reconversion to tuberculin negativity is not indicative of a loss of immunity; the protection afforded by the vaccine persists.

Leprosy

Although uncommon in the United States, millions of people throughout the world suffer from infection by *Mycobacterium leprae*. This organism is an intracellular parasite which grows primarily in macrophages and the cells of the reticuloendothelial system, much like *Mycobacterium tuberculosis.* A slow, chronic infection is established and the host is unable to eradicate the infection. All indications are that host resistance to *Mycobacterium leprae* is similar to that against *Mycobacterium tuberculosis*.

There are several clinical forms of leprosy, two or which are the best characterized and probably represent the two ends of the clinical spectrum of leprosy. *Tuberculoid leprosy* is characterized by variable skin involvement resembling the granulomatous cutaneous lesions that may be seen in tuberculosis. Most patients have scattered skin lesions which cause little morbidity. These are granulomatous lesions with epithelioid cells, macrophages and many lymphocytes. The number of intracellular stainable organisms is low and often none may be seen. These granulomatous lesions destroy local nerves; peripheral neurologic deficits are the greatest source of morbidity in this otherwise relatively less severe form of the disease.

Lepromatous leprosy is a more destructive disease. The typical lesion is also a granuloma, but there are few lymphocytes present and many stainable intracellular organisms.[146]

The differences between these two forms of leprosy probably reflect different degrees of host resistance. T-cell reactivity is measured by a delayed hypersensitivity response to a preparation of *Mycobacterium leprae* called *lepromin*.[147] Lepromin reactivity is not as well correlated with exposure to the etiologic agent as tuberculin reactivity is with exposure to *Mycobacterium tuberculosis*. False positives are not uncommon.

Lepromin reactivity does correspond reasonably well with immunity against leprosy. Exposed individuals who are lepromin-negative appear to have a higher susceptibility to the disease than individuals who are lepromin-positive.[148] Virtually all persons who have tuberculoid leprosy are lepromin-positive, while those with the severe lepromatous form do not react. It appears that patients who develop lepromatous leprosy have both a generalized depression of immune function as well as a specific unresponsiveness to the mycobacterium out of proportion to the more general immunosuppression.[149,150]

In leprosy, immunosuppression affecting primarily cell-mediated immunity has been well documented[151] and includes: (1) decreased delayed hypersensitivity to a variety of skin test antigens;[152,153] (2) diminished ability to reject skin allografts;[154] (3) diminished *in vitro* responsiveness to mitogens and specific antigens;[155] and (4) T-cell depletion in the lymph nodes and circulation. The severity of T-cell hyporesponsiveness has been correlated with the severity of the infection.[156]

Antibody production against *Mycobacterium leprae* can be demonstrated in approximately 95 per cent of patients, but there is no evidence that this plays any role in the course of the disease. Some patients have a polyclonal hypergammaglobulinemia which may include the production of several types of autoantibodies.[157,158]

Treatment. Transfer factor derived from people with demonstrable lepromin delayed hypersensitivity has been given to lepromin-negative lepromatous patients with successful transient conversion to lepromin positivity but without obvious clinical improvement.[159] Allogeneic leukocytes have been given in repeated transfusions to lepromin-negative patients with leprosy. These infusions can be shown to correct many of the immunologic abnormalities with dramatic clinical improvement.[151] The mechanism by which these transfusions produce such marked improvement is not known.

Sarcoidosis

Sarcoidosis is a systemic disease characterized by granulomatous lesions that may occur in almost any organ of the body.[160] Because the granulomatous lesions can often resemble the lesions seen in many fungal and myocobacterial infections, sarcoidosis has long been felt to be an infectious disease. However, no organism has ever been definitively associated with the disease, and none of Koch's postulates have been fulfilled. At present the etiology of sarcoidosis remains unknown. We have chosen to discuss it here because of its similarity to these other infectious processes.

Immune dysfunction is frequently found in patients with sarcoidosis.

T-Cell Function. Decreased delayed hypersensitivity to a variety of commonly encountered antigens can be demonstrated. About two thirds of patients display cutaneous anergy. Attempts to sensitize the patients to new test antigens such as keyhole-limpet hemocyanin (KLH) and DNCB are also often unsuccessful.[161]

There have been reports of diminished numbers of circulating cells capable of forming spontaneous sheep erythrocyte rosettes.[162]

The patients' lymphocytes exhibit a decreased responsiveness to mitogens *in vitro* which parallels the severity of the disease.[163,164]

B-Cell Function. B-cell function is considered to be hyperactive in the majority of patients and is reflected in a generalized hypergammaglobulinemia and high circulating antibody titers to a wide range of specific antigens.[165-167]

The etiologic basis for these findings has not been established. It has been suggested that these patients are in a state of chronic antigenic stimulation which induces a high level of lymphocyte activity. This hypothesis would explain the hypergammaglobulinemia as well as the otherwise perplexing finding that the lymphocytes from affected patients display a high spontaneous rate of DNA synthesis *in vitro*.[168] The associated anergy might be due to a nonspecific suppression like that accompanying many viral infections. This is all highly conjectural and is predicated upon the existence of an antigen (or antigens) to which the patient is highly sensitive.

Some evidence suggests that such an antigen may exist. When the material taken from a sarcoidosis lymph node is injected intradermally into an affected patient, a sarcoid-like granuloma often develops at the injection site. This test is called the *Kveim test*. A more recent modification, called the *Kveim S test*, uses an injection of splenic tissue that is involved in the disease process. The Kveim S test has been reported to be positive in 80 per cent of patients, including many otherwise anergic patients.[160] False positive reactions are rare.

There are several reasons to believe that reaction to the Kveim reagent involves an immunologic response to an antigen or group of antigens to which the patient is highly sensitive. Passive transfer of Kveim reactivity can be accomplished using the leukocytes of some Kveim-positive individuals.[169] In addition, if the lymphocytes from a patient with sarcoidosis are stimulated *in vitro* with Kveim reagent they will respond with the production of MIF. Cells taken from individuals without sarcoidosis do not exhibit such reactivity.[170] However, we cannot be sure that the sarcoid granuloma does represent an antigen-specific immune response. The Kveim reaction evolves over four to six weeks and therefore its time course as well as the histology of the lesion are quite unlike a typical cutaneous delayed hypersensitivity reaction. Clearly, the key to understanding sarcoidosis will be the isolation of a specific antigen and/or etiologic agent.

THE IMMUNOLOGY OF FUNGAL INFECTIONS

The mechanisms of immunologic resistance to fungal infections are not well understood. Fungal infections tend to be chronic, and the ability of the host to rid itself of the infection, maintain a long-term benign relationship with the organism, or succumb to a progressive infection undoubtedly depends upon a great number of factors, many of which have not been carefully studied. The increased incidence of fungal infections in patients with T-cell deficiency states suggests a primary role for cell-mediated immunity. Disseminated fungal infections are often associated with a depression of T-cell function, but it is unclear whether this is cause or effect, that is, whether diminished cellular immunity is permissive of dissemination or a result of fungal spread. Recently, hyperactive suppressor T cells have been implicated in the T-cell immunosuppression in several patients with various mycotic infections.[171]

In this section we shall briefly examine a few types of fungal infections, and then focus on the various immunologic methods available for diagnosing fungal infections.

HISTOPLASMOSIS

The relationship between *Histoplasma capsulatum* and the infected host is very similar to the host-parasite relationship of *Mycobacterium tuberculosis* infections. Initial infection occurs via inhalation, and the organism is deposited throughout the lungs. The fungus is ingested by the cells of the reticuloendothelial system where it dwells intracellularly and establishes a chronic infection. Even benign primary infections are associated with fungal spread throughout the body. Most often these are associated with transient mild respiratory and systemic symptoms. In some individuals, especially the very young and the very old, the primary infection may produce a fulminant disseminated disease with resultant hepatosplenomegaly and lymphadenopathy. Involvement of isolated organs can produce Addison's disease, meningitis and endocarditis. Ulcers may form on the body's mucosal surfaces.[172,173]

As in tuberculosis, the otherwise healthy individual with an intact immune system is able to contain the infection within about two weeks after exposure, concomitant with the development of cell-mediated immunity. Sensitization to the organism can be detected by the development of positive cutaneous delayed hypersensitivity against an antigenic extract of the mycelial phase of the fungus termed *histoplasmin*.[174] Nearly all patients show positive reactivity within two weeks of initial exposure but the histoplasmin skin test may become negative in disseminated infections and other serious illnesses that suppress the immune system.

Antifungal antibodies may not become apparent until several weeks after delayed hypersensitivity has developed, and there is no evidence that they affect the course of the infection. In fact, high titers of antibody are often seen with severe infection and have been associated with increased mortality.

COCCIDIOIDOMYCOSIS

Coccidioidomycosis, like histoplasmosis, can be a benign illness with only influenza-like symptoms, or rarely it can disseminate to involve almost any body tissue. Within three weeks of infection with *Coccidioides immitis*, the immunocompetent host will contain the disease and develop enduring immunity. Cutaneous delayed hypersensitivity to the coccidioidin extract is considered to be evidence of T-cell sensitization.[174a,175] Patients with disseminated disease often have negative coccidioidin skin tests only to develop a positive response following successful antifungal chemotherapy.

Most patients with primary symptomatic nondisseminating disease produce IgM antifungal antibodies by the third week of infection. Complement-fixing IgG antibodies develop later in the course of infection and are rarely detectable at the time when IgM levels have peaked. The titer of complement-fixing antibodies is used as a measure of the severity of infection, and high titers are generally associated with a poor prognosis. By five months after the initial infection only 25 per cent of patients will still have detectable IgM antifungal antibodies.[176]

ASPERGILLOSIS

Aspergillus species can cause several different types of disease depending in part on the type of immune response that is mounted against the fungus.[177] *Aspergillus fumigatus* is the most common etiologic agent. This particular species is ubiquitous and most people are continually exposed to it by inhalation of fungal spores.

Atopic individuals are often hypersensitive to *Aspergillus fumigatus* and develop *allergic aspergillosis* upon inhalation of the spores. In these people, antifungal IgE provides the setting for a local immediate hypersensitivity reaction in the lungs. Atopic individuals may also have *bronchopulmonary aspergillosis* which presents with transitory pulmonary infiltrates that may result in chronic pulmonary fibrosis. These patients have preexisting anti-fungal IgE and circulating levels of antifungal antibodies, which are usually IgG. Inhalation of the spores leads to an immediate hypersensitivity reaction followed by a severe Arthus reaction due to the formation and deposition of non-IgE-containing immune complexes.

Nonatopic individuals may present with any of three different types of aspergillosis. *Extrinsic allergic alveolitis* results from precipitation of immune complexes in the regions of the alveoli. This process also represents an Arthus reaction that manifests itself five to six hours after spore inhalation. The second type of disease is the formation of *aspergillomas* ("fungus balls") resulting from growth of the fungus in damaged areas of the lungs. Lastly, immunosuppressed patients are susceptible to *disseminated systemic aspergillosis*.

CANDIDIASIS

Infection with *Candida albicans* can range from an acute, localized disease to a chronic, persistent, disseminated illness. *Candida* is an opportunistic organism and normally exists in a stable relationship with the host as part of the normal flora of the gastrointestinal tract. The most common type of infection is an acute, self-limited process confined to the oral or vaginal mucous membranes. These local infections are often preceded by local abrasions or an altered nutritive and chemical milieu. There is no evidence of immunosuppression in these patients.

Disseminated infection only occurs when the host immune defenses are compromised. Chronic mucocutaneous candidiasis (CMC), usually seen in early childhood, is marked by chronic *Candida* infection of the skin, nails and mucous membranes. The infection is superficial, and fungi are readily seen in the keratinized layer of the epidermis. The dermis usually contains a marked infiltrate dominated by lymphocytes and plasma cells.

CMC almost always accompanies a primary immunodeficiency disease in which T-cell function is depressed, such as DiGeorge's syndrome, Nezelof's syndrome or severe combined immunodeficiency.[177a] These patients usually die young, although bacterial and viral infections and not *Candida* are responsible for their death. In the absence of an underlying primary immunodeficiency disease, the natural history of CMC has not been well defined other than by the observation that the course is chronic, often lasting for decades. Many of these patients will develop a severe endocrinopathy late in their course. Most often this takes the form of polyglandular failure with associated hypothyroidism, hypoparathyroidism and Addison's disease. The association between CMC and polyglandular failure is intriguing because of the probable autoimmune etiology of the latter entity (see Chap. 15).

Most patients with CMC have an intact humoral immune system and will produce anti-*Candida* antibodies. T-cell abnormalities, however, are quite common although not universally present.[178] Some patients display cutaneous anergy to all skin test antigens including the *Candida* antigens. Their lymphocytes will not produce MIF in response to antigen exposure *in vitro*, although they can be stimulated to undergo blast transformation. Another group of patients exhibits cutaneous anergy to *Candida* but not to certain other antigens. Their lymphocytes may have any of three patterns of *in vitro* activity:[178] (1) they may neither proliferate nor produce MIF in response to antigenic stimulation, (2) they may proliferate but not elaborate MIF, and (3) they may both proliferate and produce MIF. This last group of patients, however, does not respond to the intradermal injection of exogenous MIF which produces a delayed hypersensitivity-type lesion in normal individuals. It is possible that the monocytes and macrophages of these patients are not responsive to the lymphokine.

Although there appear to be many different defects in patients with CMC, all seem to involve the axis of communication between the macrophage and the lymphocyte. Thus in some patients there may be a defect in the ability of their lymphocytes to respond to *Candida* antigens, in others a failure of their lymphocytes to produce lymphokines, and in still others an inability of their nonspecific effector cells to respond to lymphocyte-derived soluble factors.

Antifungal therapy in these patients has been generally unsuccessful. However, the use of transfer factor has produced encouraging results (see Chap. 5).

IMMUNOLOGIC METHODS IN THE DIAGNOSIS OF FUNGAL INFECTIONS*

A variety of immunologic techniques are used to facilitate the diagnosis of fungal infections. These can be divided into three general categories: (1) the detection of antifungal antibodies, (2) the detection of fungal antigens, and (3) testing for cutaneous delayed hypersensitivity against fungal antigens.[174,179]

Diagnosis of Histoplasmosis

Antibodies. Complement fixation can be used to detect two distinct antifungal antibodies:

*The various serologic tests that are mentioned in this section are discussed in Appendix C.

1. Antibody directed against a yeast-phase antigen. This antibody appears two to three weeks after exposure.

2. Antibody directed against a mycelial-phase antigen called histoplasmin. This antibody appears later and is seen in lower titers than the antibody against the yeast-phase antigen. However, the titer can be high in chronically infected individuals.

Both of these tests are reliable indicators of disease. More than 95 per cent of people with active pulmonary histoplasmosis are positive for these antibodies as are an even greater percentage of patients with chronic pulmonary disease. In general, antibody to the yeast-phase antigen correlates best with acute infections, while anti-histoplasmin antibody correlates with chronic disease. False negatives can occur. The antibodies crossreact with other fungi, limiting the specificity of these tests.

Skin Test. Histoplasmin is a commonly employed skin test antigen. Cutaneous delayed hypersensitivity is a good indication of previous exposure to the fungus. Like the tuberculin skin test it suffers from occasional false negatives. Thus, 5 per cent of patients with active pulmonary histoplasmosis are negative and about one half of the patients with disseminated disease do not react. Perhaps the major drawback of the histoplasmin skin test is that application of the test will stimulate the production of complement-fixing antibodies, confusing the interpretation of the valuable serologic studies.

Diagnosis of Coccidioidomycosis

Antibodies. Both the precipitin test and the complement-fixing test are used to diagnose this disease. IgM precipitins appear early, peak within a few weeks and may be gone within one to two months. They are thus a measure of the acuteness of an infection. IgG complement-fixing antibodies rise more slowly, peak within two to three months and remain elevated for a long time. The titer of complement-fixing antibody correlates well with the severity of the infection. It has been claimed that the presence of complement-fixing antibodies in the cerebrospinal fluid is diagnostic of active meningitis, although low cerebrospinal fluid levels may merely represent a "spill-over" from the circulation.

Skin Test. The value of the coccidioidin skin test is similar to that of the tuberculin skin test. It is generally positive within several weeks of infection. A positive reaction signifies past exposure and not active disease. Furthermore, in the face of disseminated disease, it may become negative. The coccidioidin skin test can be used to support a presumptive diagnosis of coccidioidomycosis and is particularly useful if it is known that the patient was previously skin-test-negative.

Diagnosis of Aspergillosis

Antibodies. Aspergillus precipitins can be detected with an agar gel double-diffusion test. The test has been reported to be positive in 100 per cent of patients with aspergillomas and 70 per cent of patients with allergic forms of this mycosis. Very few healthy individuals are positive, but up to 70 per cent of patients with pulmonary tuberculosis have been reported to possess these precipitating antibodies. This test should be used only to support a diagnosis of aspergilloma. Patients with disseminated aspergillosis often have no detectable antibodies.

Skin Test. Extracts of *A. fumigatus* can be used to detect cutaneous delayed hypersensitivity. Only a small percentage of patients with aspergillomas will react. The great majority of patients with allergic disease are positive to the skin test.

Diagnosis of Candidiasis

Antibodies. The most accurate and specific test involves a *Candida* protoplast antigen in a precipitin reaction. The incidence of a positive reaction is usually much higher in patients with systemic candidiasis than in patients with localized disease. Rising titers have been correlated with visceral involvement. However, this test cannot be used to absolutely distinguish systemic from localized candiasis in any particular patient.

Skin Test. Because *Candida* antigens elicit a positive skin reaction in the majority of normal people, this test has no diagnostic value.

Diagnosis of Cryptococcosis

Cryptococcosis has long been difficult to diagnose by serologic techniques, and only recently have several assays been developed which have produced promising results.

Antigens. Over 50 per cent of patients with cryptococcosis have been found to be positive for cryptococcal antigens by a latex agglutination technique. This appears to be the most specific test available. Antigen titers, especially when present in the cerebrospinal fluid, may relate to the severity of the disease, with increasing levels of detectable antigen correlating with a worsening prognosis.

Antibodies. Both an agglutination assay and an indirect fluorescent antibody assay are positive in about 40 per cent of patients. The agglutinins are more specific for Cryptococcus.

Combining all of these serologic tests, a presumptive diagnosis can be made in about 90 per cent of cases.

Diagnosis of Blastomycosis

Antibodies. The most widely available test for detecting antiblastomycosis antibodies employs a complement-fixation assay. False negatives are common and less than one half of the patients with blastomycosis give a positive result. In addition, the antigen that is used will cross-react with sera from patients with histoplasmosis and coccidioidomycosis. A significant complement-fixing titer generally indicates a mycotic infection but other procedures are required to make the specific diagnosis.

Skin Test. Blastomycosis skin testing has little clinical value. Most patients infected with *Blastomyces* do not react and crossreactivity with other fungal antigens limits the skin test's specificity.

IMMUNITY TO PARASITIC INFECTIONS

TOXOPLASMOSIS

Despite the ubiquity of parasitic infections in man, very little is known about the immunologic basis of host resistance to most parasites. One organism that has been fairly extensively studied is *Toxoplasma gondii*, a protozoan that infects approximately 50 per cent of people in this country. Most often the infection is asymptomatic or produces an influenza-like syndrome with fever, lymphadenopathy and fatigue. Congenital toxoplasmosis is a potentially serious disease affecting infants of infected mothers. It has been estimated that 40 per cent of infected mothers transmit the disease across the placenta to their fetus. Fetal death or severe central nervous system pathology may result. Most cases of congenitally acquired toxoplasmosis are asymptomatic at birth and only become apparent later in life, usually as a chorioretinitis.[180] Immune compromised adults are also susceptible to severe infections with toxoplasma. Patients on immunosuppressive therapy and with Hodgkin's disease are at an increased risk to develop disseminated toxoplasmosis, and lesions occur most commonly in the brain, lungs and heart.[181]

Toxoplasma gondii is an obligate intracellular parasite, and the immunology of toxoplasma infections is similar to that of intracellular bacterial infections. The normal host limits the infection usually within several days of exposure, but generally fails to completely abort the infection. Encysted organisms may persist in infected tissues for years or even for the lifetime of the host. Unlike intracellular bacterial infections, granulomas are not seen.

The humoral limb of the immune system does not appear to play a dominant role in combating toxoplasma infections. Passive transfer of specific antibody does not afford protection to recipient hosts in experimental animal systems.[182] However, it has been shown that antibody can reduce the active penetration of toxoplasma into macrophages and other cell lines.[183,184] Toxoplasma organisms that have reacted with antibody can be phagocytosed by macrophages and are readily digested inside the cell.[184]

Passive transfer of sensitized lymphocytes does convey protection against the organism,[182] and the cellular limb of the immune system is felt to be primarily responsible for toxoplasma immunity. Progressive toxoplasmosis has been described in patients with hypergammaglobulinemia plus antitoxoplasma antibodies but who have depressed cell-mediated immunity.[185] It has been demonstrated both in animals and in man that sensitized T cells or supernatants of sensitized T cells can activate infected macrophages to inhibit the growth of the intracellular parasite.[183,184,186-189] This phenomenon clearly resembles the role of T cells and macrophages in opposing intracellular bacterial infections. Human lymphocytes sensitized to other antigens or mitogens can also activate macrophages against toxoplasma, but not as effectively as those sensitized to toxoplasma antigens.[189]

Diagnosis of acute toxoplasmosis has always been difficult. One cannot rely upon tissue biopsy and demonstration of the organism since toxoplasma can remain encysted in host tissues for many years. Until recently physicians had to depend on recognizing the typical clinical picture in association with positive serologies, but this has not proved to be satisfactory since the clinical presentation is so nonspecific and elevated titers of antitoxoplasma antibodies may persist for a long time. Recently it was reported that circulating toxoplasma antigens can be detected in acute experimental infections in mice and rabbits.[190] This techique is now being applied to the diagnosis of human infections.

IMMUNE MECHANISMS IN OTHER PARASITIC INFECTIONS

One of the hallmarks of the immune response to most parasitic infections is the production of specific IgE.[191] IgE-secreting plasma cells can often be found at the site of infection.[192] Parasitic antigens can elicit not only the production of antiparasite antibodies but can potentiate an ongoing IgE response to an unrelated antigen.[193] It is not known to what extent and by what mechanisms IgE may contribute to the elimination of parasitic infections. Several possibilities have been suggested:

1. Local anaphylaxis has been examined in experimental infections with nematodes.[194] Basophils and mast cells infiltrate into the gut at the site of infection, where combination of parasitic antigens with IgE on the surfaces of these cells leads to degranulation with the release of vasoactive amines. These inflammatory mediators are believed to facilitate worm expulsion, an idea supported by one study which showed that anti-amine drugs could inhibit elimination of the parasites.[195] It is conceivable that the increased vascular permeability resulting from the activity of the vasoactive amines allows host defense cells to enter the lumen of the gut where they can freely attack the worms.

2. IgE directed against the worms may directly damage the parasites, but there is little evidence to support this hypothesis.

3. Another possible antiparasitic function of IgE has recently been reported in *Schistosoma mansoni* infections in Fisher rats. Peritoneal macrophages from these rats have been described to adhere to the schistosomules in the presence of anti-schistosome IgE.[196] This finding suggests that IgE may be cytophilic for macrophages in this system and thus be able to opsonize the target trematode.

Cell-mediated immunity may also play a role in opposing many parasitic infections.[197] It is not clear if the cellular limb of the immune system acts directly upon the invading organisms. Alternatively, the production of lymphocyte-mediated delayed hypersensitivity reactions could lead to a local inflammatory response at the site of infection which might alter the host tissue environment so that the infection becomes untenable and is aborted.

One interesting twist to the immunologic relationship between host and parasite is illustrated by schistosomiasis. The adult organisms live in the mesenteric vessels where they are continually exposed to antischistosome antibodies. However, these worms seem to be able to escape the effect of these antibodies by incorporating host antigens, including those of the ABO blood system, into their surface structure.[198] In this way, the worms avoid immune reactivity.

REFERENCES

1. Rosenthal, J., Hayashi, K., and Notkins, A. L.: Virus antigens on the surface of infected cells. J. Gen. Virol., *18*:195, 1973.
2. Ogra, P. L., and Karzon, D. T.: Formation and function of poliovirus antibody in different tissues. Prog. Med. Virol., *13*:156, 1971.
3. Ogra, P. L., Morag, A., and Tiku, M. L.: Humoral immune response to viral infections. *In* Notkins, A. L. (ed.): Viral Immunology and Immunopathology. P. 57. New York, Academic Press, 1975.
4. Fenner, F.: The Biology of Animal Viruses. New York, Academic Press, 1968.
5. Notkins, A. L.: Immune mechanisms by which the spread of viral infection is stopped. Cell. Immunol., *11*:478, 1974.
6. ———: Immunopathology of viral infections. Prog. Immunol., *II*:141, 1974.
7. Ogra, P. L., and Karzon, D. T.: Distribution of poliovirus antibody in serum, nasopharynx and alimentary tract following segmental immunization of lower alimentary tract with poliovaccine. J. Immunol., *102*:1423, 1969.
8. Ogra, P. L., and Karzon, D. T.: Poliovirus antibody response in serum and nasal secretions following intranasal inoculation with inactivated poliovaccine. J. Immunol., *102*:15, 1969.
9. Kasel, J. A., *et al.*: Antibody responses in nasal secretions and serum of elderly persons. J. Immunol., *102*:555, 1969.
10. Wyatt, H. V.: Poliomyelitis in hypogammaglobulinemics. J. Infect. Dis., *128*:802, 1973.
11. Svehag, S.: Formation and dissociation of virus-antibody complexes with special reference to the neutralization process. Prog. Med. Virol., *10*:1, 1968.
12. Radwan, A. I., and Burger, D.: The complement-requiring neutralization of equine arteritis virus by late antisera. Virology, *51*:71, 1973.
13. Daniels, C. A.: Mechanisms of viral neutralization. *In* Notkins, A. L. (ed.): Viral Immunology and Immunopathology. P. 79. New York, Academic Press, 1975.
14. Mandell, B.: Characterization of type 1 poliovirus by electrophoretic analysis. Virology, *44*:554, 1971.
15. Bradish, C. J., Farley, J. O., and Ferrier, H. E. W.: Studies on the nature of the neutralization reaction. Virology, *18*:378, 1962.
16. Radwan, A. I., and Burger, D.: The role of sensitizing antibody in the neutralization of equine arteritis virus. Virology, *53*:366, 1973.
17. Daniels, C. A., *et al.*: Neutralization of sensitized virus by purified components of complement. Proc. Natl. Acad. Sci. U.S.A., *65*:528, 1970.
18. Radwan, A. I., and Crawford, T. B.: The mechanisms of neutralization of sensitized equine arteritis virus by complement components. J. Gen. Virol., *25*:229, 1974.
19. Oldstone, M. B. A., Cooper, N. R., and Carson, D. L.: Formation and biologic role of polyoma virus-antibody complexes. J. Exp. Med., *140*:549, 1974.
20. Smith, J. W., Adam, E., Melnick, J. L., and Rawls, W. E.: Use of the ^{51}Cr release test to demonstrate patterns of antibody response in humans to Herpes Simplex virus types 1 and 2. J. Immunol., *109*:554, 1972.
21. Shore, S. L., *et al.*: Detection of cell-dependent cytotoxic antibody to cells infected with Herpes Simplex virus. Nature, *251*:350, 1974.
22. Woodruff, J. F., and Woodruff, J. J.: T lymphocyte interaction with viruses and virus-infected tissues. Prog. Med. Virol., *19*:120, 1975.
23. Stutman, O.: Immunodeficiency states and natural resistance. *In* Koprowski, C., and Koprowski, H. (eds.): Viruses and Immunity. P. 1. New York, Academic Press, 1975.

24. Bloom, B. A., and Rager-Zisman, B.: Cell-mediated immunity in viral infections. *In* Notkins, A. L. (ed.): Viral Immunology and Immunopathology. P. 113. New York, Academic Press, 1975.
24a. Doherty, P. C., Blanden, R. V., and Zinkernagel, R. M.: Specificity of virus-immune effector T cells for H-2K or H-2D compatible interactions: implications for H-antigen diversity. Transplant. Rev., *29*:89, 1976.
24b. Zinkernagel, R. M.: H-2 restriction of virus-specific cytotoxicity across the H-2 barrier. J. Exp. Med., *144*:933, 1976.
25. Mims, C. A.: Aspects of the pathogenesis of virus diseases. Bacteriol. Rev., *28*:30, 1964.
26. Allison, A. C.: On the role of mononuclear phagocytes in immunity against viruses. Prog. Med. Virol., *18*:15, 1974.
27. Gresser, I., and Lang, D. J.: Relationships between viruses and leucocytes. Prog. Med. Virol., *8*:62, 1966.
28. Hirsch, M. S., Zisman, B., and Allison, A. C.: Macrophages and age-dependent resistance to Herpes Simplex virus in mice. J. Immunol., *104*:1160, 1970.
29. Stevens, J. G., and Cook, M. L.: Restriction of Herpes Simplex virus by macrophages. J. Exp. Med., *133*:19, 1970.
30. Goodman, G. T., and Koprowski, H.: Innate resistance to viral infection. J. Cell Physiol., *59*:333, 1962.
31. Bang, F. B., and Warwick, A.: Mouse macrophages as host cells for the mouse hepatitis virus and the genetic bases of their susceptibility. Proc. Natl. Acad. Sci. U.S.A., *46*:1065, 1960.
32. Samuel, C. E., and Joklik, W. K.: A protein-synthesizing system from interferon treated cells that discriminates between cellular and viral mRNAs. Virology, *58*:476, 1974.
33. Wiebe, M. E., and Joklik, W. K.: The mechanism of inhibition of reovirus replication by interferon. Virology, *66*:229, 1975.
34. Sydiskis, R. J., and Schultz, I.: Interferon and antibody production in mice with Herpes Simplex skin infections. J. Infect. Dis., *116*:455, 1966.
35. Wallen, W. C., Dean, J. H., and Lucas, D. O.: Interferon and the cellular immune response. Cell. Immunol., *6*:110, 1973.
36. Green, J. A., Cooperband, S. R., and Kibrick, S.: Immune specific induction of interferon production in cultures of human blood lymphocytes. Science, *164*:1415, 1969.
37. Glasgow, L. A.: Leukocytes and interferon in the host response to viral infections. J. Bacteriol., *91*:2185, 1966.
38. Notkins, A. L.: Viral Immunology and Immunopathology. P. 149. New York, Academic Press, 1975.
39. Falcoff, R.: Some properties of virus and immune-induced human lymphocyte interferons. J. Gen. Virol., *16*:251, 1972.
40. Youngner, J. S., and Salvin, S. B.: Production and properties of MIF and interferon in the circulation of mice with delayed hypersensitivity. J. Immunol., *111*:1914, 1973.
41. Valle, M. J., Bobrove, A. M., Strober, S., and Merigan, T. C.: Immune specific production of interferon by human T cells in combined macrophage-lymphocyte cultures in response to Herpes Simplex antigen. J. Immunol., *114*:435, 1975.
42. Stobo, J., Green, I., Jackson, L., and Baron, S.: Identification of a subpopulation of mouse lymphoid cells required for interferon production after stimulation with mitogens. J. Immunol., *112*:1589, 1974.
43. Epstein, L. B., Stevens, D. A., and Merigan, T. C.: Selective increase in lymphocyte interferon response to vaccinia antigen after revaccination. Proc. Natl. Acad. Sci. U.S.A., *69*:2632, 1972.
44. Epstein, L. B., Kreth, H. W., and Herzenberg, L. A.: Flourescence-activated cell sorting of human T and B lymphocytes. Cell. Immunol., *12*:407, 1974.
45. Pathak, P. N., and Tomkins, W. A. F.: Interferon production by macrophages from adult and newborn rabbits bearing fibroma virus-induced tumors. Infect. Immunol., *9*:669, 1974.
46. Hayashi, K., Niwa, A., Rosenthal, J., and Notkins, A. L.: Detection of virus-induced membrane and cytoplasmic antigen. Intervirology, *2*:48, 1973.
47. Lodmell, D. L., Niwa, A., Hayashi, K., and Notkins, A. L.: Prevention of cell to cell spread of Herpes Simplex virus by leukocytes. J. Exp. Med., *137*:706, 1973.
48. Notkins, A. L.: Viral infections: mechanisms of immunologic defense and injury. Hosp. Pract., *9*:65, 1974.
49. Johannes, R. S., and Sever, J. L.: Subacute sclerosing panencephalitis. Ann. Rev. Med., *26*:589, 1975.
50. ——: Measles—quick and slow. Lancet, *2*:27, 1971.
51. Payne, F. E., Baublis, J. V., and Itabashi, H. H.: Isolation of measles virus from cell cultures of brain from a patient with subacute sclerosing panencephalitis. N. Engl. J. Med., *281*:585, 1969.
52. Jenis, E. H., *et al.*: Subacute sclerosing panencephalitis. Arch. Pathol., *95*:81, 1973.
53. Whitaker, J. N., Sever, J. L., and Engel, W. K.: Subacute sclerosing panencephalitis in only one of identical twins. N. Engl. J. Med., *287*:864, 1972.
54. Jabbour, J. T., *et al.*: Epidemiology of subacute sclerosing panencephalitis. J.A.M.A., *220*:959, 1972.
55. Burnet, F. M.: Measles as an index of immunological function. Lancet, *2*:610, 1958.
56. Moulias, R. L., Reinert, P., and Goust, J. M.: Immunologic abnormalities in subacute sclerosing panencephalitis. N. Engl. J. Med., *285*:1090, 1971.
57. Thurman, G. B., *et al.*: Lymphocyte activation in subacute sclerosing panencephalitis virus

and CMV infections. J. Exp. Med., *138*:839, 1973.

58. Kreth, W. H., Kackell, M. Y., and TerMeulen, V.: Demonstration of *in vitro* lymphocyte-mediated cytotoxicity against measles virus in subacute sclerosing panencephalitis. J. Immunol., *114*:1042, 1975.
59. Connolly, J. H., Allen, I. V., Hurwitz, L. J., and Millar, J. H. D.: Measles-virus antibody and antigen in subacute sclerosing panencephalitis. Lancet, *1*:542, 1967.
60. Norrby, E., and Vandvik, B.: The relationship between measles virus-specific antibodies and oligoclonal IgG in the CSF in patients with subacute sclerosing panencephalitis and multiple sclerosis. Med. Microbiol. Immunol., *160*:233, 1974.
61. Pincus, J. H., *et al.*: Antibody to type III and type IV pneumococcal polysaccharides. J. Immunol., *104*:1143, 1970.
62. Dayan, A. D.: Subacute sclerosing panencephalitis. Proc. R. Soc. Med., *67*:1123, 1974.
63. Horta-Barbosa, L., *et al.*: Some characteristics of subacute sclerosing panencephalitis measles virus. Proc. Soc. Exp. Biol. Med., *134*:17, 1970.
64. Oldstone, M. B. A., Bokisch, V. A., and Dixon, F. J.: Subacute sclerosing panencephalitis: destruction of human brain cells by antibody and complement in an autologous system. Clin. Immunol. Immunopathol., *4*:52, 1974.
65. Bollengier, F., *et al.*: Immunological study of the agent responsible for subacute sclerosing panencephalitis and the biochemical characterization of measles antibody in subacute sclerosing panencephalitis. Med. Microbiol. Immunol., *160*:173, 1974.
66. Ehrnst, A., Weiner, L., and Norrby, E.: Fluctuation and distribution of measles virus antigen in chronically infected cells. Nature, *248*:691, 1974.
67. Joseph, B. S., and Oldstone, M. B. A.: Immunologic injury in measles virus infection. J. Exp. Med., *142*:864, 1975.
68. Ahmed, A., *et al.*: Demonstration of a blocking factor in the plasma and spinal fluid of patients with subacute sclerosing panencephalitis. J. Exp. Med., *139*:902, 1974.
69. Cook, M. L., Bastone, V. B., and Stevens, J. G.: Evidence that neurons harbor latent Herpes Simplex virus. Infect. Immunol., *9*:946, 1974.
70. Stevens, J. G., and Cook, M. L.: Maintenance of latent herpetic infection. J. Immunol., *113*:1685, 1974.
71. Rawls, W. E.: Herpes Simplex virus. *In* Kaplan, A. S. (ed.): Herpes Viruses. P. 291. New York, Academic Press, 1973.
72. Oldstone, M. B. A.: Virus neutralization and virus-induced immune complex disease. Prog. Med. Virol., *19*:84, 1975.
73. Cole, G. A., and Nathanson, N.: Lymphocytic choriomeningitis. Prog. Med. Virol., *18*:94, 1974.
74. Hirsch, M. S., Murphy, F. A., and Hicklin, M. D.: Immunopathology of LCM virus infection of newborn mice. J. Exp. Med., *127*:757, 1968.
75. Gilden, D. H., Cole, G. A., Monjan, A. A., and Nathanson, N.: Immunopathogenesis of acute CNS disease produced by LCM virus. J. Exp. Med., *135*:860, 1972.
76. Cole, G. A., Nathanson, N., and Prendergast, R. A.: Requirement for O bearing cells in LCM virus-induced CNS disease. Nature, *238*:335, 1972.
77. Barker, L. F., *et al.*: Hepatitis B core antigen: immunology and electron microscopy. J. Virol., *14*:1552, 1974.
78. Bancroft, W. H., Mundon, F. K., and Russell, P. K.: Detection of additional antigenic determinants of hepatitis B antigen. J. Immunol., *109*:842, 1972.
79. Alberti, A., Realdi, G., Tremolada, F., and Cadrobbi, P.: Hepatitis B antigen on liver-cell surface in viral hepatitis. Lancet, *1*:346, 1975.
80. Bond, H. E., and Hall, W. T.: Separation and purification of HAA into morphologic types by zonal ultracentrifugation. J. Infect. Dis., *125*:263, 1972.
81. Hoofnagle, J. H., Garety, R. J., and Barker, L. F.: Antibody to hepatitis B core antigens. Am. J. Med. Sci., *270*:179, 1975.
82. Alpert, E., Isselbacher, K. J., and Schur, P. H.: The pathogenesis of arthritis associated with viral hepatitis. N. Engl. J. Med., *285*:185, 1971.
83. Wands, J. R., Mann, E., Alpert, E., and Isselbacher, K. J.: The pathogenesis of arthritis associated with acute hepatitis-B surface antigen-positive hepatitis. J. Clin. Invest., *55*:930, 1975.
84. Purcell, R. H., *et al.*: Seroepidemiological studies of transfusion associated hepatitis. J. Infect. Dis., *123*:406, 1971.
85. Gocke, D. J., *et al.*: Association between polyarteritis and Australia antigen. Lancet, *2*:1149, 1970.
86. Paronetto, F., and Popper, H.: Two immunologic reactions in the pathogenesis of hepatitis? N. Engl. J. Med., *294*:606, 1976.
87. Peterson, J. M., Drenstag, J. L., and Purcell, R. H.: Immune response to hepatitis viruses. *In* Notkins, A. L. (ed.): Viral Immunology and Immunopathology. P. 213. New York, Academic Press, 1975.
88. Paronetto, F., and Vernace, S.: Immunological studies in patients with chronic active hepatitis. Clin. Exp. Immunol., *19*:99, 1975.
89. Eddington, T. S., and Chisari, F. V.: Immunological aspects of hepatitis B virus infection. Am. J. Med. Sci., *270*:213, 1975.
90. Nowoslawski, A., *et al.*: Tissue localization of Australia antigen immune complexes in acute and chronic hepatitis and liver cirrhosis. Am. J. Pathol., *68*:31, 1972.
91. London, W. T., DiFiglia, M., Sutnick, A. L., and Blumberg, B. S.: An epidemic of hepatitis in a chronic hemodialysis unit. N. Engl. J. Med., *281*:571, 1969.
92. Soloway, R. D., *et al.*: Clinical biochemical and histological remission of severe chronic active liver disease. Gastroenterology, *63*:820, 1972.
93. Kohler, P. F., Trembath, J., Merrill, D. A., Singleton, J. W., and Dubois, R. S.: Im-

munotherapy with antibody, lymphocytes and transfer factor in chronic hepatitis B. Clin. Immunol. Immunopathol., *2*:465, 1974.

94. Irwin, G. R., Hierholzer, W. J., Cimis, R., and McCollum, R. W.: Delayed hypersensitivity in hepatitis B. J. Infect. Dis., *130*:580, 1974.
95. Dudley, F. J., Guistino, V., and Sherlock, S.: Cell mediated immunity in patients positive for HAA. Br. Med. J., *4*:754, 1972.
96. Tong, M. J., Wallace, A. M., Peters, R. L., and Reynolds, T. B.: Lymphocyte stimulation in hepatitis B infections. N. Engl. J. Med., *293*:318, 1975.
97. Notkins, A. L., Mergenhagen, S. E., and Howard, R. J.: Effect of virus infections on the function of the immune system. Ann. Rev. Microbiol., *24*:525, 1970.
98. Dent, P. B.: Immunodepression by oncogenic viruses. Prog. Med. Virol., *14*:1, 1972.
99. Wybran, J., and Fudenberg, H. H.: Thymus-derived rosette-forming cells in various human disease states. J. Clin. Invest., *52*:1026, 1973.
100. Huang, S. W., Lattos, D. B., Nelson, D. B., Reeb, K., and Hong, R.: Antibody-associated lymphocytoxin in acute infection. J. Clin. Invest., *52*:1033, 1973.
101. Woodruff, J. F., and Woodruff, J. J.: Virus-induced alterations of lymphoid tissues. Cell. Immunol., *1*:333, 1970.
102. ———: Virus-induced alterations of lymphoid tissues. Cell. Immunol., *5*:296, 1972.
103. McFarland, H. F.: The effect of measles virus infection on T and B lymphocytes in the mouse. J. Immunol., *113*:1978, 1974.
104. Wolheim, F. A., and Williams, R. C.: Studies on the macroglobulins of human serum. N. Engl. J. Med., *274*:61, 1966.
105. Von Pirquet, C. E.: Allergy. Arch. Intern. Med., *7*:383, 1911.
106. Haiden, S., Coutinho, M., Edmond, R. T. D., and Sutton, R. N. P.: Tuberculin anergy and infectious mononucleosis. Lancet, *2*:74, 1973.
107. Mangi, R. J., *et al.*: Depression of cell mediated immunity during acute infectious mononucleosis. N. Engl. J. Med., *291*:1149, 1974.
108. Soontiens, F. J. C. J., and Van Der Veen, J.: Evidence for a macrophage-mediated effect of poliovirus on the lymphocyte response to phytohemagglutinin. J. Immunol., *111*:1411, 1973.
109. Hall, C. B., and Kantor, F. S.: Depression of established delayed hypersensitivity by mumps virus. J. Immunol., *108*:81, 1972.
110. Brodeur, B. R., and Merigan, T. C.: Suppressive effect of interferon on the humoral immune response to sheep red blood cells in mice. J. Immunol., *113*:1319, 1974.
111. ———: Mechanism of the suppressive effect of interferon on antibody synthesis *in vivo*. J. Immunol., *114*:1323, 1975.
112. Hirsch, M. S., Ellis, D. A., Proffitt, M. R., and Black, P. H.: Effects of interferon on leukemia virus activation in graft versus host disease. Nature [New Biol.], *244*:102, 1973.
113. Hirsch, M. S., *et al.*: Immunosuppressive effects of interferon preparation *in vivo*. Transplantation, *17*:234, 1974.
114. Lindahl-Magnusson, P., Leary, P., and Gresser, I.: Interferon inhibits DNA synthesis induced in mouse lymphocyte suspensions by phytohaemagglutinin or by allogeneic cells. Nature [New Biol.], *237*:120, 1972.
115. Chanock, R. M., *et al.*: Current approaches to viral immunoprophylaxis. *In* Notkins, A. L. (ed.): Viral Immunology and Immunopathology. P. 291. New York, Academic Press, 1975.
116. Bellanti, J. A.: Adverse effects of viral vaccines. *In* Notkins, A. L. (ed.): Viral Immunology and Immunopathology. P. 327. New York, Academic Press, 1975.
117. Ginsberg, H. S.: Subunit viral vaccines. *In* Notkins, A. L. (ed.): Viral Immunology and Immunopathology. P. 317. New York, Academic Press, 1975.
118. Smith, C. B., Purcell, R. H., Bellanti, J. A., and Chanock, R. M.: Protective effect of antibody to parainfluenza type I virus. N. Engl. J. Med., *275*:1145, 1966.
119. Perkins, J. C., *et al.*: Comparison of protective effect of neutralizing antibody in serum and nasal secretions in experimental rhinovirus type 13 illness. Am. J. Epidemiol., *90*:519, 1969.
120. Shin, H. S., Smith, M. R., and Wood, W. B., Jr.: Heat labile opsonins to pneumococcus. J. Exp. Med., *130*:1229, 1969.
121. Almeida, J. D., and Waterson, A. P.: The morphology of virus-antibody interaction. Adv. Virus. Res., *15*:307, 1969.
122. Medhurst, F. A., Glynn, A. A., and Dourmashkin, R. R.: Lesions in *Escherichia coli* cell walls caused by the action of mouse complement. Immunology, *20*:441, 1971.
123. Gewurz, H., Shin, H. S., and Mergenhagen, S. E.: Interactions of the complement system with endotoxic lipopolysaccharide: consumption of each of the six terminal complement components. J. Exp. Med., *128*:1049, 1968.
124. Miller, M. E., Oski, F. A., and Harris, M. B.: Lazy-leucocyte syndrome. Lancet, *1*:665, 1971.
125. Johnson, R. B., and Baehner, R. L.: Chronic granulomatous disease: correlation between pathogenesis and clinical findings. Pediatrics, *48*:730, 1971.
126. Salmon, S. E., Cline, M. J., Schultz, J., and Lehrer, R. I.: Myeloperoxidase deficiency: a genetic leukocyte defect. N. Engl. J. Med., *282*:250, 1970.
127. Windhorst, D. B., Zelickson, A. S., and Good, R. A.: Chediak-Higashi syndrome. Science, *151*:81, 1966.
128. Blume, R. S., and Wolff, S. M.: The Chediak-Higashi syndrome: studies in four patients and a review of the literature. Medicine, *51*:247, 1972.
129. Wolff, S. M., *et al.*: The Chediak-Higashi syndrome: studies of host defenses. Ann. Intern. Med., *76*:293, 1972.
130. Blanden, R. V.: T cell response to viral and bacterial infection. Transplant. Rev., *19*:56, 1974.
131. Lefford, M. J.: Transfer of adoptive immunity to tuberculosis in mice. Infect. Immunol., *11*:1174, 1975.

132. Gray, D. F., and Cheers, C.: The steady state in cellular immunity 1. Chemotherapy and superinfection in murine TB. Aust. J. Exp. Biol. Med. Sci., *45*:407, 1967.
133. Coppel, S., and Youmans, G. P.: Specificity of acquired resistance produced by immunization with mycobacterial cells and mycobacterial fractions. J. Bacteriol., *97*:114, 1969.
134. Youmans, G. P.: Relation between delayed hypersensitivity and immunity in tuberculosis. Am. Rev. Respir. Dis., *111*:109, 1975.
135. Klun, C. L., Neiburger, R. G., and Youmans, G. P.: Relationship between mouse mycobacterial growth-inhibitory factor and mouse migration-inhibitory factor in supernatant fluids from mouse lymphocyte cultures. J. Reticuloendothel.Soc., *13*:310, 1973.
136. Gray, D. F., and Cheers, C.: The steady state in cellular immunity II. Immunological complaisance in murine pertussia. Aust. J. Exp. Biol. Sci., *45*:417, 1967.
137. Stead, W. W.: The new face of tuberculosis. Hosp. Pract., *4*(10):62, 1969.
138. Malaviya, A. N., Sehgal, K. L., Kumar, R., and Dingley, H. B.: Factors of delayed hypersensitivity in pulmonary tuberculosis. Am. Rev. Respir. Dis., *112*:49,1975.
139. Zeitz, S. J., Ostrow, J. H., and VanArsdel, P. P.: Humoral and cellular immunity in the anergic tuberculosis patient. J. Allergy Clin. Immunol., *53*:20, 1974.
140. Joklik, W. K., and Smith, D. T.: Mycobacterium tuberculosis. *In* Zinsser: Microbiology. Ed. 15, P. 453. New York, Meredity Corp., 1972.
141. Rothschild, H., Friedenwald, J. S., and Bernstein, C.: The relation of allergy to immunity in tuberculosis. Bull. Johns Hopkins Hosp., *54*:232, 1934.
142. Raffel, S.: Chemical factors involved in the induction of infectious allergy. Experientia, 6:410, 1950.
143. Choucroun, N.: Tubercle Bacillus antigens. Am. Rev. Tuber., *56*:203, 1947.
144. Youmans, G. P., and Youmans, A. S.: Allergenicity of mycobacterial ribosomal and ribonucleic acid preparations in mice and guinea pigs. J. Bacteriol., *97*:134, 1969.
145. ———: BCG and Vole Bacillus vaccines in the prevention of tuberculosis in adolescence and early adult life. Br. Med. J., *1*:973, 1963.
146. Shepard, C. C.: The nasal excretion of *Mycobacterium leprae* in leprosy. Int. J. Lepr., *30*:10, 1962.
147. Shepard, C. C., and Saitz, E. W.: Lepromin and tuberculin reactivity in adults not exposed to leprosy. J. Immunol., *99*:637, 1967.
148. Oharmendra: Notes on Leprosy. P. 376. New Delhi, India, Ministry of Health, 1967.
149. Godal, T., *et al.*: Evidence that the mechanism of immunological tolerance ("central failure") is operative in the lack of host resistance in lepromatous leprosy. Scand. J. Immunol., *1*:311, 1972.
150. Godal, T., Myklestad, B., Samuel, D. R., and Myrvang, B.: Characterization of the cellular immune defect in lepromatous leprosy: a specific lack of circulating *Mycobacterium leprae*-reactive lymphocytes. Clin. Exp. Immunol., *9*:821, 1971.
151. Lim, S-D., *et al.*: Immunodeficiency in leprosy. Birth Defects, *11(1)*:244, 1975.
152. Bullock, W. E.: Studies of immune mechanisms in leprosy. N. Engl. J. Med., *278*:298, 1968.
153. Turk, J. L., and Waters, M. F. R.: Cell-mediated immunity in patients with leprosy. Lancet, *2*:243, 1969.
154. Han, S. H., *et al.*: Prolonged survival of skin allografts in leprosy patients. Int. J. Lep., *39*:1, 1971.
155. Dierks, R. E., and Shepard, C. C.: Effect of phytohemagglutinin and various mycobacterial antigens on lymphocyte cultures from leprosy patients. Proc. Soc. Exp. Biol. Med., *127*:391, 1968.
156. Godal, T., Myklestad, B., Samuel, D. R., and Myrvang, B.: Characterization of the cellular immune defect in lepromatous leprosy. Clin. Exp. Immunol., *9*:821, 1971.
157. Abe, M., Chinoni, S., and Hirako. T.: Rheumatoid-factor-like substance and anti-streptolysin O antibody in leprosy serum: significance in erythema nodosum leprosum. Int. J. Lepr., *35*:336, 1967.
158. Bonomo, L., Tursi, A., Trimigliozzi, G., and Dammacco, F.: LE cells and antinuclear factors in leprosy. Br. Med. J., *2*:689, 1965.
159. Bullock, W. E., Fields, J. P., and Brandriss, M. W.: An evaluation of transfer factor as immunotherapyy for patients with lepromatous leprosy. N. Engl. J. Med., *287*:1053, 1972.
160. Siltzbach, L. E., *et al.*: Course and prognosis of sarcoidosis around the world. Am. J. Med., *57*:847, 1974.
161. James D. G., Neville, E., and Walker, A.: Immunology of sarcoidosis. Am. J. Med., *59*:388, 1975.
162. Hedfors, E., Holm, G., and Pettersson, D.: Lymphocyte subpopulation in sarcoidosis. Clin. Exp. Immunol., *17*:219, 1974.
163. Buckley, C. E., III, Nagaya, H., and Sieker, H. O.: Altered immunologic activity in sarcoidosis. Ann. Intern. Med., *64*:508, 1966.
164. Kataria, Y. P., Sagone, A. L., LoBuglio, A. F., and Bromberg, P. A.: *In vitro* observations on sarcoid lymphocytes and their correlation with cutaneous anergy and clinical severity of disease. Am. Rev. Respir. Dis., *108*:767, 1973.
165. Hirshaut, Y., *et al.*: Sarcoidosis, another disease associated with serologic evidence for Herpes-like virus infection. N. Engl. J. Med., *283*:502, 1970.
166. Byrne, E. B., Evans, A. S., Fouts, D. W., and Israel, H. L.: A seroepidemiological study of Epstein-Barr virus and other viral antigens in sarcoidosis. Am. J. Epidemiol., *97*:355, 1973.
167. Sands, J. H., Palmer, P. P., Mayock, R. L., Creger, W. P.: Evidence for serologic hyperreactivity in sarcoidosis. Am. J. Med., *19*:401, 1955.
168. Hirschhorn, K., Schreibman, R. R., Bach, F. H., and Siltzbach, L. E.: *In vitro* studies of lymphocytes from patients with sarcoidosis

and lymphoproliferative diseases. Lancet, *2*:842, 1964.

169. Lebacq, E., and Verhaegen, H.: Passive transfer of the Kveim reaction to normal subjects. *In* Levinsky, L., and Macholda, F. (eds.): Proc. 5th Int. Conf. on Sarcoidosis. P. 379. Praha, Universita Karlova, 1971.
170. Lenzini, L., Rottoli, P., Rottali, L., and Sestini, S.: Leucocyte-migration-inhibition tests with Kveim antigen in sarcoidosis. Lancet, *2*:1087, 1973.
171. Stobo, J. D., Paul, S., Van Scoy, R. E., and Hermans, P. E.: Suppressor thymus-derived lymphocytes in fungal infection. J. Clin. Invest., *57*:319, 1976.
172. United States Public Health Service: Course and prognosis of untreated histoplasmosis. J.A.M.A., *177*:292, 1961.
173. Furcolow, M. L.: Comparison of treated and untreated severe histoplasmosis. J.A.M.A., *183*:823, 1963.
174. Salvin, S. B.: Immunologic aspects of the mycoses. Prog. Allergy, *7*:213, 1963.

174a. Smith, C. E., *et al.*: The use of coccidioidin. Am. Rev. Tuber., *57*:330, 1948.

175. Rapaport, F. T., *et al.*: Transfer of delayed hypersensitivity to coccidioidin in man. J. Immunology, *84*:358, 1959.
176. Pappagianes, D., Lindsey, N. J., Smith, C. E., and Saito, M. T.: Antibodies in human coccidioidomycosis: immunoelectrophoretic properties. Proc. Soc. Exp. Biol. Med., *118*:118, 1965.
177. Pepys, J.: Pulmonary aspergillosis, farmers lung, and related diseases. *In* Samter, M., Talmage, D. W., Rose, B., Sherman, W. B., and Vaughan, J. H. (eds.): Immunological Diseases. ed. 2, p. 693. Boston, Little, Brown & Co., 1971.

177a. Kirkpatrick, C. H., *et al.*: Chronic mucocutaneous candidiasis model-building in cellular immunity. Ann. Intern. Med., *74*:955, 1971.

178. Valdimarsson, H., *et al.*: Immune abnormalities associated with chronic mucocutaneous candidiasis. Cell. Immunol., *6*:348, 1973.
179. Beuchner, H. A., *et al.*: The current status of serologic, immunologic and skin tests in the diagnosis of pulmonary mycoses. Chest, *63*:259, 1973.
180. Viens, P., and Morisset, R.: Toxoplasmosis and the compromised host. Int. J. Clin. Pharmacol., *11*:361, 1975.
181. Gleason, T. H., and Hamlin, W. B.: Disseminated toxoplasmosis in the compromised host. Arch. Intern. Med., *134*:1059, 1974.
182. Frenkel, J. K.: Adoptive immunity to intracellular infection. J. Immunol., *98*:1309, 1967.
183. Stadtsbaeder, S., Nguyen, B. T., and Calvin-Preval, M. C.: Respective role of antibodies and immune macrophages during acquired immunity against toxoplasmosis in mice. Ann. Immunol. (Inst. Pasteur), *126C*:461, 1975.
184. Jones, T. C., Len, L., and Hirsch, J. G.: Assessment in vitro of immunity against *Toxoplasma gondii.* J. Exp. Med., *141*:466, 1975.
185. Sheagren, J. N., Lunde, M. N., and Simon, H. B.: Chronic lymphadenopathic toxoplasmosis. Am. J. Med., *60*:300, 1976.
186. Reikvam, A.: Macrophage proliferation and activation during *Toxoplasma gondii* infection in mice: relationship to lymphocyte stimulation. Acta Pathol. Microbiol. Scand. [C], *84*:124, 1976.
187. Sethi, K. K., *et al.*: Immunity to *Toxoplasma gondii* induced in vitro in non-immune mouse macrophages with specifically immune lymphocytes. J. Immunol., *115*:1151, 1975.
188. Borges, J. S., and Johnson, W. D., Jr.: Inhibition of multiplication of *Toxoplasma gondii* by human monocytes exposed to T-lymphocyte products. J. Exp. Med., *141*:483, 1975.
189. Anderson, S. E., Bautista, S., and Remington, J. S.: Induction of resistance to *Toxoplasma gondii* in human macrophages by soluble lymphocyte products. J. Immunol., *117*:381, 1976.
190. Raizman, R. E., and Neva, F. A.: Detection of circulating antigen in acute experimental infection with *Toxoplasma gondii*. J. Infect. Dis., *132*:44, 1975.
191. Ogilvie, B. M.: Immunity to parasites (helminths and arthropods). Prog. Immunol., *2*(4):127, 1974.
192. Ishizaka, K., Ishizaka, T., Tada, T.: Immunoglobulin E in the monkey. J. Immunol., *103*:445, 1969.
193. Editorial: IgE, parasites, and allergy. Lancet, *1*:894, 1976.
194. Murray, M., Jarrett, W. F. H., and Jennings, F. W.: Mast cells and macromolecular leak in intestinal immunological reactions. Immunology, *21*:17, 1971.
195. Rothwell, T. L. W., Dineen, J. K., and Love, R. J.: The role of pharmacologically-active amines in resistance to *trichostrongylus colubriformis* in the guinea pig. Immunology, *21*:925, 1971.
196. Capron, A., Dessaint, J. P., and Capron, M.: Specific IgE antibodies in immune adherence of normal macrophages to *Schistosoma mansoni* schistosomules. Nature, *253*:474, 1975.
197. Larsh, J. E., and Weatherly, N. F.: Cell-mediated immunity in certain parasitic infections. Curr. Top. Microbiol. Immunol., *67*:113, 1974.
198. Smithers, S. R.: Recent advances in the immunology of schistosomiasis. Br. Med. Bull., *28*:49, 1972.

12 The Immunoproliferative Diseases

The proliferation of immunocompetent cells is clearly one of the hallmarks of the immune response to an antigenic challenge. However, like most normal physiologic processes, immune proliferation can go awry and present as a primary disease process. More and more investigators are coming to view normal (reactive) and malignant lymphocyte proliferation as merely two ends of a continuous spectrum of proliferative phenomena, and as such are felt to share a number of features in common. This perspective has enabled us to view many of the immunoproliferative disorders in terms of our understanding of their benign counterparts. Although not universally accepted at present, this approach merits our attention on several grounds:

1. The frequent difficulty in distinguishing benign from malignant lesions under the light microscope
2. The existence of what we will term intermediate proliferative states in which the lymphocyte population expands without any detectable antigenic stimulus but at the same time lacks the characteristics of a true malignancy
3. Recent experimental work in animals and clinical studies in man which suggest that malignancies may develop within a setting of benign lymphoproliferation

In this chapter we shall first briefly review the characteristics of a normal proliferative response, then examine the most commonly encountered of the intermediate proliferative states, and finally turn our attention upon the malignant immunoproliferative disorders themselves.

REACTIVE LYMPHOPROLIFERATION

The resting lymph node can be anatomically divided into two regions of distinct morphology: (1) the deep cortical follicles are populated by B lymphocytes, histiocytic phagocytes and dendritic reticulum cells. These reticulum cells are unique to the follicle and can be identified microscopically by the presence of intercellular desmosomes. (2) The paracortical areas are composed of a diffuse array of thymus-derived lymphocytes and occasional macrophages.

With the introduction of antigen, the histology of the lymph node changes dramatically. The most obvious transformation is the development of germinal centers in the primary cortical follicles.[1] The blastic changes of the small follicular B lymphocytes produce new cell types that are identifiable under the light microscope. Attempts at naming and classifying these various germinal-center cells have resulted in a confusing proliferation of nomenclature in the literature. Despite this difficulty, we can identify a pattern of progressive histologic changes that is consistent with most reported observations:

The small lymphocyte contains a large, round nucleus and a scanty rim of cytoplasm. Upon activation the cell begins to enlarge and there is an increase in the ratio of cytoplasmic to nuclear mass. The nucleus acquires a more irregular outline and often develops a prominent cleavage as the process of differentiation continues. The cell continues to enlarge and displays a more prominent nucleolus. Other large cells can be found with abundant cytoplasm that possess nuclei that are not cleaved and that may contain more than one nucleolus. One group of investigators has postulated that these cells develop from the cells with cleft nuclei.[2]

The large, metabolically active cells have been termed *immunoblasts*. They exhibit a highly positive reaction to pyronine stain, indicative of their high content of ribonucleoprotein. In addition to the increase in cytoplasm there is a proliferation of polyribosomes. The mitochondria, electron-dense in the resting lymphocyte, become electron-lucent.

The last cell type to appear is the plasma cell. It is believed that plasma cells are the differentiated progeny of the immunoblasts. Whereas all of the preceding cell types possess readily stainable surface immunoglobulin, it is still debated whether or not human plasma cells also express surface immunoglobulin.

The paracortical regions also display characteristic histologic changes. The T cells undergo blast transformation and differentiation. No plasma cells are produced, but otherwise the cytologic characteristics of these transformed T cells are virtually indistinguishable from those of the activated B cells.

Patterns of Lymphoproliferation

Different antigenic stimuli produce unique patterns of histologic reactivity in a lymph node.[3] At present we do not know why a given antigen elicits a particular type of reaction. Four basic patterns have been described.

Diffuse Pattern. An antigen can induce a diffuse cellular proliferation that can obliterate the normal follicular and sinus architecture. The most prominent histologic feature is the presence of a great abundance of immunoblasts. This reaction pattern is often caused by viruses, vaccines and drug-hypersensitivity reactions.

Follicular Pattern. A variety of antigens that can cause lymph node enlargement produce a histologic picture dominated by large, active follicles. The entire spectrum of differentiating B cells is seen, from the resting small lymphocyte to the plasma cell. This pattern frequently accompanies chronic inflammatory states such as syphilis and rheumatoid arthritis. A typical example of this common pattern is shown in Figure 12-1.

Sinus Pattern. The sinuses of the lymph node are distended and filled with reactive cells. Sinus histiocytosis is a benign disorder in which the patient presents with massive lymphadenopathy. Histology reveals the sinuses of the involved nodes to be filled with histiocytes.

Mixed Pattern. This term describes a diffuse proliferation that leaves the nodal architecture intact. Follicular hyperplasia can be clearly distinguished amidst the generalized hypercellularity. This pattern may be observed in certain infectious diseases such as toxoplasmosis and infectious mononucleosis.

An Example of Reactive Lymphoproliferation: Infectious Mononucleosis

Infectious mononucleosis is a benign, self-limited lymphoproliferative disease

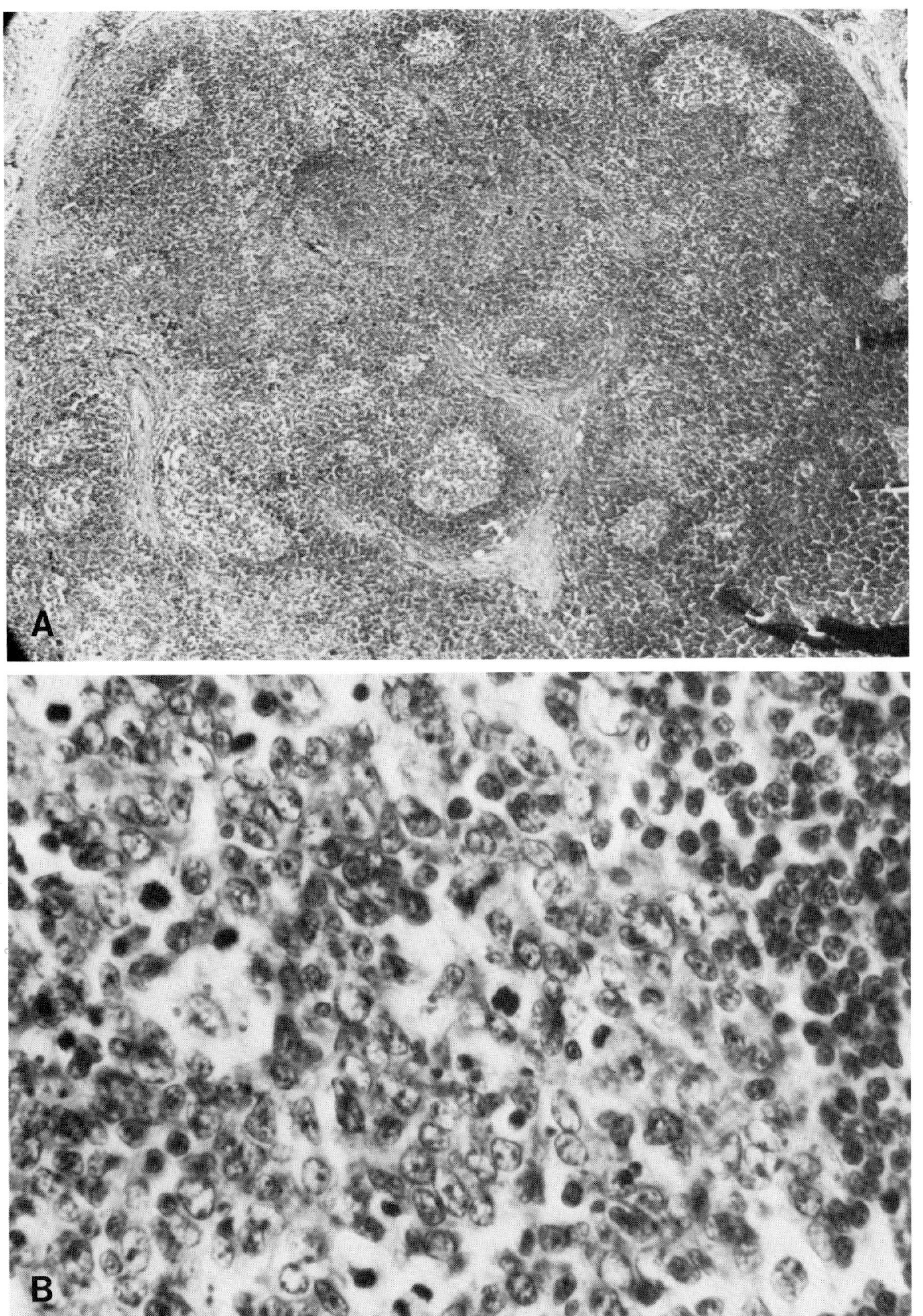

Fig. 12-1. A reactive lymph node with follicular hyperplasia. (*A*) Low-power view showing general pattern. (*B*) High-power view of the germinal center showing a mixture of cell types.

that has long puzzled investigators.[4] It can have a great variety of manifestations but is commonly marked by lymph node enlargement, fever and pharyngeal inflammation. Although the disease is self-limited, convalescence may, in unusual cases, take a year or more.

Infectious mononucleosis appears to be caused by the Epstein-Barr virus.[5] The disease is seen in previously uninfected individuals who are not immune to the virus. For this reason the attack rate is greatest in young people, especially those between 15 and 25 years of age. The details of the virology of the disease are just beginning to be understood. The Epstein-Barr virus appears preferentially to infect B lymphocytes.[6] The immune response to this infection includes the activation of T cells directed against the infected and presumably surface-altered B lymphocytes. These activated and transformed T cells are often quite prominent, appearing in the lymph nodes as well as in the peripheral blood. When present in the blood in significant numbers, they produce the picture of *atypical lymphocytosis*. The lymph nodes, especially those in the cervical region, display tremendous hyperactivity in both the B- and T-cell areas, giving rise to a mixed reactive pattern of follicular hyperplasia and proliferation in the medullary cords.

The infection is associated with the production of a variety of antibodies, many of which can be used to document the presence of the disease:

1. *Heterophil Antibody.* This is an IgM molecule that will agglutinate sheep red blood cells and is seen in the majority of cases of infectious mononucleosis. The heterophil antibody of infectious mononucleosis can be absorbed out by incubation with beef red blood cells but not by incubation with guinea pig kidney.[7]

2. *Antibodies against the Epstein-Barr virus* and against antigens expressed on virally infected cells are also produced and have been used to diagnose the infection.[8]

3. *Other Antibodies.* One of the most interesting humoral phenomena of this infection is the frequent production of IgM autoantibodies directed against the i antigen of the patient's red blood cells (see Chap. 14).[9] Other autoantibodies that have been detected include antinuclear antibodies and rheumatoid factor.

INTERMEDIATE PROLIFERATIVE STATES

There are a number of situations in which immunocompetent cells proliferate without any immediately obvious relationship to a specific antigenic stimulation, but either whose course or histology distinguishes them from true malignancies. In each of the instances cited below, however, malignancies have been described to arise, a point which serves to emphasize the fine line that can separate a benign from a malignant process.

1. *Sjögren's Syndrome* (see Chap. 8). Sjögren's syndrome is characterized by an infiltration and proliferation of lymphocytes and plasma cells in the salivary and lacrimal glands. Lymphoproliferation need not be confined to these glands, and more extensive involvement can result in a type of lymph node enlargement termed pseudolymphoma.[10]

The histology of pseudolymphoma may closely resemble a true lymphoma but the condition is reversible. Several cases of true lymphomas have been reported in patients with Sjögren's syndrome, thus completing the spectrum of lymphoproliferative findings.[10,11]

2. Occasionally, hypersensitivity to the drug *diphenylhydantoin* will produce a diffuse lymph node enlargement that histologically may simulate Hodgkin's disease.[12] Clinical findings include lymphadenopathy, fever, rash and occasionally hepatosplenomegaly. Removal of the drug leads to a prompt remission. There have been reports of true lymphomas developing in patients taking this drug.[13]

3. *Immunoblastic lymphadenopathy* is a recently described lymphoproliferative entity characterized by a diffuse proliferation of immunoblastic (probably B-cell), plasmacytoid and plasma cells.[14] Symptoms include sweats, weight loss, fever and generalized lymph node enlargement. There is an associated polyclonal hypergammaglobulinemia. In 70 per cent of the cases, drug hypersensitivity has been believed to be the precipitating event.[15] The prognosis is poor, with 18 deaths occurring among the 32 reported cases. Malignant lymphoma, appearing as an uncontrolled proliferation of immunoblasts, was found in three of the terminal cases.

MALIGNANT PROLIFERATION

Etiologic Considerations

A growing body of evidence supports the notion that immunoproliferative malignancies may arise within a setting of benign lymphoproliferation. The occasional development of a true malignancy in the intermediate proliferative states is but one example. Experimental studies in animals have shown that animals subjected to a large antigenic load, usually via exposure to foreign cells or tissues, have a very high incidence of lymphoreticular malignancies.[16-19] Renal-transplant recipients have a greatly increased susceptibility to develop lymphoreticular neoplasia. The reason for this predisposition is currently the subject of intense debate (see Chap. 13), but one theory argues that these patients exist in a state of chronic antigenic stimulation both from the presence of their grafts and from an increased rate of infection due to the immunosuppressive regimens they are on.

Although it is not known for certain why benign lymphoproliferation should predispose to malignancy, there has been no dearth of hypotheses. We will briefly mention several of these (Fig. 12-2).

1. Random genetic mutation has been postulated to be responsible for malignant transformation. It would not be unreasonable to assume that actively dividing cells might be highly susceptible to genetic errors, including malignant mutations. Antigenically stimulated lymphocytes proliferate as rapidly as any cell in the body and thus would fall prey to such molecular mistakes.

Several different types of mutations could lead to uncontrolled lymphocyte proliferation. For example, lymphocytes produce soluble substances, chalones, which inhibit lymphocyte mitosis (see Chap. 5). A mutation that rendered a cell unresponsive to these factors could result in uncontrolled proliferation. Both a human lymphoblast and a lymphocytic lymphoma cell line have been found to produce these factors but to be insensitive to their inhibitory effects.[20,21]

2. There is a considerable body of evidence implicating viruses in animal carcinogenesis. Although the importance of viruses in human malignancy is less certain, there are examples—the association between the Epstein-Barr virus and Burkitt's lymphoma being the best known—in which a viral presence is strongly implicated in carcinogenesis. Resting lymphocytes are usually not welcome hosts for viral replication, but stimulated lymphocytes that have undergone blast transformation readily support infections by a number of viruses (see Chap. 11). Chronic stimulation, producing a continuous supply of a large population of activated lymphocytes, might create a vulnerable target for oncogenic viruses.

3. The oncogene hypothesis postulates that host cells contain a gene, or possibly a few genes, that carry the requisite information for neoplastic transformation. The "oncogene" could be part of the genome of an endogenous virus that is passed from parent to progeny. It has been suggested that activated lymphocytes may occasionally derepress this oncogene, leading to malignant transformation.[22] There is evidence that a chronic

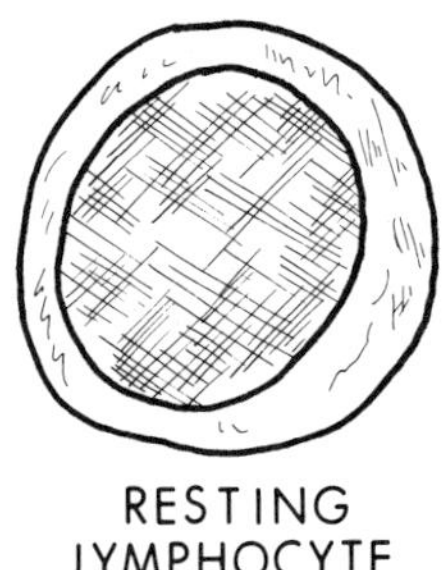

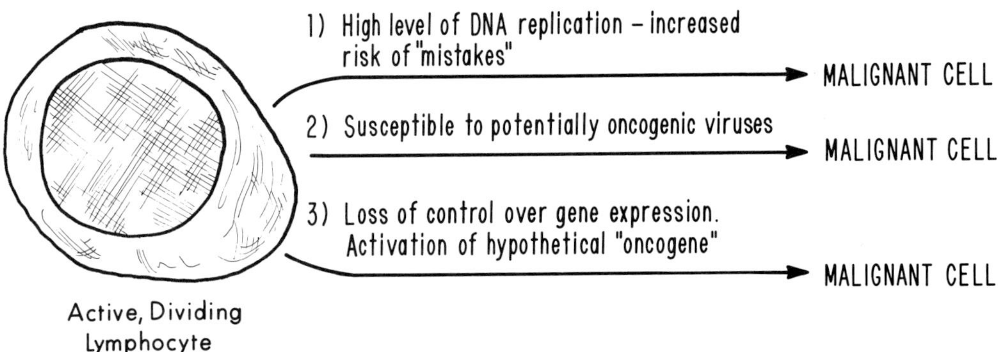

Fig. 12-2. Hypothetical schemes of the possible relationships between lymphoproliferation and oncogenesis.

graft-versus-host reaction in mice, which is associated with a high incidence of lymphomas, induces the expression of a latent malignant tumor virus in the host cells.[22,23]

THE NON-HODGKIN'S LYMPHOMAS

Table 12-1 outlines the current histologic classification of the non-Hodgkin's lymphomas. This classification has been extremely useful clinically and has provided good correlations with prognosis and survival. Several investigators have attempted to further define these disorders on immunologic grounds.[2] Each histologic type of lymphoma is postulated to correspond to a malignancy of one particular kind of immunocompetent cell (Table 12-2).

Of the two general classes of malignant lymphoma, nodular and diffuse, the immunologic restatement has been applied most successfully to the nodular lymphomas. Accordingly, the nodular appearance of these lymphomas may be directly related to the normal reactive lymph node follicles. Though histologic differences have been described, malignant nodules may be difficult to distinguish from benign reactive follicles. One clue that the nodules may correspond to normal follicles is the consistent finding of reticulum cells containing desmosomes in the nodules of the nodular lymphomas.

The histologic classification of the non-Hodgkin's lymphomas is based on the overall appearance of involved nodes as well as cytologic appearances. Thus, on a morphologic basis, two major cell types, lymphocytes and histiocytes, have been felt to be involved in these proliferations. The histiocyte has classically been defined on a morphologic basis and has been

Table 12-1. Histologic Classification of the Non-Hodgkin's Lymphomas

Type of Lymphoma	*Description Based on Morphologic Criteria*
Lymphocytic lymphoma	1. Well differentiated, nodular 2. Well differentiated, diffuse 3. Poorly differentiated, nodular 4. Poorly differentiated, diffuse
Histiocytic lymphoma	1. Nodular 2. Diffuse
Mixed histiocytic-lymphocytic lymphoma	1. Nodular 2. Diffuse
Undifferentiated lymphoma	

considered to be related to the phagocytic cells of the normal lymph node. Four major types of lymphomas have been described: lymphocytic, mixed lymphocytic-histiocytic, histiocytic, and undifferentiated.

Lymphocytic Lymphomas

The lymphocytic lymphomas have been described as being either well differentiated (about 10% of cases) or poorly differentiated (about 90% of cases). These may be unfortunate designations because they derive from assumptions based on traditional morphologic criteria and may not reflect the true state of differentiation of the involved cells.

Well-differentiated lymphocytic lymphoma cells look virtually identical to the small resting lymphocyte (Fig. 12-3A). These monomorphous cells possess stainable surface immunoglobulin in almost all cases, indicative of a B-cell origin. This type of lymphocytic lymphoma is usually diffuse and only rarely nodular.

Poorly differentiated lymphocytic lymphoma is the most common histologic type of lymphoma occurring in the adult (Fig. 12-3B). In contrast to the well-differentiated form, there is a marked preponderance of the nodular pattern. The malignant cells are also B cells and express stainable surface immunoglobulin. However, their appearance is quite different from that of the well-differentiated lymphoma cells. These cells are usually pleomorphic and lack the monotonous character of the cells of well-differentiated lymphocytic lymphoma. Careful examination reveals that they resemble the cells of a normal germinal center undergoing antigen-induced blast transformation. Cleft nuclei and prominent nucleoli are often present. Thus the cells of poorly differentiated lymphocytic lymphoma appear to be related to activated

Table 12-2. Correlation Between Immunologic and Histologic Classifications of the Non-Hodgkin's Lymphomas*

Immunologic Classification	*Histologic Classification*
B-cell lymphomas Small lymphocyte lymphomas	Well-differentiated lymphocytic lymphoma
Follicular center cell types	Poorly differentiated lymphocytic lymphoma
	Mixed histiocytic-lymphocytic lymphoma
Other	
Histiocytic-type lymphomas	Histiocytic lymphoma
Others	

*The arrows indicate where the majority of each histologic type of lymphoma would be classified immunologically. The text will discuss the correlation between histologic and immunologic characteristics in detail.

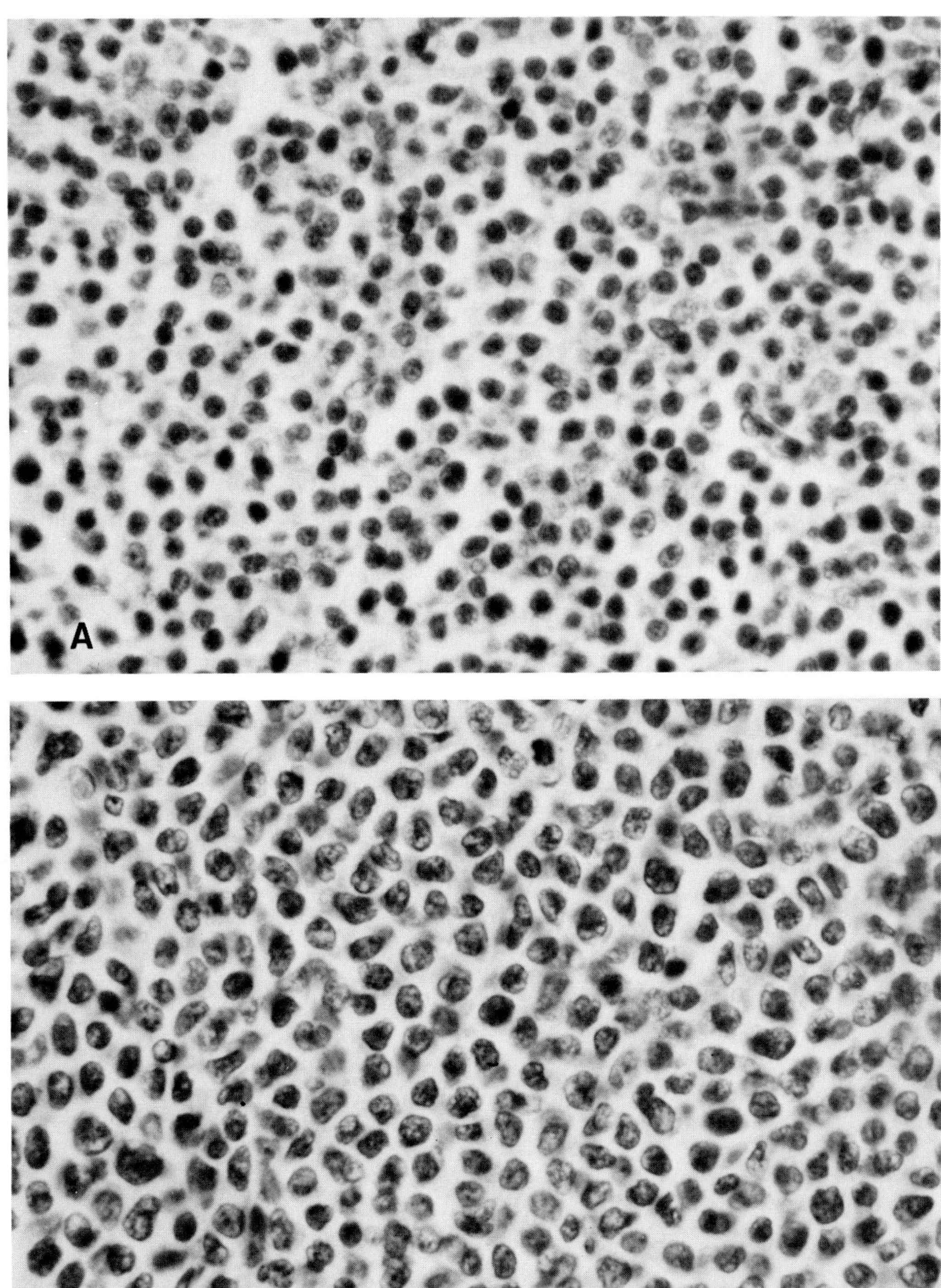

Fig. 12-3. (A) Lymph node from a patient with well-differentiated lymphocytic lymphoma. (B) Lymph node from a patient with poorly differentiated lymphocytic lymphoma.

B cells and may represent a more differentiated cell than the resting lymphocyte analogue of well-differentiated lymphocytic lymphoma.

It is important to emphasize that it is not known for certain that the well-differentiated lymphocytic lymphoma cell represents a malignancy of the small B lymphocyte, nor that the poorly differentiated lymphocytic lymphoma cell is a malignancy of the more differentiated germinal-center cell. This does appear to be a useful model, however, and may offer some unique insights into the behavior of these disease entities:

1. Within the normal lymph node, the small B lymphocyte is not a rapidly dividing cell, whereas the more differentiated germinal-center cells are actively proliferating. If these growth properties are applicable to the malignant counterparts of these cells, we would expect the well-differentiated lymphocytic lymphoma cell to remain a more slowly dividing cell than the poorly differentiated cell. This hypothesis may explain the longer survival time of patients with well-differentiated lymphocytic lymphoma.

2. Poorly differentiated lymphocytic lymphoma occurs predominantly as a nodular lymphoma. Well-differentiated lymphocytic lymphoma can display either a diffuse or, much less commonly, a nodular pattern. In the normal follicle, the small B lymphocyte remains at the periphery and mingles to a varying degree with the more diffuse medullary and paracortical areas. On the other hand, the more differentiated germinal-center cells are more strictly localized to the follicles. If poorly differentiated lymphocytic lymphoma is a malignancy of the germinal-center cells, it is reasonable that it would be more often seen in a nodular form.

3. Both types of lymphocytic lymphoma can be associated with a leukemic phase at some time during their course. The normal circulating B cell is a small lymphocyte and it is somewhat unusual to see germinal-center cells or blast forms in the circulation under normal circumstances. This observation may reflect either differing intrinsic properties of these various cell types or different controls upon the migration and circulation of the B cell at various stages in its differentiation. Whatever the reason for the differential propensity to circulate, it is interesting that the small lymphocyte of well-differentiated lymphocytic lymphoma is apparently more likely to circulate (and produce a leukemic phase of the disease) than is the B cell of poorly differentiated lymphocytic lymphoma.

The cells of well-differentiated lymphocytic lymphoma and of the leukemic phase that may develop during the course of well-differentiated lymphocytic lymphoma are morphologically similar to the peripheral blood cells of chronic lymphocytic leukemia. Nevertheless, it is not known if these disorders are simply different presentations of the same basic disease entity. The leukemic phase of poorly differentiated lymphocytic lymphoma has been called, by some, lymphosarcoma-cell leukemia to distinguish it from the far more common chronic lymphocytic leukemia. The immunologic classification of chronic lymphocytic leukemia and lymphosarcoma leukemia was discussed in Chapter 3.

Histiocytic Lymphomas

Histiocytic lymphomas may also present with either a nodular or a diffuse pattern (Fig. 12-4). The term "histiocytic" lymphoma was determined on a purely morphologic basis because the features of the cells resembled those of histiocytes, the phagocytic cells of the node. However, evidence of phagocytic capabilities and other histiocytic functions has generally been lacking. In addition, further scrutiny reveals that the malignant cells

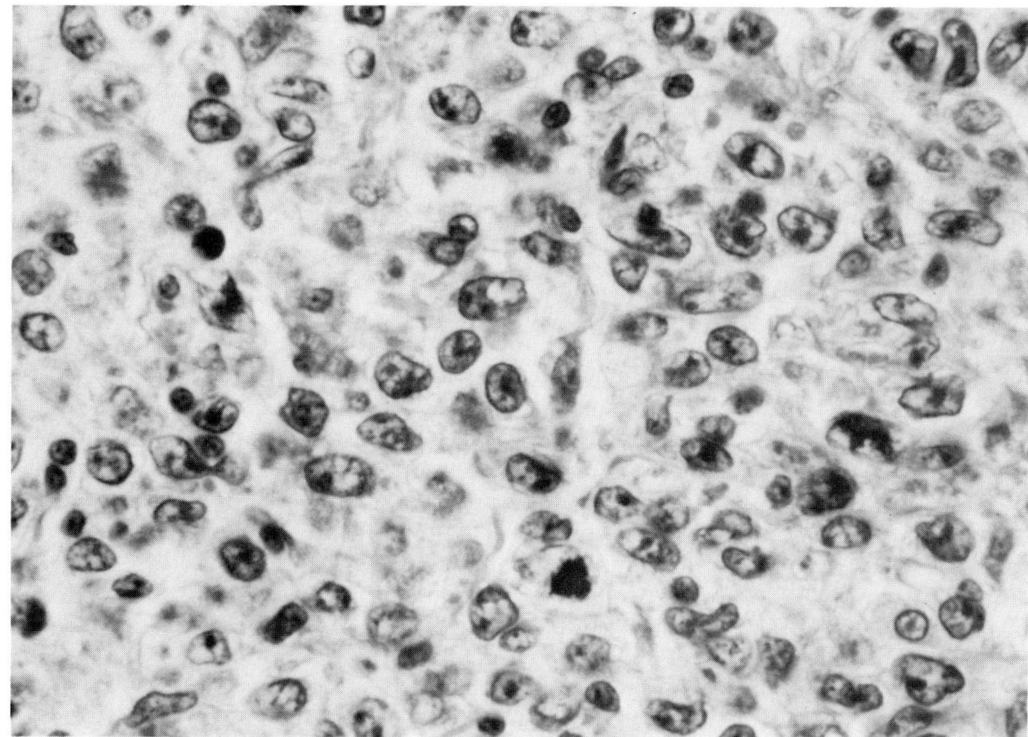

Fig. 12-4. Lymph node from a patient with histiocytic lymphoma.

bear considerable similarity to antigen-transformed lymphocytes.

The malignant cells are larger than circulating lymphocytes and contain vesicular nuclei, nucleoli and abundant cytoplasm which may be pyroninophilic. This description can fit a histiocyte or an immunoblast. Under the electron microscope, normal histiocytes have a well-organized system of organelles; the immunoblast has a much more monotonous cytoplasm. Electron microscopic studies of many cases of histiocytic lymphoma have demonstrated that the cytoplasm of the malignant cell resembles that of an immunoblast.[24] Furthermore, the cells of some cases of histiocytic lymphoma have easily detectable surface immunoglobulin, suggesting a B-cell origin.[25] These observations are strongly suggestive that at least some of the cases heretofore considered histiocytic lymphomas may instead represent malignancies of lymphocyte-derived cells.

Mixed Histiocytic-Lymphocytic Lymphomas

These lymphomas contain cells of both small lymphocyte and large "histiocyte" morphologies (Fig. 12-5). They are usually nodular. If the histiocytic cells are truly immunoblasts, then mixed lymphomas would represent germinal-center lymphocyte-derived neoplasms in which a limited degree of normal differentiation is preserved. It is interesting in this regard that most cases of mixed lymphomas eventually acquire a predominantly "histiocytic" appearance.

Undifferentiated Lymphoma

Burkitt's lymphoma is described as an undifferentiated lymphoma because it has

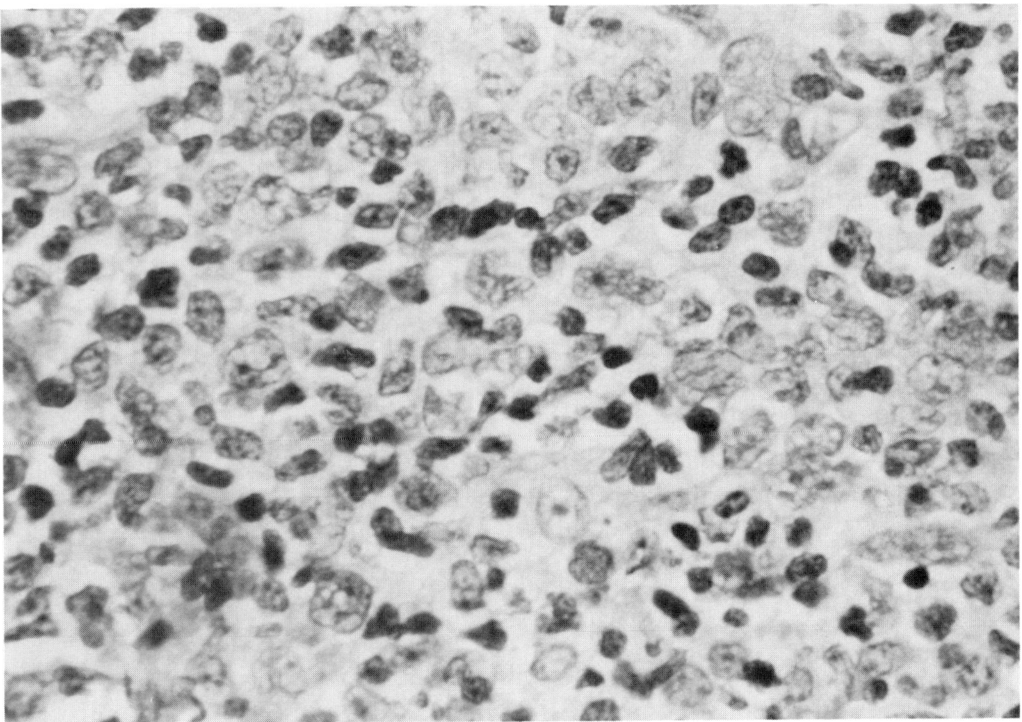

Fig. 12-5. Lymph node from a patient with mixed histiocytic-lymphocytic lymphoma.

been felt to lack morphologic characteristics of either histiocytic or lymphocytic differentiation (Fig. 12-6). This tumor is endemic in the tropical regions of Africa and New Guinea. It is predominantly a disease of childhood and most commonly involves the jaw bones. It is rare to see a leukemic phase. The Epstein-Barr virus has been implicated as the causative agent.[26]

Histologically, the tumor consists of sheets of small, relatively uniform cells. Mitoses are frequent. The sheets of abnormal cells are often interspersed with large clear macrophages. The presence of these cells lends the biopsy specimen its "starry sky" appearance.

The morphologic appellation of "undifferentiated" is probably misleading in light of recent studies which show that the malignant cells possess surface immunoglobulin.[27] As with the other B-cell malignancies, the cells seem to derive from a single clone.

A small percentage of the non-Hodgkin's lymphomas appears to consist of T cells as defined by surface markers. We do not yet know whether the clinical course of such lymphomas is any different than the far more common B-cell lymphomas.

Immune Defects in Patients with Non-Hodgkin's Lymphomas and Lymphocytic Leukemia

Patients with lymphoma and those with chronic lymphocytic leukemia (CLL) have a notoriously increased incidence of infections of all kinds, notably bacterial or due to usually nonpathogenic organisms such as opportunistic fungi.[28-30] The increased rate and severity of infections in these patients correlate with the extent of their immune depression.[28]

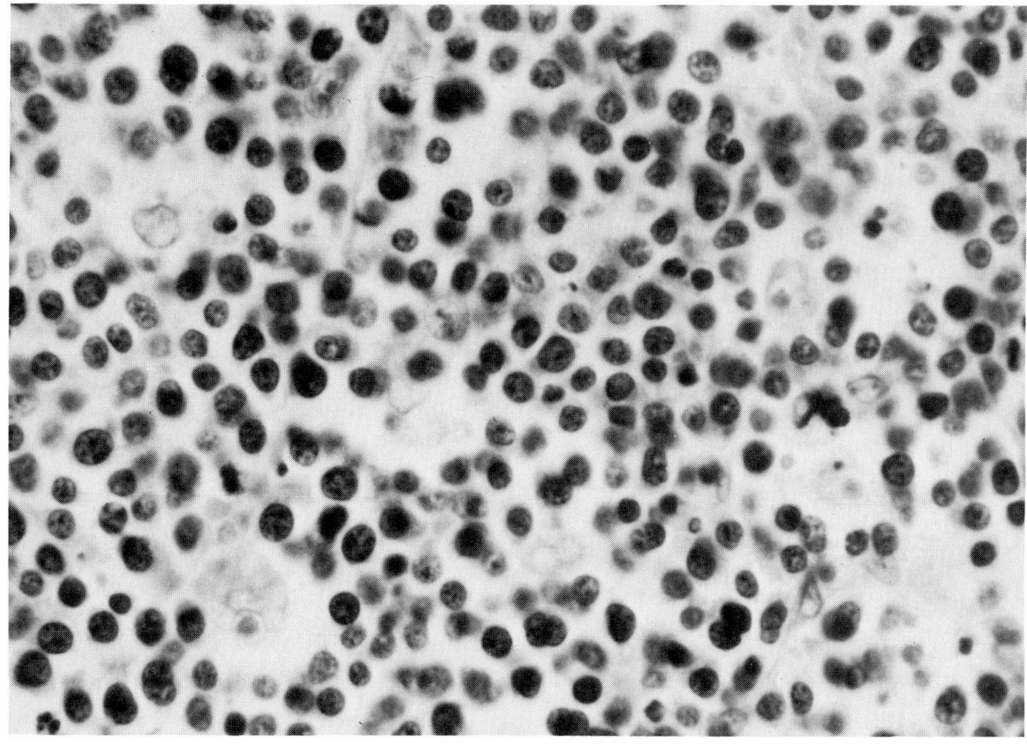

Fig. 12-6. Lymph node from a patient with undifferentiated lymphoma.

Abnormalities of immunoglobulin production are by far the most common immunologic abnormalities in patients with non-Hodgkin's lymphomas,[31] a finding consistent with the B-cell nature of these diseases. Hypergammaglobulinemia is common, and monoclonal immunoglobulin spikes may be present.[32] The latter finding is presumably a reflection of immunoglobulin production by a single clone of proliferating neoplastic cells. Hypogammaglobulinemia has been reported in 15 per cent or more of patients with non-Hodgkin's lymphomas. Most commonly this takes the form of a selective IgM deficiency but other selective and combined deficiencies can occur.[33] The origin of the hypogammaglobulinemia in these patients is not known.

Although serum immunoglobulin levels are a useful measure of humoral abnormality, the production of specific antibodies is a much finer probe of immunocompetency. Thus, some patients with non-Hodgkin's lymphomas have depressed levels of antiviral complement-fixing antibody titers.[34] The increased susceptibility to bacterial infections, notably by the streptococcus and pneumococcus, provides further evidence for a diminished ability to produce antigen-specific antibody.

Most studies have failed to detect any compromise in cell-mediated immunity with the exception of the finding of delayed allograft rejection in a few patients.[35]

Abnormalities of immune function in patients with chronic lymphocytic leukemia are very common. It has been reported that approximately one half of all patients with CLL are hypogammaglobulinemic, often to a severe extent.[28,36] This may be at least partially responsible for their increased susceptibility to infections. Many patients exhibit a decreased ability to produce antibodies against specific antigens.[37]

One prominent humoral abnormality is the production of IgG antibodies directed against erythrocyte antigens which may lead to hemolytic anemia in greater than 10 per cent of all patients with CLL.[38,39] It is not known why chronic lymphocytic leukemia is so often the setting for the production of these autoantibodies. The antibodies are polyclonal and there is no evidence that they are produced by the monoclonal proliferating clone of leukemic lymphocytes.

Peripheral blood lymphocytes from patients with CLL exhibit diminished responses to the T-cell mitogen PHA.[40,41] However, it is not known whether this finding reflects an intrinsic T-cell defect or whether it is the result of the dilution of T cells by the large number of abnormal leukemic lymphocytes. Otherwise, there is little evidence to support a significant deficiency in cell-mediated immunity in these patients. In fact, some patients have been described who appear to have exaggerated delayed hypersensitivity responses.[42]

CLL lymphocytes, believed to be derived from B cells, also display a subnormal response to B-cell mitogens, suggesting an immune defect in the malignant cell population.[41] One study has suggested that there is a serum inhibitory factor that depresses B-cell and T-cell mitogen responsiveness.[43]

HODGKIN'S DISEASE

Hodgkin's disease is a malignant lymphoproliferative disorder that arises in the lymph nodes. Diagnosis depends upon the presence of the distinctive Sternberg-Reed giant cell in the appropriate histologic setting (Fig. 12-7). Many abnormal cells can be identified in addition to the Sternberg-Reed cell, and investigators still disagree about which of these cells constitutes the malignant entity in Hodgkin's disease. An inflammatory reaction accompanies the presence of these abnormal cells.

Hodgkin's disease has been classified into four histologic types, each reflecting a unique relationship between the abnormal cells and the reactive elements. The latter are mostly lymphocytes which can be observed in different stages of reactive transformation. Neutrophils, eosinophils and plasma cells may also be present. The classification of Hodgkin's disease is as follows:[44]

1. *Lymphocyte Predominance.* Lymphocytes greatly outnumber the abnormal cells.
2. *Mixed Cellularity.* There is a more equal proportion of malignant-appearing cells and lymphocytes.
3. *Lymphocyte Depletion.* There are many abnormal cells and few lymphocytes.
4. *Nodular Sclerosis.* Malignant-appearing cells and lymphocytes appear in islands surrounded by bands of fibrous tissue.

The normal architecture of involved lymph nodes is usually obliterated by the disease process. Each histologic picture usually involves the entire node diffusely and follicular structures are rarely seen.

As with the non-Hodgkin's lymphomas, we can look at the different cell types of Hodgkin's disease in terms of their relationship to normal immune cells and attempt to apply this understanding to the different patterns of disease.

The Sternberg-Reed cell has long been considered to be a malignant histiocyte on morphologic grounds. It is a bizarre cell with a characteristic "owl's eye" appearance produced by binuclearity with a prominent nucleolus in each nucleus. The cells are large but the nuclear-to-cytoplasmic ratio is relatively high. It is not uncommon to observe mitoses. Ultrastructural studies have supported the histiocytic origin of the Sternberg-Reed

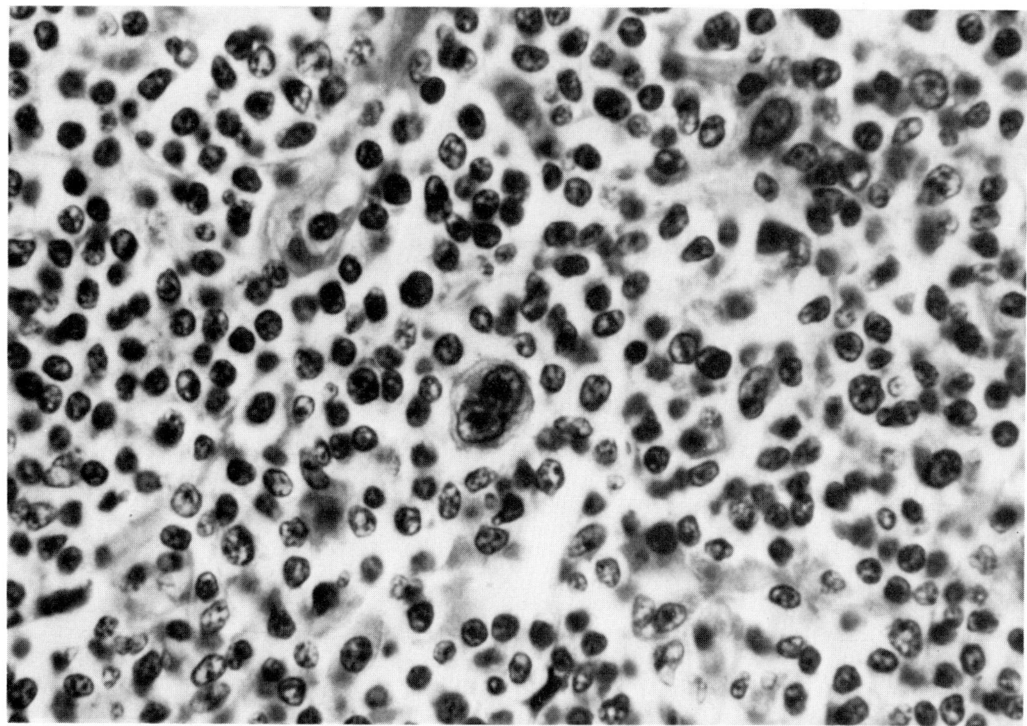

Fig. 12-7. Lymph node from a patient with Hodgkin's disease showing a Sternberg-Reed cell.

cell,[45] but other studies have questioned this view. Histiocytes can be distinguished from lymphocytes by histochemical demonstration of hydrolytic enzymes present only in the former. Sternberg-Reed cells lack these enzymes and thus appear histochemically related to lymphocyte-derived cells.[46] There are reports that Sternberg-Reed cells contain both cytoplasmic and surface immunoglobulin,[47,48] and some investigators have suggested that the Sternberg-Reed cell may be a B-cell-derived blast. The question of the origin of the Sternberg-Reed cell is still not resolved, and it is certainly not impossible that in some cases it represents a malignant histiocyte and in others a malignant B cell.

A useful, although speculative, model for the interpretation of the histologic findings in Hodgkin's disease views the process as a struggle between the proliferation of malignant cells and the response of the immune and inflammatory systems. The histology may vary depending upon which adversary seems to be gaining the upper hand. According to this model, nodular sclerosis can be viewed as a relatively successful attempt to contain the malignancy with an effective inflammatory response. There are few Sternberg-Reed cells and the histologic picture is dominated by reactive cells and the scars of fibrosis. Nodular sclerosis has a good five-year survival rate.[49]

The other three types of Hodgkin's disease are even more graphic illustrations of the postulated contest between the two opposing forces. There is a definite inverse relationship between the prominence of abnormal cells and the number of surrounding lymphocytes. Patients with lymphocyte depletion carry a much worse prognosis than those with lymphocyte predominance; mixed cellularity falls in between.[49] Patients with

Hodgkin's disease have been observed to progress toward an end stage of lymphocyte depletion. Thus, one might speculate that without therapeutic intervention, the immune/inflammatory forces almost always lose the battle as the malignant cells outpace the host's attempts at containment, and death results.

The majority of lymphocytes in the nodes of Hodgkin's disease are T cells and the population of reactive cells is similar to that seen in normally reactive nodes.[50] One can postulate that the malignant cells in Hodgkin's disease present an immunogenic target to the host immune system (tumor cells can express new surface antigens) and thus can further predict that the lymphocyte-predominance form is the product of a significant antitumor response. The relationship between the reactive T cells and the altered B cells in infectious mononucleosis may serve as a model for this process (see earlier in the chapter).

Immune Defects in Patients with Hodgkin's Disease

It appears that the immune system in patients with Hodgkin's disease is progressively overwhelmed and suppressed, although the mechanisms by which this occurs have not been successfully elucidated. It has been known for quite some time that the immune system can be severely deficient in patients with Hodgkin's disease. In contrast with the other lymphomas, Hodgkin's disease is characterized by deficient cellular immunity. This can be demonstrated *in vivo* by:

1. Anergy to skin test antigens.[44,51,52] According to one study, approximately one third of patients with stage 1, 2 or 3A Hodgkin's disease display cutaneous anergy while greater than two thirds of patients with advanced disease are anergic.[52] Other reports have found a lesser incidence of cutaneous anergy.[51]

2. Inability to become sensitized to new antigens[44]

3. Diminished ability to reject skin allografts[53]

These defects are progressive, in step with the progress of the disease, and may contribute to the high incidence and severity of infections. Although the majority of infections are bacterial, it is not uncommon for these patients to contract viral, fungal and parasitic infections as well, often with organisms that are usually of low virulence.

Decreased T-cell function *in vitro* is also evident. The most carefully studied example has been the lymphocyte-proliferative response to PHA. Careful analysis of dose-response curves to PHA has revealed T-cell defects, even in patients with early-stage Hodgkin's disease, which become more severe with advancing disease.[52,54,55]

Defects in the inflammatory response have also been observed. Patients with Hodgkin's disease fail to mobilize neutrophils and monocytes effectively at sites of injury.[56] Some patients with Hodgkin's disease have been found to possess a serum factor that prevents neutrophil and monocyte migration to a variety of chemotactic agents.[57] It is possible that macrophage dysfunction, perhaps on the basis of inhibitory serum substances, may make a significant contribution to many aspects of the abnormal cellular immunity in these patients.

Peripheral lymphocytopenia also tends to progress as the malignancy expands. It has been suggested that this may represent a type of immune exhaustion from chronic antigenic stimulation.[58] Autoimmune destruction of lymphocytes has also been offered as a pathogenetic mechanism. A majority of patients with Hodgkin's disease have been reported to possess autoantibodies to their own lymphocytes.[59] These can be cytotoxic and have been termed lymphocytotoxins. Their maximum activity *in vitro*, however, occurs at temperatures between 10 and 20 degrees C. and thus their importance *in vivo* remains to be established. Lymphocytotoxins have been described in two patients with immunodeficiency presenting with lymphopenia and immunologic defects much like those of Hodgkin's disease.[60] Although a direct etiologic relationship between lymphocytotoxin production and the immune deficiency has not been established, it would not be an unreasonable expectation since the administration of antilymphocyte serum to humans can cause lymphopenia and functional immune deficits (see Chap. 16).[61]

LYMPHOPROLIFERATIVE DISEASES WITH T-CELL CHARACTERISTICS

The majority of lymphoproliferative malignancies appear to be of B-cell origin. There are, however, a group of lymphoproliferative syndromes that are now being referred to as the *cutaneous T-cell lymphomas* and which are exciting a great deal of interest. As the name implies, these disorders are characterized by a proliferation of malignant cells with T-cell characteristics. The major clinical feature is one of skin infiltration by the abnormal cells. Two such syndromes have been traditionally recognized, mycosis fungoides and Sezary's syndrome. We shall see that these may represent a single disease entity.

Mycosis Fungoides

Mycosis fungoides is a rare lymphoma of the skin which carries a grave prognosis; approximately 50 per cent of patients die within four years of biopsy diagnosis.[62] In its early stages there is a nonspecific infiltration of inflammatory cells into the skin, and a definitive diagnosis cannot be made on biopsy. Mononuclear cells dominate the lesion, and neutrophils and eosinophils may also be prominent. The infiltrating lymphocytes cannot be diagnosed as malignant at this time. The skin lesions progressively thicken and plaques develop. The cytologic picture now assumes a more characteristic appearance, and the diagnosis becomes apparent. Mononuclear cells continue to be the major cell type present, and they may appear in bizarre forms. Included among these unusual monocytes are very large cells with darkly staining nuclei which are extraordinarily convoluted and serpentine. These are called *mycosis cells* (Fig. 12-8), and are considered to be characteristic of mycosis fungoides although they have been described in other situations as well. Clusters of abnormal cells form Pautrier's microabscesses in the epidermis. Skin tumors develop, ulcers may form, and eventually the disease process spreads to the peripheral lymph nodes and the viscera, and death ensues.[62]

Sezary's Syndrome

Sezary's syndrome is a chronic lymphoid leukemia associated with erythroderma, edema and intense pruritus.[63] The skin lesions are identical to those of mycosis fungoides except that tumor formation and ulceration are less common. The dermis is heavily infiltrated with malignant-appearing cells and epidermal invasion can result in the formation of Pautrier's microabscesses. The histologic appearance of the skin cannot be distinguished from that of mycosis fungoides. Lymph node enlargement and hepatosplenomegaly are common, and leukocyte counts can be very high. The leukemic cell is a large cell with marked nuclear convolutions, called the Sezary cell; it is indistinguishable from the tissue-bound mycosis cell.[63]

The great similarity between mycosis fungoides and Sezary's syndrome has led to the suggestion that they represent different manifestations of a single disease process. Sezary's syndrome may be viewed as the leukemic variant of the

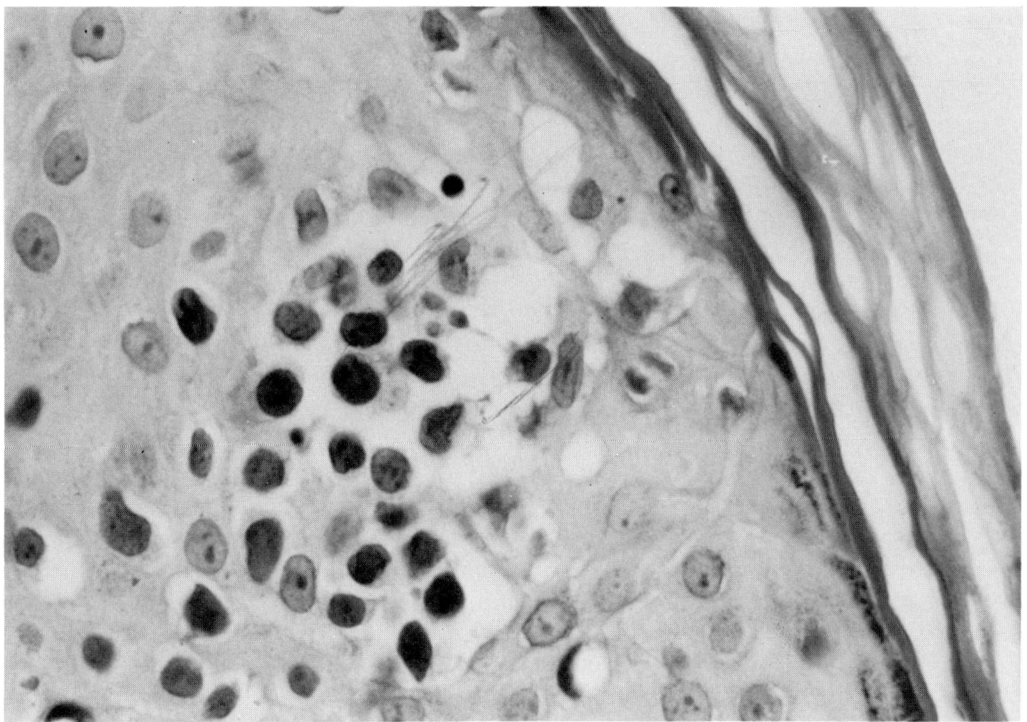

Fig. 12-8. Several mycosis cells (large cells with a convoluted nucleus) are seen within a Pautrier's abscess in the skin of a patient with mycosis fungoides.

basic cutaneous lymphoma of mycosis fungoides. We shall therefore explore these disorders as if they were one, a perspective that has gained the support of many workers in the field.[63,64]

The Sezary (Mycosis) Cell[65]

The Sezary cell has been shown to be lymphocytic in origin. Surface marker characterization has revealed the presence of human T-cell antigenic markers and the ability to form spontaneous rosettes with sheep red blood cells.[66,67] Easily detectable surface immunoglobulin is not present. For these reasons mycosis fungoides and Sezary's syndrome have been referred to as the cutaneous T-cell lymphomas.

Two forms of the Sezary cell have been identified, a large cell and a smaller cell.[68] The small cell is the same size as a normal resting lymphocyte or the malignant cell of chronic lymphocytic leukemia. It can be distinguished from these other cells by the characteristic convoluted nucleus although electron microscopy is often required to make this distinction. The existence of large and small Sezary cells may be related to specific defects in the normal cell cycle. Thus, in some studies, the small cell has been shown to possess the normal diploid chromosome number whereas the large cell may be tetraploid.[63] In addition, the small cell contains less intracellular DNA polymerase than the larger Sezary cell. It has therefore been hypothesized that the small cell is locked in the G1 (pre-DNA replication) phase of the cell cycle. The large cell, on the other hand, may have successfully completed DNA replication but is unable to enter mitosis because of an inability to move beyond the G2 (postreplication) phase. We do wish to emphasize that there is little direct evidence as yet to support these contentions.

The Relation of the Cutaneous T-Cell Lymphomas to Benign Cutaneous T-Cell Proliferation

Just as the lymphomas with B-cell characteristics may bear a relationship to the normal process of B-cell differentiation, the cutaneous T-cell lymphomas may possess correlates in normal T-cell reactivity. The existence of a spectrum of benign cutaneous T-cell disorders suggests that the transition between a typical immune response and a lymphoproliferative neoplasm may be a subtle one. These diseases have been termed the *benign dermal lymphocytic reticuloses.*[69] Histologic examination of the cells in psoriasis, lichen planus and cutaneous vasculitis has revealed cells that are extremely similar to the malignant cells of Sezary's syndrome and mycosis fungoides.[70] In the benign lymphocytic reticuloses, however, there is no compelling reason to believe that these bizarre cells are malignant.

Among the nonmalignant dermatoses that have been examined for a possible relationship to the cutaneous lymphomas are lymphomatoid papulosis and parapsoriasis en plaques. Lymphomatoid papulosis is a clinically benign disorder which histologically appears malignant.[71] Many of the infiltrating cells have the morphologic appearance of Sezary's cells and have recently been defined as T cells.[72] Parapsoriasis en plaques is characterized by a mononuclear cell infiltrate which includes Sezary-like cells.[73] This last observation is especially intriguing since parapsoriasis en plaques is considered to be a premalignant state from which mycosis fungoides may develop.[73a]

These observations suggest that the conditions that give rise to Sezary's syndrome and mycosis fungoides may share much in common with certain benign cutaneous lymphoproliferative disorders. Once again, we must consider the possibility that malignant lymphoproliferation is an exaggerated and/or uncontrolled proliferative response bearing a close relationship to benign proliferation.

Disease Manifestations Associated with the T-Cell Nature of these Disorders

One of the goals of immunologically classifying the lymphoproliferative diseases is the possibility of understanding some of the manifestations of each disorder in light of the known characteristics of the normal, benign counterparts of the malignant cells. Despite the recent advances in immunologic classification of the T-cell lymphomas, this goal has not been readily obtained. Nevertheless, certain characteristics of the normal T cell may explain certain features of these malignant T-cell disorders.

The normal T cell is a migratory cell and comprises the majority of the recirculating pool of lymphocytes. Although it is a mobile cell, it traverses a somewhat limited portion of the body. For example, the normal T cell is much less abundant in the bone marrow than the B lymphocyte. It is perhaps not surprising, therefore, that the marrow is relatively spared in the cutaneous T-cell lymphomas, even in severe cases with high peripheral leukocyte counts.

The reasons for the cutaneous involvement in these T-cell lymphomas are more obscure. The predilection of T-cell malignancies for involving the skin is illustrated by the 2 per cent of patients diagnosed as having chronic lymphocytic leukemia who present with an exfoliative erythroderma indistinguishable from that of Sezary's syndrome.[74] In one study, examination of the malignant cells of these patients revealed that they were T cells.[75] The cells in some of these patients displayed convoluted nuclei and appeared indistinguishable from the small-cell variety of Sezary's syndrome. Some patients with T-cell chronic lymphocytic leukemia and erythroderma do not have these distinctive lymphocytes and may have a different type of T-cell malignancy. More likely is the possibility that we are once again dealing with a spectrum of disease since careful study of the malignant cells of mycosis fungoides has revealed a gradation of nuclear contours from conspicuously convoluted to nearly rounded.[76]

Several theories have been advanced to explain the apparent predisposition of T-cell lymphoproliferative diseases for involving the skin:

1. We have already emphasized the possible role of chronic antigenic stimulation in providing a fertile setting for malignant lymphoproliferation. One of the responses to antigenic challenge in the cutaneous tissues is a typical delayed hypersensitivity response, involving the migration and proliferation of T cells. Thus the T-cell population might be susceptible to chronic stimulation by cutaneous antigens. No particular antigen has been identified in the malignant or premalignant T-cell lesions, but the possibility that these disorders arise from chronic inflammation is an attractive one.

2. There are several reasons to believe that a special relationship exists between the T cell and the skin: (1) epithelial cells are one of the few nonlymphoid cells capable of stimulating allogeneic lymphocytes in a mixed lymphocyte reaction. These cells must therefore express "LD" antigens in a manner similar to lymphocytes (see Chap. 9).[77] (2) Mouse epithelial cells express the θ antigen, a T-cell surface marker.[78] (3) Nude mice lack mature thymuses as well as cutaneous hair.[79]

We can conclude very little from these observations at present. However, they do suggest that the skin bears a unique but recondite relationship to the T lymphocyte.

Immune Abnormalities in the Cutaneous T-Cell Lymphomas

Dramatic immunodeficiency states such as those which occur in Hodgkin's disease are *not* seen in the cutaneous T-cell syndromes. Patients with premalignant lesions such as lymphomatoid papulosis do not exhibit any clinically overt immune defects. Most patients with mycosis fungoides also appear to be immunologically normal and only rarely display anergy to skin test antigens.[63] Incubation of the patient's lymphocytes with skin test antigens *in vitro* may reveal a subnormal response.[63]

Immunodeficiency is more apparent in patients with the Sezary variant. They display cutaneous anergy in addition to decreased responsiveness of their peripheral blood lymphocytes to antigens and mitogens *in vitro*.[63] Serum from affected patients will not block the functions of normal lymphocytes, but there are reports that an extract obtained from Sezary cells can inhibit the migration of monocytes and macrophages. It is analogous to a similar substance described in patients with other types of malignant lymphomas.

T helper function and B-cell function appear normal in this patients. Patients with cutaneous T-cell lymphomas rarely present with hypogammaglobulinemia, in marked contrast to many patients with B-cell lymphoproliferative diseases. In fact, IgA and IgE levels are often elevated.[82] These immunoglobulin classes are considered to be highly dependent upon T-cell helper function (see Chap. 6). The ability to mount antigen-specific antibody responses also appears to be well preserved. It is possible that T helper cells are selectively spared by the disease process or that the malignant cells maintain the ability to provide helper function. In one instance, Sezary cells were able to restore the ability of B cells taken from a patient with a primary T-cell deficiency and panhypogammaglobulinemia to secrete immunoglobulin *in vitro*.[83]

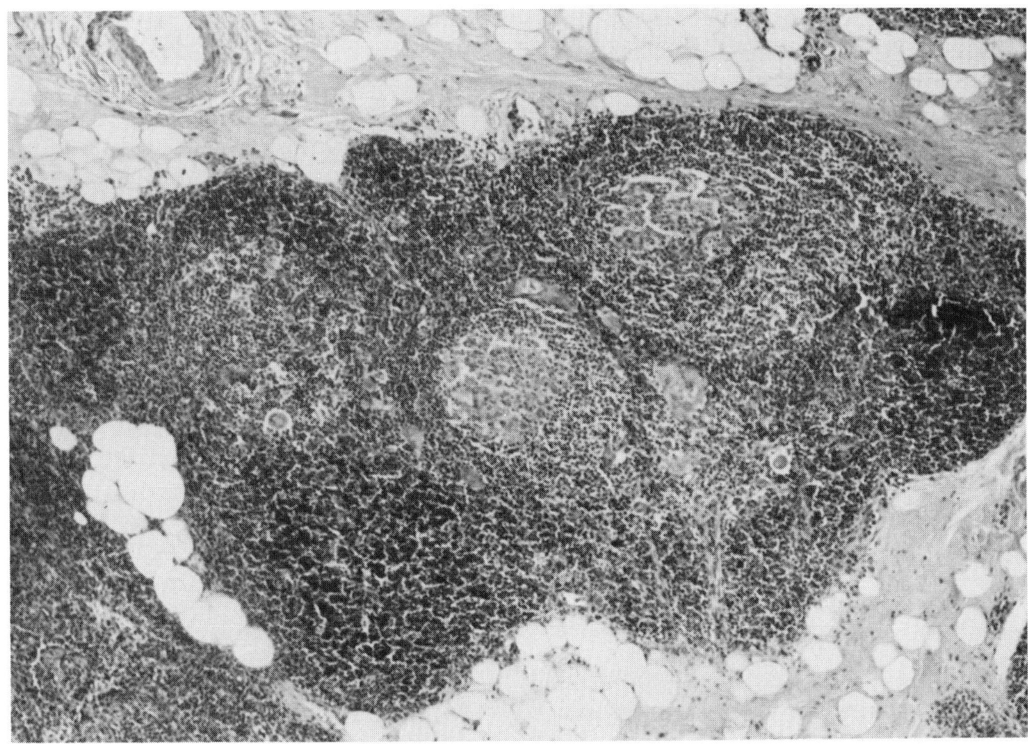

Fig. 12-9. Hyperplasia of the thymus illustrating the presence of germinal centers within the gland.

PROLIFERATIVE DISEASES OF THE THYMUS

Just as there are immunodeficiency disorders associated with thymic hypoplasia (Chap. 10), there are also several diseases associated with cellular proliferation within the thymus. Thymic proliferation can present as thymic hyperplasia or thymoma.

THYMIC HYPERPLASIA

Thymic hyperplasia might more accurately be termed thymic dysplasia since the thymus often maintains its normal size. The characteristic histologic finding is the presence of proliferating germinal centers (Fig. 12-9). This is a distinctly abnormal finding; B cells and plasma cells are not normally found in the thymus. The presence of germinal centers in the thymus is associated with a number of systemic diseases most prominent of which is myasthenia gravis. Approximately 60 to 70 per cent of patients with myasthenia gravis have thymic hyperplasia.[84] Other disorders that are sometimes associated with thymic hyperplasia include systemic lupus erythematosus, rheumatoid arthritis, hypogammaglobulinemia, aplastic anemia and others.[85]

The appearance of germinal centers in the thymus is thought to represent B-cell reactivity against an antigenic challenge within the thymus.[86] Ectopic germinal centers can occur in other sites and in other situations as well. For example, the inflamed synovium of rheumatoid arthritis may become so filled with germinal centers and infiltrating lymphocytes that it resembles a lymph node.[87]

An experimental model for the development of thymic germinal centers has utilized the injection of antigen directly into animal thymuses.[86] The response to the antigenic challenge begins with a proliferation of epithelial cells. The antigen is phagocytosed, most likely by the cells of the Hassall's corpuscles. Lymphocytes and plasma cells appear around the corpuscles and within one month full-blown proliferating germinal centers can be detected. If this model is an accurate reflection of the source of spontaneously generating germinal centers, a basic question which emerges is: what is the antigen that induces thymic hyperplasia in the various disease states listed above? We shall return to this issue below.

THYMOMA

There have been more than one thousand cases of *thymoma* reported in the literature. Some thymomas are clearly malignant while others are benign. It is not known, however, if the malignant lesions develop out of previously benign lesions.[88] Four histologic types have been identified: epithelial, lymphocytic, mixed lymphoepithelial and spindle cell.[89] The spindle cells are believed to be of epithelial origin, and comprise the highest percentage of thymomas.[90]

In a large review of patients with thymoma, it was found that over 70 per cent suffered from an associated systemic disease.[91] These included, in decreasing order of occurrence, myasthenia gravis, hematologic abnormalities, extrathymic cancer, hypogammaglobulinemia, polymyositis, systemic lupus erythematosus and other immunologic disorders. This list is very similar to the list of diseases associated with thymic hyperplasia, and raises the issue of whether thymic hyperplasia and thymoma are in some way related.

Diseases Associated with Thymoma

1. Diseases in which abnormal immunologic phenomena are seen:
   - Myasthenia gravis
   - Pure red cell aplasia
   - Hypogammaglobulinemia
   - Systemic lupus erythematosus
   - Polymyositis
2. Cancer
3. Endocrine disorders:
   - Cushing's disease
   - Hyperthyroidism
   - Addison's disease

It has been suggested that the appearance of germinal centers precedes the development of thymomas in myasthenia gravis.[92] Thymomas are usually seen late in the disease process, and germinal-center proliferation can be seen in the normal, surrounding, nonthymomatous thymic tissue. Some recent work has failed to support the concept of the evolution of thymomas out of a setting of germinal-center proliferation. One report has indicated that patients with thymic hyperplasia and those with thymoma may be separable on the basis of HLA typing.[93] The former group showed a high association with the HLA-B8 allele, whereas the latter had an association, albeit less impressive, with HLA-A3. The existence of two distinct populations of patients would undermine the notion that thymic hyperplasia will progress to thymoma.

THYMIC PROLIFERATION AND AUTOIMMUNE DISEASE

Autoimmune diseases are the most common type of disorders associated with thymic proliferation. In Chapter 8 we saw that there are essentially two ways in which tolerance to self-antigens might be broken and autoimmunity result: by bypassing the block in immune reactivity, for example, by challenging the host with an antigen that crossreacts with a host constituent, and by a loss of suppressive mechanisms. Utilizing these principles, it is apparent that the thymus could be involved in extrathymic autoimmunity in the following ways:

1. Autoimmune phenomena could be directed against thymic antigens which crossreact with antigens on other tissues.

2. Thymic dysfunction could result in the loss of dynamic controls over autoreactivity; for example, the loss of thymic-dependent T suppressor cells or the stimulation of autoreactive clones of lymphocytes within the thymus.

Myasthenia Gravis

Myasthenia gravis is a chronic disease that is characterized by neuromuscular dysfunction leading to various degrees of weakness and fatigability. The muscles most commonly affected are the facial, ocular, laryngeal, pharyngeal and respiratory muscles. A generalized weakness of voluntary muscles may occur in advanced disease and primarily affects the proximal musculature.

Myasthenia gravis has the highest association of any disease with thymic proliferation. Sixty-five per cent of myasthenic patients have thymic hyperplasia with germinal-center proliferation and another 10 per cent have thymomas. As many as 45 per cent of patients with thymomas have myasthenia.[91]

Autoimmunity in Myasthenia Gravis. Myasthenia gravis is associated with several autoimmune phenomena which may be of pathogenic significance in the development of the clinical syndrome. The production of autoantibodies against muscle acetylcholine receptors in particular has been implicated in the disease process. A majority of patients with myasthenia gravis have been reported to have serum antibodies directed against their own acetylcholine receptors.[94]

A myasthenia-like syndrome can be experimentally induced in animals by injecting them with purified acetylcholine receptors. This has been demonstrated in rabbits injected with receptors from the electric eel *Electrophus electricus*[95] and in rats injected either with electric eel receptors or syngeneic rat muscle acetylcholine receptors.[95a] These animals develop weakness and fatigability, and electromyography shows evidence of decreased neuromuscular transmission.[95a] In rats with experimental autoimmune myasthenia gravis, one can detect autoantibodies to muscle acetylcholine receptors both in the serum and complexed to the receptor moieties. The antibodies do not appear to bind precisely to the acetylcholine binding site. Perhaps most importantly, the complete clinical syndrome can be transferred from animal to animal by purified IgG taken from sera of rats with experimental autoimmune myasthenia gravis.[95b]

There is also some evidence implicating cellular autoimmunity in myasthenia. Lymphocytes taken from a majority of patients with myasthenia gravis exhibit blast transformation when challenged with purified acetylcholine receptors *in vitro*. The degree of stimulation may correlate with disease activity. Normal lymphocytes or lymphocytes taken from patients with other neuromuscular disorders are much less reactive in this system.[96]

Other autoantibodies are present in myasthenia, including antibodies directed against striated muscle fibers, thymic tissue and occasionally antithyroid and antinuclear antibodies.[97] However, these antibodies are not specific for myasthenia, and suggest only a general malfunction of the immune system. Cell-mediated hypersensitivity directed against autologous muscle fibers has also been demonstrated.[98]

How do these autoimmune phenomena relate to the thymic proliferation seen so commonly in these patients? It has been known for some time that thymic epithelial cells crossreact with muscle cells.[99] Since myasthenia patients often have antithymic antibodies, investigators have suggested that the primary autoantigen may be the thymus itself. This view is supported by the experimental finding that immunization with thymic tissue, producing an autoimmune thymitis, results in a myasthenic neuromuscular disorder in animals.[100] Thus, it would be satisfying to find a crossreactive mechanism that could account for the appearance of the potentially pathogenic antiacetylcholine receptor antibodies. So far, this has not been done. One possibility derives from the presence of acetylcholine receptors on lymphocytes (see Chap. 4). There is one report that thymic lymphocytes from myasthenic patients with thymic hyperplasia will stimulate a proliferative response by the patient's own peripheral lymphocytes.[101] One could speculate that the receptors on thymic lymphocytes might be the primary antigenic targets for the autoreactive clones. One difficulty with this hypothesis is that the neuromuscular dysfunction of myasthenia gravis involves the nicotinic acetylcholine receptors, whereas the lymphocyte receptors appear to be muscarinic.[102]

The crossreactive mechanism is certainly not the only way in which the thymus or thymic cells could be implicated in the disease. Thymic dysfunction could lead to a loss of T suppressor cells or a release of self-reactive clones. At present there is no evidence to allow us to choose among these mechanisms.

Attributing the pathogenesis of myasthenia gravis to the presence of antithymic autoimmune phenomena or an escape from immune regulation merely shifts the blame from the neuromuscular junction to the thymus, leaving still unanswered the question of why a person should develop thymic dysfunction or autoimmunity in the first place. The suggestion that a viral mechanism may be involved[102a] has not yet found experimental support.

Thymectomy in Myasthenia Gravis. Thymectomy has been used as a treatment for myasthenia gravis for almost half a century. Although its efficacy was suspect for a long time,[103] recent studies have affirmed its utility and thymectomy has become an established and successful mode of treatment.[103] The success of thymectomy provides convincing evidence for the involvement of the thymus in the disease process.

One of the reasons for the early confusion about the relative merits of thymectomy may have been due to the typical delay in remission following thymectomy; the disease symptoms may not abate for many years. Patients with an acute onset of the disease tend to have few germinal centers in their thymuses and remit promptly following thymectomy. Many of these patients exhibit a normalization of their EMG findings immediately after thymectomy. The later a patient presents in the course of his disease, the greater are the number of thymic germinal centers and the later the onset of remission postoperatively.[104] Remissions have been observed to occur as late as ten years post-thymectomy.

Other Disorders Associated with Thymic Proliferation

Patients with thymoma often present with varying degrees of immunodeficiency. Hypogammaglobulinemia is most common but deficits in cell-mediated immunity have also been described.[105] Hematologic abnormalities include various cytopenias. Anemia is most common and may be autoimmune in nature.[105]

Five per cent of patients with thymoma develop *pure red cell aplasia*, and up to 50 per cent of adults who acquire pure red cell aplasia have thymomas.[106] Some patients have been cured of their red cell aplasia by thymectomy.[107] As in myasthenia, remission occurs at longer intervals post-thymectomy the more severe the thymic pathology. This suggests an etiologic relationship between thymic disease and pure red cell aplasia. An autoimmune basis for this disease has been postulated. Antibodies have been found which are reactive against autologous erythroblasts and erythropoietin.[108,109] Immunosuppressive agents have been successfully used in some of these patients.[110]

In one large study of 146 patients with thymomas, 21 per cent developed extrathymic malignancies when followed over 20 years. In contrast, only 8 per cent of 177 patients with parathyroid adenomas developed a second malignancy.[111] This is a preliminary hint that the thymus, and hence the immune system, may have a special relationship to cancer (see Chap. 13).

MULTIPLE MYELOMA

Multiple myeloma is an extremely aggressive disease characterized by a malignant proliferation of plasma cells. These cells are believed to arise from the uncontrolled proliferation of a single clone of immunocompetent cells. With rare exceptions, the malignant plasma cells secrete a single, homogeneous molecular species of immunoglobulin. These monoclonal proteins are detected as a sharp spike on serum or urine electrophoresis, and are generally comprised of intact immunoglobulin molecules or light chains (Fig. 12-10).

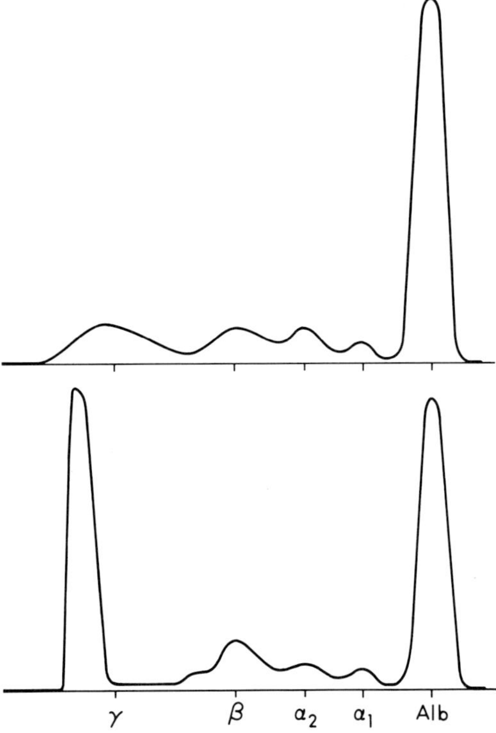

Fig. 12-10. Serum electrophoresis. Above, a normal pattern. The pattern below was obtained from a patient with multiple myeloma. The large γ spike represents the monoclonal immunoglobulin produced by the malignant plasma cells. Note the relative hypogammaglobulinemia in the rest of the γ region.

Patients can be classified according to the nature of their myeloma proteins:[112-115]

1. In 50 per cent of patients, the myeloma protein is IgG.

2. Twenty-five per cent of patients have a monoclonal IgA component.

3. Twenty per cent of patients produce high levels of monoclonal kappa or lambda light chains. This form of myeloma is often referred to as "light-chain disease."

4. IgE and IgD myelomas are uncommon. IgM myelomas are extremely rare, although large quantities of monoclonal IgM are encountered in patients with Waldenström's macroglobulinemia (see below).

5. Occasionally, patients with plasma-cell proliferation present without any evidence of a monoclonal spike on either serum or urine electrophoresis. Since no abnormal protein component can be demonstrated, these are considered to be cases of nonsecreting multiple myeloma.

The diagnosis of multiple myeloma is established by the identification of large numbers of plasma cells in the bone marrow and the demonstration of a monoclonal protein in the serum or urine (except in the rare cases of nonsecreting myeloma). Monoclonal protein spikes can be detected in the serum of about 70 per cent of patients, and urine spikes are present in 40 to 50 per cent of myeloma patients. The peripheral blood reveals a normal or depressed leukocyte count with a relative lymphocytosis; plasma cells can be found in many patients, and terminally the periphery may be flooded by an outpouring of malignant cells. Anemia is present in almost all patients, and thrombocytopenia occurs in about one third.

Multiple myeloma has a wide spectrum of clinical involvement.[116] Most characteristic are lytic bone lesions and nephrotoxicity, the latter being most common in patients producing excess light chains. These light chains are detected in the urine as Bence Jones proteins and are believed to interfere with normal tubular function. Other factors, including hypercalciuria, hyperuricosuria and dehydration, may also contribute to the renal involvement of multiple myeloma. Neurologic, hemorrhagic and arthritic complaints are also common, and cryoglobulinemia and amyloidosis may be present.

Certain manifestations of multiple myeloma appear to be variably associated with the different immunoglobulin classes of the myeloma proteins.[114,115] The hyperviscosity syndrome, although most commonly associated with macroglobulinemia, may occur in multiple myeloma and is seen most often in IgG myeloma. Monoclonal IgG_3 is present in a greater-than-expected percentage of these patients. IgG myeloma is also associated with a severe depression of normal immunoglobulin levels, especially normal IgG. These patients have a high incidence of infection.

IgA myeloma appears to have a relatively high incidence of associated amyloidosis. Hyperviscosity may also develop. The plasma cells of these patients often display a distinct morphology and have been referred to as *flame cells*. The flamelike appearance is due to the high carbohydrate content of IgA, so that the accumulation of intracellular immunoglobulin stains red with routine marrow stains. Flame cells are encountered less frequently in the other types of myeloma.

Light-chain myeloma is associated with a high incidence of severe renal disease. Monoclonal IgD spikes may be associated with an increased incidence of plasmacytomas. Some observers feel that nonsecreting myeloma carries the worst prognosis, but this has not been widely confirmed.

Patients with multiple myeloma generally have a significantly depressed level of normal immunoglobulins. The number of peripheral lymphocytes bearing normal surface immunoglobulin isotypes as detected with standard immunofluorescent antisera is also decreased.[117,118] However, a large percentage of circulating cells appear to carry surface immunoglobulin that can be detected with antisera directed against the idiotype of the monoclonal serum immunoglobulin (why this immunoglobulin should not be detected by usual immunofluorescent techniques

Table 12-3. Special Characteristics of the Different Classes of Myeloma

Class of Myeloma	*Percentage of Total Patients*	*Special Clinical Manifestations*
IgG	50%	Hyperviscosity, decreased levels of normal Ig, increased severity and number of infections
IgA	25%	Amyloidosis, hyperviscosity, flame cells in the marrow
Light chain disease	20%	Severe renal disease
IgD	Rare	Increased incidence of plasmacytomas
IgE	Rare	
Nonsecreting	Rare	May carry worst prognosis

is unclear).[117,118] Trypsinization of these lymphocytes removes the surface molecules, but within 18 hours the cells have regenerated immunoglobulin of the same idiotypic specificity, suggesting that the surface immunoglobulin is synthesized by the cells and not merely picked up from the serum.[119] It is thus possible that the plasma-cell accumulation that characterizies multiple myeloma reflects the proliferation and differentiation of a single clone of precursor lymphocytes. An alternative hypothesis is that the malignant plasma cells secrete a factor which "instructs" the peripheral lymphocytes to synthesize the monoclonal immunoglobulin. RNA has been suggested to subserve this role.[119]

Recent work has implicated suppressor cells in the pathogenesis of the hypogammaglobulinemia commonly seen in multiple myeloma. There is no evidence that these are T suppressor cells, and preliminary analysis has suggested that phagocytic mononuclear cells may be responsible.[120] Associated with the hypogammaglobulinemia is an increased susceptibility to bacterial infection. Pneumococcal pneumonia can be very severe and is a frequent cause of death. Herpes zoster infections are also common, but otherwise viral infection is not a major problem. Cell-mediated immunity is generally intact.

The events leading to the development of multiple myeloma are not known. As with the B-cell lymphomas, chronic stimulation has been offered as a possible pathogenetic mechanism. This view is supported by several observations in animal systems:

1. C3H strain mice develop plasmacytomas in regions of cecal ulceration.[121,122]

2. Plasma-cell tumors are readily induced in Balb/c mice by intraperitoneal injection of adjuvants.[123,124] Viruslike particles have been detected in these tumors, as well as in those of the C3H mouse.[125,126]

3. Some of the monoclonal proteins produced by these animal tumors possess antibody reactivity to bacterial antigens.[127] Others have been found to be capable of reacting with various natural and synthetic antigens.

Evidence in man is suggestive but less convincing. Plasma-cell dyscrasias have been found to occur in settings of chronic inflammatory disease and nonreticular neoplasms.[128] In addition, human monoclonal proteins have been described that have specific antibody activity.[129-131] Perhaps in some instances these antibody molecules are the product of a plasma-cell response to a specific antigen, but due either to the persistence of the antigen or some abnormality in the proliferating clone, these cells escaped the normal regulatory mechanisms and gave rise to a malignancy.

WALDENSTRÖM'S MACROGLOBULINEMIA

Macroglobulinemia occurs most frequently in elderly individuals. Common findings include anemia, a bleeding diathesis with or without thrombocytopenia, the presence of an IgM spike in the serum, and a marrow infiltrate of lymphocytoid-plasma cells.[132,133] Terminally, these abnormal cells can be found in the peripheral circulation. As many as one half of affected patients may have lymphadenopathy and/or hepatosplenomegaly.

The monoclonal IgM spike can contribute to morbidity in a number of ways:[132,133]

1. *Hyperviscosity Syndrome.* Vascular occlusion and sludging due to the high concentration of IgM can contribute to renal, neurologic and hematologic complications.[134]

2. *The monoclonal IgM can coat the surfaces* of platelets and clotting factors and prevent their normal function, contributing to the bleeding tendency in these patients.

3. *Cryoglobulinemia* is not uncommon in macroglobulinemia. The manifestations of cryoglobulinemia were discussed in Chapter 7.

Although 19S IgM is by far the predominant abnormal serum protein in these patients, 7S IgM, μ heavy chains and heavy-chain fragments can be found as well.[135,136] Bence Jones proteins are present in at least 20 per cent of patients.[133]

The precise nature of the malignant cell is not known, and the typical description of a "lymphocytoid-plasma cell" reflects our ignorance as to its origin as much as its true morphologic description. A brief discussion of the surface characteristics of the malignant cells in Waldenström's macroglobulinemia can be found in Chapter 3.

BENIGN MONOCLONAL GAMMOPATHY

Benign monoclonal gammopathy (BMG) is now recognized as a relatively common entity in which otherwise healthy individuals are found to possess a monoclonal immunoglobulin spike in their serum. The incidence of BMG increases with age and is present in about 3 per cent of people over 70 years of age. In contrast to multiple myeloma, the concentration of the monoclonal serum component in BMG remains constant for many years.[112]

BMG is asymptomatic, is not progressive, and does not require treatment. The serum spike can be IgG, IgM or IgA. Bence Jones proteinuria is only rarely detected. The bone marrow appears essentially normal, with a slight increase in the percentage of plasma cells the only suspicious feature.

The major importance of BMG is the necessity to distinguish it from multiple myeloma. BMG will never be confused with flagrant, advanced multiple myeloma with lytic bone lesions and greatly increased numbers of plasmacytoid cells in the marrow. However, the distinction from early myeloma is often difficult and occasionally impossible to make. At present, the only way to make the diagnosis of BMG is to watch the patient and wait.

Whereas almost all patients with multiple myeloma have a depression in their normal serum immunoglobulin levels, most patients with BMG have normal titers of immunoglobulin.[112] Examination of the surface markers on the peripheral blood lymphocytes of patients with BMG reveals normal numbers of B and T cells. The number of cells bearing immunoglobulin with the same idiotype as the serum spike is not abnormally increased. These findings are in contrast to those in patients with multiple myeloma who often possess a diminished percentage of normal B cells and a great preponderance of cells expressing surface immunoglobulin with the same idiotype as the immunoglobulin spike.[117]

The reason for the generation of the monoclonal spike and its failure to progressively increase in concentration remains unknown. Possibilities include the spontaneous production of a hyperactive clone that nevertheless remains susceptible to normal homeostatic controls, or the vigorous response of a single clone of cells to a specific antigenic challenge. Such monoclonal antibody responses to antigens are not common in man, but have been described to occur against certain infectious agents. In these cases, unlike BMG, the monoclonal antibody is present only transiently.[137]

THE HEAVY-CHAIN DISEASES

The heavy-chain diseases are extremely rare disorders characterized by the presence of an abnormal immunoglobulin heavy chain in the serum.[138] A broad, abnormal protein band can often be observed on routine serum electrophoresis, but it is not unusual to be unable to detect any abnormal band. In the latter instance the diagnosis is then made by immunoelectrophoresis. Despite the apparently heterogeneous character of the protein band, it is believed that the heavy-chain diseases represent the expansion of a single clone of abnormal cells. The heterogeneity is probably due to the tendency of these abnormal proteins to polymerize, the variable amount of carbohydrate attached to each chain and variations in amino acid content. Heavy-chain diseases of the α, γ and μ classes have been described.

The heavy chains which are produced in these diseases are not complete proteins, but, as we shall see, are missing a polypeptide segment. With the exception of the rare μ-chain disease, light chains are not detected in the serum. These observations suggest that there are two basic intracellular defects in heavy-chain disease: (1) the synthesis of abnormal heavy chains and (2) the failure of light-chain synthesis. These two processes could be linked theoretically if one hypothesizes that normal heavy-chain synthesis is required for light-chain synthesis to occur. However, this point is purely speculative.

Alpha Heavy-Chain Disease

Alpha heavy-chain disease is the most common of the heavy-chain diseases.[139] It is almost always associated with a malignant lymphoma of the small intestine, a disease occurring predominantly in the Mediterranean area. The mesenteric nodes are involved in the malignant process, and the lamina propria of the small intestine is infiltrated with lymphocytes and plasma cells. These cells have been shown to be actively synthesizing the abnormal protein. Other lymphoid organs, including the peripheral lymph nodes and spleen, are usually spared except in advanced cases. Marrow invasion may occur, and terminally one may see abnormal cells in the blood and throughout the body tissues. A less common variety of alpha-chain disease involves predominantly the respiratory tract.

Clinically, alpha-chain disease presents as a intestinal lymphoma. Malabsorption is the most frequent and serious complication. Weakness, weight loss and lymphadenopathy and hepatosplenomegaly may also be present. Anemia, thrombocytopenia and leukocytosis with eosinophilia are frequently encountered.

The histology of the involved nodes is nonspecific, usually displaying a variable lymphocyte and plasma-cell infiltrate. In some patients the lymph node histology may closely resemble that of Hodgkin's disease or histiocytic lymphoma. Early biopsy reveals cells that appear nonmalignant, and some observers feel that the disease undergoes a long, premalignant phase during which antibiotic therapy may abort the disease process.[140] Spontaneous remissions have been reported. Nevertheless, partly because of the difficulty in making an early diagnosis (a sharp peak is virtually never seen, and only 50% of the patients display an abnormal broad band on serum electrophoresis[141]), and partly because of the aggressive nature of the malignancy, the prognosis is poor, with most patients dying within four years of diagnosis.

All of the patients that have been described in the literature have had abnormal α_1 heavy chains; no case of a patient with α_2 heavy-chain disease has been reported. This is a tantalizing clue to the nature of the cell involved in the disease process but at present its meaning is elusive.

The molecular weight of the abnormal α_1 polypeptide ranges between 29,000 and 34,000, that is, somewhere between one half and three quarters of the molecular weight of an intact α_1 chain.[138] The molecule consists of an intact hinge region and Fc portion, and is missing virtually all of the Fd piece (which includes the variable and CH_1 domains; Fig. 12-11), suggesting that there may be a failure at

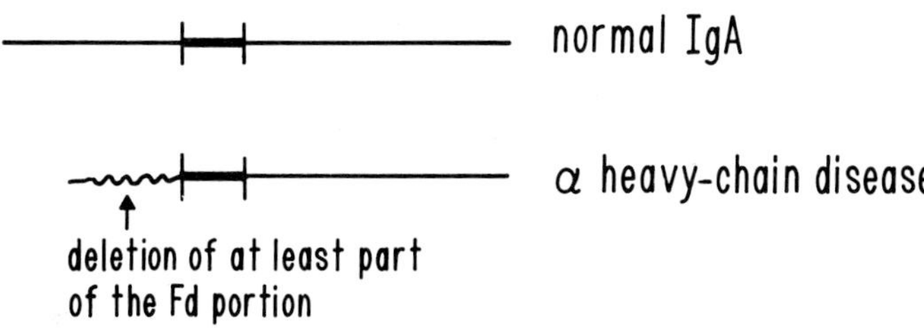

Fig. 12-11. Alpha heavy-chain disease. A schematic of the abnormal heavy chain.

the level of DNA translocation resulting in the deletion of specific genetic regions. The amino terminal portion of the abnormal polypeptide consists of a heterogeneous array of several amino acids before normal synthesis is resumed at the hinge region. This finding may reflect abnormal synthesis and/or intracellular proteolysis of the remnant of the Fd portion.

Gamma Heavy-Chain Disease

Gamma heavy-chain disease usually occurs in a setting of chronic disease, especially tuberculosis, rheumatoid arthritis, Sjögren's syndrome, myasthenia gravis, systemic lupus erythematosus, hypereosinophilic syndrome and thyroiditis. It presents like a malignant lymphoma with lymph node enlargement the most common clinical sign.[142] Fever, anemia and hepatosplenomegaly are also frequent features of the disease. The bone marrow and lymph nodes reveal a marked increase in plasma cells, lymphocytes and eosinophils. Serum electrophoresis may reveal a broad, heterogeneous band or a sharp peak. Frequently, however, a concentrated urine sample must be examined in order to detect an abnormal protein. Hypoalbuminemia and hypogammaglobulinemia are always present. The immune response of these patients is compromised, accounting for their frequent infections.

Heavy chains of the γ_1 subclass predominate, but other subclasses of γ heavy chains have also been described. These polypeptides are rich in carbohydrates and their molecular weights are variable. Four types of γ heavy chains have been described in these patients. A given patient will have only one of the first three types, and may additionally have type 4 (Fig. 12-12):[138]

1. *Type 1.* A partial deletion of the Fd portion of the molecule with resumption of normal synthesis at the hinge region (at residue 216). Often there is a variable number of uncharacteristic residues preceding residue 216, at which point normal synthesis resumes. This is the most common type of abnormal γ chain.
2. *Type 2.* The γ chain lacks only the hinge region (residues 216 to 232).
3. *Type 3.* Deletion of the Fd and hinge regions with resumption of normal synthesis around residue 230.
4. *Type 4.* Some proteins appear to be the result of enzymatic cleavage of types 1 through 3.

Mu Heavy-Chain Disease

The most rare of all the heavy-chain diseases is μ heavy-chain disease. It has been described almost solely in patients with long-standing chronic lymphocytic leukemia.[143] The presence of vacuolated plasma cells in the marrow has been associated with the presence of the disease. In this disorder both μ-chain fragments and free light chains have been found, suggesting a defect in the region of attachment of the heavy and light polypeptides to each other. However, analysis of one abnormal μ chain has revealed the region of interchain bridging to be intact.[144] Why light-chain synthesis continues in μ-chain disease but not in α- or γ-chain disease is not known.

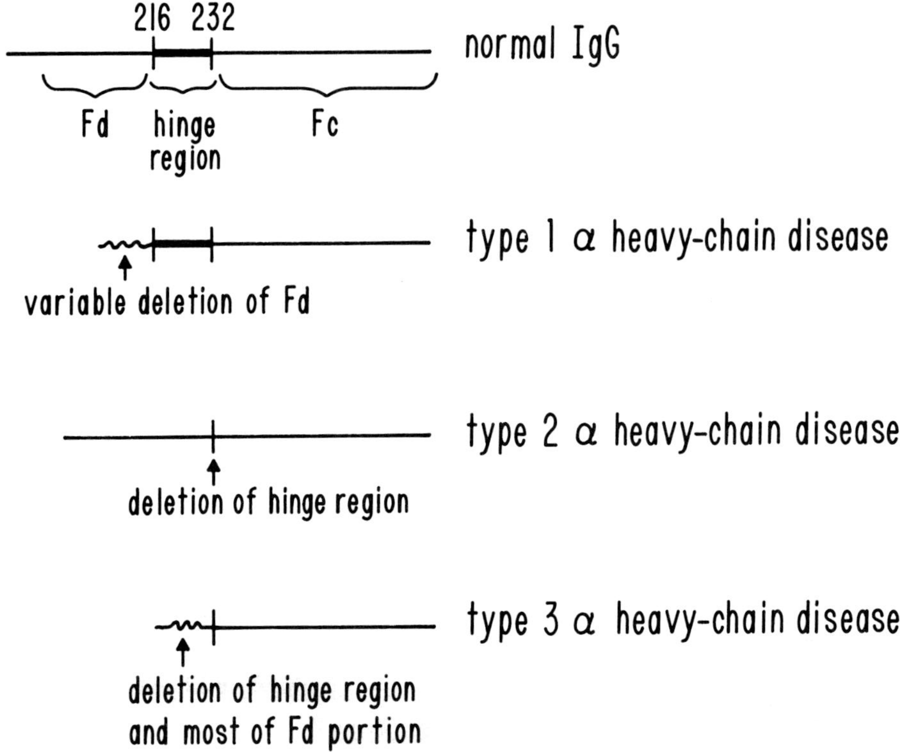

Fig. 12-12. Gamma heavy-chain disease. The three types of abnormal γ heavy chains.

AMYLOIDOSIS

Amyloidosis is a systemic disease characterized by the deposition of a proteinaceous material—amyloid—in various organs throughout the body. Clinical symptomatology results from the destruction and replacement of tissue parenchyma by this material and may include evidence of congestive heart failure, orthostatic hypotension, the nephrotic syndrome, malabsorption, peripheral neuropathy, and the carpal tunnel syndrome. Hepatosplenomegaly and macroglossia are also frequently encountered.[145]

Amyloidosis can be divided into a number of clinical subtypes:[146]

1. Primary amyloidosis occurs in individuals without any associated or underlying disease process.

2. Amyloidosis is not uncommonly seen in patients with multiple myeloma and other plasma-cell dyscrasias.

3. Secondary amyloidosis is the term used to describe the occurrence of amyloidosis in patients with some underlying disease. There are mostly chronic illnesses and include neurologic disorders, lymphoreticular malignancies, leprosy and rheumatoid arthritis. As many as 20 to 60 per cent of patients with long-standing rheumatoid arthritis have detectable amyloid deposits.

4. Amyloidosis can occur in a familial form, notably in patients with familial Mediterranean fever.

5. Amyloid deposits can frequently be seen in senile plaques within the brain, blood vessels and other organs of elderly individuals.

6. Amyloid has been detected in endocrine glands in patients with hormonal

disorders such as medullary carcinoma of the thyroid and diabetes mellitus.

The Chemical Nature of Amyloid

Amyloid is recognized by its characteristic green birefringence when involved tissues are stained with congo red dye and viewed under polarized light. It is composed of long fibrils arranged in a β-pleated sheet conformation. A minor doughnut-shaped structure called P component can also be found in some amyloid deposits.

Biochemical and immunologic analysis of the major fibrillar component of amyloid has revealed that there are several types of proteins capable of eliciting the characteristic staining by which amyloid is defined:

1. The amyloid found in patients with primary amyloidosis or with amyloidosis associated with multiple myeloma is derived from fragments of immunoglobulin light chains.[147] Usually, these fragments consist of the variable portion plus some fraction of the constant region of the light chain, although occasionally intact light chains have been detected. The majority of light-chain-derived amyloid fibrils are fragments of λ chains.

Fifty per cent of patients with primary amyloidosis and 75 per cent of patients with amyloidosis associated with multiple myeloma have monoclonal serum spikes.[145] Amyloid present in patients with Bence Jones proteinuria has been reported to possess the same amino acid sequence as the Bence Jones protein.[148]

Amyloid fibrils can be formed in the laboratory by subjecting immunoglobulin light chains to proteolysis at an acid pH. Not all immunoglobulin light chains can be converted to amyloid fibrils, and it is believed that only certain immunoglobulin light chains are amyloidogenic both *in vitro* and *in vivo*. It has been further suggested that some immunoglobulin light chains may have a greater affinity for tissue deposition than others.[149]

2. The amyloid fibrils of patients with secondary amyloidosis do not appear to be related to immunoglobulin light chains, although small amounts of light-chain-derived protein may sometimes be present in these amyloid deposits. The major fibrillar component has been termed the AA protein (amyloid A). An antigenically related substance termed SAA (serum A-related protein) can be demonstrated in the serum of these patients, and is believed to be the precursor of the AA protein.[150] It has a molecular weight of approximately 180,000[151] but its precise chemical nature has not been determined. The concentration of SAA is markedly elevated in most patients with secondary amyloidosis, but also rises with infection, neoplasia, chronic illness, pregnancy and aging.

3. Insulin and glucagon can both be altered biochemically to form β-pleated sheets. This observation may explain the origin of the amyloid deposits in the endocrinopathies. In addition, thyrocalcitonin has been found in the amyloid deposits of medullary carcinoma of the thyroid.[152]

The Pathogenesis of Amyloid

Experiments carried out *in vitro* have demonstrated that amyloid fibrils can be produced by the proteolysis of several different types of proteins, including immunoglobulin light chains. Proteolysis has therefore been postulated to be responsible for the generation of amyloid fibrils *in vivo* (Fig. 12-13). The macrophage has been implicated as the site of *in vivo* proteolysis and amyloid formation.[153] Amyloid deposits are typically found surrounding phagocytic cells, and amyloid material can be found within macrophage lysosomes.[154]

If the macrophage is responsible for the production of amyloid, then one can imagine several mechanisms by which amyloid formation could occur *in vivo*: (1) aberrant macrophage metabolism of

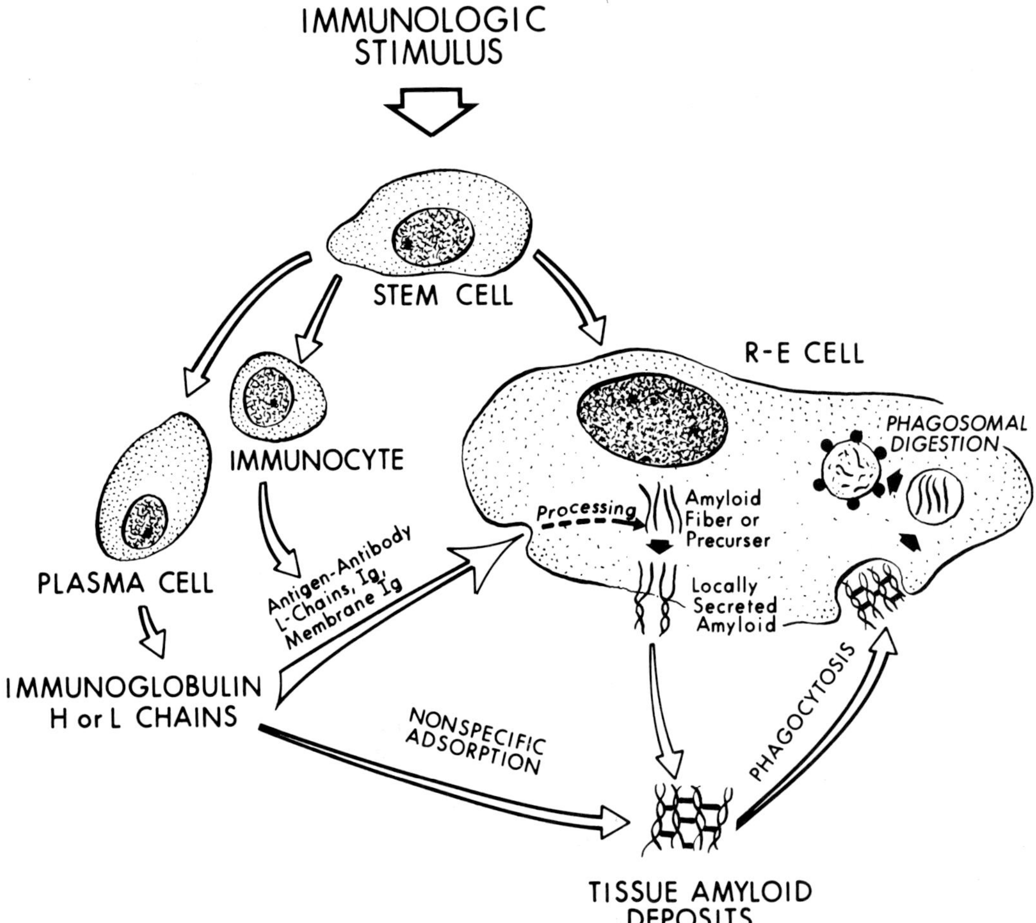

Fig. 12-13. A possible pathogenesis of amyloid formation. (Cohen, H. J., *et al.*: Resolution of primary amyloidosis during chemotherapy. Ann. Intern. Med., *82*:466, 1975.)

normal proteins; (2) abnormal proteins presented to the macrophage for processing and/or disposal; and (3) the presence of large amounts of material that overwhelm or distort the macrophage's capacity for normal protein metabolism with the resultant production of amyloid fibrils.

There is no convincing evidence to support either of the first two postulated mechanisms. Most observers favor the third hypothesis since there is evidence in both primary and secondary amyloidosis for the existence of an increased quantity of an amyloid-related material that is either not present or present in only very low levels in normal people. In patients with myeloma-associated amyloidosis and in the 50 per cent of patients with primary amyloidosis who have a serum spike, the high concentration of monoclonal protein could theoretically overwhelm the normal catabolic mechanisms of the body's phagocytes and lead to the formation of amyloid. The origin of primary amyloidosis not associated with a detectable serum spike remains a mystery.

In patients with secondary amyloidosis, the serum substance SAA is present in high concentrations and is believed to be the amyloidogenic material. The study of secondary amyloidosis has been greatly aided by the development of an animal model. Many animal species, including several strains of mice, develop amyloidosis while receiving repeated injections of casein.[155] The development of amyloidosis in these animals can be accelerated by immunosuppression, suggesting that the inability of the immune system to properly handle the casein may predispose to amyloid formation. Decreased cellular immunity[156] and humoral hyperactivity[157] have been described in these animals. Thymosin treatment restores their T-cell function and reduces the incidence and severity of their disease.[158] It is of considerable interest that amyloidosis is not uncommonly seen in human patients with various immunodeficiency diseases.[159]

It does not appear that native casein itself is deposited as the amyloid fibril in these experimental systems. Characterization of the amyloid material in guinea pigs injected with casein has revealed an amino acid sequence very nearly identical to the AA protein found in human patients with amyloidosis.[160] Similarly, murine serum precursor SAA appears closely to resemble human SAA.[161] In casein-injected mice, SAA behaves like an acute-phase reactant. During the acute rise in SAA, the amount of protein AA detectable in liver tissue rises as well.[161] It thus appears either that casein is transformed into SAA (unlikely in view of the many different conditions that are associated with a rise in SAA) or that repeated injections of casein somehow trigger the rise in SAA titers.

Studies in humans have shown that SAA is present in very low concentrations in normal sera, but is increased in the sera of patients with amyloidosis, in patients having diseases that predispose to amyloidosis, and during acute inflammation.[162] It has therefore been postulated that SAA in humans is either an acute-phase reactant or is a component of normal tissues that is released into the circulation following injury with an associated inflammatory response.[163] In support of the latter interpretation is the finding by indirect immunofluorescence of SAA-like material in human fibroblasts.[163] If this report is confirmed, then a possible source of SAA and hence of the AA protein will have been identified.

REFERENCES

1. Cottier, H., Odartchenko, N., and Schindler, R.: Germinal Centers in Immune Responses. New York, Springer-Verlag, 1967.
2. Lukes, R. J., and Collins, R. D.: Immunologic characterization of human malignant lymphomas. Cancer, *34*:1488, 1974.
3. Dorfman, R. F., and Warnke, R.: Lymphadenopathy simulating the malignant lymphomas. Hum. Pathol., *5*:519, 1974.
4. McKinney, A. A., and Cline, W. S.: Infectious mononucleosis. Br. J. Haematol., *27*:367, 1974.
5. Henle, W., and Henle, G.: Epstein-Barr virus and infectious mononucleosis. N. Engl. J. Med., *288*:263, 1973.
6. Carter, R. L.: Infectious mononucleosis: model for self-limiting lymphoproliferation. Lancet, *1*:846, 1975.
7. ———: Antibody formation in infectious mononucleosis. Br. J. Haematol., *12*:259, 1966.
8. Horwitz, C. A., Henle, W., Henle, G., and Schmitz, H.: Clinical evaluation of patients with infectious mononucleosis and development of antibodies to the R component of the Epstein-Barr virus-induced early antigen complex. Am. J. Med., *58*:330, 1975.
9. Troxel, D. B., Innella, F., and Cohen, R. J.: Infectious mononucleosis complicated by hemolytic anemia due to anti-i. Am. J. Clin. Pathol., *46*:625, 1966.
10. Anderson, L. G., and Talal, N.: The spectrum of benign to malignant lymphoproliferation in Sjögrens Syndrome. Clin. Exp. Immunol., *10*:199, 1972.
11. ———: Sjögren's Syndrome with lymphadenopathy. Am. J. Med., *57*:801, 1974.
12. Saltzstein, S. L., and Ackerman, L. V.: Lymphadenopathy induced by anticonvulsant drugs and mimicking clinically and pathologically malignant lymphomas. Cancer, *12*:164, 1959.
13. Hyman, G. A., and Sommers, S. C.: The development of Hodgkin's Disease and lymphoma during anticonvulsant therapy. Blood, *28*:416, 1966.
14. Lukes, R. J., and Tindle, B. H.: Immunoblastic lymphadenopathy: a hyperimmune entity resembling Hodgkin's Disease. N. Engl. J. Med., *292*:1, 1975.
15. Schultz, D. R., and Yunis, A. A.: Immunoblastic lymphadenopathy with mixed cryoglobulinemia. N. Engl. J. Med., *292*:8, 1975.
16. Metcalf, D.: Reticular tumours in mice sub-

jected to prolonged antigenic stimulation. Br. J. Cancer, *15*:769, 1961.

17. Balls, M., and Ruben, L. N.: The induction of lymphosarcoma in *Xenopus laevis* by cancerous and normal tissues of *Rana pipiens*. Ann. N.Y. Acad. Sci., *126*:274, 1965.
18. Howard, J. G., Michie, D., and Simonsen, M.: Splenomegaly as a host response in graft-versus-host disease. Br. J. Exp. Pathol., *42*:478, 1961.
19. Armstrong, M. Y. K., *et al.*: Chronic allogeneic disease II. Development of lymphomas. J. Exp. Med., *132*:417, 1970.
20. Smith, R. T., Bausher, J. A. C., and Adler, W. H.: Studies of an inhibitor of DNA synthesis and a nonspecific mitogen elaborated by human lymphoblasts. Am. J. Pathol., *60*:495, 1970.
21. Hersh, E. M., and Drewinko, B.: Specific inhibition of lymphocyte blastogenic responses to mitogens by a factor produced by cultured human malignant lymphoma cells. Cancer Res., *34*:215, 1974.
22. Schwartz, R. S.: A new concept of immunoregulation and its application to leukemia and lymphoma. Tumori, *59*:383, 1973.
23. Hirsch, M. S., *et al.*: Leukemia virus activation in chronic allogeneic disease. Proc. Natl. Acad. Sci. U.S.A., *67*:1914, 1970.
24. Levine, G. D., and Dorfman, R. F.: Nodular lymphoma: an ultrastructural study of its relationship to germinal centers and a correlation of light and electron microscopic findings. Cancer, *35*:148, 1975.
25. Morris, M. W., and Davey, F. R.: Immunologic and cytochemical properties of histiocytic and mixed histiocytic-lymphocytic lymphomas. Am. J. Clin. Pathol., *63*:403, 1975.
26. O'Connor, G. T.: Persistent immunologic stimulation as a factor in oncogenesis, with special reference to Burkitt's Tumor. Am. J. Med., *48*:279, 1970.
27. Klein, E., *et al.*: Surface IgM-kappa specificity on a Burkitt lymphoma cell *in vivo* and in derived culture lines. Cancer Res., *28*:1300, 1968.
28. Vitmann, J. E., Fish, W., Osserman, E., and Gellhorn, A.: The clinical implications of hypogammaglobulinemia in patients with chronic lymphocytic leukemia and lymphocytic lymphosarcoma. Ann. Intern. Med., *51*:501, 1959.
29. Parkhurst, G. F., and Vlahides, G. D.: Fatal opportunistic fungus disease. J.A.M.A., *202*:131, 1967.
30. Miller, D. G.: Patterns of immunological deficiency in lymphomas and leukemias. Ann. Intern. Med., *57*:703, 1962.
31. ———: Patterns of immunological deficiency in lymphomas and leukemias. Ann. Intern. Med., *57*:703, 1962.
32. Moore, D. F., Migliore, P. J., Shullenberger, C. C., and Alexanian, R.: Monoclonal macroglobulinemia in malignant lymphoma. Ann. Intern. Med., *72*:43, 1970.
33. Hobbs, J. R.: Secondary antibody deficiency. Proc. R. Soc. Med., *61*:883, 1968.
34. Millian, S. J., Miller, D. G., and Schaeffer, M.: Viral complement-fixing antibody in patients with Hodgkin's Disease, lymphosarcoma, reticulum cell sarcoma and chronic lymphatic leukemia. Cancer, *18*:674, 1965.
35. Miller, D. G., Lizardo, J. G., and Snyderman, R. K.: Homologous and heterologous skin transplantation in patients with lymphomatous disease. J. Natl. Cancer Inst., *26*:569, 1961.
36. Zacharski, L. R., and Linman, J. W.: Chronic lymphocytic leukemia versus chronic lymphosarcoma cell leukemia. Am. J. Med., *47*:75, 1969.
37. Cone, L., and Uhr, J. W.: Immunological deficiency disorders associated with chronic lymphocytic leukemia and multiple myeloma. J. Clin. Invest., *43*:2241, 1964.
38. Troup, S. B., Swisher, S. N., and Young, L. E.: The anemia of leukemia. Am. J. Med., *28*:751, 1960.
39. Damashek, W., and Gunz, F.: Leukemia. Ed. 2, p. 235. New York, Grune & Stratton, 1964.
40. Holm, G., Perlmann, P., and Johansson, B.: Impaired phytohemagglutinin-induced cytotoxicity *in vitro* of lymphocytes from patients with Hodgkin's Disease or chronic lymphatic leukemia. Clin. Immunol., *2*:351, 1967.
41. Smith, J. L., Cowling, D. C., and Barker, C. R.: Response of lymphocytes in chronic lymphocytic leukemia to plant mitogens. Lancet, *1*:229, 1972.
42. Weed, R. I.: Exaggerated delayed hypersensitivity to mosquito bites in chronic lymphocytic leukemia. Blood, *26*:257, 1965.
43. Utsinger, P. D.: Impaired T-cell transformation in chronic lymphocytic leukemia (CLL): demonstration of a blastogenesis inhibitory factor. Blood, *46*:883, 1975.
44. Aisenberg, A. C.: Malignant lymphoma. N. Engl. J. Med., *288*:883, 1973.
45. Frajola, W. J., Greider, M. H., and Bouroncle, B. A.: Cytology of the Sternberg-Reed cell as revealed by the electron microscope. Ann. N.Y. Acad. Sci., *73*:221, 1958.
46. Roulet, F. C. (ed.): The Lymphorecticular tumors in Africa P. 304. New York, S. Krager, 1964.
47. Garvin, A. J., Spicer, S. S., Parmley, R. T., and Munster, A. M.: Immunohistochemical demonstration of IgG in Reed-Sternberg and other cells in Hodgkin's Disease. J. Exp. Med., *139*:1077, 1974.
48. Leech, J.: Immunoglobulin-positive Reed-Sternberg cells in Hodgkin's Disease. Lancet, *2*:265, 1973.
49. Butler, J. J.: Relationship of histologic findings to survival in Hodgkin's Disease. Gann, *15*:275, 1973.
50. Bukowski, R. M. Noguchi, S., Hewlett, J. S., and Deodhar, S.: Lymphocyte subpopulations

in Hodgkin's Disease. Am. J. Clin. Pathol., *65*:31, 1976.

51. Young, R. C., Corder, M. P., Haynes, H. A., DeVita, V. T.: Delayed hypersensitivity in Hodgkin's Disease. Am. J. Med., *52*:63, 1972.
52. Ziegler, J. B., Hansen, P., and Penny, R.: Intrinsic lymphocyte defect in Hodgkin's Disease: analysis of the phytohemagglutinin dose-jresponse. Clin. Immunol. Immunopathol., *3*:451, 1975.
53. Kelly, W. D., Good, R. A., and Varco, R. L.: Anergy and skin homograft survival in Hodgkin's Disease. Surg. Gynec. Obstet., *107*:565, 1958.
54. Matchett, K. M., Huang, A. T., and Kremer, W. B.: Impaired lymphocyte transformation in Hodgkin's diseajse. J. Clin. Invest., *52*:1908, 1973.
55. Levy, R., and Kaplan, H. S.: Impaired lymphocyte function in untreated Hodgkin's Disease. N. Engl. J. Med., *290*:181, 1974.
56. Rebuck, J. W., Monto, R. W., Monaghan, E. A., and Riddle, J. M.: Potentialities of the lymphocyte with an additional reference to its dysfunction in Hodgkin's Disease. Ann. N.Y. Acad. Sci., *73*:8, 1958.
57. Ward, P. A., and Berenberg, J. L.: Defective regulation of inflammatory mediators in Hodgkin's Disease. N. Engl. J. Med., *290*:76, 1974.
58. Hong, R.: Immunodeficiency: enigmas and speculations. Prog. Clin. Immunol., *2*:1, 1974.
59. Girifoni, V., Del Giacco, S., Tognella, S., and Manconi, P. E.: Lymphocytotoxins. Lancet, *1*:293, 1971.
60. Kretschmer, R., August, C. S., Rosen, F. S., and Janeway, C. A.: Recurrent infection, episodic lymphopenia and impaired cellular immunity. N. Engl. J. Med., *281*:285, 1969.
61. James, K.: Anti-lymphocytic antibody: review. Clin. Exp. Immunol., *2*:615, 1967.
62. Epstein, E. H., Jr., Levin, D. L., Croft, J. D., Jr., and Lutzner, M. A.: Mycosis fungoides. Medicine, *51*:61, 1972.
63. Lutzner, M., *et al.*: Cutaneous T-cell lymphomas: the Sezary syndrome, mycosis fungoides, and related disorders. Ann. Intern. Med., *83*:534, 1975.
64. ———: Weekly clinicopathological exercise: Sezary's syndrome. N. Engl. J. Med., *293*:598, 1975.
65. ———: Symposium on the Sezary cell. Mayo Clin. Proc., *49*:513–596, 1974.
66. Brouet, J. C., Flandrin, G., and Seligmann, M.: Indications of the thymus-derived nature of the proliferating cells in six patients with Sezary's syndrome. N. Engl. J. Med., *289*:341, 1973.
67. Broome, J. D., *et al.*: Leukemic cells with membrane properties of thymus-derived (T) lymphocytes in a case of Sezary's syndrome: morphologic and immunologic studies. Clin. Immunol. Immunopathol., *1*:319, 1973.
68. Lutzner, M. A., *et al*: Cytogenetic, cytophotometric, and ultrastructural study of large cerebriform cells of the Sezary syndrome and description of a small-cell variant. J. Natl. Cancer Inst., *50*:1145, 1973.
69. Winkelman, R. K.: Clinical studies of T-cell erythroderma in the Sezary syndrome. Mayo Clin. Proc., *49*:519, 1974.
70. Flaxman, B. A., Zelazny, G., and Van Scott, E. J. Nonspecificity of characteristic cells in mycosis fungoides. Arch. Dermatol., *104*:141, 1971.
71. Macaulay, W. L.: Lymphomatoid papulosis. Arch. Dermatol., *97*:23, 1968.
72. Schneiderman, R., Edelson, M., Lutzner, M., Gullino, M., and Green, I.: Lymphomatoid papulosis: immunologic and ultrastructural studies. Clin. Res., *23*:455, 1975.
73. Lutzner, M. A., Hobbs, J. W., and Horvath, P.: Ultrastructure of abnormal cells. Arch. Dermatol., *103*:375, 1971.

73a. Fleischmajer, R., Pascher, F., and Sims, C. F.: Parapsoriasis en plagues and mycosis fungoides. Dermatologica, *131*:149, 1965.

74. Scott, R. B.: Leukemia. Lancet, *1*:1162, 1957.
75. Edelson, R. L., *et al.*: Preferential cutaneous infiltration by neoplastic thymus-derived lymphocytes. Ann. Intern. Med., *80*:685, 1974.
76. Edelson, R. L., *et al.*: Morphologic and functional properties of the atypical T lymphocytes of the Sezary syndrome. Mayo Clin. Proc., *49*:558, 1974.
77. Main, R. K., Cochrum, K. C., Jones, M. J., and Kountz, S. L.: DNA synthesis in mixed cultures of rat leukocytes and allogeneic dissociated skin cells. Proc. Natl. Acad. Sci. U.S.A., *68*:1165, 1971.
78. Scheid, M., Boyse, E. A., Carswell, E. A., and Old, L. J.: Serologically demonstrable alloantigens of mouse epidermal cells. J. Exp. Med., *135*:938, 1972.
79. Pantelouris, E. M.: Absence of thymus in a mouse mutant. Nature, *217*:370, 1968.
80. Yoshida, T., Edelson, R., Cohen, S., and Green, I.: Migration inhibitory activity in serum and cell supernatants in patients with Sezary syndrome. J. Immunol., *114*:915, 1975.
81. Cohen, S., Fisher, B., Yoshida, T., and Bettigole, R. E.: Serum migratory-inhibitory activity in patients with lymphoproliferative diseases. N. Engl. J. Med., *290*:882, 1974.
82. Blaylock, W. K., Clendenning, W. E., Carbonne, P. P., and Van Scott, E. J.: Normal immunologic reactivity in patients with the lymphoma mycosis fungoides. Cancer, *19*:233, 1966.
83. Waldmann, T. A., *et al.*: The role of suppressor cells in the pathogenesis of common variable hypogammaglobulinemia and the immunodeficiency associated with myeloma. Fed. Proc., *35*:2067, 1976.
84. Castleman, B., and Norris, E. H.: the pathology of the thymus in myasthenia gravis. Medicine, *28*:27,1949.
85. Mackay, I. R., and deGail, P.: Thymic "germi-

nal centers" and plasma cells in systemic lupus erythematosus. Lancet, *2*:667, 1963.

86. Sherman, J. D., Adner, M. M., and Damashek, W.: Experimental production of germinal follicles in the thymus. Ann. N.Y. Acad. Sci., *124*:105, 1965.
87. Castleman, B.: The pathology of the thymus gland in myasthenia gravis. Ann. N.Y. Acad. Sci., *135*:496, 1966.
88. Batata, M. A., *et al.*: Thymomas: clinicopathologic features, therapy, and prognosis. Cancer, *34*:389, 1974.
89. Bernatz, V. E., Harrison, E. G., and Clagett, D. T.: Thymoma: a clinicopathologic study. J. Thorac. Surg., *42*:424, 1961.
90. Jeunet, F. S., and Good, R. A.: Thymoma, immunologic deficiencies and hematological abnormalities. Birth Defects, *4*:192, 1968.
91. Souadjian, J. V., Enriquez, P., Silverstein, M. N., and Pepin, J. M.: The spectrum of diseases associated with thymoma. Arch. Intern. Med., *134*:375, 1974.
92. Papatestas, A.E., *et al.*: Studies in myasthenia gravis: effects of thymectomy. Am. J. Med., *50*:465, 1971.
93. Fritze, D., *et al.*: HL-A antigens in myasthenia gravis. Lancet, *1*:240, 1974.
94. Appel, S. H., Almon, R., and Levy, N.: Acetylcholine receptor antibodies in myasthenia gravis. N. Engl. J. Med., *293*:760, 1975.
95. Patrick, J., and Lindstrom, J.: Autoimmune response to acetylcholine receptor. Science, *180*:871, 1973.

95a. Lindstrom, J. M., Einarson, B. L., Lennon, V. A., and Seybold, M. E.: Pathological mechanisms in experimental autoimmune myasthenia gravis I. Immunogenicity of syngeneic muscle acetylcholine receptor and quantitative extraction of receptor and antibody-receptor complexes from muscles of rats with experimental autoimmune myasthenia gravis. J. Exp. Med., *144*:726, 1976.

95b. Lindstrom, J. M., *et al.*: Pathological mechanisms in experimental autoimmune myasthenia gravis II. Passive transfer of experimental autoimmune myasthenia gravis in rats with anti-acetylchoine receptor antibodies. J. Exp. Med., *144*:739, 1976.

96. Richman, D. P., Patrick, J., and Arnason, B.: Cellular immunity in myasthenia gravis. N. Engl. J. Med., *294*:694, 1976.
97. Beutner, E. H., Witebsky, E., Ricken, D., and Adler, R. H.: Studies on autoantibodies in myasthenia gravis. J.A.M.A., *182*:46, 1962.
98. Alpert, L. I., *et al.*: Studies in myasthenia gravis: cellular hypersensitivity to skeletal muscle. Am. J. Clin. Pathol., *58*:647, 1972.
99. Van der Geld, H., and Osterhuis, H. J. G. H.: Autoantibodies and myasthenia gravis: epithelial cells of the thymus. Ann. N.Y. Acad. Sci., *135*:631, 1966.
100. Goldstein, G., and Whittingham, S.: Experimental autoimmune thymitis. Lancet, *2*:315, 1966.
101. Abdou, N. I., *et al.*: The thymus in myasthenia gravis: evidence for altered cell populations. N. Engl. J. Med., *291*:1271, 1974.
102. Hadden, J. W., *et al.*: Cyclic GMP in cholinergic and mitogenic modulation of lymphocyte metabolism and proliferation. Fed. Proc., *32*:1022(A), 1973.

102a. Schwartz, R. S., and Datta, S. K.: Infectious(?) myasthenia. N. Engl. J. Med., *291*:1304, 1974.

103. Eaton, L. M., and Clagett, O. T.: Thymectomy in the treatment of myasthenia gravis. J.A.M.A., *142*:963, 1950.
104. Genkins, G., Papatestas, A. F., Horowtiz, S. H., and Kornfeld, P.: Studies in myasthenia gravis: early thymectomy. Am. J. Med., *58*:517, 1975.
105. Mongan, E. S., Kern, W. A., and Terry, R.: Hypogammaglobulinemia with thymoma, hemolytic anemia, and disseminated infection in cytomegalovirus. Ann. Intern. Med., *65*:548, 1966.
106. ———: Pure red cell aplasia. Br. J. Haematol., *25*:1, 1973.
107. Schmid, J. R., *et al.*: Thymoma associated with pure red-cell agenesis. Cancer, *18*:216, 1965.
108. Krantz, S. B., Moore, W. H., and Zaentz, S. D.: Studies on red cell aplasia. J. Clin. Invest., *52*:324, 1973.
109. Jepson, J. H., and Lowenstein, L.: Panhypoplasia of the bone marrow: demonstration of a plasma facjtor with anti-erythropoietin-like activity. Can. Med. Assoc. J., *99*:99, 1968.
110. Zucker, S., Likhite, V. V., Weintraub, L. R., and Crosby, W. H.: Remission in pure red blood cell aplasia following immunosuppressive therapy. Arch. Intern. Med., *134*:317, 1974.
111. Souadjian, J. V., Silverstein, M. N., and Titus, J. L.: Thymoma and cancer. Cancer, *22*:1221, 1968.
112. Ritzmann, S. E., *et al.*: Idiopathic (asymptomatic) monoclonal gammopathies. Arch. Intern. Med., *135*:95, 1975.
113. Kyle, R. A.: Multiple myeloma. Mayo Clin. Proc., *50*:29, 1975.
114. A Cooperative Study by Acute Leukema Group B: Correlation of abnormal immunoglobulin with clinical features of myeloma. Arch. Intern. Med., *135*:46, 1975.
115. Hobbs, J. R.: Immunochemical classes of myelomatosis. Br. J. Haematol., *16*:599, 1969.
116. Zawadzki, Z. A., and Edwards, G. A.: Clinical significance of monoclonal immunoglobulinemia. Bull. Rheum. Dis., *25*:810, 1975.
117. Lindstrom, F. D . Hardy, W. R., Eberle, B. J., and Williams, R. C., Jr.: Multiple myeloma and benign monoclonal gammapathy: differentiation by immunofluorescence of lymphocytes. Ann. Intern. Med., *78*:837, 1973.
118. Abdou, N. I., and Abdou, N. L.: The monoclonal nature of lymphocytes in multiple myeloma. Ann. Intern. Med., *83*:42, 1975.
119. Chen, Y., Bhoopalam, N., Yakulis, V., and Heller, P.: Changes in lymphocyte surface immunoglobulins in myeloma and the effect of

an RNA-containing plasma factor. Ann. Intern. Med., *83*:625, 1975.
120. Broder, S., *et al.*: Impaired synthesis of polyclonal (non-paraprotein) immunoglobulins by circulating lymphocytes from patients with multiple myeloma. N. Engl. J. Med., *293*:887, 1975.
121. Dunn, T. B.: Plasma-cell neoplasms beginning in the ileocecal area in strain C_3H mice. J. Natl. Cancer Inst., *19*:371, 1957.
122. Pilgrim, H. I.: the relationship of chronic ulceration of the ileocecal junction to the development of reticuloendothelial tumors in C_3H mice. Cancer Res., *25*:53, 1965.
123. Potter, M., and Robertson, C. L.: Development of plasma-cell neoplasms in Balb/c mice after intraperitoneal injection of paraffin-oil adjuvant, heat-killed staphylococcus mixtures. J. Natl. Cancer Inst., *25*:847, 1960.
124. Potter, M., and Boyce, C. R.: Induction of plasma-cell neoplasms in strain Balb/c mice with mineral oil and mineral oil adjuvants. Nature, *193*:1086, 1962.
125. Dalton, A. J., Potter, M., and Merwin, R. M.: Some ultrastructural characteristics of a series of primary and transplanted plasma-cell tumors of the mouse. J. Natl. Cancer Inst., *26*:1221, 1961.
126. Parsons, D. F., *et al.*: Electron microscopy of plasma-cell tumors of the mouse. J. Biophys. Biochem. Cytol., *9*:353, 1961.
127. Potter, M., and Leon, M. A.: three IgA myeloma immunoglobulins from the Balb/c mouse: precipitation with pneumococcal C polysaccharide. Science, *162*:369, 1968.
128. ———: Plasma cell dyscrasias. Am. J. Med., *44*:256, 1968.
129. Eisen, H. N., *et al.*: A myeloma protein with antibody activity. Cold Spring Harbor Symp. Quan. Biol., *32*:75, 1967.
130. Metzger, H.: Characterization of a human macroglobulin: a Waldenström macroglobulin with antibody activity. Proc. Natl. Acad. Sci. U.S.A., *57*:1490, 1967.
131. Farhangi, M., and Osserman, E. F.: Myeloma with xanthoderma due to an IgG λ monoclonal antiflavin antibody. N. Engl. J. Med., *294*:177, 1976.
132. Ritzmann, S. E., Thurm, R. H., Truax, W. E. and Levin W. K.: The syndrome of macroglobulinemia. Arch. Intern. Med., *105*:939, 1960.
133. Waldenström, J. G.: Monoclonal and Polyclonal Hypergammaglobulinemia Nashville, Vanderbilt University Press, 1968.
134. Bloch, K. J., and Maki, D. G.: Hyperviscosity syndromes associated with immunoglobulin abnormalities. Semin. Hematol., *10*:113, 1973.
135. Solomon, A., and McLaughlin, C. L.: Biosynthesis of low molecular weight (7S) and high molecular weight (19S) immunoglobulin M. J. Clin. Invest., *49*:150, 1970.
136. Bhoopalam, N., Lee, B. M., Yakulis, V. J., and Heller, P.: IgM heavy chain fragments in Waldenström's macroglobulinemia. Arch. Intern. Med., *128*:437, 1971.
137. Snapper, I., and Kahn, A.: Myelomatosis. Baltimore, University Park Press, 1971.
138. Fragione, B., and Franklin, E. C.: Heavy chain diseases: clinical features and molecular significance of the disordered immunoglobulin structure. Semin. Hematol., *10*:53, 1973.
139. Seligmann, M.: Immunochemical, clinical and pathological features of α-chain disease. Arch. Intern. Med., *135*:78, 1975.
140. Roge', J., *et al.*: Alpha-chain disease cured with antibiotics. Br. Med. J., *4*:225, 1975.
141. Seligmann, M., and Mihaesco, E.: Current knowledge of alpha chain disease. Adv. Exp. Med., Biol., *45*:365, 1973.
142. Franklin, E. C., Frangione, B., and Cooper, S.: Heavy chain discases. Ann. N.Y. Acad. Sci., *190*:457, 1971.
143. Franklin, E. C.: Mu-chain disease. Arch. Intern. Med., *135*:71, 1975.
144. Franklin, E. C., Frangione, B., and Prelli, F.: The defect in mu heavy chain disease protein GLI. J. Immunol., *116*:1194, 1976.
145. Kyle, R. A., and Bayrd, E. D.: Amyloidosis: review of 236 cases. Medicine, *54*:271, 1975.
146. Franklin, E. C.: Amyloidosis. Bull. Rheum. Dis., *26*:832, 1975.
147. Glenner, G. G.: Current concepts on the formation and composition of amyloid. Ann. Clin. Lab. Sci., *5*:257, 1975.
148. Terry, W. D., *et al.*: Structural identity of Bence-Jones and amyloid fibril proteins in a patient with plasma cell dyscrasia and amyloidosis. J. Clin. Invest., *52*:1276, 1973.
149. Ossermann, E. F., Takatsuki, K., Talal, N.: The pathogenesis of "amyloidosis." Semin. Hematol., *1*:3, 1964.
150. Husby, G., and Natwig, J. B.: A serum component related to nonimmunoglobulin amyloid protein AS, a possible precursor of the fibrils. J. Clin. Invest., *53*:1054, 1974.
151. Sipe, J. D., Ignaczak, T. F., Pollock, P. S., and Glenner, G. G.: Amyloid fibril protein AA: purification and properties of the antigenically related serum component as determined by solid phase radioimmunoassay. J. Immunol., *116*:1151, 1976.
152. Tashjian, A. H., Wolfe, H. J., Voekel, E. F.: Human calcitonin. Am. J. Med., *56*:840, 1974.
153. Cohen, H. J., Lessin, L. S., Hallal, J., and Burkholder, P.: Resolution of primary amyloidosis during chemotherapy. Ann. Intern. Med., *82*:466, 1975.
154. Shirahama, T., and Cohen, A. S.: Intralysosomal formation of amyloid fibrils. Am. J. Pathol., *81*:101, 1975.
155. Scheinberg, M. A., and Cathcart, E. S.: Casein-induced experimental amyloidosis. Immunology, *27*:953, 1974.
156. Baumal, R., Wilson, B., and Pass, E.: Experimental murine amyloidosis: a model system for studying amyloid formation. Can. Med. Assoc. J., *113*:512, 1975.

157. Scheinberg, M. A., and Cathcart, E. S.: Casein-induced experimental amyloidosis. Immunology, *31*:443, 1976.
158. Scheinberg, M. A., Goldstein, A. L., and Cathcart, E. S.: Thymosin restores T cell function and reduces the incidence of amyloid disease in casein-treated mice. J. Immunol., *116*:156, 1976.
159. Mandema, E., Ruinen, L., Scholten, J. H., and Cohen, A. S. (eds.): Amyloidosis. Amsterdam, Excerpta Medica Foundation, 1968.
160. Skinner, M., Cathcart, E. S., Cohen, A. S., and Benson, M. D.: Isolation and identification by sequence analysis of experimentally induced guinea pig amyloid fibrils. J. Exp. Med., *140*:871, 1974.
161. McAdam, K. P. W. J., and Sipe, J. D.: Murine model for human secondary amyloidosis: genetic variability of the acute-phase serum protein SAA response to endotoxins and casein. J. Exp. Med., *144*:1121, 1976.
162. Rosenthal, C. J., and Franklin, E. C.: Variation with age and disease of an amyloid A protein-related serum component, J. Clin. Invest., *55*:746, 1975.
163. Linder, E., Anders, R. F., and Natvig, J. B.: Connective tissue origin of the amyloid-related protein SSA. J. Exp. Med., *144*:1336, 1976.

13 Tumor Immunology

In 1909, Paul Ehrlich proposed that the immune system was responsible not only for defending against microbial invasion, but also for eliminating altered host constituents from the body.[2] It was eventually realized that cancer cells might represent such altered constituents and thus become antigenic targets for the immune system. The modern formulation of this idea evolved through the efforts of Thomas,[2] Burnet,[3] and Good,[4] and has been termed the *immune surveillance theory*. Its essential postulate is that a normally functioning immune system continually polices the body against neoplastic growths by destroying newly arising tumors. Malignant transformation is considered to be a fairly common event, and but for the intervention of the immune system numerous malignancies might rapidly emerge.

Recent findings in the laboratory, as well as a reinterpretation of clinical data, have forced a reappraisal of the concept of immune surveillance. At present, the relationship between the immune system and cancer is the center of much controversy.

TUMOR ANTIGENS

Tumor cells express many of the same surface antigens—for example, transplantation antigens—as normal cells. However, most tumor cells also express antigens that are not found on equivalent normal cells but that are specific to the malignant clone. These antigens are called *tumor-specific antigens*, or TSA (Fig. 13-1).

The existence of tumor-specific antigens was first demonstrated in animals. Mice were immunized with methylcholanthrene-induced sarcoma cells taken from a syngeneic animal. The growing tumor was then removed and the mice were challenged with a second inoculum of sarcoma cells. The immunized mice rapidly rejected the tumor challenge, thus demonstrating the immunogenicity of the tumor cells (Fig. 13-2).[5]

The first tumor-specific antigen associated with a virally induced malignancy was detected in the same manner on a mouse tumor induced by a polyoma virus.[6] Because this method for detecting tumor-specific antigens measures tumor rejection by a preimmunized host, tumor antigens have been frequently referred to as *tumor-specific transplantation antigens* (TSTA).

Following these initial successes, many laboratories attempted to define tumor-specific transplantation antigens on a great variety of different animal tumors. Two major conclusions emerged from this work:

1. All tumors induced by a given virus

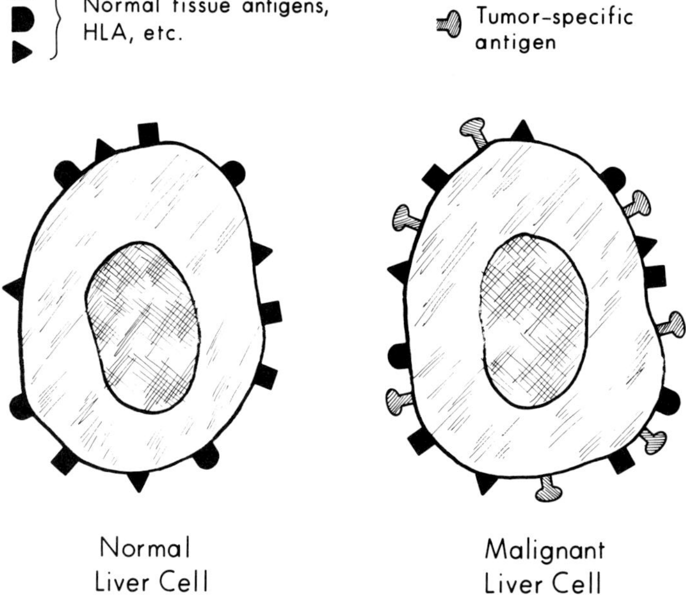

Fig. 13-1. Tumor cells express normal cell-surface antigens as well as tumor-specific antigens (TSA).

share certain antigenic determinants called "group-specific TSTA." Tumors induced by a particular chemical agent, no matter how similar their histologic appearance, are antigenically distinct. They are said to express "individual TSTA" (Fig. 13-3).[7] These are not absolute rules; weak crossreacting antigens may appear on some chemically induced tumors, and individual antigens may be found on some virally induced tumors. A given tumor may express both group-specific and individual tumor antigens.

2. Tumors vary widely in their immunogenicity. In general, tumors induced experimentally *in vivo* with chemical or viral agents are highly immunogenic, whereas tumors arising spontaneously *in vivo* are poorly immunogenic.[8]

The low immunogenicity of spontaneously arising tumors originally suggested that in a normal setting (that is, without the introduction of an experimental carcinogenic agent) only tumors capable of avoiding immune reactivity could grow successfully in an immunocompetent host. This view was consistent with the immune surveillance hypothesis according to which tumors that are highly immunogenic should be readily destroyed by

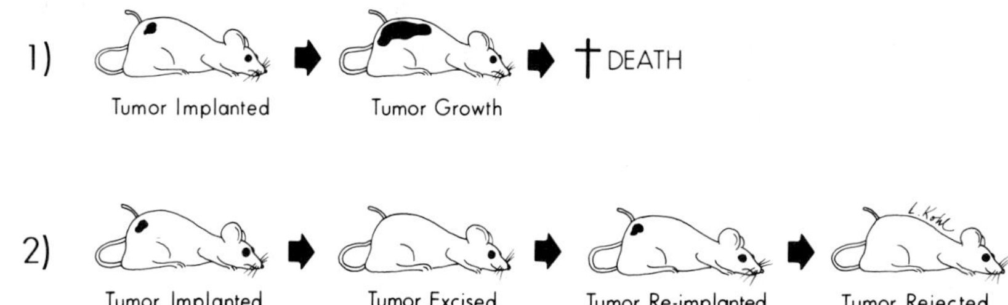

Fig. 13-2. (1) A tumor implant grows and kills the recipient animal. (2) When excision of a tumor implant is followed by reimplantation, the immunized animal is able to reject the tumor mass.

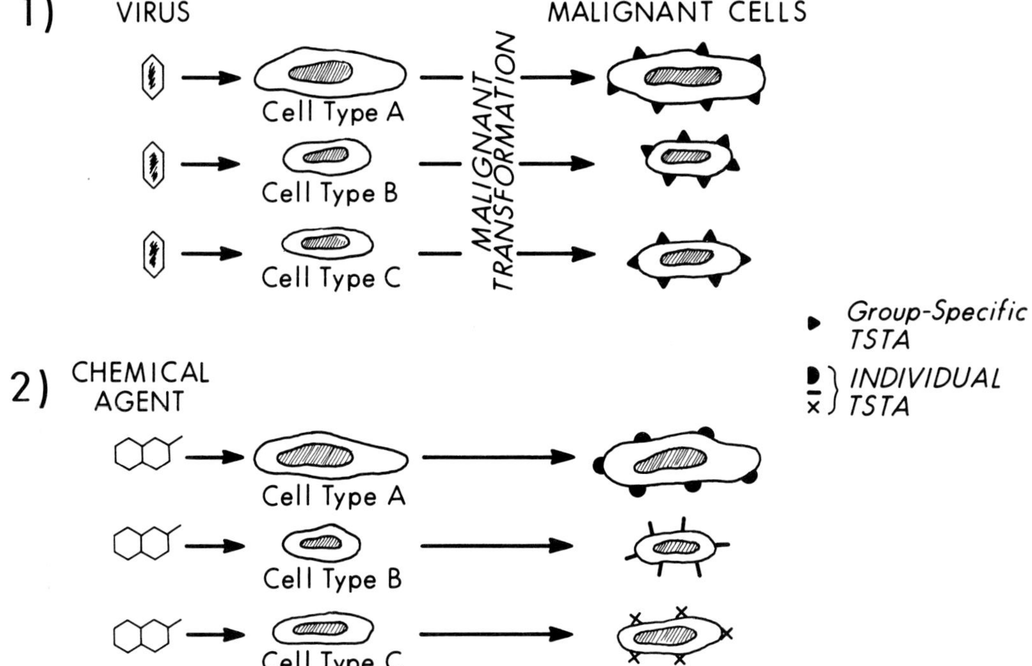

Fig. 13-3. (1) Different tumors induced by the same viral agent all share certain determinants called group-specific TSTA. (2) Different tumors induced by the same chemical agent are antigenically distinct.

the immune system. This process of eliminating all but tumors of low immunogenicity was termed *immunoselection*.

In vitro experiments have failed to support the concept of immunoselection. Tumors arising spontaneously *in vitro* appear to be as poorly immunogenic as tumors arising spontaneously *in vivo* in the presence of the host immune system.[9] This result suggests that the immune system may not be responsible for selecting out poorly immunogenic tumors. Tumors induced by chemical carcinogens *in vitro* are highly immunogenic, and the immunogenicity of the tumor is dose-related.[10] It therefore appears that the nature and the dose of the oncogenic agent, rather than the influence of the immune system, determine the immunogenicity of a tumor. Spontaneously arising tumors may therefore be poorly immunogenic because of the characteristics of naturally occurring oncogenic agents and events, such as the activation of C-type viruses or somatic mutation. Experimental carcinogens induce tumors of high immunogenicity.

The antigenicity of human tumors has been difficult to prove since transplantation experiments are ethically prohibited. Indirect evidence of host sensitization to autologous tumors includes reports of cutaneous delayed hypersensitivity to tumor extracts,[11] and the presence of immune complex renal disease resulting from the deposition of antibody-tumor antigen complexes in rare patients.[12,13] In order to evaluate more directly human immunity to human tumors, *in vitro* assays for antitumor immunity have been developed. The two most commonly employed tests are the colony-inhibition assay and the microcytotoxicity assay.

In the *colony-inhibition assay* (Fig. 13-4), tumor cells are plated on the bot-

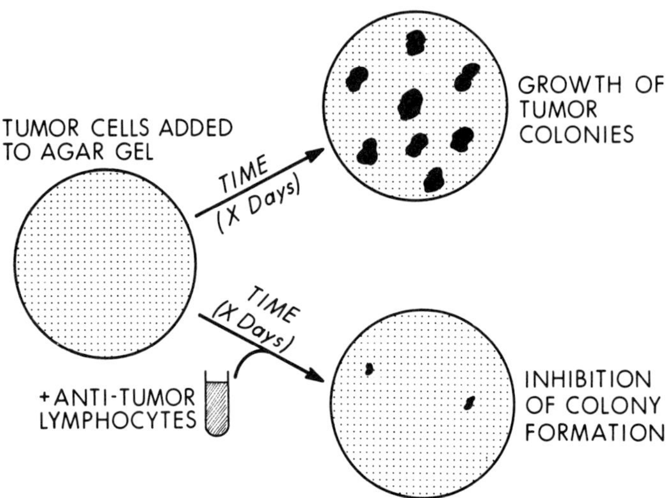

Fig. 13-4. The colony-inhibition assay. Tumor cells are dispersed in an agar gel and will proliferate to form colonies of tumor cells. The addition of sensitized lymphocytes reduces the number of tumor colonies, and the per cent of reduction is an index of colony inhibition.

tom of a container or dispersed in an agar gel. The neoplastic cells proliferate and form a readily detectable colony. In order to measure immunologic reactivity against the tumor, lymphocytes from the tumor-bearing host are added to the culture and the number of tumor-cell colonies formed in the presence of lymphocytes is compared to suitable controls. The result is recorded as a per cent of inhibition of colony formation.[14]

The *microcytotoxicity assay* requires fewer cells and a shorter incubation time since it is not necessary to wait several days for tumor cells to grow out into colonies. Lymphocytes and the target cells are cultured together and the degree of cytotoxicity is measured,[15,16] usually by monitoring the release of an intracellular label.

Based upon these *in vitro* techniques, there are now many reports that immunocompetent cells can kill or inhibit the growth of autologous tumor cells.[17,18] Much of the early work indicated that the effect was specific: lymphocytes from a given donor were cytotoxic against cells of the host's own tumor or a histologically related tumor, but would not kill cells from histologically unrelated tumors.[17] For example, lymphocytes taken from a patient with melanoma would react against melanoma cells from many donors but not against colon carcinoma cells. Lymphocytes taken from healthy individuals were unreactive.

More recent results have questioned these findings. Human lymphocytes taken from healthy, non-cancer-bearing donors have been shown to be cytotoxic for a variety of human tumor-cell types *in vitro*.[19,20] This phenomenon has also been studied in animal systems and has been referred to as *natural cell-mediated cytotoxicity*. Natural cytotoxicity may reflect host sensitization to common viral antigens, perhaps associated with oncogenic viruses, which may be expressed on tumor cells.[21] Still other investigators have reported that lymphocytes from tumor-bearing patients are cytotoxic to a variety of unrelated tumors.[22] These results seriously question the many reports of specific tumor sensitization, and a reevaluation of this work will be necessary.

MECHANISMS OF CYTOTOXICITY

The methods by which immunocompetent cells can destroy tumor cells have been studied entirely *in vitro*. It remains to be determined whether these results have any applicability to the tumor-host relationship *in vivo*.

T Cells

It would seem reasonable to assume that tumor-cell cytotoxicity might be primarily a result of T-killer-cell activity since the destruction of antigenically foreign cells—as in transplantation immunity—is so clearly a property of the T-cell population. There have, however, been only scattered reports of T-cell-mediated tumor-cell cytotoxicity in animal systems and in humans.[23] At present, the role of the T cell in antitumor immunity is uncertain.

Non-T Lymphocytes

Other populations of human lymphocytes have been implicated in tumor-cell destruction. These cells have not been well characterized but do not appear to be T cells by conventional surface analysis.[24]

Lymphocytes taken from cancer-free *unsensitized* nude mice possessing little or no T-cell function have been shown to be cytotoxic against syngeneic and allogeneic tumors.[21] These "naturally cytotoxic" lymphocytes do not resemble B cells, T cells or macrophages, nor do they appear to partake in antibody-dependent cytotoxicity. Normal mice have been found to possess cytotoxic cells for mouse leukemia cells that also cannot be classified as either T or B cells.[25] It is possible that the cells responsible for natural cytotoxicity are a population separate from those involved in presensitized tumor killing. How these cells act and what subpopulation of cells they represent remain unknown.

Antibody

There are two ways in which antibody could theoretically contribute to tumor-cell destruction:

1. *Complement Fixation*. Antitumor antibody and complement components have been detected on the surface of some human tumors,[26] but this finding alone gives us little information as to the cytotoxic potential of complement-fixing antibody. Complement-fixing antitumor antibodies can be detected *in vivo*, but usually only when the tumor load is low, and may disappear as the tumor enlarges or with tumor recurrence.

2. *Antibody-Dependent Cell-Mediated Cytotoxicity (ADCC)*. ADCC has only recently been studied as a possible mediator of *in vitro* tumor-cell cytotoxicity. There are already several reports that suggest a role for ADCC *in vitro*,[27,28] and further work may soon permit an accurate assessment of the relative contribution of this mechanism to tumor killing.

The Macrophage

Increasing consideration is being given to the macrophage as a possibly important component in the host reaction to a tumor. Macrophages can be activated for tumor destruction by lymphocytes exposed to tumor tissue.[29] The mechanism of macrophage killing is unknown, although in most instances direct contact between the macrophage and the target cells seems to be required.[29,30] Phagocytosis does not seem to play a major role. Tumor destruction by macrophages has been primarily demonstrated in experimental situations where the tumor is allogeneic to the macrophage population.[31,32] In syngeneic systems, which more closely reflect the clinical situation, cytostasis, the inhibition of cell proliferation with only minimal cell destruction, may be more significant.[33,34] In some situations the macrophages appear to be directed specifically against the immunizing tumor and will spare unrelated tumor cells.[35,36] In other systems, macrophage activity has been observed to be more nonspecific and can be directed against a variety of tumors.[35,37]

TUMOR EVASION OF THE IMMUNE SYSTEM

There are several mechanisms by which a tumor appears to be able to avoid interaction with a potentially damaging immune system:

1. *Sneaking Through*. Several reports have described situations in which large inocula of immunogenic tumor cells fail to grow in a syngeneic or even allogeneic recipient, but where smaller doses grow and eventually overwhelm the host.[38-40] The mechanism of "sneaking through" is unknown, but its existence questions the importance of the immune system in destroying newly arising tumors.

2. *Antigenic Modulation*. There are a few descriptions in the literature of instances in which tumor cells have been serially passed in immunized hosts and have lost their surface antigenicity. This phenomenon appears to depend on a functioning intact immune system.[41-43] It is not certain how often intrinsic antigenic modulation versus the mere masking of surface antigens by antitumor antibody may occur.

3. *Immunosuppression by the Tumor*. An aggressive tumor can contribute to host immunosuppression by directly invading lymphoid tissues or by secreting soluble substances that inhibit immune reactivity. Immunosuppressive factors have been described in the serum of cancer patients, in the medium of tumor-cell cultures and in extracts of tumor cells. The specific targets of these substances and the mechanisms by which immunosuppression occurs are currently being defined. One possibility is that tumors may secrete factors that depress macrophage function.[44] Tumors can suppress reticuloendothelial function, but this may be due in part to a decline in nonspecific opsonins normally present in the serum.[45]

It is well known that the presence of a cancer can significantly reduce an individual's capacity to mount an immune response against a wide variety of antigens. The anergy associated with Hodgkin's disease and the decreased synthesis of normal immunoglobulin in multiple myeloma are just two examples. A degree of immunosuppression has been found in almost all cancer patients that have been studied. The most frequently explored parameter of immune competence has been the ability to manifest a positive skin test to dinitrochlorobenzene (DNCB), a measure of delayed hypersensitivity. Almost all healthy individuals will mount a positive response manifested as an induration reaction to an application of DNCB on the skin two to three weeks after they have been first sensitized to the agent. This is not true for many cancer patients.[46] Negative responses frequently can be seen in patients with a primary tumor only, a primary tumor with regional spread and a primary tumor with distal metastases. In general, an increase in tumor burden is associated with a decreased percentage of patients responding to DNCB.[47] The persistence of DNCB anergy has been associated with poor prognosis and rapid progression of the disease.[48] Interestingly, similar correlations are not found with antigens with which the individual has previously come into contact, such as mumps and *Candida*,[46,47] indicating that responsiveness to new antigens, such as DNCB, may be the more accurate prognostic indicator.

ENHANCEMENT, BLOCKING AND IMMUNOSTIMULATION

The results of a number of experiments are now challenging many traditionally held views concerning the interaction between tumors and the immune system. There is a growing body of evidence that the immune system may be an ineffective antitumor antagonist, and in certain situations may even contribute to tumor

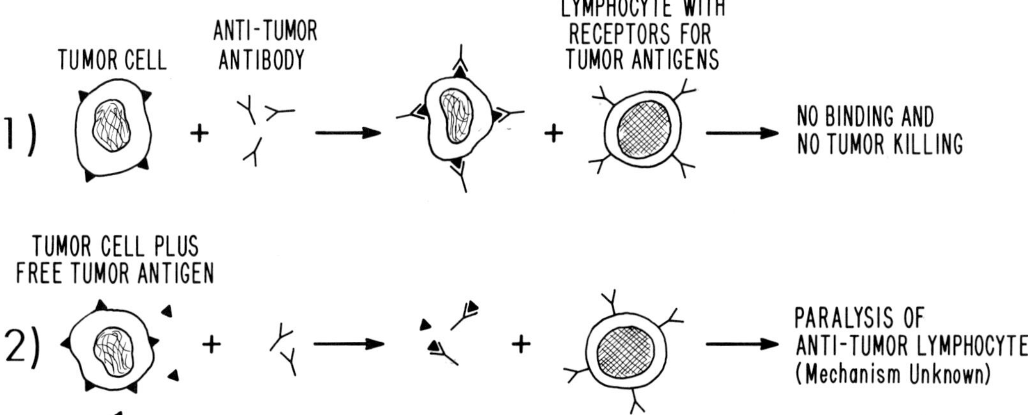

Fig. 13-5. Two postulated mechanisms of blocking and enhancement. (1) Antibody coats the surface antigens on the tumor cell blocking access of immunocompetent cells to the target. (2) Antibody-tumor antigen complexes paralyze the lymphocyte population.

growth. The following paragraphs will attempt to summarize this work.

In early attempts at immunizing animals against a particular tumor, it was occasionally observed that initial immunization actually enhanced the growth of a subsequent tumor challenge.[49] This phenomenon was termed *immunologic enhancement*. Enhancement could be transferred to other hosts with the serum of tumor-immunized animals and was felt to be due to tumor-specific antibody.[50]

A similar phenomenon has since been demonstrated *in vitro* using autologous serum and lymphocytes. In performing the colony-inhibition assay, it was found that addition of the cancer patients' serum to the culture system blocked lymphocyte reactivity against autologous tumor cells.[51] Blocking activity has been attributed to free antigen shed by the tumor cells, free antibody, and complexes of antigen and IgG.[51-54]

Two mechanisms have been offered as explanations for blocking and enhancement (Fig. 13-5):

1. *Masking*. The covering up of antigenic sites on the surface of tumor cells by free antibody may prevent access of immunocompetent cells to the target antigens.

2. *Central Blockade*. Free antigen or antigen-antibody complexes could directly inhibit lymphocyte activity, perhaps by delivering a tolerogenic signal to the lymphocyte.

Serum taken from human cancer patients in remission or postsurgery has been found to possess "unblocking" activity,[51] that is, the ability to remove the inhibitory effect of blocking sera. The phenomenon of unblocking has been attributed to antibody, but this conclusion has not been confirmed. The mechanism of unblocking is unknown, but it has been suggested that it is due to the clearance of blocking antigen or antigen-antibody complexes from the lymphocyte surface, thereby freeing the lymphocytes to respond.

Evidence has also been accumulating that the cellular limb of the immune system may be capable of encouraging tumor growth (Fig. 13-6). Spleen cells from tumor-immunized mice were mixed with target tumor cells and inoculated into thymectomized, x-irradiated hosts. When the inoculum contained large numbers of sensitized splenic lymphocytes, prolifera-

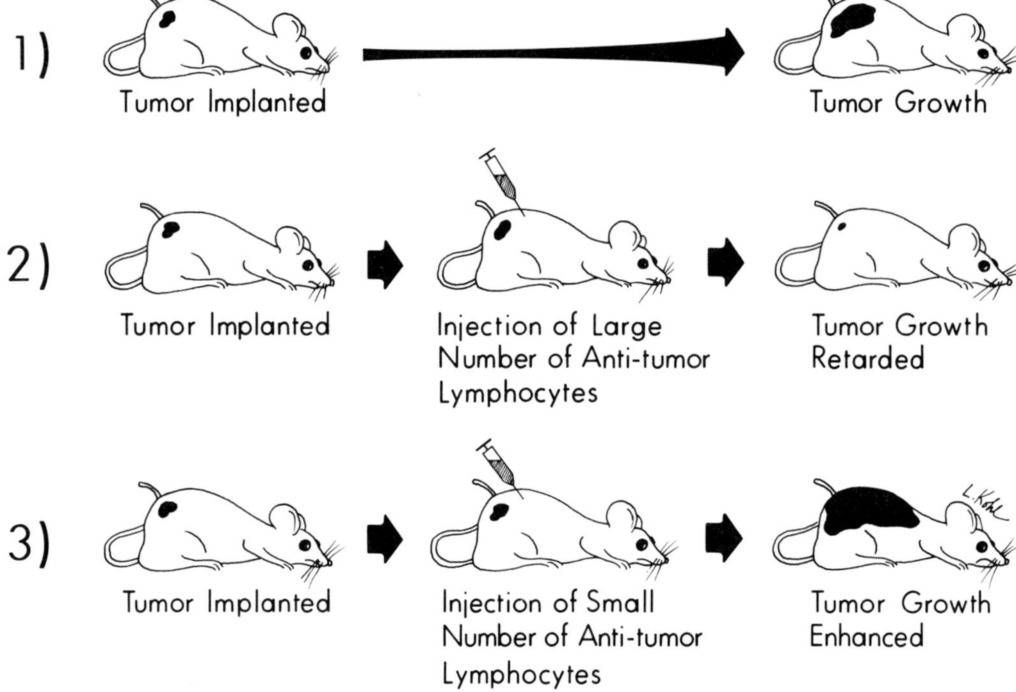

Fig. 13-6. Immunostimulation. (1) Growth of a tumor implant. (2) Large numbers of sensitized lymphocytes retard tumor growth. (3) Small numbers of sensitized lymphocytes enhance tumor growth beyond that seen in (1).

tion of the tumor cells in the recipient animal was retarded. However, small numbers of sensitized lymphocytes enhanced tumor growth beyond that attained when no spleen cells were added.[55,56] Similar observations have since been made *in vitro*[57,58] and *in vivo*.[59,60] This phenomenon has been referred to as immunostimulation. These results are especially important because it is precisely when a tumor is small, and the immune response is just getting under way, that most investigators have thought that the immune system would be most effective in destroying a tumor. These experiments indicate that small numbers of sensitized lymphocytes may instead enhance tumor growth. The mechanism of this effect is unknown, but the observation that low concentrations of lymphocytotoxin may be stimulatory for tumor growth offers one possibility.[61]

An analysis of the data we have examined thus far might lead one to conclude that the immune system is capable of responding to most tumors but that this response may be less than adequate at curtailing tumor growth. However, we must emphasize that most of this data comes from *in vitro* studies and *in vivo* systems that have been subjected to profound experimental manipulation, and one must be very cautious in extrapolating from these systems to the tumor *in situ*.

STUDIES IN VIVO

Perhaps the most relevant data concerning the relationship between tumors and the immune system comes from clinical observations of animals and humans with defective immune systems. These individuals provide us with an outstanding opportunity to evaluate the impact of the immune system on oncogenesis *in vivo*.

Animal Studies

Neonatal thymectomy, treatment with antilymphocyte serum and x-irradiation increase the susceptibility of animals to tumorigenesis. However, the increase in tumor susceptibility is seen predominantly with virally induced neoplasms and much less so with chemically induced and spontaneously arising tumors.[62-64] A similar phenomenon is seen with the nude (athymic) mouse. This animal lacks virtually all aspects of T-cell function, including T-killer-cell activity, T-helper-cell activity (TSTA are T-dependent antigens) and presumably T-cell macrophage-activating ability.* In a study of several thousand nude mice observed over their normal life span, no spontaneously arising tumors have been observed.[65] These animals are also not unusually susceptible to chemical carcinogens but are highly susceptible to viral oncogenesis.[65-67]

The implication from these animal studies is that the immune system may not be critical in eliminating neoplastic growths from the body. If the immune surveillance theory were true as originally stated, one would expect that immunosuppressed animals should be susceptible to all types of tumors, not just those induced by experimental viruses. Instead, the above observations can be interpreted to suggest that the major antitumor effect of the immune system may be the removal or destruction of oncogenic viruses. This is a very different concept than that expressed by the immune surveillance theory. According to the latter, neoplastic transformation is considered to be a fairly common event, and the immune system is responsible for directly destroying newly arising tumors. The observations in the nude mouse and other immunosuppressed animals suggest that spontaneous oncogenesis is not common, and the role of the immune system may be more to protect the body against invasion by tumorigenic viruses than to destroy neoplastic cells.

Human Studies

Two to 10 per cent of children afflicted with immunodeficiency disorders develop malignancies, a rate 100 to 1000 times greater than that of the normal population.[68] However, this increased incidence of cancer applies only to a restricted range of malignancies including primarily lymphomas.[69] Similarly, renal-graft recipients receiving immunosuppressive therapy have an increased rate of malignancy nearly 200 times greater than that of the normal population,[69] but about one half of these malignancies are lymphoreticular in origin.[69,70]

In our discussion of lymphoreticular malignancies in Chapter 12 we described how the lymphorecticular system appears to be unusually susceptible to malignant transformation in a setting of chronic antigenic stimulation. A kidney-graft recipient on immunosuppression is subjected to a powerful antigenic load, and it is possible that the elements of the immune system which remain intact in these immunosuppressed patients are subjected to continual antigenic stimulation leading eventually to a lymphorecticular malignancy. This concept is supported by the evidence that a graft-versus-host reaction can induce lymphomas in mice and both a graft-versus-host and a mixed lymphocyte reaction can induce the appearance of oncogenic viruses.[71-73] It is also of interest that the majority of the nonlymphorecticular malignancies in these patients are cancers in which viral agents are strongly implicated in the pathogenesis.[74]

---

*It is necessary to emphasize, however, that there is no evidence that the macrophage system in the nude mouse is less than competent. It is thus possible that critical elements of anti-tumor immunity remain intact in these animals.

Thus, as in the animal studies, it appears that a deficient immune system in man predisposes to only certain types of malignancies, and these may be explained by the failure of the immune system to eliminate oncogenic agents, especially viruses, from the immunocompromised host. A deficient surveillance system would lead one to predict an increase in all types of cancer, and this does not occur. The role of the immune system in defense against cancer may thus be less one of surveillance against neoplastic cells and more one of the elimination of cancer-inducing agents from the body.

TUMOR IMMUNOTHERAPY

Immunotherapy in neoplastic disease involves the use of immunologic manipulations in an attempt to destroy a tumor. Tumor immunotherapy is presently under study in extensive clinical trials and its place in the overall approach to treating human cancer is only now being evaluated.

MODALITIES OF IMMUNOTHERAPY

Immunoprophylaxis

In certain animals the development of leukemia has been traced directly to the presence of particular viruses. Chemically altered viruses or attenuated viral strains have been given to these animals as vaccines. These vaccines have provided remarkable protection against the development of leukemia upon subsequent challenge with a fully active virus. This has been shown in mice vaccinated with formalin-treated leukemia virus[75] and in chickens given an attenuated vaccine of a Marek's disease virus.[76] Marek's disease is a lymphoproliferative and inflammatory disease of domestic fowl caused by a herpes virus. Vaccines have now been used successfully in protecting millions of chickens against Marek's disease. Vaccines have also prevented leukemia in cats[77] and malignant lymphoma in marmosets.[78] Leukemia vaccines have not yet been tried in humans since no virus has been definitively implicated as an etiologic agent in human leukemia. It would be absolutely essential to insure that the vaccine was both inactive and capable of conveying immunity to the recipient.

Active Immunotherapy

This form of immunotherapy has been the most extensively studied and thus far has been the most successful. Active immunotherapy can take two forms; nonspecific immunotherapy, where nonspecific stimulants are used to boost the patient's overall immune response including that against his tumor, and specific immunotherapy, where the cancer patient is given tumor cells bearing antigens that crossreact with his tumor. In some of the more successful studies, a combination of specific and nonspecific modes of therapy has been used.

Two types of active, nonspecific immunotherapy have been employed. In one, the antigen DNCB is applied topically to superficial lesions of squamous-cell or basal-cell carcinoma. The patient's lymphocytes respond to the DNCB and, in the ensuing inflammatory response, the tumor cells are destroyed as well. More than 90 per cent of superficial basal cell and squamous cell carcinomas can be destroyed by this delayed hypersensitivity reaction.[79]

The second type of active, nonspecific immunotherapy employs adjuvants. Two in particular are being subjected to extensive clinical and experimental studies, BCG and *C. parvum*.

BCG is a live, attenuated strain of *Mycobacterium bovis*.[80] BCG vaccinations in animals produce a generalized enhancement of immune responsiveness against a great variety of antigens. The effects of BCG include enhanced antigen clearance and phagocytosis, increased humoral immunity, accelerated rejection of transplants and increased resistance to infection.[81] BCG's antitumor activity was first demonstrated by the retardation of transplanted tumor growth in animals infected with the mycobacterium.[82] BCG was shown to prevent the growth of tumor transplants if given several days prior to transplantation, and to inhibit the growth of already established tumors.[80] In some instances, it could also be stimulatory to tumor growth.[83] Systemic BCG inoculation has proved to be less successful than the direct injection of the agent into the tumor site. Mixing tumor cells with the inoculum appears to be especially effective in experimental protocols.

The mechanisms of BCG's antitumor activity have yet to be determined. BCG injection elicits a granulomatous inflammatory reaction that may destroy tumor cells as "innocent bystanders." BCG's ability to stimulate nonspecifically the immune system, that is, to act as an adjuvant, is also likely to be an important factor. Mechanisms of adjuvanticity were discussed in Chapter 2.

There was historical precedent for the use of bacteria and bacterial products in the treatment of human cancer in the work of Dr. William B. Coley done at the end of the last century. He had noted that one patient with recurrent inoperable sarcoma of the neck had experienced a nearly miraculous recovery after two attacks or facial erysipelas.[84] Coley proceeded to inoculate cancer patients with heat-killed or filtered cultures of streptococci with mixed but encouraging results. These inocula became known as Coley's toxins.[85] Because the results were inconsistent, work with Coley's toxins was not pursued, but the precedent for nonspecific adjuvant therapy had been set.

BCG has been used predominantly in two settings: in treating acute leukemia, and in treating cutaneous neoplasms. The effectiveness of BCG in the treatment of leukemia is controversial. Following conventional therapy in order to maintain minimal residual tumor volume and to get the patient into remission, BCG has been used in combination with additional chemotherapy in order to maintain remission. The first reports describing this mode of treatment in acute lymphoblastic leukemia were very encouraging. More than one third of treated patients were maintained in long-term remission by this regimen.[86] Subsequent studies have tempered this enthusiasm,[87] and the role of BCG in the treatment of acute lymphoblastic leukemia must be considered uncertain. Claims of clinical benefit in acute myelogenous leukemia[88] and chronic myelocytic leukemia[89] using BCG have also been made. The efficacy of such therapy is currently being evaluated in clinical trials.

The greatest success with BCG has been in the treatment of cutaneous tumors, notably melanoma. In a review of several studies done prior to 1974,[80] 58 per cent of tumor nodules injected with BCG were observed to regress versus only 14 per cent of noninjected lesions. In patients who became PPD-positive following BCG injection, 90 per cent of injected lesions regressed. Other reports have been equally encouraging.[90] A small percentage of noninjected lesions in patients receiving BCG also regressed. Unfortunately, visceral metastases almost never respond to this form of therapy, and long-term survivors are limited to patients with disease confined to the skin, subcutaneous tissues and regional lymph nodes. Other skin lesions, including basal- and squamous-cell carcinoma, mycosis fungoides, Kaposi's sarcoma, reticulum-cell sarcoma, lymphangiosarcoma and cutaneous metastases of both breast and colon cancer appear to be susceptible to local injection of BCG as well.[80]

BCG has been given to a great number of children in Europe as a vaccine against tuberculosis. Some epidemiologic studies of these children suggest that BCG may have a prophylactic effect against developing childhood leukemia.[91] Other statistical surveys have failed to confirm this finding.[92]

BCG therapy is not without its difficulties. Systemic reactions, with fever, chills and malaise, though rare, may occur. The risk of systemic infection is particularly great in patients immunosuppressed by chemotherapy. Repeated injections of BCG have been associated with hypersensitivity and anaphylaxis. Most importantly, one must be aware of the danger of inducing blocking and enhancement with this nonspecific immunostimulant. BCG is an unstable, living vaccine whose efficacy depends on the number of live organisms it contains. For all of these reasons, some investigators have sought for other nonspecific stimulants.

Corynebacterium parvum, the gram-negative anaerobe, is easily standardized and is given in nonviable form. It is being increasingly employed in experimental protocols. *C. parvum* seems to act primarily by stimulating macrophage function; its effect on T-cell immunity is less clear.[93,94] *C. parvum* is most effective as an antitumor agent when it is injected directly into the tumor site,[95] and it may work well in combination with chemotherapy.[96] Significant regression of established large tumors in mice has been described.[97] *C. parvum* used in combination with chemotherapy has had important clinical effects in patients with lung cancer and disseminated disease.[98] Toxicity has occasionally been encountered in some animals given *C. parvum* systemically. Local injections do not appear to have toxic side effects.

Other adjuvants are receiving initial trials as of this writing. Two in particular are noteworthy:

1. Levamisole is a synthetic antihelminthic drug which has been found to have significant effects on tumor immunity. It appears to be able to boost a patient's faltering cellular immunity, but not to potentiate a normal response. It may therefore be valuable in combination with chemotherapy. In a study of women with stage three (nonresectable) breast cancer first treated with x-irradiation, levamisole increased the 30-month survival rate from 35 per cent to 90 per cent.[99] One of the great advantages to levamisole is that it can be taken orally.

2. MER is a methanol extraction of killed tuberculin bacilli. It is therefore safer and easier to manipulate than BCG. In a series of animal studies, MER has been shown to be as potent as BCG against a variety of tumors.[100]

In many studies, tumor cells have been added to the nonspecific stimulants in the inoculum. These can either be killed or inactivated autologous or allogeneic tumor cells.[80] The hope is that in combination with BCG or some other adjuvant the tumor antigens will become potently immunogenic and induce a rejection reaction against the patient's own tumor. Cells treated with neuraminidase exhibit heightened immunogenicity,[101] and thus may be especially effective in inducing regression. Neuraminidase removes terminal sialic acid residues from membrane glycoproteins. This may affect immunogenicity in many ways, such as by decreasing the negative surface charge, by increasing susceptibility to phagocytosis, or by exposing neoantigens on the cell's surface.[101] Attaching concanavalin A to tumor-cell membranes has also been shown to increase tumor-cell immunogenicity (perhaps via its activity as a mitogen), and administration of concanavalin-A-treated cells can lead to tumor regression in animals.[102] One of the reasons cell-surface modification may be successful in tumor therapy may be its selective enhancement of cellular over humoral reactivity. This result may be due to crossreactivity at the cellular but not the humoral level between the modified cells and the patient's tumor cells.

Similar findings have been seen with the carboxymethylated derivative of lysozyme[103] and the acetoacetylated derivitive of flagellin,[104] both of which show cellular crossreactivity with the original unmodified proteins but not humoral crossreactivity.

Passive Immunotherapy

The earliest attempts at immunotherapy involved raising antisera to a patient's cancer in an animal and then injecting the antisera back into the patient. Passive transfer of antibody was attempted throughout the early part of the century and has since been abandoned as being of no demonstrable benefit. From our discussion of the role of the humoral response in tumor immunology, this is not particularly surprising. It has been suggested, however, that antitumor antibody may be useful if attached to chemotherapeutic agents as a means of specifically guiding the drug to the site where its actions are desired.[105]

In Vitro Stimulation of the Patient's Lymphocytes

Attempts have been made to expose a patient's lymphocytes to his own tumor cells[106] or to PHA[107] *in vitro* and then to inject the activated cells back into the patient. This technique has not been extensively pursued.

Adoptive Transfer

Instead of trying to manipulate the patient's own immune system, some investigators have attempted to transfer cells or cell extracts from healthy individuals. There are essentially three types of adoptive transfer that have been tried.

Leukocyte Transfer. In one large study, peripheral blood from patients with chronic myelocytic leukemia was given to 52 patients with various malignancies whose course was complicated by neutropenia and infection.[108] In 50 per cent of the recipients a transient graft was established. In combination with chemotherapy, nine out of 24 recipients with acute leukemia achieved partial or complete remission. All of them developed signs and symptoms of graft-versus-host disease. It is possible that destruction of the patient's leukemic cells by the graft may have played a role in achieving remission.

Bone Marrow Transplant. This form of adoptive transfer is aimed at providing a more permanent graft than simple leukocyte transfer, since stem cells as well as mature cells are given to the patient. Bone marrow transplant has been predominantly used for patients with aplastic anemia and other bone marrow defects with the hope of supplying normal marrow elements, and for patients with immunodeficiency diseases or cancer. It is a complex and hazardous procedure. The graft must become permanently established in order to supply the needed hematologic elements. The great danger is graft-versus-host disease. If the GVH reaction can be suppressed, stem cells will be able to mature and may emerge tolerant to host constituents, thus removing the danger of GVH disease. To illustrate the hazards of the procedure, in one study[109] bone marrow transplants given to 21 leukemic patients resulted in 15 successful takes. All were complicated by graft-versus-host disease. Eleven patients died, and only four became successfully established chimeras. With an identical twin donor the danger is much less[110] and the procedure is often successful.

Success may be possible with intensive management through the GVH crisis. In one report, a 19-year-old boy with acute myelogenous leukemia received an ABO-incompatible HLA-compatible allogeneic bone marrow transplant and suffered a near fatal GVH reaction. He had eleven severe viral and bacterial infections associated with diminished lymphoid tissue, decreased immunoglobulin levels, and decreased cellular reactivity. With vigorous treatment of every complication the patient survived and was well through three years post-transplant.[111]

Transfer Factor

Aside from a few scattered reports of clinical benefit,[112] little is known about the possible role of transfer factor in cancer therapy.

ONCOFETAL MARKERS

An oncofetal marker is an antigen that is found in both fetal and malignant tissue.[113] Most are expressed on the cell surface and some can be found free in the serum as well. Oncofetal markers have now been described in a great variety of tumors, including tumors induced experimentally by viruses and chemicals and spontaneous tumors arising in animals and man. Oncofetal markers are considered to be normal fetal antigens expressed by the malignant cell as a result of the transformation process. Their existence supports the notion that cancer represents a "dedifferentiation" of the involved cell to a more primitive state. In the following discussion we shall be focusing on those oncofetal markers that are expressed on the tumor-cell surface.

Since oncofetal antigens are not normally expressed in the adult, one can ask whether they provoke an immune response on the part of the host, and whether such a response might be of protective value. A study in the early 1900's demonstrated that immunizing an animal with embryonic cells could lead to rejection of a subsequently transplanted tumor which in nonimmunized hosts grew and killed the recipient animal.[114] There have been some later reports confirming this finding, although it has often been necessary to irradiate the embryonic cells in order for the preimmunization to be successful (the embroyonic cells might otherwise mature and lose their fetal characteristics).[113-115] Many other workers, however, have performed similar types of experiments and have found that fetal antigens do not contribute significantly to tumor destruction, are not protective, and in some circumstances may even have an enhancing effect.[113,116-118] Oncofetal antigens therefore do not appear to be tumor-specific transplantation antigens (TSTA), as shown both by the inability of immunization with fetal tissue to lead to tumor rejection and by the failure of fetal antigens and TSTA to crossreact serologically.

Although not powerful enough to provoke a rejection reaction, fetal antigens can be immunogenic in their host. In one study, 70 per cent of patients with localized digestive-system cancers were found to have anti-carcinoembryonic-antigen antibodies. These antibodies did not appear to be of any protective value. Antibodies were not found in patients with widely metastasizing cancer, suggesting that disseminated cancer may act as an antibody sink, and, indeed, these patients had very high levels of circulating carcinoembryonic antigen.[119] Other investigators have failed to demonstrate anti-carcinoembryonic-antigen antibody production.[120,121] The immunogenicity of oncofetal antigens is thus still controversial.

The importance of oncofetal antigens does not lie in their protective value for the host, but rather as markers for monitoring the various cancers with which they are associated. We shall briefly describe the two most carefully studied of these markers.

Carcinoembryonic Antigen (CEA)

Human CEA was discovered in 1965[122] and found to be associated with fetal and embryonic gut, pancreas and liver, as well as malignancies of the esophagus, stomach, small intestine, colon, rectum and pancreas.[123] Over 90 per cent of patients with malignancies of the colon or pancreas are CEA positive.[124] CEA is a glycoprotein with a molecular weight of approximately 200,000,[125] and may be related to the ABO blood group antigens.[126] It is found on the plasma membrane and is synthesized by the tumor cell.[127]

CEA initially caused great excitement as a potentially simple and accurate diagnostic test for gastrointestinal malignancies. However, these hopes were dimmed by the finding of elevated levels of CEA in patients with colonic polyps,[128] ulcerative colitis, Crohn's disease,[129] severe alcoholic cirrhosis, uremia,[130] and other types of malignancies. CEA has also been detected in normal colonic tissue, although at a much lower concentration than in comparable malignant tissue.[131] High levels are generally found only in advanced malignancies. Early curable carcinomas only rarely have greatly elevated CEA levels,[113,132-134] and therefore its use as a diagnostic tool for early malignancy has been disappointing.

The value of CEA determination lies in its relationship to disease progression. Changing CEA titers appear to correlate with progression or remission of the disease.[135] Very high levels of CEA are almost invariably associated with the presence of metastases.[136] It has been suggested that the elevation of CEA titers in ulcerative colitis may be transient, and persistence of high levels of the antigen may be a sign of malignant transformation, a not uncommon development in patients with ulcerative colitis.[137]

Alpha-Fetoprotein (αFP)

Fetuin, an alpha globulin found in the serum of fetal calves but not that of adults, was described in 1944.[138] A similar protein was detected immunologically in serum from human fetuses.[139] The human antigen was named alpha-fetoprotein and has since been found to be chemically distinct from fetuin.[140] Its protein core bears a striking structural resemblance to albumin, although it possesses carbohydrate groups as well and is therefore a glycoprotein.[141] αFP is made in the yolk sac, fetal tissues including the liver and kidney, the placenta and possibly the gastrointestinal tract.[142] In the adult it can have two sources: malignancies of entodermal origin such as liver tumors, and gonadal tumors.[140,143,144] A majority of patients with either of these disorders are αFP-positive.[113,144,145] Higher levels are seen with hepatocellular cancer than with other malignancies or benign diseases.[113] There does not appear to be a correlation between the absolute level of αFP and prognosis.[146]

Like CEA, αFP is not very disease-specific. Elevated levels are also seen in tumors of nonhepatic origin that have metastasized to the liver, in various forms of liver disease such as hepatitis and cirrhosis, and in ataxia telangiectasia.[140,147] High levels of αFP in amniotic fluid may predict neural-tube malformations.[140]

REFERENCES

1. Ehrlich, P.: Ned. Erste Helf, No. 5, Tijdschr. Geneeskd. 1909.
2. Thomas, L.: *In* Lawrence, H. S. (ed.): Cellular and Humoral Aspects of the Hypersensitive States. P. 529. New York, Harper & Row, 1959.
3. Burnet, F. M.: Somatic mutation and chronic disease. Br. Med. J. *1*:338, 1965.
4. Good, R.: *In* Smith, R. T., and Landy, M. (eds.): Immune Surveillance, P. 437, New York, Academic Press, 1970.
5. Foley, E. J.: Antigenic properties of methylcholanthrene-induced tumors in mice of the strain of origin. Cancer Res., *13*:835, 1953.
6. Sjögren, H. O., Hellström, I., and Klein, G.: Transplantation of polyoma virus-induced tumors in mice. Cancer Res., *21*:329, 1961.
7. Currie, G. A.: Cancer and the Immune Response. Baltimore, Williams & Wilkins, 1974.
8. Prehn, R. T.: *In* Smith, R. T., and Landy, M. (eds.): Immune Surveillance, P. 457. New York, Academic Press, 1970.

9. ———: Do tumors grow because of the immune response of the host? Transplant. Rev., *28*:34, 1976.
10. ———: Relationship of tumor immunogenicity to concentration of the oncogen. J. Natl. Cancer Inst., *55*:189, 1975.
11. Herberman, R. B.: Delayed hypsersensitivity skin reactions to antigens on human tumors. Cancer, *34*: (Suppl.): 1469, 1974.
12. Loughridge, L. W., and Lewis, M. G.: Nephrotic syndrome in malignant disease of non-renal origin. Lancet, *1*:256, 1971.
13. Lee, J. C., Yamauchi, H., and Hopper, J., Jr.: The association of cancer and the nephrotic syndrome. Ann. Intern. Med., *64*:41, 1966.
14. Hellström, I.: A colony inhibition (CI) technique for demonstration of tumor cell destruction by lymphoid cells *in vitro*. Int. J. Cancer, *2*:65, 1967.
15. Brunner, K. T., Mauel, J., Cerottini, J.-C., and Chapuis, B.: Quantitative assay of the lytic action of immune lymphoid cells on ^{51}Cr-labelled allogeneic target cells *in vitro*; inhibition by isoantibody and by drugs. Immunology, *14*:181, 1968.
16. Takasugi, M., and Klein, E.: A microassay for cell-mediated immunity. Transplantation, *9*:219, 1970.
17. Hellström, I., Hellström, K. E., Sjögren, H. O., and Warner, G. A.: Demonstration of cell-mediated immunity to human neoplasms of various histological types. Int. J. Cancer, 7:1, 1971.
18. Hellström, I., Hellström, K. E., Pierce, G. E., and Yang, J. P. S.: Cellular and humoral immunity to different types of human neoplasms. Nature, *220*:1352, 1968.
19. Takesugi, M., Mickey, M. R., and Terasaki, P. I.: Reactivity of lymphocytes from normal persons on cultured tumor cells. Cancer Res., *33*:2898, 1973.
20. Jeejeebhoy, H. F.: Immunological studies of women with primary breast carcinoma. Int. J. Cancer, *15*:867, 1975.
21. Herberman, R. B., Nunn, M. E., and Lavrin, D. H.: Natural cytotoxic reactivity of mouse lymphoid cells against syngeneic and allogeneic tumors. Int. J. Cancer, *16*:216, 230, 1975.
22. Takasugi, M., Mickey, M. R., and Terasaki, P. I.: Studies on specificity of cell-mediated immunity to human tumors. J. Natl. Cancer Inst., *53*:1527, 1974.
23. Wybran, J., Hellström, I., Hellström, K. E., and Fudenberg, H. H.: Cytotoxicity of human rosette-forming blood lymphocytes on cultivated human tumor cells. Int. J. Cancer, *13*:515, 1974.
24. deVries, J. E., Cornain, S., and Rümke, P.: Cytotoxicity of non-T versus T-lymphocytes from melanoma patients and healthy donors on short- and long-term cultured melanoma cells. Int. J. Cancer, *14*:427, 1974.
25. Kiessling, R., Klein, E., Pross., H., and Wigzell, H.: "Natural" killer cells in the mouse II: cytotoxic cells with specificity for mouse maloney leukemia cells characteristic of the killer cell. Eur. J. Immunol., *5*:117, 1975.
26. Irie, K., Irie, R., and Morton, D. L.: Evidence for *in vivo* reaction of antibody and complement to surface antigens of human cancer cells. Science, *186*:454, 1974.
27. Hakala, T. R., and Lange, P. H.: Serum induced lymphoid cell mediated cytotoxicity to human transitional cell carcinomas of the genitourinary tract. Science, *184*:795, 1974.
28. Pollack, S., Heppner, G., Brawn, R. J., and Nelson, K.: Specific killing of tumor cells *in vitro* in the presence of normal lymphoid cells and sera from hosts immune to the tumor antigens. Int. J. Cancer, *9*:316, 1972.
29. Evans, R., and Alexander, P.: Cooperation of immune lymphoid cells with macrophages in tumor immunity. Nature, *228*:620, 1970.
30. Hibbs, J. B., Jr., Lambert, L. H., Jr., and Remington, J. S.: Possible role of macrophage mediated nonspecific cytotoxicity in tumor resistance. Nature [New Biol.], *235*:48, 1972.
31. Cruse, J. M., Whitten, H. D., Lewis, G. K., and Watson, E. S.: Facilitation of macrophage-mediated destruction of allogeneic fibrosarcoma cells by tumor-enhancing IgG2 *in vitro*. Transplant. Proc., *5*:961, 1973.
32. denOtter, W., Evans, R., Alexander, P.: Cytotoxicity of murine peritoneal macrophages in tumor allograft immunity. Transplantation, *14*:220, 1972.
33. Keller, R.: Cytoastatic elimination of syngeneic rat tumor cells *in vitro* by nonspecifically activated macrophages. J. Exp. Med., *138*:625, 1973.
34. Evans, R.: Macrophages in syngeneic animal tumors. Transplantation, *14*:468, 1972.
35. Evans, R., and Alexander, P.: Mechanism of immunologically specific killing of tumor cells by macrophages. Nature, *236*:168, 1972.
36. VanLoveren, H., and denOtter, W.: Macrophages in solid tumors 1. Immunologically specific effector cells. J. Natl. Cancer Inst., *53*:1057, 1974.
37. Piessens, W. F., Churchill, W. H., and David, J. R.: Macrophages activated *in vitro* with lymphocyte mediators kill neoplastic but not normal cells. J. Immunol., *114*:293, 1975.
38. Humphreys, S. R., Glynn, J. P., Chirigos, M. A., and Golden, A.: Further studies on the homograft response in BALB/c mice with L1210 leukemia and a resistent subline. J. Natl. Cancer Inst., *28*:1053, 1962.
39. Bonmassar, E., Henconi, E., Goldin, A., and Cudkowicz, G.: Escape of small numbers of allogeneic lymphoma cells from immune surveillance. J. Natl. Cancer Inst., *53*:475, 1974.
40. Marchant, J.: Sarcoma induction in mice by methylcholanthrene. Br. J. Cancer, *23*:383, 1969.
41. Old, L. J., Stockert, E., Boyse, E. A., and Kim, J. H.: Antigenic modulation: loss of TL antigen

from cells exposed to TL antibody. Study of the phenomenon *in vitro*. J. Exp. Med., *127*:523, 1968.
42. Fenyö, E. M., Klein, E., Klein, G., and Swiech, K.: Selection of an immunoresistant maloney lymphoma subline with decreased concentration of tumor-specific surface antigens. J. Natl. Cancer Inst., *40*:69, 1968.
43. Aoki, T., and Johnson, P. A.: Suppression of gross leukemia cell-surface antigens: a kind of antigenic modulation. J. Natl. Cancer Inst., *49*:183, 1972.
44. Synderman, R., and Pike, M. C.: An inhibitor of macrophage chemotaxis produced by neoplasms. Science, *192*:370, 1976.
45. Levy, M. H., and Wheelock, E. F.: The role of macrophages in defense against neoplastic disease. Adv. Cancer Res., *20*:131, 1974.
46. Pinsky, C. M.: *In* Smith, R. T., and Landy, M. (eds.): Immunobiology of the Tumor-Host Relationship. P. 301. New York, Academic Press, 1975.
47. Eilber, F. R., Nizze, J. A., and Morton, D. L.: Sequential evaluation of general immune competence in cancer patients: correlation with clinical course. Cancer, *35*:660, 1975.
48. Lee, Y.-T. N., Sparks, F. C., Eilber, F. R., and Morton, D. L.: Delayed cutaneous hypersensitivity and peripheral lymphocyte counts in patients with advanced cancer. Cancer, *35*:748, 1975.
49. Snell, G. D., Cloudman, A. M., Failor, E., and Douglass, P.: Inhibition and stimulation of tumor homoiotransplants by prior injections of lyophilized tumor tissue. J. Natl. Cancer Inst., *6*:303, 1946.
50. Kaliss, N.: Immunological enhancement of tumor homografts in mice: a review. Cancer Res., *18*:992, 1958.
51. Hellström, K. E., and Hellström, I.: Lymphocyte-mediated cytotoxicity and blocking serum activity to tumor antigen. Adv. Immunology, *18*:209, 1974.
52. Robins, R. A., and Baldwin, R. W.: Tumor-specific antibody neutralization of factors in rat hepatoma-bearer serum which abrogate lymph-node-cell cytotoxicity. Int. J. Cancer, *14*:589, 1974.
53. Sjögren, H. O., Hellström, I., Bansal, S. C., and Hellström, K. E.: Suggestive evidence that the "blocking antibodies" of tumor-bearing individuals may be antigen-antibody complexes. Proc. Natl. Acad. Sci. U.S.A., *68*:1372, 1971.
54. Baldwin, R. W., Price, M. R., and Robins, R. A.: Significance of serum factors modifying cellular immune responses to growing tumors. Br. J. Cancer, *28*(Suppl. 1):37, 1973.
55. Prehn, R. T.: Immunomodulation of tumor growth. Am. J. Pathol., *77*:119, 1974.
56. ———: The immune reaction as a stimulator of tumor growth. Science, *176*:170, 1972.
57. Kall, M. A., and Hellström, I.: Specific stimulatory and cytotoxic effects of lymphocytes sensitized *in vitro* to either alloantigens or tumor antigens. J. Immunol., *114*:1083, 1975.
58. Fidler, I. J.: *In vitro* studies of cellular-mediated immunostimulation of tumor growth. J. Natl. Cancer Inst., *50*:1307, 1973.
59. Umiel, T., and Trainin, N.: Immunological enhancement of tumor growth by syngeneic thymus-derived lymphocytes. Transplantation, *18*:244, 1974.
60. Treves, A. J., Carnaud, C., Trainin, N., Feldman, M., and Cohen, I. R.: Enhancing T lymphocytes from tumor-bearing mice suppress host resistance to a syngeneic tumor. Eur. J. Immunol., *4*:722, 1974.
61. Kolb, W. P., and Granger, G. A.: Lymphocyte *in vitro* cytotoxicity: characterization of mouse lymphotoxia. Cell. Immunol., *1*:122, 1970.
62. Law, L. W.: Studies of thymic function with emphasis on the role of the thymus in oncogenesis. Cancer Res., *26*:551, 1966.
63. Allison, A. C., and Taylor, R. B.: Observations on thymectomy and carcinogenesis. Cancer Res., *27*:703, 1967.
64. Haughton, G., and Whitmore, A. C.: Genetics, the immune response and oncogenesis. Transplant. Rev., *28*:75, 1976.
65. Rygaard, J., and Povlsen, C. O.: The nude mouse vs the hypothesis of immunological surveillance. Transplant. Rev., *28*:43, 1976.
66. Stutman, O.: Tumor development after polyoma infection in athymic nude mice. J. Immunol., *114*:1213, 1975.
67. ———: Tumor development after 3-methylcholanth in immunologically deficient athymic-nude mice. Science, *183*:534, 1974.
68. Good, R. A.: Immunodeficiency in developmental perspective. Harvey Lect., *67*:1, 1971.
69. Penn, I.: Malignant Tumors in Organ Transplant Recipients. New York, Springer-Verlag, 1970.
70. Möller, G., and Möller, E.: The concept of immunological surveillance against neoplasia. Transplant. Rev., *28*:3, 1976.
71. Schwartz, R. S., and Beldotti, L.: Malignant lymphomas following allogenic disease: transition from an immunological to a neoplastic disorder. Science, *149*:1511, 1965.
72. Hirsch, M. S., *et al.*: Activation of leukemia viruses by graft-versus-host and mixed lymphocyte reactions *in vitro*. Proc. Natl. Acad. Sci. U.S.A., *69*:1069, 1972.
73. Hirsch, M. S.: Immunological activation of oncogenic viruses: interrelationship of immunostimulation and immunosuppression. Johns Hopkins Med. J., *3*(Suppl.):177, 1974.
74. Schwartz, R. S.: Immunosuppression and neoplasia. Prog. Immunol., *11*(V 5):229, 1974.
75. Friend, C.: Immunological relationships of a filterable agent causing a leukemia in adult mice 1. The neutralization of infectivity by specific antisera. J. Exp. Med., *109*:217, 1959.
76. Churchill, A. E., Payne, L. N., and Chubb, R.

C.: Immunization against Marek's disease using a live attenuated virus. Nature, *221*:744, 1969.

77. Jarrett, W., Mackey, L., Jarrett, O., Land, H., and Hood, C.: Antibody response and virus survival in cats vaccinated against feline leukemia. Nature, *248*:230, 1974.
78. Laufs, R., and Steinke, H.: Vaccination of non-human primates against malignant lymphoma. Nature, *253*:71, 1975.
79. Holmes, E. C., Eilber, P. R., and Morton, D. L.: Immunotherapy of malignancy in humans: current status. J.A.M.A., *232*:1052, 1975.
80. Bast, R. C., Zbar, B., Borsos, T., and Rapp, H. J.: BCG and cancer. N. Engl. J. Med., *290*:1413, 1458, 1974.
81. Hanna, M. G., Jr.: Immunologic aspects of BCG-mediated regression of established tumors and metastases in guinea pigs. Semin. Oncology, *1*:319, 1974.
82. Old, L. J., Clarke, D. A., and Benacerraf, B.: Effect of bacillus calmette-Guerin infection on transplanted tumors in the mouse. Nature, *184*:291, 1959.
83. Weiss, D. W.: Nonspecific stimulation and modulation of the immune response and of states of resistance by the methanol-extraction residue fraction of tubercle bacilli. Natl. Cancer Inst. Monog., *35*:157, 1972.
84. Coley, W. B.: Contribution to the knowledge of sarcoma. Ann. Surg., *14*:199, 1891.
85. Nauts, H. C., Fowler, G. A., and Bogatko, F. H.: A review of the influence of bacterial infection and of bacterial products on malignant tumors in man. Acta Med. Scand., *145*(Suppl):276, 1953.
86. Mathe, G., *et al.*: Active immunotherapy for acute lymphoblastic leukemia. Lancet, *1*:697, 1969.
87. Treatment of acute lymphoblastic leukemia. Preliminary report to the medical research council by the leukemia committee and the working party on leukemia in childhood. Br. Med., J., *4*:189, 1971.
88. Powles, R.: Immunotherapy of acute myelogenous leukemia in man. Natl. Cancer Inst. Monogr., *39*:243, 1973.
89. Sokal, J. E., August, C. W., and Grace, J. T., Jr.: Immunotherapy of chronic myelocytic leukemia. Natl. Cancer Inst. Monogr., *39*:195, 1973.
90. Morton, D. L., *et al.*: BCG immunotherapy of malignant melanoma. Ann. Surg., *180*:635, 1974.
91. Davignon, L., Lemonde, P., Robillard, P., and Frappier, A.: BCG vaccination and leukaemia mortality. Lancet, *2*:638, 1970.
92. Kinlen, L. J., and Pike, M. C.: BCG vaccination and leukemia. Lancet, *2*:398, 1971.
93. Adlam, C., and Scott, M. T.: Lympho-reticular stimulatory properties of *Corynebacterium parvum* and related bacteria. J. Med. Microbiol., *6*:261, 1972.
94. Howard, J. G., Scott, M. T., and Christie, G. H.: Cellular mechanisms underlying the adjuvant activity of *Corynebacterium parvum* interactions of activated macrophages with T and B lymphocytes. Ciba Found. Symp., *18*:101, 1973.
95. Scott, M. T.: *Corynebacterium parvum* as a therapeutic antitumor agent in mice II. Local injection. J. Natl. Cancer Inst., *53*:861, 1974.
96. Currie, G. A., and Bagshawe, K. D.: Active immunotherapy with *Corynebacterium parvum* and chemotherapy in murine fibrosarcomas. Br. Med. J., *1*:541, 1970.
97. Fisher, B., Wolmark, N., Saffer, E., and Fisher, E. R.: Inhibitory effect of prolonged *Corynebacterium parvum* and cylophosphamide administration on the growth of established tumors. Cancer, *35*:134, 1975.
98. Israel, L.: Preliminary results of nonspecific immune therapy for lung cancer. Cancer Chemother. Rep. Part 3, *4*(2):283, 1973.
99. Rojas, A. F., Mickiewicz, E., Feierstein, J. N., Glait, H., and Olivari, A. J.: Levamisole in advanced human breast cancer. Lancet, *1*:211, 1976.
100. Weiss, D. W.: Immunological intervention in neoplasia. Johns Hopkins Med. J., *3*(Suppl): 131, 1974.
101. Simmons, R. L., Rios, A., and Ray, P. K.: Immunogenicity and antigenicity of lymphoid cells treated with neurominidase. Nature [New Biol.], *231*:179, 1971.
102. Wunderlich, J. R., Martin, W. J., and Fletcher, F.: Enhanced immunogenicity of syngeneic tumor cells coated with concanavalin A. Fed. Proc., *30*:246, 1971.
103. Thompson, K., Harris, M., Benjamini, I. E., Mitchell, G., and Noble, M.: Cellular and humoral immunity: a distinction in antigenic recognition. Nature [New Biol.], *238*:20, 1972.
104. Parish, C. R.: Immune response to chemically modified flagellin 1. Induction of antibody tolerance to flagellin by acetoacetylated derivatives of the protein. J. Exp. Med., *134*:1, 1971.
105. Rubens, R. D.: Antibodies as carriers of anticancer agents. Lancet, *1*:498, 1974.
106. Moore, G. E., and Moore, M. B.: Autoinoculation of cultured human lymphocytes in malignant melanoma. N.Y. State J. Med., *69*:460, 1969.
107. Cheema, A. R., and Hersh, E. M.: Local tumor immunotherapy with *in vitro* activated autocthonous lymphocytes. Cancer, *29*:982, 1972.
108. Schwarzenberg, L., *et al.*: Study of factors determining the usefulness and complications of leukocyte transfusions. Am. J. Med., *43*:206, 1967.
109. Mathé, G., *et al.*: Immunogenetic and immunological problems of allogeneic haemopoietic radio-chimeras in man. Scand. J. Haematol., *4*:193, 1967.
110. Fass, L., *et al.*: Studies of immunological reactivity following syngeneic or allogeneic marrow grafts in man. Transplantation, *16*:630, 1973.

111. Bleyer, W. A., Blaese, R. M., Bujak, J. S., Herzig, G. P., and Graw, R. G., Jr.: Long-term remission from acute myelogenous leukemia after bone marrow transplantation and recovery from acute graft-versus-host reaction and prolonged immunoincompetence. Blood, *45*:171, 1975.
112. LoBuglio, A. F., and Neidhart, J. A.: A review of transfer factor immunotherapy in cancer. Cancer, *34*:1563, 1974.
113. Costanza, M. E., and Nathanson, L.: Carcinofetal antigens. Prog. Clin. Immunol., *2*:191, 1974.
114. Schöne, G.: Munch. Med. Wochensch., *51*:1, 1906.
114a. Buttle, G. A. H., and Frayn, A.: Effect of previous injection of homologous embryonic tissue on the growth of certain transplantable mouse tumors. Nature, *215*:1495, 1967.
115. Hanna, M. G., Jr., Tennant, R. W., and Coggin, J. H. L.: Suppressive effect of immunization with mouse fetal antigens on growth of cells infected with Rauscher leukemia virus and in plasma-cell tumors. Proc. Natl. Acad. Sci. U.S.A., *68*:1748, 1971.
116. Ting, R. C.: Failure to induce transplantation resistance against polyoma tumor cells with syngeneic embryonic tissues. Nature, *217*:858, 1968.
117. Lausch, R. N., and Rapp, F.: Tumor-specific antigens and expression of fetal antigens in mammalian cells. Prog. Exp. Tumor Res., *19*:45, 1974.
118. Parmiani, G., and Lembo, R.: Effect of antiembryo immunization on methylcholanthrene-induced sarcoma growth in BALB/C mice. Int. J. Cancer, *14*:55, 1974.
119. Gold, P.: Circulating antibodies against carcinoembryonic antigens of the human digestive system. Cancer, *20*:1663, 1967.
120. Collatz, E.,vonKleist, S., and Burtin, P.: Further investigations of circulating antibodies in colon cancer patients: on the autoantigenicity of the carcinoembryonic antigens. Int. J. Cancer, *8*:298, 1971.
121. LoGerfo, P., Herter, F. P., and Bennett, S. J.: Absence of circulating antibodies to carcinoembryonic antigen in patients with gastrointestinal malignancies. Int. J. Cancer, *9*:344, 1972.
122. Gold, P., and Freedman, S. O.: Demonstration of tumor-specific antigens in human colonic carcinomata by immunological tolerance and absorption techniques. J. Exp. Med., *121*:439, 1965.
123. ———: Specific carcinoembryonic antigens of the human digestive system. J. Exp. Med., *122*:467, 1965.
124. Moore, T. L., Kupchik, H. Z., Marcon, N., and Zamcheck, N.: Carcinoembryonic antigen assay in cancer of the colon and pancreas and other digestive tract disorders. Am. J. Dig. Dis., *16*:1, 1971.
125. Terry, W. D., Henkart, P. A., Coligan, J. E., and Todd, C. E.: Structural studies of the major glycoprotein in preparations with carcinoembryonic antigen activity. J. Exp. Med., *136*:200, 1972.
126. Simmons, D. A. R., and Perlmann, P.: Carcinoembryonic antigen and blood group substances. Cancer Res., *33*:313, 1973.
127. Laing, C. A., Heppner, G. H., Kopp, L. E., and Calabresi, P.: Detection of carcinoembryonic antigen in the media of cultures of carcinomatous cells of digestive-system origin. J. Natl. Cancer Inst., *48*:1909, 1972.
128. Burton, P., Martin, E., Sabine, M. C., and von Kleist, S.: Immunological study of polyps of the colon. J. Natl. Cancer Inst., *48*:25, 1972.
129. Rule, A. H., Straus, E., Vandevoorde, J., and Janowitz, H. D.: Tumor-associated (CEA-reacting) antigen in patients with inflammatory Boucl disease. N. Engl. J. Med., *287*:24, 1972.
130. LoGerfo, P., Krupey, J., and Hansen, H. J.: Demonstration of an antigen common to several varieties of neoplasia. N. Engl. J. Med., *285*:138, 1971.
131. Martin, F., Martin, M. S., Bordes, M., and Bourgeaux, C.: The specificity of carcinofoetal antigen of the human digestive tract tumors. Eur. J. Cancer, *8*:315, 1972.
132. LoGerfo, P., LoGerfo, F., Herter, F., Barker, H. G., and Hansen, H. J.: Tumor-associated antigen in patients with carcinoma of the colon. Am. J. Surg., *123*:127, 1972.
133. Laurence, D. J. R., *et al.*: Role of plasma carcinoembryonic antigen in diagnosis of gastrointestinal, mammary, and bronchial carcinoma. Br. Med. J., *3*:605, 1970.
134. Costanza, M. E., Das, S., Nathanson, L., Rule, A., and Schwartz, R. S.: Carcinoembryonic antigen: report of a screening study. Cancer, *33*:583, 1974.
135. Skarin, A. T., Delwiche, R., Zamcheck, N., Lakich, J. J., and Frei, E., III: Carcinoembryonic antigen: chemical correlation with chemotherapy for metastatic gastrointestinal cancer. Cancer, *33*:1239, 1974.
136. Booth, S. N., *et al.*: Carcinoembryonic antigen in management of colorectal carcinoma. Br. Med. J., *4*:183, 1974.
137. Moore, T. L., Kantrowitz, P. A., and Zamcheck, N.: Carcinoembryonic antigen (CEA) in inflammatory bowel disease. J.A.M.A., *222*:944, 1972.
138. Pederson, K. O.: Fetuin, a new globulin isolated from serum. Nature, *154*:575, 1944.
139. Bergstrand, C. G., and Czar, B.: Demonstration of a new protein fraction in serum from the human fetus. Scand. J. Clin. Lab. Invest., *8*:174, 1956.
140. Adinolfi, A., Adinolfi, M., and Lessof, M. H.: Alpha-feto-protein during development and in disease. J. Med. Genet., *12*:138, 1975.
141. Ruoslahti, E., Pihko, H., and Seppälä, M.: Immunochemical purification and chemical properties. Expression in normal state and in

malignant and non-malignant liver disease. Transplant. Rev., *20*:39, 1974.

142. Gitlin, D., Perricelli, A., and Gitlin, G. M.: Synthesis of α-fetopecotein by liver, yolk sac, and gastrointestinal tract of the human conceptus. Cancer Res., *32*:979, 1972.
143. Alpert, M. E., Uriel, J., and deNechaud, B.: Alpha$_1$ fetoprotein in the diagnosis of human hepatoma. N. Engl. J. Med., *278*:984, 1968.
144. Smith, J. B., and O'Neill, R. T.: Alpha-fetoprotein: occurrence in germinal cell and liver malignancies. Am. J. Med., *51*:767, 1971.
145. Purves, L. R., Bersohn, I., Path, F. C., and Geddes, E. W.: Serum alpha-feto-protein and primary cancer of the liver in man. Cancer, *25*:1261, 1970.
146. Purves, L. R., McNab, M., Geddes, E. W., and Bersohn, I.: Serum-alpha-foetoprotein and primary hepatic cancer. Lancet, *1*:921, 1968.
147. Waldmann, T. A., and McIntire, K. R.: Serum-alpha fetoprotein levels in patients with atoxia-telangiectasia. Lancet, *2*:1112, 1972.

14 Immunohematology

Landsteiner first demonstrated the existence of antigens on the surface of red blood cells and showed that they differed from individual to individual.[1] This work was done at the turn of the century, and many antigen systems, some of extraordinary complexity, have since been identified on most of the formed elements of the blood. The red cell has long been the major focus of this work, and only recently has the analysis of leukocyte and platelet antigens been approached successfully.

ANTIGENS OF THE RED BLOOD CELL SURFACE

Many different genetically controlled systems of antigens have been identified on the red blood cell surface. Each of these defines a set of histocompatibility antigens similar to the HLA system. However, the number of blood-group alleles within most of these systems is relatively restricted compared to the remarkable polymorphism of the HLA system, with the noted exceptions of the highly polymorphic Rh and Kell antigen systems.

We will begin our discussion of immunohematology with a brief look at several of the major blood-group systems. Our purpose is to convey a basic understanding of the most important surface antigens of the red cell so that we may then be able to appreciate the immunologic aspects of transfusion reactions and erythrocyte autoimmunity. Complete discussions of these antigen systems can be found in several excellent textbooks of immunohematology.[2-4] It must be emphasized that, despite extensive knowledge about the intricacies of these antigen systems, there is at present little understanding of the intrinsic, physiologic roles that these surface molecules may play.

The ABO Blood Group

The antigens of the ABO blood group were the first system of red blood cell surface antigens to be discovered. In some very elegant experiments, Landsteiner was able to show that different individuals expressed different antigens on their red cells.[1] He first obtained blood from a number of individuals and separated the serum from the red cells. Next, he mixed each person's cells with the serum from every other individual and looked for agglutination. Agglutination signified that a person's serum contained antibodies against the added cells, as depicted in Figure 14-1.

Following this simple methodology, investigators were able to define four

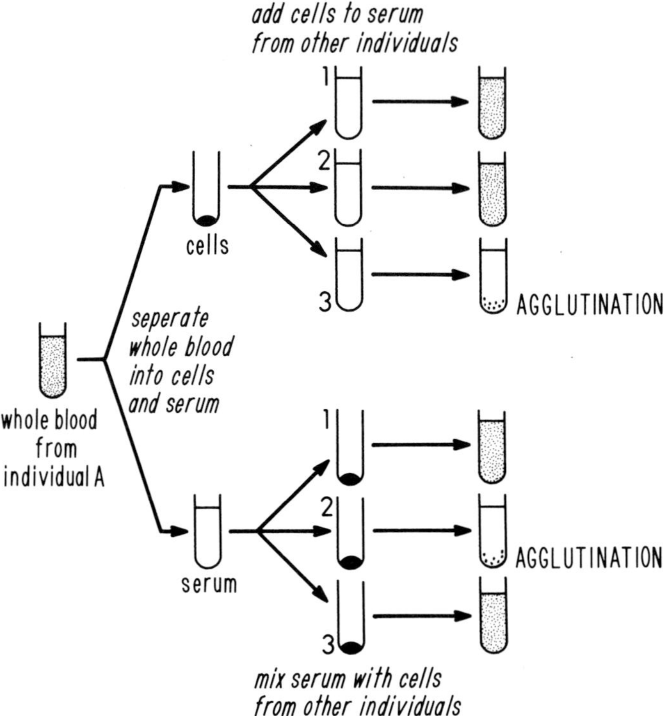

Fig. 14-1. Red-cell antigens and antibodies. Above: red cells from individual A are mixed with serum obtained from other people. The presence of agglutination in the third test tube indicates that person 3 possesses antibodies against the red cells of individual A. Below: serum from individual A is mixed with red cells from these same people. Agglutination in the second test tube identifies the presence of antibodies in A's serum directed against the red cells of individual 2.

groups of individuals according to their patterns of agglutination (Table 14-1). It was recognized that these four groups derived from the expression or lack of expression of two red-cell surface antigens, called A and B. Type A people express the A antigen only, type B people express the B antigen only, and type AB individuals have both antigens on their red cells. Type O people have neither detectable A nor B antigen.

There is a reciprocal relationship between the antigen present on a person's red cells and the type of antibody present in that individual's serum. People will not normally make antibodies against their own red-cell antigens, and thus, for example, type A individuals possess anti-B antibodies but not anti-A antibodies. Type B individuals will possess only anti-A antibodies. Type O people will produce antibodies against both A and B antigens, and type AB people will possess neither antibody.

Table 14-1. The Four ABO Blood Groups

Blood Group	*Red-Cell Antigens*	*Serum Antibodies*
A	A	Anti-B
B	B	Anti-A
AB	A and B	——
O	Neither A nor B	Anti-A and Anti-B

Landsteiner's methodology has since been used—with various modifications—to detect other red-cell antigen systems. This technique illustrates a basic principle of immunohematology: *all red-cell antigens are defined by their ability to react with specific antisera*. Thus a person with type A blood is said to possess the A antigen because his cells react with anti-A antisera. It is the antisera that defines the antigen.

The genetic basis of the ABO system was established by numerous family studies.[5] There is a single genetic locus having any of three possible alleles: A, B or O. O represents the lack of either A or

B and is a "silent" allele. An individual inherits one allele from each of his parents. There are thus six possible genotypes: AA, AB, AO, BB, BO and OO. The alleles are codominant; that is, the gene product of each allele is expressed on the red-cell surface. Thus, AA individuals react only with anti-A antisera and are considered to have type A blood. AO individuals also react with anti-A antisera and thus are also detected as type A. Individuals carrying both A and B genes (AB) will express both antigens and have type AB blood. Since the O gene is silent, only those people who are homozygous for O (OO) will fail to react with anti-A and anti-B antisera and are called type O. Thus, typing with anti-A and anti-B antisera defines four ABO phenotypes (Table 14-2).[5a]

This scheme was worked out over 50 years ago. Since then much greater complexity has become apparent. Many antigenic variants of both A and B have been described, but these are very rare and are

Table 14-2. ABO Genotypes and Phenotypes*

Genotype	*Phenotype*	*Frequency of Phenotype in Britain*
AA	A	} 42%
AO	A	
BB	B	} 8%
BO	B	
AB	AB	3%
OO	O	47%

*From Dobson, A. M., and Ikin, E. W.: The ABO blood groups in the United Kingdom; frequencies based on a very large sample. J. Pathol. Bacteriol., *58*:221, 1946.

of little importance in clinical medicine. One exception is the existence of A_1 and A_2 variants of the A antigen.[6] These are both common in the general population; the majority of people with type A blood possess the A_1 antigen. Both A antigens react with the usual anti-A antisera. However, anti-A absorbed with type A_2 cells still retains some reactivity with A_1 cells, whereas the reverse is not true (Fig. 14-2). This finding has been interpreted to mean that the A antigen may be composed of more than one antigenic determinant and that A_2 individuals lack an A antigenic determinant which is present in A_1 individuals.

We have referred to the O gene as a silent gene and have implied that type O blood is without a surface antigen. This is true only when anti-A and anti-B antisera are used to define the red-cell antigens present. In fact, O individuals *do* possess a surface antigen called the H antigen. The H antigen is present on the red cells of type A, B, AB and O individuals. Type O individuals express the largest amount of cell-surface H antigen (Fig. 14-3).

The H antigen is a precursor for both the A and B antigens.[7] The A and B genes are alleles that code for two different enzymes, each of which modifies the H antigen in a particular way to produce either the A or B antigen, respectively. This scheme allows us to understand the different antigens associated with each blood type. Type O individuals possess only the H antigen. Type A individuals can modify the H antigen into the A anti-

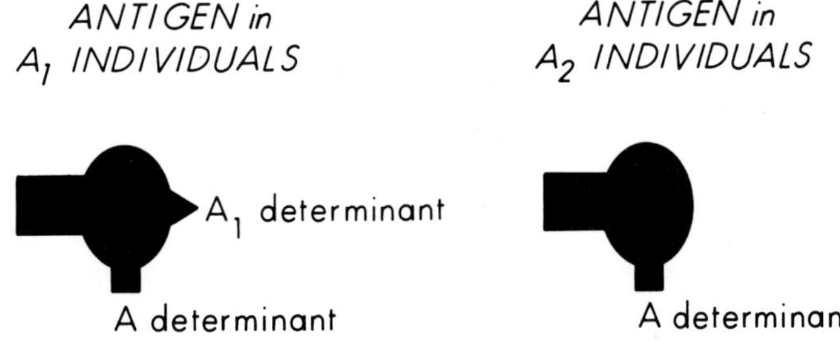

Fig. 14-2. Schematic interpretation of the A antigen. Type A_1 individuals possess an antigen expressing both the A and A_1 determinants. Type A_2 individuals possess an antigen with only the A determinant.

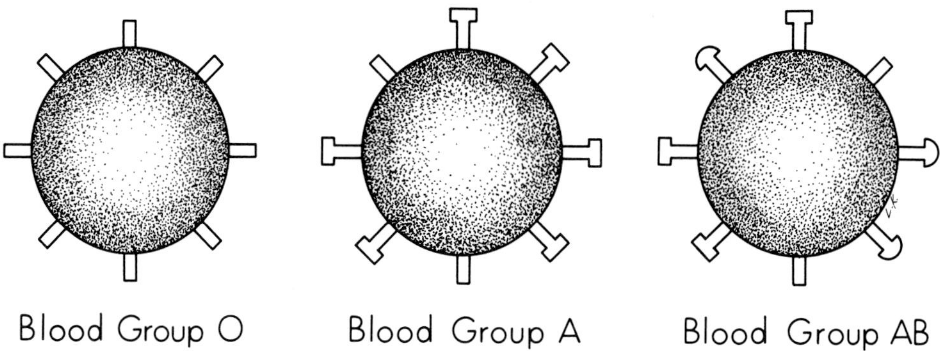

Fig. 14-3. ABH antigens on the erythrocytes of individuals with different blood types. Group 0: red cells possess only the H antigen. Group A: red cells possess the H and A antigens. Group AB: red cells possess the H, A and B antigens.

gen and will express both unmodified H antigen and A antigen on their red cells. Type B individuals will similarly express the H and B antigens. The presence of both A and B alleles in an individual will result in the expression of all three antigens: H, A and B.

Very rarely a person is found whose cells lack the H antigen. Such an individual would be considered to be type O when his cells are tested with anti-A and anti-B antisera. Only more sensitive screening can reveal the failure to express the H antigen. This rare blood type is called "Bombay."[8] Either HH or Hh genotypes will result in the production of H antigen, and only the homozygous hh individuals have the Bombay phenotype. Because the H substance is the precursor for the A and B antigens, Bombay-type individuals can have the A and/or B genetic alleles but still be unable to produce the A or B antigens for lack of sufficient precursor substance for the A- or B-coded enzymes to modify (see Table 14-3).

Over the past several years, our understanding of the ABH system has evolved greatly with the elucidation of the biochemical structure of the various antigens. This work represents one of the most exciting stories in immunohematology. The chemical structures of these antigens are the best characterized of all the different blood group system antigens.[7,9]

A four-residue polysaccharide precursor

Table 14-3. The H Gene and ABO Phenotypes

With the Genotype HH or Hh		*With the Genotype hh (Bombay)*	
ABO Genotype	*ABO Phenotype*	*ABO Genotype*	*ABO Phenotype*
OO	O	OO	O
AA or AO	A	AA or AO	O
BB or BO	B	BB or BO	O
AB	AB	AB	O

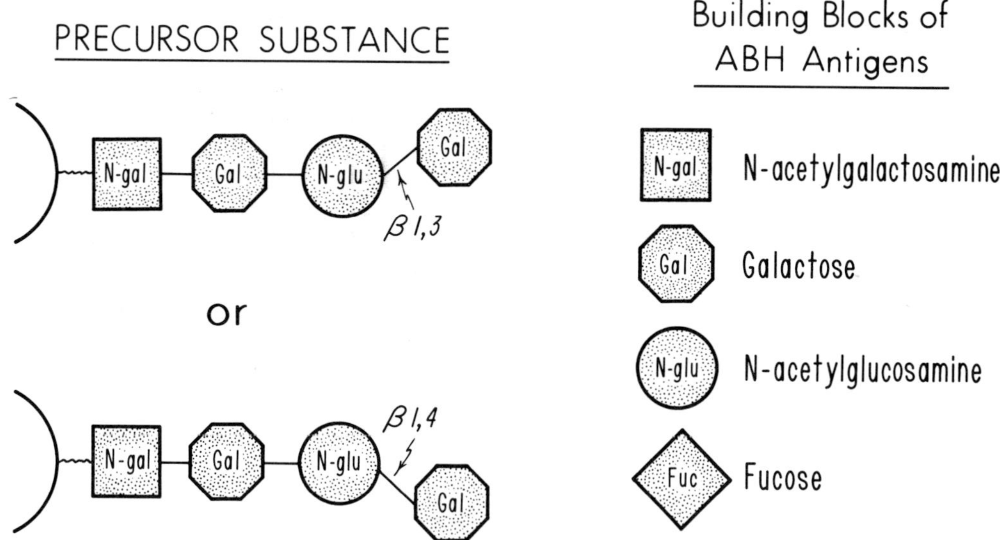

Fig. 14-4. Chemical structure of the terminal portion of the precursor substance for the ABH antigens. Note the two different types of terminal glycosidic linkages.

forms the backbone of the A, B and H antigens and is shown below (Fig. 14-4). This tetrasaccharide is attached to a red-cell-membrane sphingolipid and serves as the precursor substance for the H gene product. Note that the terminal galactose can be joined to the N-acetylglucosamine by either a 1,3 or 1,4 glycosidic linkage.

The H gene codes for a fucosyl transferase that adds a fucose to the terminal galactose of the precursor substance (Fig. 14-5). This five-residue molecule is the H antigen. The biochemical pathway ends here in type O individuals.

The A and B genes code for enzymes which each add a single substrate to the

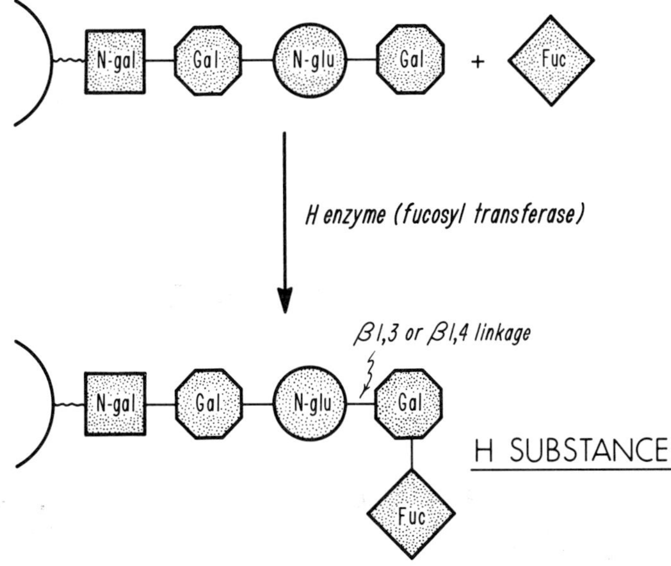

Fig. 14-5. Production of the H antigen. The H enzyme fucosyl transferase adds a fucose to the terminal galactose of the precursor substance.

terminal galactose of the H antigen (Fig. 14-6). The A gene codes for a transferase that adds N-acetylgalactosamine, thereby creating the A antigen. The B gene codes for a different transferase that adds a galactose to the H antigen. Type AB people will express both A and B antigens on the surface of their red cells. In these individuals, the two transferases compete for the available H antigen, converting some to A and some to B.

The Soluble Blood-Group Antigens: ABO, Lewis and Secretor Systems

Some of the same four-residue polysaccharide precursor which forms the backbone of the A, B and H antigens can also be found in the serum and secretions of all normal individuals as part of a soluble glycoprotein. This extracorpuscular precursor substance is modified into a variety of soluble blood-group antigens. Four systems of genetic alleles are involved: the Lewis system, the secretor system, the Hh system and the ABO system. The precise location of the cells that produce the soluble precursor substance and that make the soluble enzymes that modify it is not known. However, the appropriate enzymes (i.e., the H, A and B transferases) can be found in a wide variety of tissues as well as in the plasma and bodily secretions.

The Lewis System. The soluble blood-group antigens, and the Lewis system in particular, provide an example of a unique type of red-cell antigen—an *extrinsic* antigen. Thus, the Lewis antigens are not assembled as part of the red-cell membrane as are most other erythrocyte antigens. Rather, they are produced throughout the body as soluble antigens that passively adsorb onto the surface of the mature red cells.[10] Thus, for example, red

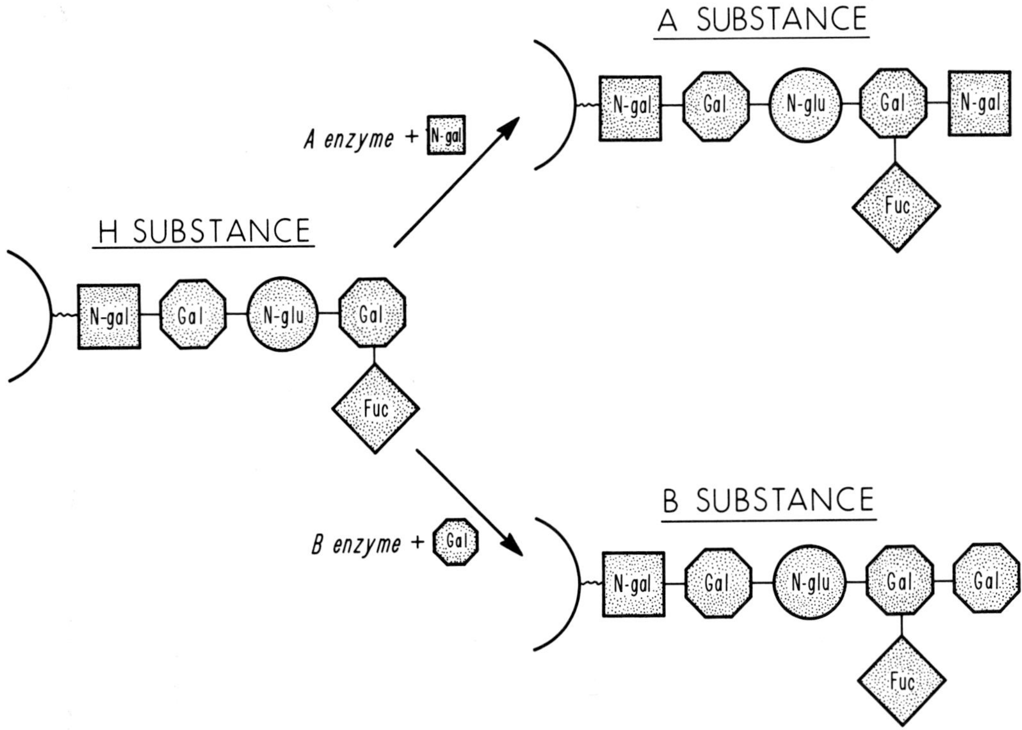

Fig. 14-6. Production of the A and B antigens. The A enzyme adds N-acetylgalactosamine to the galactose of the H antigen, the B enzyme adds galactose to the H antigen as shown.

cells that do not express the Lewis a antigen can be placed in the serum of a person who is positive for the Lewis a antigen and acquire the capacity to react with anti-Lewis-a antisera (Fig. 14-7).[11]

The Lewis system, like the H system, enzymatically modifies the tetrasaccharide precursor substance.[12] This soluble precursor substance is found in virtually all body fluids except the cerebrospinal fluid. It is present in two forms, reflecting the two possible type of terminal glycosidic linkages, 1,3 and 1,4.

The Lewis gene (Le) codes for a fucosyl transferase. It is inherited as a dominant trait. There is also a silent allele that is written as le. An individual with either the Le/Le or Le/le genotype will produce the enzyme and will be able to modify the soluble precursor. Only the homozygous le/le person makes no enzyme and is called Lewis-negative. Approximately 10 per cent of the Caucasian population is Lewis-negative (le/le).

Unlike the H gene fucosyl transferase, the Lewis enzyme adds the fucose to the penultimate saccharide, the N-acetylglucosamine (Fig. 14-8). Furthermore, the Lewis enzyme has a marked proclivity to modify the 1,3 form of the precursor substance, unlike the H enzyme which will act equally well on both forms. The product of this modification is called the Lewis a antigen (Le^a). The Lewis a antigen is found free in the serum and other secretions and can passively adsorb onto the surface of red cells. However, this is a relatively weak and reversible association. Any red cell can adsorb the Le^a soluble antigen, and thus a red cell can possess the Le^a, H and A/B antigens, depending upon the genetic constitution of the individual.

The Secretor System. The A, B and H antigens can also be found as soluble substances. Like the Lewis antigens, these arise as a result of the enzymatic modification of the soluble precursor substance. The soluble antigens found in any person are a reflection of his ABO blood type. Thus, for example, a type A person can have soluble H and A substance but will not have soluble B substance. However, merely because a person has type A or type B blood does not mean that he will necessarily possess soluble A or B or H substance. In the northern European population about 80 per cent of people possess soluble H, A or B substance. These people were originally called "secretors" because they were presumed to possess the ability to secrete these antigens into the body fluids. However, as we shall see, "secretor" gene function has

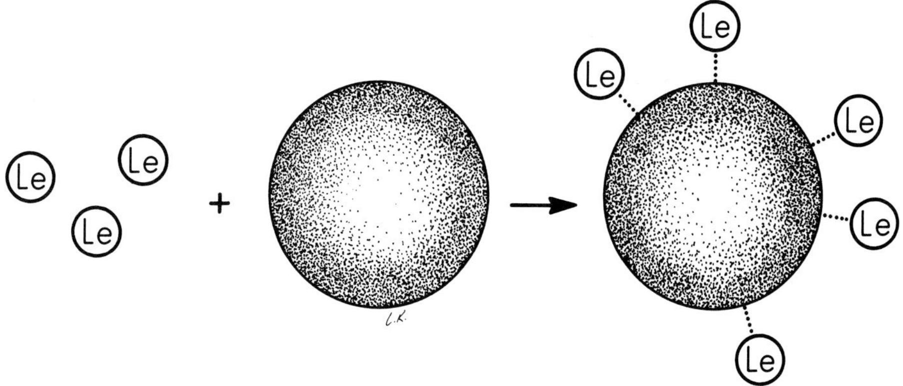

Fig. 14-7. The soluble red-cell antigens. The Lewis antigens are free in the serum and attach to the red cell by passive adsorption. The ABH antigens, on the other hand, are intrinsic to the red-cell surface (but can exist in soluble form also—see text).

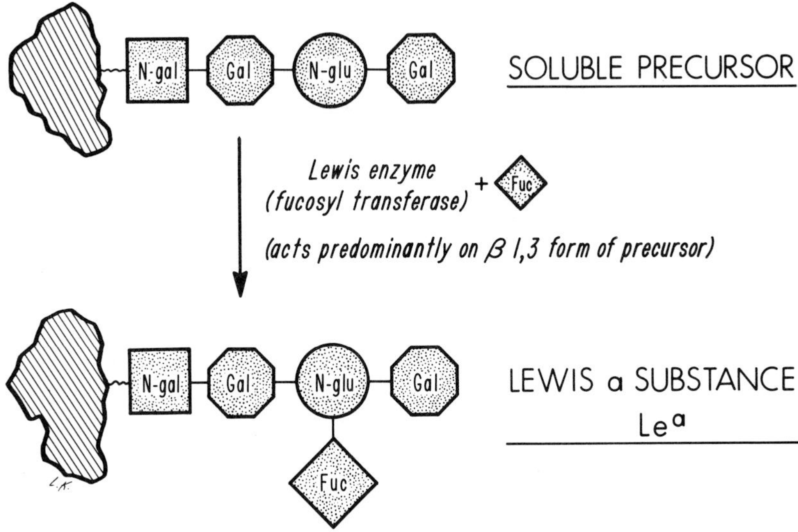

Fig. 14-8. Formation of the Lewis a antigen. The Lewis enzyme fucosyl transferase adds fucose to the N-acetylglucosamine of the precursor substance to form the Lewis a antigen.

nothing to do with the ability to secrete the blood-group antigens. The 20 per cent of people who do not produce these soluble antigens still possess the appropriate *intrinsic* ABH antigens on their red cells.

Secretor function is inherited as a dominant trait. Individuals with either the genotype Se/Se or Se/se are secretors while only the homozygous se/se individuals are nonsecretors.

The secretor gene functions as a permissive gene; no secretor gene product has been identified. The presence of the secretor gene allows the H enzyme to modify the soluble precursor substance. The site of this reaction *in vivo* has not been determined. Because of its permissive action the presence of an Se gene will result in the production of soluble H antigen. The H enzyme acts on both forms of soluble precursor substance.

If an individual has both the Le gene and an Se gene, the H enzyme will also transform the soluble Le^a antigen by adding a fucose to the terminal galactose (Fig. 14-9). This new molecule is called the Lewis b antigen (Le^b).[13] Thus, an Le-positive Se-positive individual will convert the Lewis a antigen to the Lewis b antigen and will only have Lewis b antigen to adsorb onto his red cells. Only a person who is Le-positive and a nonsecretor (se/se) will possess the Lewis a antigen, both in his secretions and on his erythrocytes (Fig. 14-10).

Once having made the H antigen, a person possessing the Se gene will be able to convert the soluble H substance to a soluble A or B antigen if that person carries either the A or B allele (Fig. 14-11). Thus, for example, a person who is blood type O and Lewis-positive and secretor-positive will have the Lewis b and the H antigens on his red cells and as soluble substances. A person who is blood type A and Lewis-positive and secretor-positive will have A antigen and Lewis b antigen on his red cells and as soluble substances. Table 14-4 summarizes the genetic interactions of the different soluble blood-group systems and the ultimate phenotypes they can produce.

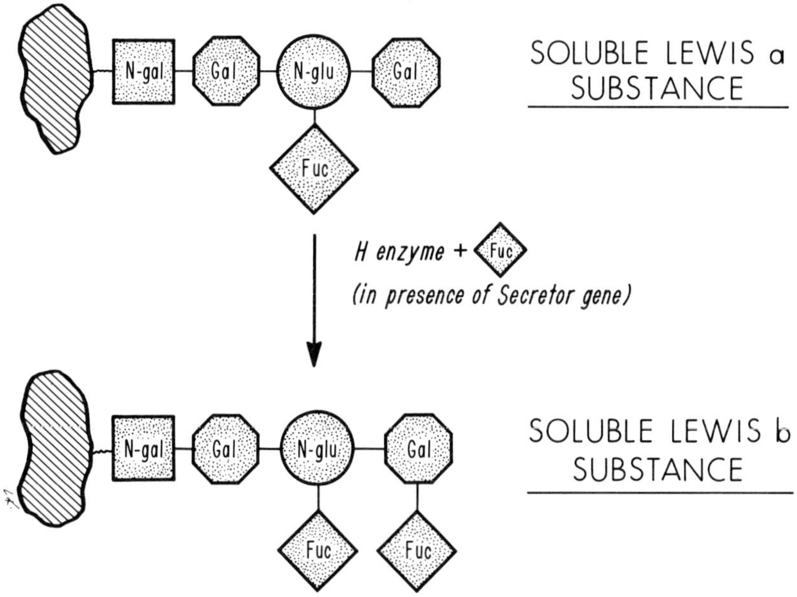

Fig. 14-9. Formation of the Lewis b antigen. The presence of a secretor gene allows the H enzyme to add a fucose to the terminal galactose of the Lewis a antigen, creating the Lewis b antigen.

The Rh System

In 1940, Landsteiner and Wiener showed that rabbit antiserum that had been raised by injecting rabbits with blood of the rhesus monkey agglutinated the red cells of 85 per cent of Caucasians from New York.[14] These individuals were termed Rh-positive and the remaining 15 per cent were referred to as Rh-negative. At that time a human red-cell antigen that was responsible for a case of hemolytic disease of the newborn (see later in this chapter) was also detected.[15] At first it was believed that the anti-rhesus-antigen antisera was directed against this antigen, and thus the culpable antigen was termed the Rh antigen. Subsequently the antigen responsible for the majority of cases of hemolytic disease of the newborn was found not to be the same antigen that reacted with the rhesus antisera. However, the appellation "Rh" has stuck and is used to refer to the antigen system we will now briefly describe.

The Rh system plays a prominent role in many clinical settings, including hemolytic disease of the newborn, some autoimmune hemolytic anemias and, occasionally, transfusion reactions. The Rh antigens are proteins in contrast to the polysaccharide antigens of the ABO and Lewis systems.

The genetic basis of the Rh system is still the center of great controversy. Two theories of inheritance have been proposed:

According to the first theory,[16] the Rh system is viewed as consisting of three closely linked genetic loci each coding for separate molecules (Fig. 14-12). These are termed the D, C and E loci. The major antigen is coded for by the D locus and is the only allelic gene product of this locus. Thus a person either carries the D gene and expresses the D antigen on his red cells or he does not; there is no "d" antigen. About 85 per cent of the European population is D-positive.

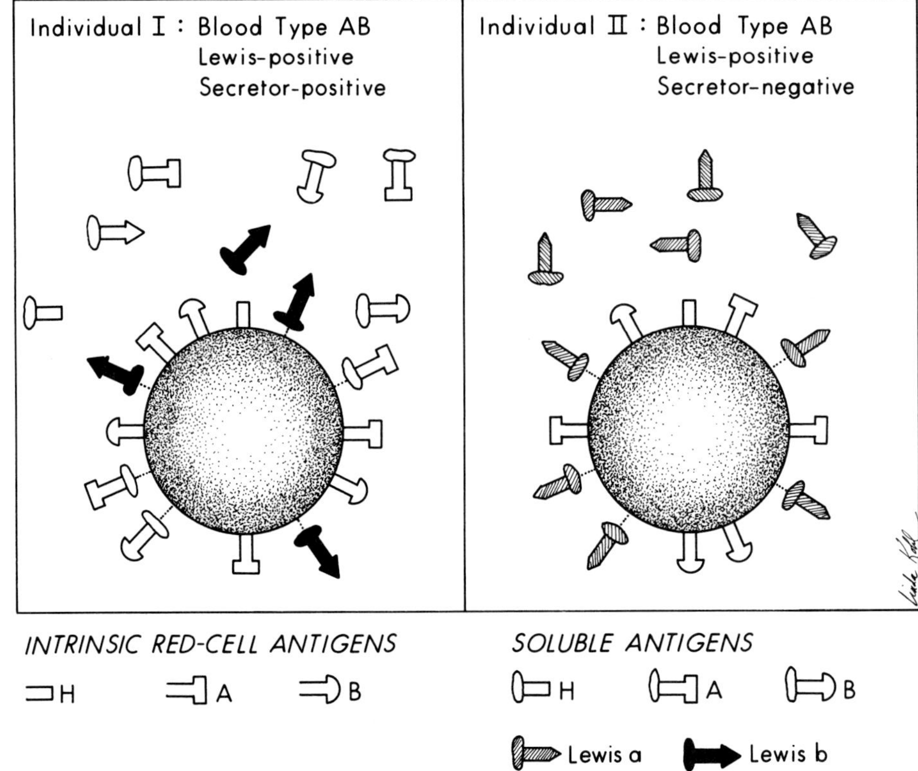

Fig. 14-10. Soluble and intrinsic red-cell antigens. Individual I possesses A, B and H intrinsic red-cell antigens. He is also Lewis-positive and secretor-positive so that he has Lewis b antigen in his serum as well as soluble H, A and B antigens. These can all be adsorbed onto his red cells. Individual II also possesses A, B and H antigens. However, he is Lewis-positive and secretor-negative, and therefore has only the Lewis a antigen in his serum.

The other loci have several alleles, each of which appears to code for a particular antigenic gene product. The C locus has two common allelic products, the C and c antigens, as well as other, much more unusual antigens. The third locus codes for the E and e allelic products. The gene products of these alleles can be detected on the surface of red cells by using specific antisera.

According to this first theory, each individual inherits one allele at each of these three closely linked loci from each of his parents. Thus, for example, a person may inherit the gene complex DCe from one parent and Dce from the other. His red cells will then react with anti-D, anti-C, anti-c and anti-e antisera.

This first theory postulates the existence of three genes, each with two alleles. Hence, there are eight possible genotypic combinations on each chromosome, and 36 complete phenotypes are possible for a given cell (8 × 8 minus duplications).

Another way to generate an equal number of phenotypes is to postulate the existence of a single Rh gene with eight possible allelic forms. This is precisely the approach taken by the second theory of Rh inheritance.[17] This second theory postulates the existence of only a single Rh gene on each chromosome (Fig. 14-13). Each of the eight alleles codes for a single surface antigen which has several distinct determinants. Each determinant can be defined by a unique antibody and each Rh

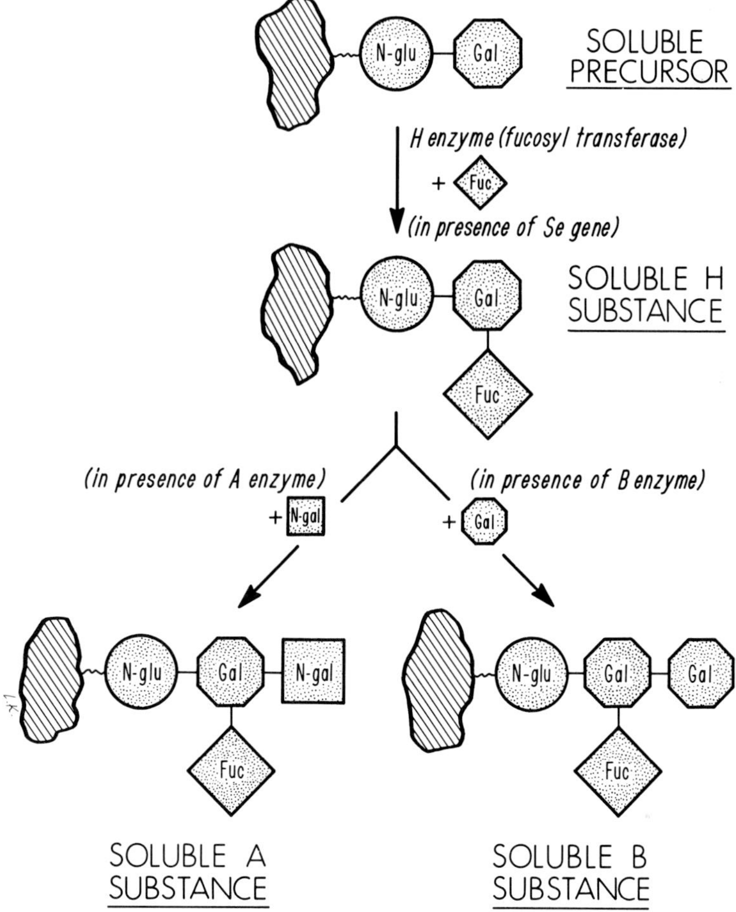

Fig. 14-11. The production of soluble H, A and B antigens.

antigen (possessing more than one determinant) can be identified by its reaction with a unique set of antideterminant antisera. Each antigen has been given a particular Rh designation and corresponds to a particular pattern of DCE-locus antigens as described by the first theory.[2,4] Thus, for example, the Rh_1 surface antigen reacts with anti-D, anti-C and anti-e antisera, the Rh_2 reacts with anti-D, anti-c and anti-E, and so on. Whereas the first theory postules a silent d gene, there is no compelling reason to expect a "d" antigen according to the second theory. Thus, a person carrying the r^y allele expresses the rh^y antigen which contains the C and E determinants but no D determinant.

Table 14-4. Antigens in the Saliva and on the Red Cell as a Function of Secretor and Lewis Genotypes in a Person with Blood Type A

Genotype Lewis	*Genotype* Secretor	*Saliva (Soluble Antigens)*	*Red Cell (Soluble and Intrinsic Antigens)*
Le/Le or Le/le	se/se	Le^a	Le^a, A, H
le/le	se/se	None	A, H
Le/Le or Le/le	Se/Se or Se/se	Le^b, H, A	Le^b, A, H
le/le	Se/Se or Se/se	H, A	A, H

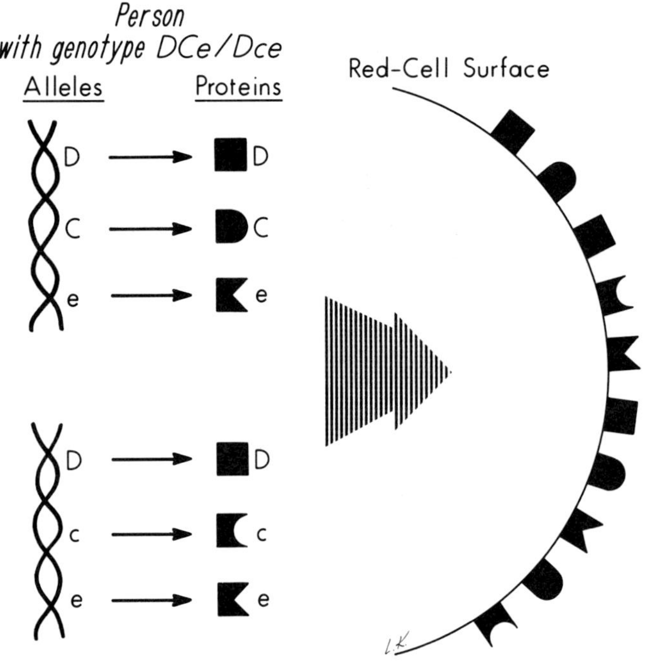

Fig. 14-12. The three-gene theory of the Rh system. An individual possesses two sets of three separate genes, each coding for a separate molecule which is expressed on the red-cell surface.

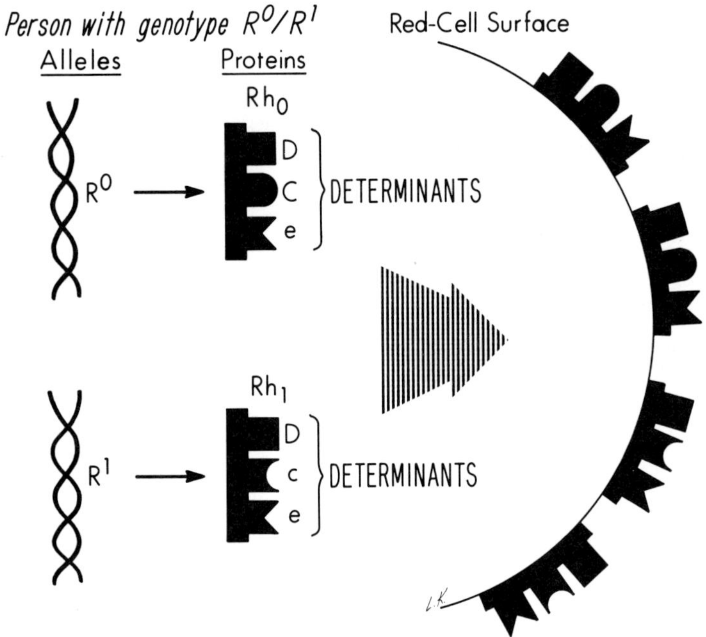

Fig. 14-13. The one-gene theory of the Rh system. Each individual possesses two alleles of a single gene that codes for one surface molecule. Each molecule, however, is complex and possesses three distinct antigenic determinants.

The Rh antigen has not been isolated and studied and thus there is no way to choose between these theories at present. We must emphasize that the D determinant, whether a separate molecule or only a determinant on a larger molecule, is the most significant Rh determinant in clinical medicine. The others are rarely of clinical importance.

The Ii System

During development from fetal life to about 18 months of age there is an increase in the amount of I antigen present on the red-cell population with a concomitant decrease in i antigen. From 18 months on, the normal individual maintains his peak reactivity with anti-I antisera and displays only a residuum of anti-i reactivity.[18] Only rare individuals remain strongly i-positive and I-negative into adult life. The I and i genes do not appear to be alleles and may in fact bear little genetic relationship to each other. It also appears that the I and i antigens are not single antigens but probably represent multiple determinants.

The MN System

Within this system two major polysaccharide antigens have been defined, M and N, and three phenotypes exist: M, MN and N. It was originally believed that this was a diallelic system with two codominant alleles, M and N. More recent evidence has indicated that this system is more complex. It appears that the N substance serves as a substrate for the M gene product.[19] Thus individuals possessing the M gene modify the N antigen to produce the M antigen. The allele of M is felt to be silent as is the O allele of the A or B gene. An individual with only one M gene does not transform all of the N antigen to M and appears phenotypically as MN. A person who is homozygous for M (M/M) transforms virtually all of the N to M and is detected as blood type M (Fig. 14-14). We must emphasize that this model has not been proved and our understanding of this system lags considerably behind that of the ABO system.

The P System

This system consists of two genetic alleles coding for the antigens P_1 and P_2. Rarely, a person may lack both of these antigens and is designated as p. The P_1 antigen has been defined chemically as a glycosphingolipid globoside. The determinant portion of the antigen has the formula D - galactosyl - α (1→4) - D - galactosyl - β (1→4) - N - acetyl - D - glucosamine.[20]

The Kell System

There are two major antigens in this system: K and k. Three genotypes are pos-

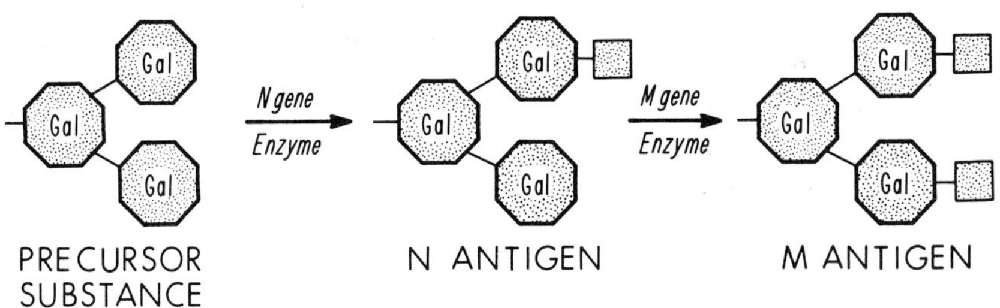

Fig. 14-14. Tentative scheme for the structure of the M and N antigens. The N antigen is believed to be the precursor of the M antigen.

sible: KK, Kk and kk. Less than 10 per cent of the population has the K gene in either a homozygous or heterozygous fashion. Therefore, transfusion with K-positive blood can theoretically be immunogenic to about 90 per cent of the population. The Kell antigens are potently immunogenic. Rare individuals who have neither the K nor k antigens have been detected and are referred to as K_0. Some patients with chronic granulomatous disease (see Chap. 11) have red cells that fail to react with or weakly react with antibodies to Kell antigens.[21] In addition to the K antigens, a number of other antigens have been included in the Kell system, notably Kp^a and Kp^b, and Js^a and Js^b.

The Kidd System

This diallelic system codes for two possible antigens, Jk^a and Jk^b. The three phenotypes Jk^a, Jk^b and Jk^aJk^b are all common, and only rare individuals lack both antigens.

The Duffy System

This is also a diallelic system and the antigens are designated Fy^a and Fy^b. Individuals negative for both antigens are quite unusual in the Caucasian population but attain a frequency of 70 per cent in the African Negro population.

Other antigen systems have been described but are beyond the range of this brief introduction.

Chemical Nature of the Red-Cell Antigens

The red-cell antigens can be grossly divided into two chemical groups, polysaccharides and proteins. The polysaccharide antigens include the A, B, H, M, N, I, i and P antigens. Many of these antigens are physically associated with the glycophorin molecule, one of the major red-cell-membrane components. The protein antigens include the Rh, Kell, Kidd and Duffy antigens.

ANTIBODY REACTIONS WITH RED BLOOD CELLS

The presence of antibodies directed against erythrocyte antigens is most commonly detected by assaying red-cell agglutination *in vitro*. Agglutination results because of the di- or multivalent nature of all immunoglobulin molecules. When the combining site of a single antibody attaches to identical determinants on the surfaces of adjacent red cells, the cells are agglutinated.

In order for an antibody to cross-link two red cells, it must overcome the negative surface charge that normally repels one cell from another.[22] This "zeta potential" is a result of the characteristics of the red-cell surface and the medium in which the cells are resting (Fig. 14-15). Many factors determine the ability of an antibody to successfully bridge the zeta potential. The large, pentameric 19S IgM molecule can easily bridge the zeta potential between two erythrocytes suspended in physiologic saline. On the other hand, the small 7S IgG molecule is often incapable of agglutinating red cells suspended in saline (Fig. 14-16). For this reason, IgM molecules are referred to as saline agglutinins, or complete agglutinins. The term "complete" refers to the ability of an antibody to act as an agglutinin without the use of any special procedures to help the antibody overcome the zeta potential. Incomplete agglutinins are unable to agglutinate red cells without experimental intervention. IgG is most often an "incomplete agglutinin"; however, there are important exceptions and IgG directed against certain red-cell antigens (such as A or B) can act as a complete agglutinin.

There are several techniques which can be employed to increase the susceptibility of red cells to agglutination by incomplete antibodies. These involve either reducing the zeta potential or effectively "stretching" the agglutinin bridge. Suspension of the target erythrocytes in a col-

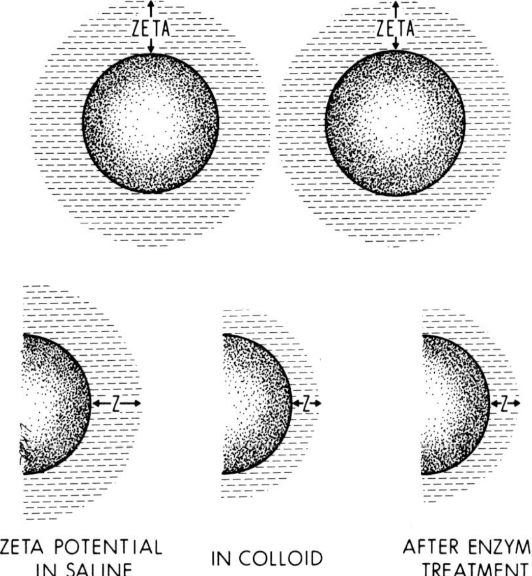

Fig. 14-15. The zeta potential. The size of the charge cloud that surrounds an erythrocyte is reduced in colloidal media and also by enzymatic treatment of the red cells.

loidal medium (such as albumin solutions) reduces the zeta potential and often permits IgG molecules to agglutinate cells. Treatment of the surface of red cells with enzymes may also alter the zeta potential, but the use of this technique is limited by the enzymatic destruction of certain red-cell antigens, thereby precluding the detection of IgG directed against those determinants.

One of the most useful methods for detecting the presence of antibodies against erythrocyte antigens is the Coombs' test.[23] It employs anti-immunoglobulin antisera as the test reagent. The anti-immunoglobulin antibodies bind to red-cell-bound antibody and essentially provide a longer bridge so that the mutually repulsive erythrocytes can be agglutinated (Fig. 14-17). This particular type of

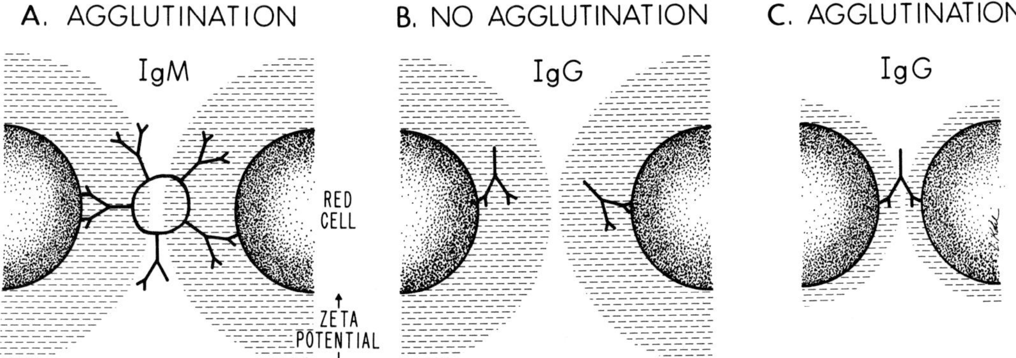

Fig. 14-16. Red-cell agglutination. (A) IgM can agglutinate red cells even in the presence of the large zeta potential present in saline. (B) IgG cannot bridge the zeta potential when the cells are suspended in saline. (C) Reduction of the zeta potential by placing the cells in a colloidal medium allows IgG to bridge the charge clouds and agglutinate the cells.

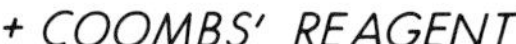

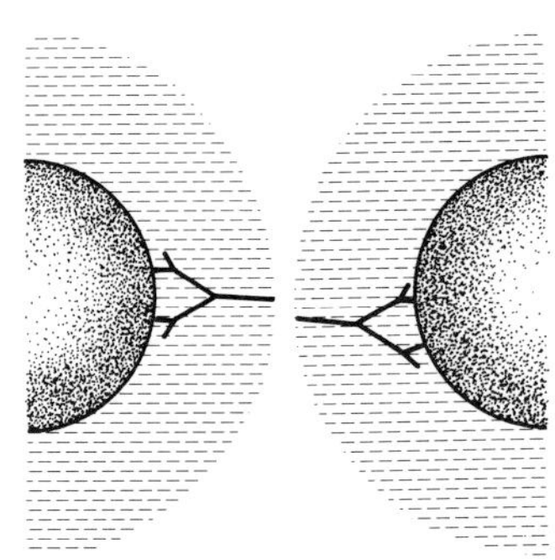

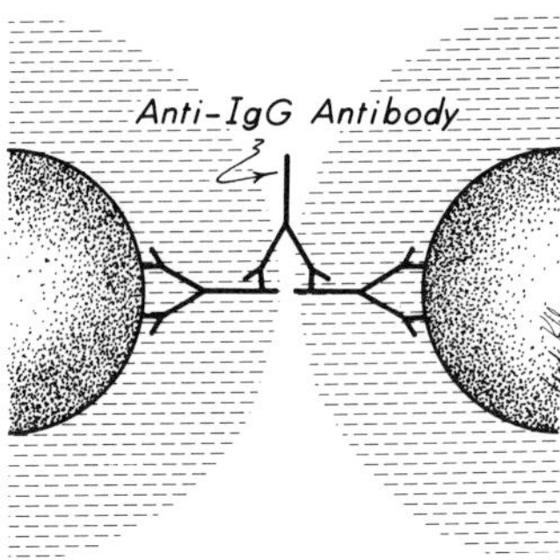

Fig. 14-17. The direct Coombs' test. IgG cannot agglutinate red cells in saline. The addition of anti-IgG antibody (Coombs' reagent) allows the bridging of the zeta potential and results in red-cell agglutination.

Coombs' test is called the direct Coombs' test. A variation of this procedure, the indirect Coombs' test, is used to detect free antierythrocyte antibodies in a patient's serum. In the indirect Coombs' test, a test-cell suspension is first mixed with the patient's serum, and then anti-immunoglobulin antiserum is added to detect if any antibodies have bound to the red cell (Fig. 14-18). The class of the offending antibodies can be determined in either variation of the Coombs' test by employing anti-immunoglobulin antiserum that is class-specific.

Other factors may modify the ability of IgG to act as a red-cell agglutinin. The red-cell surface can be pictured as a rugged terrain marked by numerous peaks and crevices. It is possible, although it has not been proved, that certain antigens may be predominantly located on the crests of surface prominences and therefore be readily cross-linked by IgG molecules. Antigen buried in surface crevices might defy the ability of the small IgG molecule to link adjacent cells.[4]

When antibody is reacted against many of the red-cell antigens, those antigens migrate and patch on the red-cell surface. This patching process may be important in allowing the agglutination of red cells.[24,25] For instance, IgG can induce patching of the A or B antigens while anti-D (anti-Rh_0) IgG does not lead to antigen movement. It is thus interesting that anti-D IgG is virtually always an incomplete agglutinin while anti-ABO IgG is able to agglutinate red cells.

IgA is rarely implicated as an antibody against erythrocyte antigens. When IgA has been present, it has behaved most often as an incomplete agglutinin.

Additional characterization of antibodies to erythrocyte antigens can be obtained by examining the "thermal amplitude" of the antibody–red-cell interaction. This has permitted the identification of warm-reacting and cold-reacting antibodies. Warm-reacting antibodies are maximally reactive at normal physiologic temperatures around 37° C. Cold-reacting antibodies bind most intensely with the target red cells at temperatures below 31°, and often as low as 4° C. These antibodies dissociate from the erythrocyte when the temperature is raised. Cold-reacting antibodies are directed against polysaccharide antigens, whereas protein antigen-antibody reactions are almost always optimal at warm temperatures. The distinction between warm- and cold-reacting antibodies is especially important in autoimmune hemolytic anemia (see below).

It is worthwhile to emphasize at this

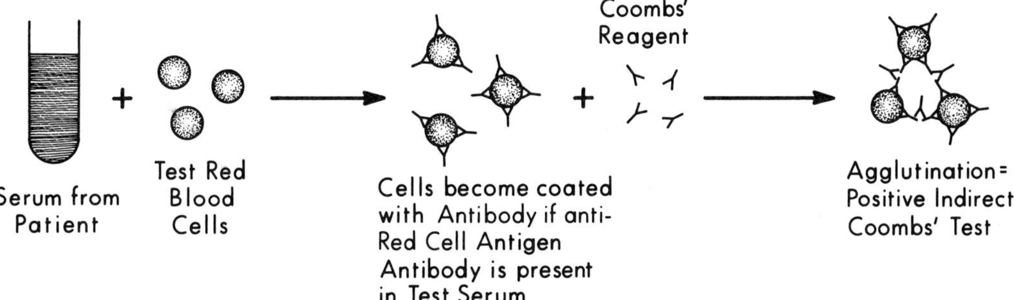

Fig. 14-18. The indirect Coombs' test. Patient's serum is added to the test red cells. If antibody is present it will coat the red cells, and the addition of the Coombs' reagent will agglutinate the cells.

point that the preference of cold-reacting antibodies for polysaccharide antigens and warm-reacting antibodies for protein antigens is only one of several distinctions between the types of antibodies elicited by these two classes of red-cell antigens. Antibodies directed against polysaccharide antigens are most often IgM although they can include IgG, while the typical antibodies directed against the protein antigens are IgG. These and other differences between the polysaccharide and protein antigens are summarized in Table 14-5.

SITUATIONS IN WHICH ANTIBODIES AGAINST ERYTHROCYTE ANTIGENS CAN BE FOUND

Naturally Occurring Isoantibodies

All people with competent immune systems possess circulating antibodies against several red-cell antigens. These naturally occurring antibodies are isoantibodies (or isoagglutinins) because they are directed against blood-group antigens not present on the cells of the host. For example, a person with type A blood has anti-B isoantibodies in his serum. Type O individuals have both anti-A and anti-B isoantibodies, and type AB people have neither.

Naturally occurring isoantibodies are virtually always directed against polysaccharide antigens. ABO isoantibodies are the most significant naturally occurring antibodies in clinical medicine. They are strongly reactive at physiologic temperatures. An ABO transfusion mismatch can have fatal consequences, and the existence of these isoantibodies provides the fundamental reason for strict blood-typing before transfusion. Type AB individuals possess no isoantibodies and are often referred to as "universal recipients"; they will not react against type A, B, AB or O blood. Since almost all people carry the H antigen, O blood cells can almost always be safely given, and type O individuals have appropriately been termed "universal donors." However,

Table 14-5. Protein and Polysaccharide Red-Cell Antigens

	Polysaccharide Antigens	*Protein Antigens*
Antigen systems	ABH, MN, Ii, P	Rh, Kell, Kidd, Duffy
Class of antibody response elicited	Primarily IgM	Primarily IgG
Warm-reacting antibodies	Yes	Yes
Cold-reacting antibodies	Yes	No
Naturally occurring isoantibodies	Yes	Rare
Transfusion reactions	Often immediate	Often delayed

since type O blood contains anti-A and anti-B antibody, and since it is unusual to give red blood cells washed free of serum in transfusion, in practice one would rather give type A blood to a type A recipient than type O blood.

Naturally occurring isoantibodies directed against other red-cell polysaccharide antigens also exist. Lewis-negative (le/le) individuals can possess antibodies against both the Le^a and Le^b antigens. Anti-Lewis antibodies rarely cause significant hemolytic reactions, perhaps because the Lewis antigens will dissociate from the red cell more readily than the intrinsic antigens.

Naturally occurring isoantibodies of the MN system are usually cold-reacting complete agglutinins. Less commonly they are active at physiologic temperatures and can then cause transfusion reactions. Cold-reacting anti-P_1 antibody is frequently found in P_2 individuals. The rare type p individuals possess antibodies against both P_1 and P_2.

What stimulates the production of naturally occurring isoantibodies? By definition, a person possessing naturally occurring isoantibodies to a given red-cell antigen has not been previously exposed to erythrocytes bearing that antigen. The most popular explanation is that bacterial cell walls may have antigens in common with the red-cell surface, and that isoantibodies result from immune stimulation by these crossreacting bacterial antigens. ABO antigens have indeed been found to crossreact with certain bacterial antigens, but this by no means confirms the theory.[26]

Isoantibodies Arising from Immunization

Direct immunization with red-cell antigens usually results either from a mismatched transfusion or the leakage of fetal cells into the maternal circulation during pregnancy and delivery. These isoantibodies are predominantly IgG once the response has become established. Isoantibodies against certain red-cell antigen systems can only be formed by direct immunization; naturally occurring isoantibodies to antigens other than those of the ABO, P, MN and Lewis systems are extremely rare.

Transfusions which are incompatible for a given antigen do not always result in isoimmunization. Even the highly immunogenic D antigen of the Rh system is associated with a frequency of immunization of only 50 per cent upon single transfusion into a D-negative individual. A single transfusion with red cells bearing the K antigen of the Kell system will immunize only 5 per cent of K-negative individuals. Other red-cell antigens are even less immunogenic (see Table 14-6).[26a]

Autoantibodies

Occasionally, individuals may make antibodies against their own red-cell antigens. These autoantibodies may often be no more than serologic curiosities and of

Table 14-6. Immunogenicity of Some Red-Cell Antigens*

Antigen	*Frequency of Immunization After One Transfusion into an Antigen-Negative Recipient*
Rh antigens	
D	>50.00%
c	2.05%
E	1.69%
e	0.56%
C	0.11%
Kell antigens	
K	5.00%
k	1.50%
Duffy antigens	
Fy^a	0.23%
Kidd antigens	
Jk^a	0.07%
Jk^b	0.03%

*From Sturgeon, P.: Erythrocyte antigens and antibodies. *In* Williams, W. J., Beutler, E., Erslev, A. J., and Rundles, R. W. (eds.): Hematology. P. 1272. New York, McGraw-Hill, 1972.

no clinical consequence. However, they can occasionally be responsible for a serious and life-threatening hemolytic anemia with varying manifestations depending upon the characteristics of the autoantibody. We will discuss the autoimmune hemolytic anemias later in this chapter.

THE EFFECTS OF ANTIBODY ON RED CELLS

Antibodies against erythrocyte antigens can have various effects on the target red cells, ranging from none to erythrocyte agglutination and destruction. Agglutination can lead to small-vessel occlusion and is responsible for many of the symptoms of cold agglutinin disease (see below). Erythrocyte destruction is responsible for the major symptoms of transfusion reactions, isoimmune hemolysis and autoimmune hemolytic anemias. There are several ways in which antibody that binds to red cells can mediate their destruction.

Immune Adherence and Opsonization

IgG-coated red cells can attach to macrophage Fc receptors and be promptly phagocytosed.[27] Since aggregated IgG attaches most efficiently to Fc receptors on phagocytic cells, red cells coated with a high density of IgG are phagocytosed most rapidly. In general, the amount of red-cell-bound IgG correlates with the rate of erythrocyte destruction.[28] Cells coated with a low density of antibody are preferentially destroyed in the spleen where the circulatory dynamics allow maximal interaction between the coated red cells and the phagocytic cells.[3] Cells coated with a higher density of immunoglobulin may be phagocytosed in the liver as well.

Opsonized red cells are not always destroyed following attachment to phagocytic cells. Sometimes the cells may remain attached long enough for phagocytes to remove part of the red-cell membrane. The cell that is released has a reduced ratio of surface area to volume and is called a *spherocyte* (Fig. 14-19). These cells are mechanically and osmotically fragile. Spherocyte formation occurs predominantly in the spleen. Only IgG antibodies can induce spherocyte formation since only IgG can mediate immune adherence. Spherocytes are most commonly seen in IgG autoimmune hemolytic anemia.

Although experiments *in vitro* suggest that red-cell phagocytosis via opsonization is a significant mechanism of erythrocyte destruction, opsonization may not be as important *in vivo* as originally believed. Free IgG has been shown to competitively inhibit the binding of IgG-coated red cells to phagocytes bearing Fc receptors. Since IgG is present in large amounts in normal serum, inhibition of immune adherence may occur *in vivo*. However, it is possible that the dynamics of the spleen are such as to maximize the opportunities for immune adherence, and thus partially negate this effect.

Antibody-Dependent Cell-Mediated Cytotoxicity

Several investigators have shown that IgG-coated red cells can be destroyed *in vitro* by the process of antibody-dependent cell-mediated cytotoxicity.[29,30] Whether or not this mechanism is of any importance in hemolysis *in vivo* is currently unknown.

Complement Fixation

When the complement system was first experimentally investigated, it was demonstrated that activation of the complete complement pathway could result in red-cell lysis. The importance of complement-mediated red-cell lysis *in vivo*, however, remains to be convincingly shown. For example, normal human red cells have been found to be highly resistant to lysis by human complement.

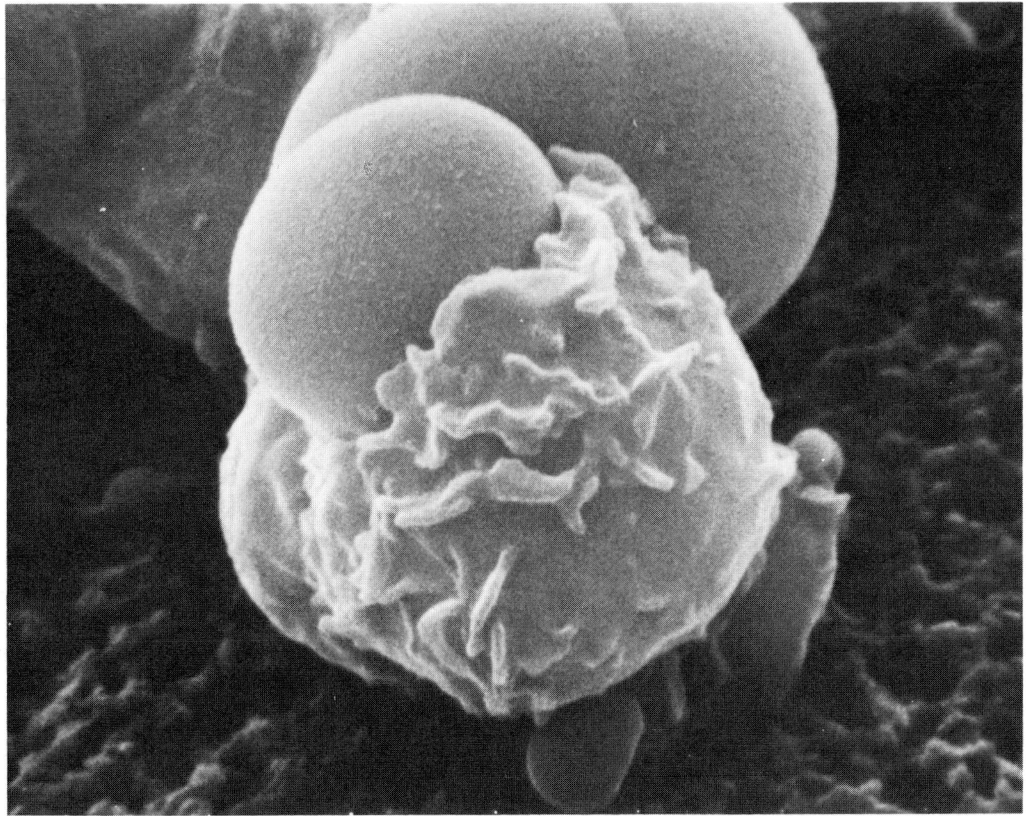

Fig. 14-19. Scanning electron micrograph of the production of a red-cell spherocyte. (Courtesy Dr. W. F. Rosse.)

However, at present there is no other mechanism available to account for IgM-mediated red-cell destruction.

In order for IgG to activate complement, the antibodies must be bound to the red-cell surface in close proximity to each other. Rh antigens are relatively sparsely distributed on the cell surface, and anti-Rh antibodies only rarely can fix complement. The ABH antigens, on the other hand, are more densely represented. It has been estimated that several thousand anti-A IgG molecules per cell are required for complement fixation while fewer than 100 IgM molecules will suffice.[31] Another way to view the spatial requirements for complement fixation by IgG is to take into consideration the phenomenon of antibody-induced antigen aggregation (surface patching). It has been proposed that IgG–red-cell antigen complexes that patch (such as A and B) will provide the appropriate complement-fixing topography while nonpatching antigens (such as the D antigen of the Rh system) will not.

Although there are adherence receptors for complement components on phagocytic cells, red cells coated solely with complement do not appear to be phagocytosed. Complement alone is not effective at opsonizing red cells. However, there is some evidence that IgG opsonization is enhanced by the presence of complement on the opsonized target.

A direct Coombs' test using anticomplement antisera measures the presence of red-cell-bound complement by agglutination of red cells. Positive agglutination can be taken as presumptive evidence for the presence of antibodies against erythrocyte antigens at some time in the patient's course. It is not unusual to fail to detect any immunoglobulin on the surface of red cells which nevertheless can be demonstrated to have bound complement. This could be due to any of the following:

1. Low-affinity antibody may bind to red cells, fix complement and then dissociate, leaving behind only the activated complement components.
2. Cold-reactive antibodies may attach reversibily to red cells in the extremities where the body temperature is low. They may then fix complement only to dissociate when the cells are rewarmed. The complement components will remain on the cells.
3. Low amounts of immunoglobulin may be present on the red cells and remain below the limits of detectability of the assay.
4. Complement may be present on the red-cell surface due to activation of the properdin complement pathway.

RED-CELL IMMUNITY IN CLINICAL MEDICINE

TRANSFUSION REACTIONS

An immediate immune hemolytic reaction is the greatest hazard of an incompatible blood transfusion.[3] This catastrophic situation can be prevented by carefully screening the recipient for preformed antibody against the donor red cells. Nevertheless, transfusion reactions still occur when emergency transfusions have to be given without allowing time for crossmatching, or due to clerical errors in the handling of blood. Preformed antibodies combine with transfused cells and produce either intravascular hemolysis (often seen with ABO incompatibility) or extravascular destruction of the antibody-coated cells by the reticuloendothelial system.

Signs and symptoms of immediate transfusion reactions include fever, nausea, vomiting, low back pain and hypotension. Pathologic bleeding due to a consumption of coagulation factors may occur. When a transfusion reaction is recognized, the transfusion must be stopped immediately. Steps should be taken to prevent bleeding and to maintain an effective circulating volume and diuresis aimed primarily at protecting the kidneys.

Transfusion reactions may occur as long as three days to two weeks after a transfusion is given. Such delayed hemolytic reactions are usually mild and probably most often occur subclinically. On occasion, however, a full-blown picture resembling an acute reaction may occur. Delayed reactions are believed to be the result of an anamnestic response to a pre-

Table 14-7. Transfusion Reactions

Type	*Clinical Signs*	*Mechanisms*
Immediate (minutes to hours)		
Hemolytic	Fever, back pain, nausea, vomiting, hypotension, consumptive coagulopathy, acute renal failure	Antibody-mediated destruction of incompatible erythrocytes
Febrile	Fever, chills	Bacterial pyrogens, sensitivity to donor platelets and leukocytes
Allergic	Pruritus, urticaria, bronchospasm, anaphylaxis	Immune sensitivity to foreign serum protein—seen in IgA-deficient patients with anti-IgA antibodies
Delayed (4–14 days)		Delayed development of anti-donor antibodies

viously encountered red-cell antigen. These people presumably avoid acute reactions because they possess very low, undetectable levels of antibody at the time of the crossmatching and transfusion. The Rh, Kidd and Duffy antigens are most often responsible for delayed hemolytic reactions.

HEMOLYTIC DISEASE OF THE NEWBORN

If a pregnant woman possesses isoantibodies against paternal antigens expressed on fetal blood cells, destruction of the fetal cells can ensue, producing a hemolytic anemia with erythroid hyperplasia, splenomegaly and hyperbilirubinemia due to hemoglobin catabolism. This syndrome is referred to as *erythroblastosis fetalis* or *hemolytic disease of the newborn*. The severity of this disorder is determined by the extent of hemolysis of the fetal red blood cells. High levels of unconjugated bilirubin can damage neural tissue and produce the neurologic syndrome of kernicterus. The fetus and neonate are especially susceptible to the damaging effects of bilirubin since their immature livers have only a limited capacity to conjugate bilirubin and their immature blood-brain barrier cannot serve as an adequate defense.

Although ABO incompatibility between mother and fetus is very common, ABO incompatibility is rarely the cause of newborn hemolysis. There are several reasons for this:

1. In order for hemolysis of fetal blood cells to occur, antibody must pass from the mother to the fetus. Only IgG can pass across the placenta. Since naturally occurring isoantibodies in type A and B individuals are predominantly IgM, there is little danger of fetal hemolysis in type A or B mothers. ABO-incompatible fetal red blood cell hemolysis occurs almost exclusively with women of blood type O, who do possess significant titers of IgG anti-A and anti-B isoantibodies.

2. The ABO antigens are only poorly expressed on fetal red cells. This may render fetal cells relatively resistant to the effects of IgG ABO isoantibodies.

The major offending antigen in hemolytic disease of the newborn is the D (or Rh_o) antigen. Naturally occurring Rh antibodies probably do not exist, and therefore immunization of an Rh-negative mother with Rh-positive cells must first take place. This occurs most commonly from a previous pregnancy; Rh hemolytic disease of the newborn is virtually never seen in a first pregnancy unless the mother has been sensitized by a previous transfusion. There have been two significant contributions toward reducing the incidence of erythroblastosis fetalis.

Specific testing has allowed the early recognition of Rh-negative women and alerted physicians to avoid sensitization with transfusions of Rh-positive blood.

Specific immunotherapy arose from the observation that maternal-fetal ABO incompatibility protected against maternal immunization by Rh-positive fetal cells (Fig. 14-20). This phenomenon has been felt to be due to the rapid clearance of ABO-incompatible cells by naturally occurring isoantibodies, thereby preventing sensitization of the maternal immune system to the Rh determinant. Injection of concentrated human anti-Rh_o IgG into mothers just after the delivery of an Rh_o-incompatible baby was begun with the hope of inducing just such a rapid clearance of immunogenic cells from the maternal circulation. This procedure has been remarkably successful in preventing Rh sensitization, and has contributed greatly to reducing the incidence of hemolytic disease of the newborn. However, despite its success, the exact mechanism for the protection it affords is still not totally clear (see also p. 120).

AUTOIMMUNE HEMOLYTIC DISEASE[32-34]

Disorders due to the presence of autoantibodies against erythrocyte antigens

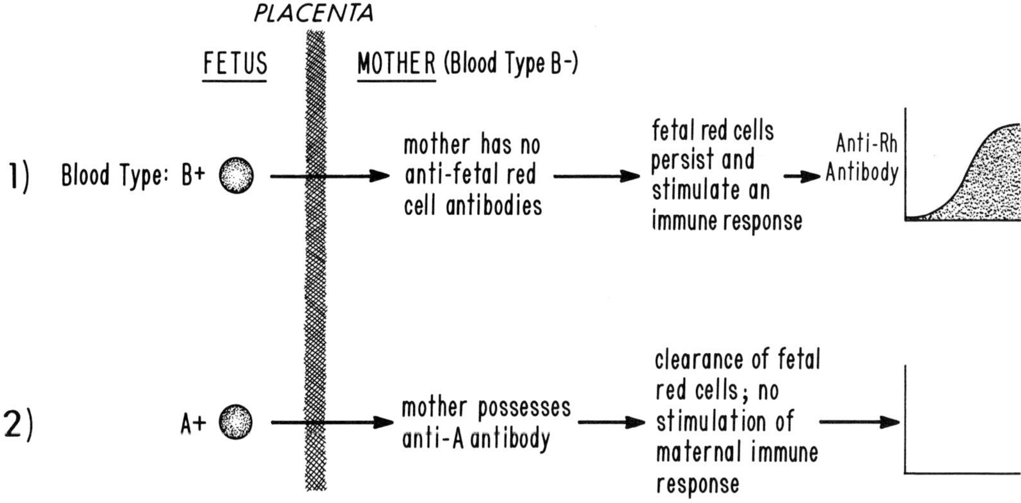

Fig. 14-20. ABO incompatibility protects against maternal Rh immunization. (1) Fetal red cells that are ABO-compatible survive in the maternal circulation long enough to stimulate the production of anti-Rh antibodies. (2) ABO-incompatible cells are rapidly destroyed in the maternal circulation because of the presence of naturally occurring isoantibodies, thus diminishing the chance of Rh-incompatible cells eliciting anti-Rh antibody production.

have been classified according to the thermal characteristics of the antibody (warm versus cold) and according to whether the disease is idiopathic or associated with the presence of another disease, most often lymphoreticular malignancies, autoimmune diseases and infectious diseases (Table 14-8).

Warm Autoantibodies

Most cases of autoimmune hemolytic anemia are associated with warm-reacting autoantibodies. A majority of patients with autoimmune hemolytic anemia have an associated disease, and probably only about 20 per cent of patients have a primary or idiopathic variety. Warm-reacting autoimmune hemolytic anemia can be a life-threatening disease, and mortality rates of greater than 50 per cent have been recorded, although this figure strongly reflects the associated prognosis of the underlying disease. Among patients with idiopathic autoimmune hemolytic anemia, the mortality is less than 40 per cent.[35]

IgG autoantibodies are the most frequent. Warm-reacting IgM and IgA autoantibodies are far less common and when present usually occur together with IgG antibody.[36] By using specific antisera against immunoglobulin and complement components, four patterns of red-cell coating can be identified:[37]

Table 14-8. Autoimmune Hemolytic Disease

Antibody Class	*Warm-reacting*	*Cold-reacting*
IgG	Common. There is spherocyte formation and splenic sequestration. Targets are the Rh and "universal" antigens.	Rare, e.g., the Donath-Landsteiner antibody. There is paroxysmal cold hemoglobinuria with intravascular hemolysis. Targets are the P antigens.
IgM	Rare	Common. Spherocytes are rarely seen. Targets are the I and i antigens.

1. Only immunoglobulin is detected on the red-cell surface: this is observed in 20 to 50 per cent of patients. There is usually little evidence of intravascular hemolysis, whereas spherocytosis is very common.
2. Both immunoglobulin and complement are fixed to the red-cell surface: this occurs in 30 to 50 per cent of patients.
3. In a similar percentage of cases, complement alone may be present.
4. Rarely, neither immunoglobulin nor complement can be detected on the red cells. Such patients may have extensive hemolysis but its immune nature is unclear.

Serum titers of autoantibodies do not strictly correlate with the degree of hemolysis, and remissions may occur without any demonstrable serologic changes.

Spherocytes are commonly seen with warm-reacting autoantibodies, presumably because of the ability of IgG molecules to opsonize the red cells, resulting in partial phagocytosis. This finding is in contrast to IgM cold-reacting autoimmune anemia where spherocytosis is rare. Opsonization of the erythrocytes by IgG is believed to be responsible for the significant splenic sequestration that is often seen.[38]

It has proved difficult to define the antigens against which the autoantibodies are directed. Most early reports of warm-reacting autoantibody specificity implicated the Rh antigens as the targets.[33] However, these reports could account for only about one third of all patients with warm-reacting autoimmune hemolysis. More recently it has been found that many of the remaining cases appear to involve specificities that are common to almost all normal red cells and hence remained unclassified for a long time. A significant percentage of these antibodies have been shown to have specificity for an almost universally present, undefined component of the Rh system.[39,40] This conclusion has been reached on the basis of the failure of these antisera to react with a very rare type of red cell (Rh null) which lacks all Rh-system determinants.

Cold Autoantibodies

Cold-reacting autoantibodies directed against erythrocyte antigens are usually associated with only minimal or mild hemolysis, although in certain situations they may predictably cause extensive hemolysis (see below). The infrequency of severe hemolysis is almost certainly due to the antibodies' maximal reactivity at temperatures below 31° C. However, it is important to remember that the peripheral cutaneous microcirculation can normally reach temperatures of 30° C. and can be even further reduced by exposure to the cold. Vascular occlusion in the extremities due to autoagglutination can cause numbness and Raynaud's phenomenon.

Acute transient elevations in levels of cold-reacting antibodies are most often seen after infections, especially infectious mononucleosis and atypical pneumonias. The i antigen is frequently the target in cold hemolysis associated with infectious mononucleosis. These cases are only rarely associated with an overt hemolytic anemia.

More than 50 per cent of cold-reacting hemolytic disease has been classified as "chronic idiopathic" or "chronic cold agglutinin" disease, and primarily affects elderly patients. The majority of patients with chronic cold agglutinin disease have a bone marrow lymphocytosis. The cold agglutinin molecule is an IgM, and is usually either monoclonal or of greatly restricted heterogeneity. The agglutinin virtually always possesses κ light chains. With rare exceptions, the target is the I antigen.

Occasionally, chronic cold agglutinin disease is associated with a lymphoreticular malignancy. Frequently, the antibody in these patients is directed against the i antigen.[32]

Cold-reacting antibodies are almost always IgM agglutinins. These antibodies attach to the red cell at cold temperatures, and dissociate as the cells are rewarmed. Complement fixation varies among different antibodies. Because the antibodies are IgM, immune adherence does not occur and spherocytes are rarely seen.

The unique thermal basis of these antibodies does not appear to be a characteristic of the antibody molecules themselves. Instead, it is the expression of the antigenic target that appears to be cold-dependent.[41] Both the I and i antigens are part of the glycophorin molecule, the major glycoprotein of human red-cell surfaces. By isolating glycophorin from the membrane, investigators have shown that the cold-reacting antibodies can bind to their target determinants at all temperatures, including the normal physiologic temperature of 37° C. Thus, these antibodies are clearly capable of reacting at warm temperatures. The most likely explanation is that the glycophorin molecule is held in a temperature-dependent conformation within the red-cell membrane. Only at cold temperatures are the glycophorin I and i determinants made available for interaction with these autoantibodies (Fig. 14-21).

Uncommonly, cold-reacting antibodies are IgG. Donath-Landsteiner antibodies are examples of such cold-reacting IgG molecules. The Donath-Landsteiner antibodies readily fix complement and are responsible for the clinical syndrome of *paroxysmal cold hemoglobinuria*. This is a rare syndrome in which patients experience a sudden onset of signs and symptoms referable to acute hemolysis, including fever, pain in the extremities and the back, jaundice, abdominal cramps and hemoglobinuria, all following exposure to the cold. Paroxysmal cold hemoglobinuria was initially described in association with syphilis, but acute episodes following viral infections and a chronic idiopathic variety have since been recognized.

Donath-Landsteiner antibodies react

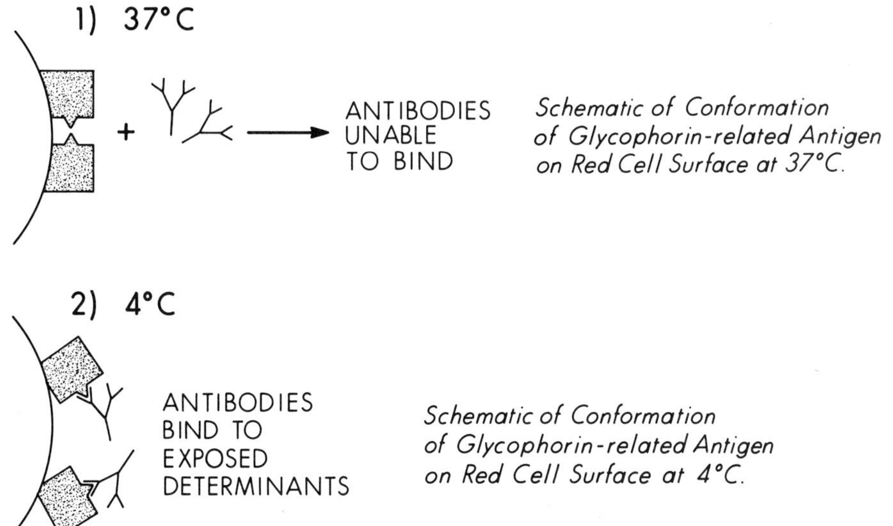

Fig. 14-21. Schematic of the molecular basis of cold-reacting antibodies. (1) At 37° C. the conformation of the glycophorin molecule "hides" the target determinants from the serum antibody. (2) At 4° C. the conformation of glycophorin changes so that the target antigens are now "exposed" and can react with antibody.

against antigens of the P system and lead to a biphasic hemolytic reaction *in vitro*.[42] The antibodies bind to the red cell only at cold temperatures and can fix the early components of complement. The complement sequence can only be completed, with attendant hemolysis, when the reaction mixture is warmed. The P antigen, like the I antigen, has been found to be present on the red-cell-membrane glycophorin molecule which may explain the temperature-dependent character of the Donath-Landsteiner antibodies.[41]

DRUG-INDUCED HEMOLYTIC ANEMIA

Between 15 and 20 per cent of all cases of acquired immune hemolytic anemia are drug-induced. Four mechanisms of drug-induced hemolytic anemia have been recognized (Table 14-9):[43]

Drugs Associated with Hemolytic Anemia with a Positive Direct Coombs' Test

Fuadin	Quinine
Quinidine	Antihistamine
P-Aminosalicylic acid	Chlorpromazine
Penicillin	Cephalothin
Sulfonamides	Mefenamic acid
Isoniazid	Insulin
α-Methyldopa	Rifampicin
L-Phenylalanine mustard	L-Dopa
Sulfonylurea drugs	Phenacetin

1. Drug-antibody complexes can be passively adsorbed onto the red-cell surface and fix complement. This process can produce extensive intravascular hemolysis and is called the innocent bystander reaction. Most drugs which can cause a hemolytic anemia seem to do so by this mechanism.

2. Penicillin readily combines with proteins of the red-cell membrane. Almost all patients who receive large doses of penicillin will have the drug attached to their red cells. Once on the red-cell surface the benzylpenicilloyl moiety acts as a hapten and can become a target of the immune response. Because of the high frequency of penicillin exposure, the majority of the population in the United States has circulating antibodies against penicillin. These are primarily IgM.

A very small percentage of patients receiving massive doses of penicillin will develop a hemolytic anemia. These patients have a positive direct Coombs' test, and the antibody involved is IgG. Complement fixation rarely occurs, and red-cell destruction probably takes place via erythrophagocytosis. The hemolytic anemia resolves after the cessation of drug administration. The high titers of antipenicillin IgG that are present in these patients do not correlate with the

Table 14-9. Drug-Induced Immune Hemolytic Anemia

Mechanism	*Example of Drug*	*Direct Coombs' Test*	*Clinical Findings*
Innocent bystander	Quinidine, sulfonamides, etc.	Often complement positive only; occasionally IgG positive	1. Small drug doses 2. Acute intravascular hemolysis 3. Often with renal failure
Drug as hapten	Penicillin	Strongly positive IgG	1. Large doses 2. Subacute extravascular hemolysis
Membrane alteration with nonspecific adsorption to red-cell-surface	Cephalosporins	Positive IgG, complement and other serum proteins	
Uncertain	Aldomet	IgG positive; rarely complement positive	Gradual onset of hemolytic anemia

(Modified from Garratty, G., and Petz, L. D.: Drug-induced hemolytic anemia. Am. J. Med., *53*:398, 1975)

presence or absence of the more common penicillin allergies.

3. The cephalosporins may induce a positive direct Coombs' test in a manner similar to penicillin. However, another suggestion has been made based upon the observation that normal serum proteins will nonspecifically coat cephalothin-sensitized red blood cells. It has been proposed that the celphalosporins can modify the red-cell membrane so that it becomes "sticky" to serum proteins, including immunoglobulin. These immunoglobulin molecules will produce a positive Coombs' test even though they are not acting as specific antibodies.

4. Alpha-methyldopa is an antihypertensive drug that will induce a positive direct Coombs' test in 10 to 15 per cent of patients taking it in high doses. Less than 1 per cent of patients taking alpha-methyldopa will develop a hemolytic anemia. When they do, the offending immunoglobulin is IgG. The pathogenesis of the hemolysis is unknown, but it has been postulated that alpha-methyldopa alters antigens of the red cell so that they become immunogenic to the host. There have been reports that the antibody bound to the red cell may have some specificity for the Rh blood group antigens.

In summary, four possible mechanisms of drug-induced hemolytic anemia have been proposed: passive adsorption of immune complexes; binding of the drug to the red cell where it acts as the target antigen; nonspecific surface modification; and specific antigenic modulation. Only the first two mechanisms have been adequately demonstrated.

PLATELET IMMUNITY

Immune-mediated thrombocytopenia may be even more common than immune hemolytic anemia, but very little is known about the immunology of antiplatelet reactions. An innocent bystander mechanism involving the adsorption of drug-antibody complexes onto the platelet surface has been described, notably with the drugs quinidine and quinine (see Chap. 7). In addition, certain disease states have now been associated with the production of antiplatelet antibodies (see below).

Several platelet-specific antigens have been described, although, with only one exception, their clinical importance has not been established. The exception is the platelet antigen Pl^{A1} present on the platelets of 98 per cent of the population.[44] Pl^{A1}-positive individuals can be divided into two groups, those whose platelets absorb a large amount of Pl^{A1} antibody on serologic testing, and those whose platelets absorb about one half of the amount of the first group. People in the maximally reactive group are felt to be homozygous for the Pl^{A1} allele, whereas those in the second group are believed to be heterozygotes. The latter group expresses only half the amount of Pl^{A1} antigen plus a second antigen Pl^{A2} coded for by an alternate allele. The 2 per cent of the population that are negative for Pl^{A1} are homozygous for Pl^{A2}.

Isoimmune Neonatal Thrombocytopenia

This disease is analogous to hemolytic disease of the newborn. Immunization of the mother against paternal antigens present on the fetal platelets results in the production of IgG that crosses the placenta and attacks the platelets of the fetus.[45] Most often the mother is Pl^{A1}-negative and the maternal antibodies are directed against the Pl^{A1} antigen on the fetal platelets. The affected infant presents with a variable degree of thrombocytopenia with bleeding abnormalities reflecting the level of the newborn's circulating platelets. The thrombocytopenia clears over the first few weeks of life as the maternal antibodies are catabolized.

Idiopathic Thrombocytopenic Purpura

Increased platelet destruction of unknown etiology has been referred to as idiopathic thrombocytopenic purpura (ITP). It now appears that ITP may be a true autoimmune disease. In children, the disease often presents acutely following a viral infection. In adults, the disease is more often chronic and is sometimes seen in association with systemic diseases such as systemic lupus erythematosus and lymphoma. The immunoglobulin present on the platelet surface is IgG, but a target antigen has not been defined.[46,47] The platelets are coated with a large amount of IgG and this may lead to platelet sequestration and destruction by the reticuloendothelial system and the spleen in particular.[48]

NEUTROPHIL IMMUNITY

Neutrophils express many surface antigens, some of which are shared by other tissues (such as the HLA antigens) and some of which are specific to the cell line. Definition of these neutrophil-specific antigen systems is just beginning.[49] Thus far, three major antigens have been described by using maternal serum obtained after incompatible pregnancies. NA1 and NA2 are coded for by the NA locus, and NB1 is coded for by the NB locus. The maternal antibodies are IgG and can cross the placenta. They appear to be responsible for the disease *isoimmune neonatal neutropenia.*[50] Infants with this unusual syndrome usually present with marked neutropenia and infection. The neutropenia is transient since the sole source of antibody is the mother; however, the disease can be so severe that not all infants survive.

Antineutrophil antibodies have recently been implicated in *idiopathic neutropenia*. Patients have been described who possess autoantibodies against their own neutrophils.[51] The auto-IgG appears capable of successfully opsonizing the neutrophils for phagocytosis by mononuclear cells. In one child, the autoantibody has been shown to be directed against the NA2 antigen.[52] Treatment of this child with steroids resulted in a concomitant drop in the anti-NA2 titer and a rise in the neutrophil count.

Felty's syndrome is defined by the triad of rheumatoid arthritis, splenomegaly and neutropenia. An immune etiology for the neutropenia was originally suggested by the observation that plasma taken from a patient with this syndrome could produce a fall in the leukocyte count of healthy recipients.[53] Large quantities of IgG have since been detected on the surface of the neutrophils of patients with Felty's syndrome.[54,55] There is little evidence that excessive neutrophil destruction occurs in these patients, and the significance of these antibodies remains undefined. The neutropenia is more likely due to a maturational arrest of neutrophil precursors, and it is possible that the neutrophil antibodies may prevent proper development of the granulocyte precursors. We must emphasize that it is still not certain whether these are true autoantibodies directed against a neutrophil antigen.

Splenectomy is often of value in this syndrome, and the neutrophil count frequently returns to normal postoperatively.[55] It has long been suggested that the spleen produces a humoral substance which is responsible for the neutropenia.[56] A marked decrease in the amount of neutrophil-bound IgG has been noted postsplenectomy in certain patients, suggesting that the IgG may, at least in part, be produced within the spleen.[57]

REFERENCES

1. Landsteiner, K.: Über Agglutinationserscheinungen normalen menschlichen Blutes. Wien. Klin. Wochenschr., *14*:1132, 1901.
2. Race, R. R., and Sanger, R.: Blood Groups in Man. Ed. 6. Oxford, Blackwell Scientific Publications, 1975.
3. Mollison, P. L.: Blood Transfusion in Clinical Medicine. Ed. 5. Oxford, Blackwell Scientific Publications, 1972.

4. Zmijewski, C. M., and Fletcher, J. L.: Immunohematology. Ed. 2. New York, Meredith Corp. 1972.
5. Bernstein, F.: Ergebnisse einer biostatischen zusammenfassenden Betrachtung über die erblichen Blutstrukturen des Menschen. Klin. Wochenschr., *3*:1495, 1924.

5a. Dobson, A. M., and Ikin, E. W.: The ABO blood groups in the United Kingdom; frequencies based on a very large sample. J. Pathol. Bacteriol., *58*:221, 1946.

6. Friedenreich, V.: Ueber die Serologie der Untergruppen A_1 und A_2. Z. Immunitaetsforsch., *71*:283, 1931.
7. Watkins, W. M.: Blood-group substances. Science, *152*:172, 1966.
8. Levine, P., Robinson, E., Celano, M., Briggs, O., and Falkinburg, L.: Gene interaction resulting in suppression of blood group substance B. Blood, *10*:1100, 1955.
9. Morgan, W. T. J.: A contribution to human biochemical genetics; the chemical basis of blood-group specificity. Proc. R. Soc. Lond. [Biol.], *151*:308, 1960.
10. Grubb, R.: Observations on the human group system Lewis. Acta Pathol. Microbiol. Scand., *28*:61, 1951.
11. Sneath, J. S., and Sneath, P. H. A.: Transformation of the Lewis groups of human red cells. Nature, *176*:172, 1955.
12. Watkins, W. M.: Relationship between structure, specificity, and genes within the ABO and Lewis blood-group systems. P. 443. Stockholm, Proc. 10th Cong. Int. Soc. Blood Trans., 1964.
13. Grubb, R.: Correlation between Lewis blood group and secretor character in man. Nature, *162*:933, 1948.
14. Landsteiner, K., and Wiener, A. S.: An agglutinable factor in human blood recognized by immune sera for rhesus blood. Proc. Soc. Exp. Biol. Med., *43*:223, 1940.
15. Levine, P., and Stetson, R. E.: An unusual case of intragroup agglutination. J.A.M.A., *113*:126, 1939.
16. Race, R. R., and Sanger, R.: Blood Groups in Man. Ed. 2. Oxford, Blackwell Scientific Publications, 1954.
17. Weiner, A. S.: Genetic theory of the Rh blood types. Proc. Soc. Exp. Biol. Med., *54*:316, 1943.
18. Marsh, W. L.: Anti-i: a cold antibody defining the Ii relationship in human red cells. Br. J. Haematol., *7*:200, 1961.
19. Springer, G. F., and Huprikar, S. V.: On the biochemical and genetic basis of the human blood-group MN specificities. Haematologia, *6*:81, 1972.
20. Naiki, M., and Marcus, D. M.: Human erythrocyte P and P^k blood group antigens: identification as glycosphingolipids. Biochem. Biophys. Res. Commun., *60*:1105, 1974.
21. Giblett, R. R., *et al.*: Kell phenotypes in chronic granulomatous disease: a potential transfusion hazard. Lancet, *1*:1235, 1971.
22. Pollack, W., *et al.*: A study of the forces involved in the second stage of hemagglutination. Transfusion, *5*:158, 1965.
23. Coombs, R. R. A., Mourant, A. E., and Race, R. R.: A new test for the detection of weak and "incomplete" Rh agglutinins. Br. J. Exp. Pathol., *6*:255, 1945.
24. Nicolson, G. L.: The relationship of a fluid membrane structure to cell agglutination and surface topography. Ser. Haematol., *6*:275, 1975.
25. Romano, E. L., Stolinski, C., and Hughes-Jones, N. C.: Distribution and mobility of the A, D and C antigens on human red cell membranes: studies with a gold-labelled antiglobulin reagent. Br. J. Haematol., *30*:507, 1975.
26. Eisler, M.: Über die Blutantigene in paratyphus-und dysentere Shigabakterrein. Z. Immunitaetsforsch., *73*:37, 1937.

26a. Sturgeon, P.: Erythrocyte antigens and antibodies. *In* Williams, W. J., Beutler, E., Erslev, A. J., and Rundles, R. W. (eds.): Hematology. P. 1272. New York, McGraw-Hill, 1972.

27. Huber, H., *et al.*: IgG subclass specificity of human monocyte receptor sites. Nature, *229*:419, 1971.
28. Rosse, W. F.: Quantitative immunology of immune hemolytic anemia. J. Clin. Invest., *50*:734, 1971.
29. Perlmann, P., Perlmann, H., and Wigzell, H.: Lymphocyte mediated cytotoxicity *in vitro*: induction and inhibition by humoral antibody and nature of effector cells. Transplant. Rev., *13*:91, 1972.
30. Pollack, S. B., Nelson, K., and Grausz, J. D.: Separation of effector cells mediating antibody-dependent cellular cytotoxicity (ADC) to erythrocyte targets from those mediating ADC to tumor targets. J. Immunol., *116*:944, 1976.
31. Rosse, W. F.: The detection of small amounts of antibody on the red cell in autoimmune hemolytic anemia. Ser. Haematol., *7*:358, 1974.
32. Dacie, J. V.: Autoimmune hemolytic anemia. Arch. Intern. Med., *135*:1293, 1975.
33. ———: The Hemolytic Anemias. Part 2. New York, Grune & Stratton, 1962.
34. ———: Aspects of autoimmune hemolytic anemias. Ser. Haematol., *7*(3):303–426, 1974.
35. Pirofsky, B., and Bardana, E. J., Jr.: Autoimmune hemolytic anemia I: clinical aspects. Ser. Haematol., *7*:367, 1974.
36. Engelfriet, C. P., Borne, A., Beckers, D., and Van Loghem, J. J.: Autoimmune hemolytic anemia: serological and immunochemical characteristics of the autoantibodies; mechanisms of cell destruction. Ser. Haematol., *7*:328, 1974.
37. Rosse, W. F.: The antiglobulin test in autoimmune hemolytic anemia. Ann. Rev. Med., *26*:331, 1975.
38. Brown, D. L.: The Behavior of phagocytic cell receptors in relation to allergic red cell destruction. Ser. Haematol., *7*:348, 1974.
39. Wiener, W., and Vos, G. H.: Serology of acquired hemolytic anemias. Blood, *22*:606, 1963.
40. Leddy, J. P., Peterson, P., Yeaw, M. A., and Bakemeier, R. F.: Patterns of serologic specificity of human γG erythrocyte autoantibodies. J. Immunol., *105*:677, 1970.
41. Lau, F. O., and Rosse, W. F.: The reactivity of

red blood cell membrane glycophorin with "cold-reacting" antibodies. Clin. Immunol. Immunopathol., *4*:1, 1975.

42. Hinz, C. F., Jr.: Serologic and physiochemical characterization of Donath-Landsteiner antibodies from six patients. Blood, *22*:600, 1963.
43. Garratty, G., and Petz, L. D.: Drug-induced hemolytic anemia. Am. J. Med., *58*:398, 1975.
44. Shulman, N. R., Marder, V. J., Hiller, M. C., and Collier, E. M.: Platelet and leukocyte isoantigens and their antibodies: serologic, physiologic and clinical studies. Prog. Hematol., *4*:222, 1964.
45. Pearson, H. A., Shulman, N. R., Marder, V. J., and Cone, T. E., Jr.: Isoimmune neonatal thrombocytopenic purpura: clinical and therapeutic considerations. Blood, *23*:154, 1964.
46. Shulman, N. R., Marder, V. J., and Weinrach, R. S.: Similarities between known antiplatelet antibodies and the factor responsible for thrombocytopenia in idiopathic purpura: physiologic, serologic, and isotopic studies. Ann. N.Y. Acad. Sci., *124*:499, 1965.
47. Aster, R. H., and Keene, W. R.: Site of platelet destruction in idiopathic thrombocytopenic purpura. Br. J. Haematol., *16*:61, 1969.
48. Dixon, R., Rosse, W. R., and Ebbert, L.: Quantitative determination of antibody in idiopathic thrombocytopenic purpura. N. Engl. J. Med., *292*:230, 1975.
49. Lalezari, P., and Radel, E.: Neutrophil-specific antigens: immunology and clinical significance. Semin. Hematol., *11*:281, 1974.
50. Boxer, L. A., Yokoyama, M., and Lalezari, P.: Isoimmune neonatal neutropenia. J. Pediatr., *80*:783, 1972.
51. Boxer, L. A., Greenberg, M. S., Boxer, G. J., and Stossel, T. P.: Autoimmune neutropenia. N. Engl. J. Med., *93*:748, 1975.
52. Lalezari, P., Jiang, A. F., Yeagen, L., and Santorineou, M.: Chronic autoimmune neutropenia due to anti-NA2 antibody. N. Engl. J. Med., *93*:744, 1975.
53. Calebresi, P., Edwards, E. A., and Schilling, R. F.: Fluorescent antiglobulin studies in leukopenic and related disorders. J. Clin. Invest., *38*:2091, 1959.
54. Rosenthal, F. D., Beeley, J. M., Gelsthorpe, K., and Doughty, R. W.: White-cell antibodies and the aetiology of Felty's Syndrome. Q. J. Med., *43*:187, 1974.
55. Barnes, C. G., Turnbull, A. L., and Vernon-Roberts, B.: Felty's Syndrome. Ann. Rheum. Dis., *30*:359, 1971.
56. Dameshek, W.: Editorial. Blood, *1*:173, 1946.
57. Logue, G.: Personal communication.

15 Other Immunologic Disorders

IMMUNE DERMATOLOGIC DISEASES

Systemic and Discoid Lupus Erythematosus

The deposition of immune complexes along vessel walls may cause a vasculitis that frequently affects the cutaneous vessels, and as a result areas of erythema, urticaria and infiltrative palpable purpura can develop. Cutaneous immune complex vasculitis may occur in hypersensitivity angiitis, mixed cryoglobulinemia and lupus erythematosus.[1]

Approximately 50 per cent of patients with SLE have cutaneous manifestations at some time during the course of their illness. Pigmentary changes, telangiectasias, scarring, atrophy and cutaneous photosensitivity may be present to varying degrees. There is another group of patients with identical skin lesions but without any manifestations of systemic disease. Lupus erythematosus limited to the skin has been termed *discoid lupus erythematosus* (DLE). The great majority of patients with DLE do not go on to develop SLE.

Immunofluorescence studies on biopsies of skin lesions of patients with both SLE and DLE reveal immunoglobulin and complement distributed in a band just beneath the dermal-epidermal junction (Fig. 15-1).[2] IgG is the major immunoglobulin present, although IgM and occasionally IgA can also be detected. There is evidence for the activation and deposition of components of both the classical and properdin complement pathways.[3]

SLE with cutaneous involvement can often be distinguished from DLE by biopsy of uninvolved areas of skin. In 50 to 60 per cent of patients with SLE there is a band of immunoglobulin visible by immunofluorescence at the dermal-epidermal junction of otherwise normal skin. This finding is referred to as a positive band test. Patients with DLE almost never have a positive band test.[4]

The immunoglobulin is deposited at the dermal-epidermal junction as immune complexes. Acid elution studies have demonstrated that much of the measurable antibody activity is directed against nuclear antigens.[5] The deposition of anti-DNA–DNA complexes has also been implicated in the vascular disease and renal disease of SLE (see Chap. 7).[6] Antibody directed against basement-membrane antigens can also be eluted from the skin biopsy despite the absence of detectable circulating anti-basement-membrane antibodies in patients with SLE.[5]

There are two possible mechanisms by which immune complexes could deposit beneath the epidermal basement mem-

Table 15-1. The Immune Dermatologic Diseases

Disease	*Results of Immunofluorescence Studies*	*Antigenic Target*
Systemic lupus erythematosus	Ig and complement at dermal-epidermal junction in affected and often normal skin	Deposition of immune complexes containing nuclear antigens
Discoid lupus erythematosus	Ig and complement at dermal-epidermal junction of involved skin only	Deposition of immune complexes containing nuclear antigens
Pemphigus	Ig and complement in intercellular spaces of epidermis	Glycocalyx of keratinocytes
Bullous pemphigoid	Linear deposition of Ig and complement along basement membrane	Basement membrane
Dermatitis herpetiformis	Granular deposition of IgA and components of the properdin pathway	Unknown

brane: (1) circulating immune complexes may filter through the basement membrane and become trapped there, much as immune complexes are trapped by the renal basement membrane; (2) a true Arthus phenomenon may occur in which free antinuclear antibody in the dermis combines with nuclear antigens released from the rapidly proliferating epidermis.[7]

It is not known if these immune complexes are actually responsible for the cutaneous lesions. In fact, the only available evidence suggests that they are not:

1. Immune complexes are present in

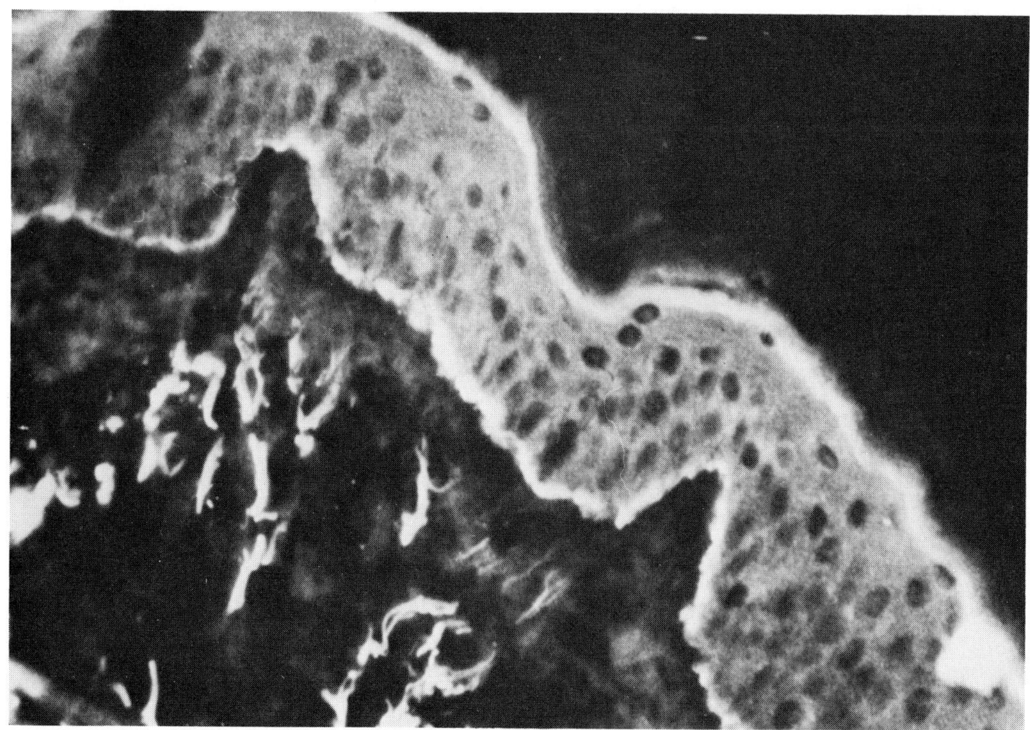

Fig. 15-1. Immunofluorescense of IgG at the dermal-epidermal junction in the skin of a patient with SLE. (Courtesy of Dr. Mitchell Sams.)

clinically uninvolved skin of a majority of patients with SLE (a positive band test). There is, in fact, an inverse correlation between the presence of immunoglobulin in normal skin of patients with SLE and the occurrence of chronic destructive skin lesions.[7]

2. The cellular infiltrate in cutaneous lupus lesions is predominantly lymphocytic and is thus more reminiscent of a cell-mediated immune process than the nonspecific inflammatory response that one would expect with an antibody-mediated process.[8]

Despite the uncertain pathogenic nature of the cutaneous immune complexes, their presence conveys significant prognostic information about the patient. Thus, despite the inverse correlation between a positive band test and the presence of destructive *skin lesions*, a positive band test has been found to correlate significantly with the presence of *renal disease* and *hypocomplementemia*, the latter often being evidence of severe, destructive immune complex disease. In general, a positive band test does not augur well for a patient with SLE.[9]

Pemphigus

Pemphigus is a cutaneous disease characterized by widespread bullae and erosions of the skin and mucous membranes that typically has its onset between the fifth and seventh decades of life. The bullae are flabby and break easily. The ability to spread the bullae by locally applied pressure is a characteristic finding that is termed Nikolsky's sign. The abnormality in pemphigus is the loss of the intercellular integrity of the prickle-cell layer of the epidermis (acantholysis). Pemphigus is a serious disease and if untreated is almost uniformly fatal.

Recent findings have implicated immune mechanisms in the pathogenesis of pemphigus. The majority of patients possess antibodies in their sera that are reactive with antigen in the intercellular cement of the prickle-cell layer of the epidermis. The precise antigenic target has been reported to be the glycocalyx of the keratinocytes.[10] Immunofluorescence of skin biopsy material reveals immunoglobulin and complement in the intercellular spaces of the epidermis (Fig. 15-2).[11] The immunoglobulin is predominantly IgG. More than 90 per cent of patients have positive immunofluorescence for immunoglobulin and complement in biopsies of their lesions and adjacent areas.[12,13]

These antibodies may be responsible for the acantholysis. The titer of the antibody is correlated with the severity of the disease, and the areas of antibody deposition within the epidermis correlate with the areas of blister formation.[14,15] For example, pemphigus vulgaris and pemphigus foliaceus, two variants of pemphigus, both exhibit intraepidermal bullae and antibodies against antigen in the epidermal intercellular substance. However, the lesions of pemphigus foliaceus are more superficial and the blisters form between the outer layers of the epidermis. Patients with pemphigus foliaceus have been found to possess antibodies against antigens that are restricted to the very superficial subcorneal intercellular substance;[16] the antibodies of pemphigus vulgaris are not limited in their reactivity to only the superficial epidermis. This association between the site of antibody reactivity and the site of the bullous lesions argues strongly on behalf of an immune etiology for pemphigus but does not rule out the possibility that antibody production is secondary to a preexisting intraepidermal lesion.

Bullous Pemphigoid

Bullous pemphigoid is a chronic, relatively benign disorder characterized by numerous tense bullae. Unlike pemphigus the bullae are subepidermal, forming at the dermal-epidermal junction. Skin biopsy reveals the linear deposition

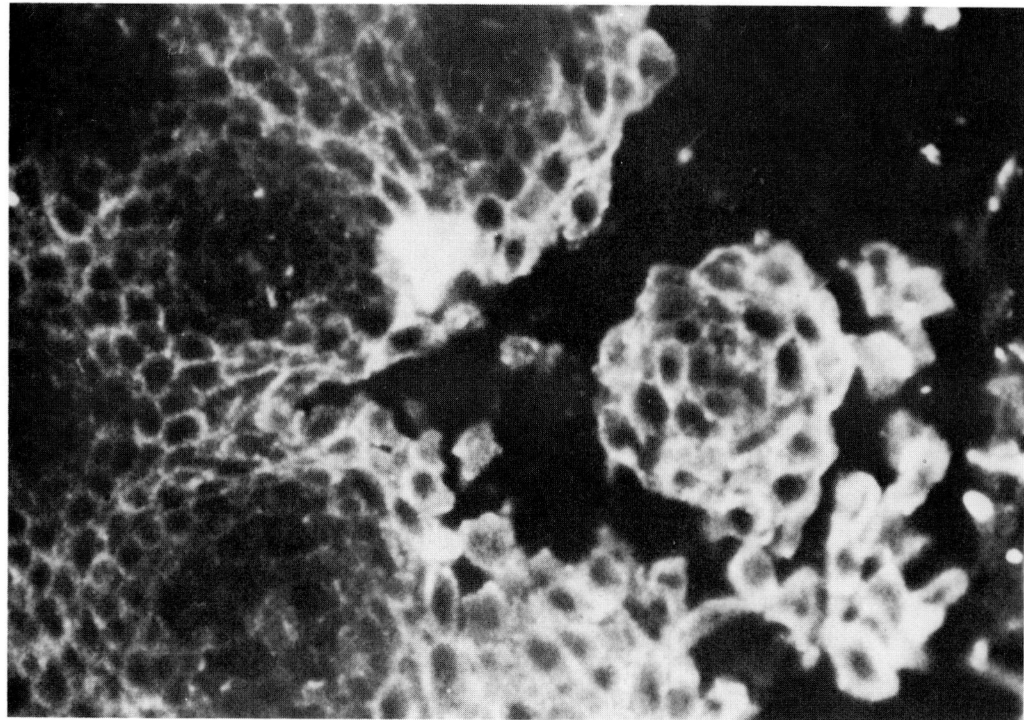

Fig. 15-2. Intercellular distribution of IgG in the epidermis of a patient with pemphigus. (Courtesy of Dr. Mitchell Sams.)

of IgG and complement along the basement membrane and circulating anti-basement membrane antibodies are detectable in the serum.[17] Thus, as in pemphigus, autoantibodies are present at the precise site in the skin where the bullae develop.

The finding of a linear deposition pattern of immunofluorescence is significant (Fig. 15-3). Whereas immune complex deposition has a characteristic granular appearance on immunofluorescence, the so-called "lumpy-bumpy" appearance, a smooth, linear array is usually associated with the presence of antibody directed against the tissue itself. In bullous pemphigoid, the antigenic target is the cutaneous basement membrane. The distinction between a linear and "lumpy-bumpy" deposition pattern is an important one to keep in mind when interpreting immunofluorescence studies.

As in pemphigus, it is still uncertain whether these antibodies are responsible for the lesions. A causal relationship is even more questionable in bullous pemphigoid since (1) there is a poor correlation between antibody titer and disease activity, and (2) one can detect antibody bound to the basement membrane of unaffected tissues.[18]

Dermatitis Herpetiformis

Dermatitis herpetiformis is a chronic disease distinguished by the presence of subepidermal bullae and intense pruritus. The site of blister formation is thus similar to that of bullous pemphigoid on a microscopic level. Immunoglobulin and complement deposit at the dermal-epidermal junction and are most prominent at the tip of the dermal papillae. Although the cutaneous localization of immunoglobulin is similar to that of bullous

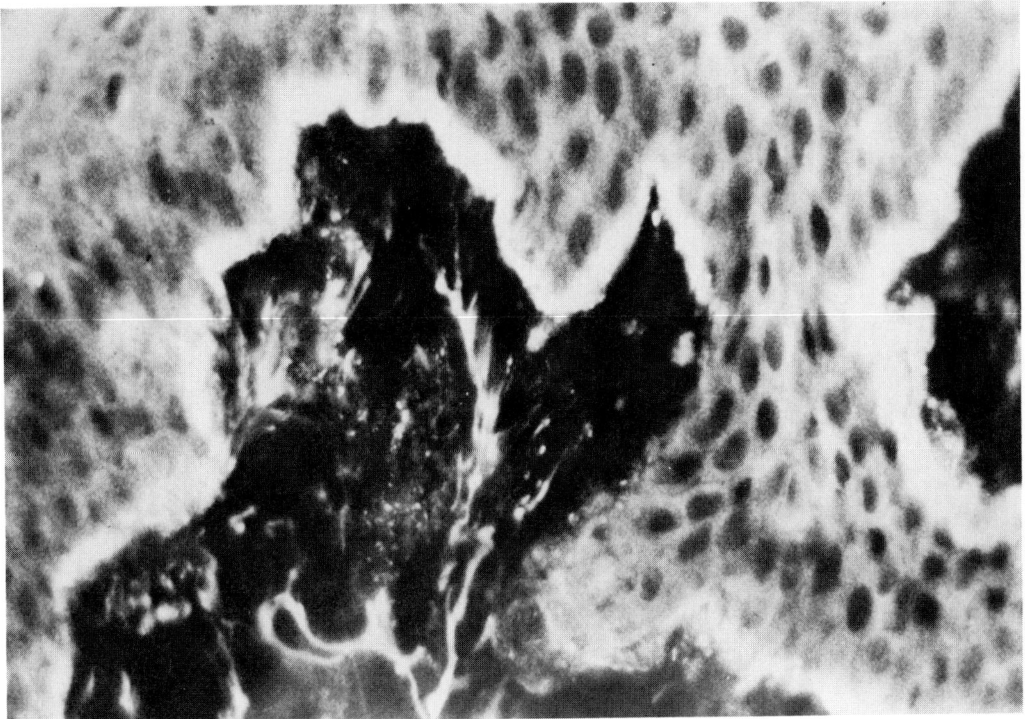

Fig. 15-3. Linear deposition of IgG along the basement membrane of the skin in a patient with bullous pemphigoid. (Courtesy of Dr. Mitchell Sams.)

pemphigoid, the pattern of immunofluorescence is quite distinct (Fig. 15-4). In bullous pemphigoid there is a linear array of immunoglobulin staining suggesting reactivity against a local antigen in the region of the basement membrane. In dermatitis herpetiformis the immunoglobulin deposition is most often granular, suggestive of immune complex deposition.[19] Circulating 10S complexes have been described in these patients.[20] A second distinction is especially noteworthy: although IgG and IgM can occasionally be detected by immunofluorescence, IgA is always the major—and sometimes the sole—immunoglobulin present.[21]

IgA deposits can be found in unaffected skin in these patients, indicating that the presence of immunoglobulin alone may not be sufficient to cause vesicle formation. However, complement activation by IgA may relate to disease activity.[22] IgA can only activate complement via the properdin pathway, and there is evidence that components of the properdin pathway are activated and deposited in the skin of these patients.[23]

The most perplexing feature of this disease is the abundance of immunoglobulin of the IgA class in the skin of these patients. IgA is predominantly a secretory immunoglobulin and ordinarily has little business being in the cutaneous tissues. Some data has emerged over the past several years which may help to explain this enigma. Many patients with dermatitis herpetiformis have high circulating levels of IgA, and investigators have found that jejunal biopsy tissue of these patients produces significantly greater-than-normal amounts of IgA *in vitro*.[24,25] Almost all patients with dermatitis herpetiformis display jejunal lesions that are indistin-

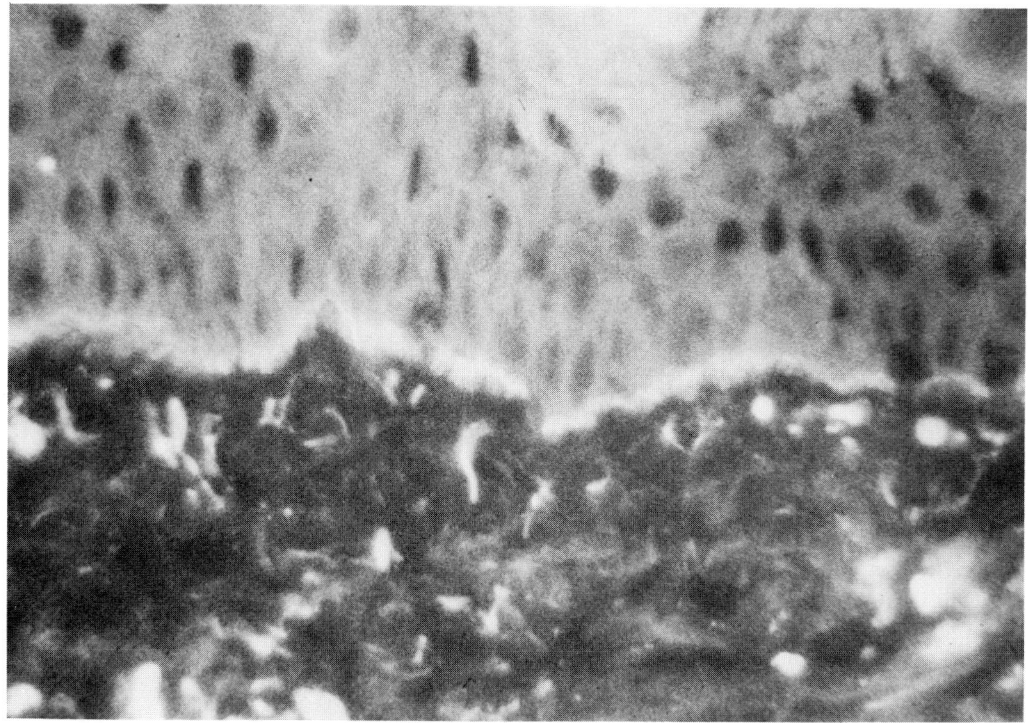

Fig. 15-4. Granular deposition of IgA along the basement membrane of the skin in a patient with dermatitis herpetiformis. (Courtesy of Dr. Mitchell Sams.)

guishable from those of gluten-sensitive enteropathy (celiac disease).[26] We still do not know precisely how the presence of gastrointestinal lesions relates to the cutaneous disease, but this finding may allow us to understand the cutaneous disease as a secondary process rather than a primary skin disorder. It is perhaps not surprising that in an attempt to understand the association of IgA with skin disease, we may end up examining the immunopathology of the gastrointestinal tract.

GLUTEN-SENSITIVE ENTEROPATHY (GSE)

Gluten-sensitive enteropathy, or celiac disease, is a disorder of the intestinal mucosa characterized by villous atrophy (observed as flattening of the small bowel mucosa) and an inflammatory infiltrate in the lamina propria. Numerous plasma cells are present in the mucosal infiltrate.[27] Patients with GSE often first present to their physicians with signs and symptoms of malabsorption and malnutrition. The malabsorption can be attributed, at least in part, to the loss of mucosal absorptive surfaces. It has been known for several years that the mucosal lesion of GSE is due to the ingestion of wheat protein. The responsible moiety is in the gluten fraction of the protein, and the mucosal lesions can be healed by adherence to a gluten-free diet.[28]

An immunologic basis for the disease was first suspected when antigluten antibodies were detected in the serum and intestinal secretions of these patients.[29] However, it has been difficult to establish whether these antibodies are pathogenic or are produced secondarily to an underlying disease process. These patients also display circulating antibodies against other dietary proteins, which may suggest that the abnormal antibodies arise in response to altered processing or absorption of food particles.[30]

In an attempt to understand the role of antibodies in this disease, an *in vitro* experimental model has been developed in which jejunal biopsy tissue is cultivated in short-term culture.[31,32] In this system, normal biopsy tissue will exhibit an increase in alkaline phosphatase content over a 48-hour incubation period. This rise is felt to correlate with continuing maturation of the epithelial cells. The deep cells of the crypts differentiate and migrate up the walls of the crypts, eventually forming a mature brush border. Cultured biopsies taken from patients with active GSE exhibit subnormal initial levels of alkaline phosphatase, considered to reflect the lack of normal enterocyte maturation. After 48 hours in culture, however, the enzyme level rises dramatically. This is believed to be due to the "release" of the mucosa from a local toxic environment present in patients with active disease. The addition of gluten peptides to the culture medium can prevent the rise in alkaline phosphatase in the GSE specimens, but not in normal biopsy tissue. Thus, as *in vivo*, gluten seems to have a toxic effect on the intestinal cells of patients with GSE.

In order to determine whether the gluten is directly toxic to the epithelium, biopsy specimens of patients with GSE in remission have been studied. In these experiments, gluten peptides would not inhibit the rise in alkaline phosphatase over the 48-hour culture period. However, if the remission biopsy material is cultured in the presence of both gluten and tissue from patients with active GSE, the rise in alkaline phosphatase in the remission tissue does not occur. This result suggests that the toxicity of gluten peptides is mediated via the induction of soluble endogenous substances in the tissue of patients with active GSE, and not via a direct toxic action of the gluten itself.

It is felt that the endogenous substance stimulated by gluten is locally produced antigluten antibody. Although this has not been proved conclusively, there is enough suggestive evidence to make this an attractive postulate. Patients with GSE produce large amounts of immunoglobulin in their intestinal mucosa when challenged with gluten.[33] The immunoglobulin is predominantly of the IgM and IgA classes. A large percentage of these immunoglobulin molecules have antibody activity against gluten.[34] Administration of gluten to a patient with GSE results in the deposition of IgA and complement in the basement membrane of the gastrointestinal mucosa. Immunofluorescence studies have revealed a relationship between the deposition of these substances and subsequent evidence of tissue damage.[35]

Even if immunopathologic mechanisms are involved in GSE, it is curious that only certain people develop gluten sensitivity. Genetic analysis may provide some insight into this problem. Eighty per cent of patients with GSE possess the HLA-B8 gene locus compared to only 20 per cent of the normal population.[36] Patients with dermatitis herpetiformis who have the jejunal changes of GSE also have the same high frequency of HLA-B8 as patients with GSE without dermatitis herpetiformis.[25] However, the presence of HLA-B8 is neither necessary nor sufficient for the expression of the disease, since most HLA-B8-positive people do not have GSE and not all people with GSE possess HLA-B8. It is possible that HLA-B8 may be in linkage disequilibrium with another locus that more closely relates to gluten sensitivity, and it is therefore of great interest that a recent report has found an even higher disease association with the HLA-Dw3 antigen.[37]

A model for the pathogenesis of GSE has been proposed based upon the HLA association and the antigluten immune response. This theory posits that the epithelial cells of patients with GSE possess surface molecules which are capable of binding gluten. It has, in fact, been observed that gluten binds to gut epithelial cells of GSE patients but not to cells of normal patients.[38] These surface molecules may be coded for by genes in linkage disequilibrium with HLA-B8. Binding of gluten to gut epithelial cells could have two consequences.

1. The gluten molecule might be presented in immunogenic form to the local immune system, thereby accounting for the abnormal production of antigluten antibodies.

2. Once antibodies are formed, they might bind to the attached gluten molecules, thus forming immune complexes, and initiate the many humoral mechanisms that carry such powerful destructive potential.

AUTOIMMUNE ENDOCRINE DISEASES

THYROID DISEASES

Hashimoto's Thyroiditis

Hashimoto's thyroiditis, also called chronic lymphocytic thyroiditis or autoimmune thyroiditis, is one of the most common of the so-called autoimmune diseases. It occurs most frequently in women between 30 and 50 years of age. Patients usually present with a goiter with or without evidence of thyroid dysfunction. Acutely, thyroid function may be normal or even elevated, but hypothyroidism is the invariable end result of the disease process.

Histologic study reveals a gland that is the site of intense immune reactivity (Fig. 15-5). There is a diffuse cellular infiltrate

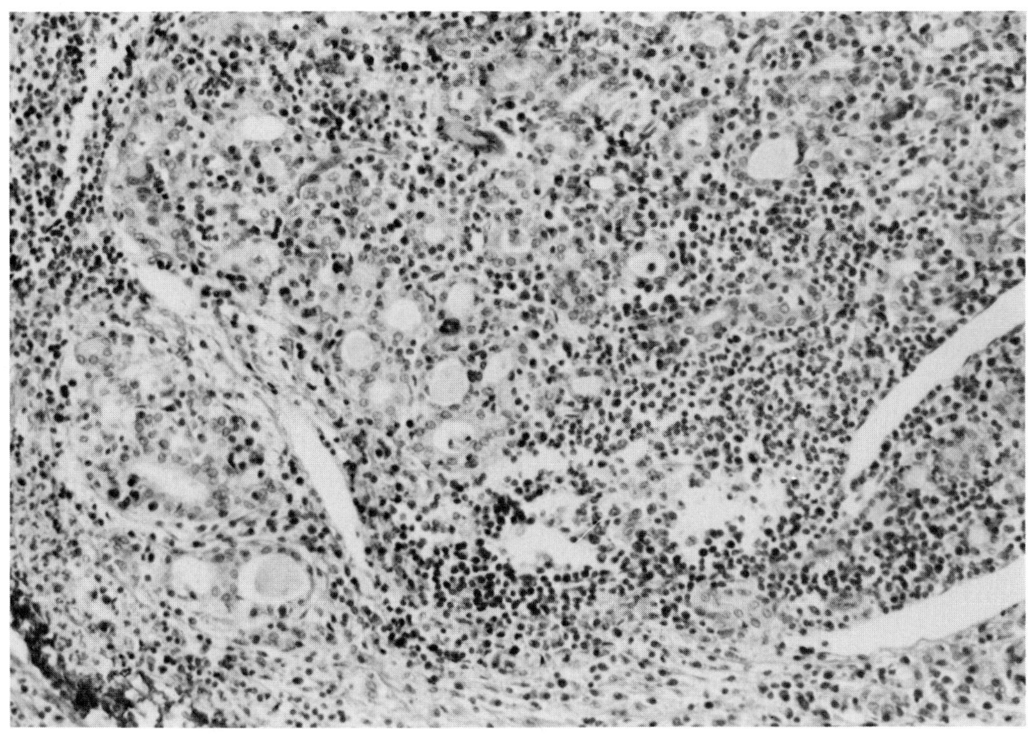

Fig. 15-5. The thyroid of a patient with active Hashimoto's thyroiditis. Note the presence of many lymphocytes and the destruction of the normal follicular architecture.

composed primarily of lymphocytes and other mononuclear cells. Plasma cells are often quite prominent and germinal centers can be seen. The normal follicular architecture is destroyed and there may be varying degrees of fibrosis.

The discovery of several autoimmune phenomena directed against thyroid antigens has lent support to the notion that Hashimoto's thyroiditis is an immunologic disease. Four thyroid antigens have been identified as targets for the circulating autoantibodies. In practice, only antibodies against the first two antigens are used for diagnostic purposes:[39]

1. *Thyroglobulin* is found circulating in normal individuals in very low levels. Increased levels can result from a hyperactive gland and a variety of processes that lead to destruction of the thyroid.[40] Normal people possess circulating B lymphocytes capable of specifically binding thyroglobulin but only rarely produce circulating antibodies to thyroglobulin in any appreciable amount.[41] Antithyroglobulin antibody can be seen in a number of thyroid diseases. Patients with Hashimoto's thyroiditis often have very high levels of this autoantibody, which is predominantly IgG. Although these patients do not have greater than normal numbers of circulating lymphocytes that can bind thyroglobulin, the lymphocytic infiltrate within the thyroid is greatly enriched for these antigen-specific cells.[42] The majority of antithyroglobulin antibody production occurs within the thyroid gland.

2. *Microsomal Cytoplasmic Antigen.* This antigen is a lipoprotein derived from the membranes of cytoplasmic vesicles. It is specific to the thyroid epithelial cells.[43]

3. *Second Colloid Antigen (CA2).* The antibody directed against this antigen produces a uniform staining of the colloid by immunofluorescence. It is not specific for Hashimoto's disease since about one half of the patients with Graves' disease, one half of the patients with de Quervain's thyroiditis, and one third of the patients with thyroid cancer possess this antibody.[39]

4. *Thyroid cell-surface antigen* is the only cell-surface antigen of the four. It may therefore be an important target for immune destruction of thyroid cells.[44]

As with all diseases associated with autoantibody production, it is essential to determine whether the antibodies are of pathogenic importance or are merely epiphenomena, perhaps reacting to cell constituents that have been altered and rendered immunogenic by an underlying disease process. This has been a particularly difficult question to answer for Hashimoto's disease. Autoantibody titers have not been reliably correlated with the severity of the disease.[39] Transplacental passage of antithyroid antibody does not produce thyroiditis in the infants of mothers with circulating antithyroid antibodies, and patients' serum can be given to animals without causing thyroid damage.[45,46] In addition, one can sometimes reduce the size of the goiter and decrease the production of antithyroid antibodies by thyroid replacement alone, suggesting that the autoantibodies may arise secondarily to an underlying glandular disease.[39]

Experimental studies in animal systems have implicated antibodies in the destructive process and may offer an explanation for the failure to transfer the disease with the serum of affected patients. Animals injected with homologous thyroglobulin in complete Freund's adjuvant can develop a thyroiditis. As in the human studies just cited, the disease cannot be transferred with the serum of these animals.[47] However, if the animals are thyroidectomized after the injection of thyroglobulin, the serum will then contain antibodies that can cause thyroid lesions in recipient animals.[48] This result suggests that the thyroid might be acting as a sink for antithyroid antibodies, and might therefore be removing antithyroid antibodies from the serum. These same investigators later confirmed that antithyroglobulin reactivity first appears in the circulation and then migrates to the thyroid gland.[49]

Circulating antigen-antibody complexes have been detected in patients with Hashimoto's disease.[50] The deposition of immune complexes along the acinar cell membrane in affected glands has been reported in a small minority of cases.[51] The nature of the antigen moiety in the complexes has not been determined, nor has it been established that these complexes are able to fix complement and produce tissue damage.

There is also evidence that IgG antithyroid autoantibodies can lyse thyroglobulin-coated cells *in vitro* in the presence of normal human lymphocytes.[52] This is the phenomenon of antibody-dependent cell-mediated cytotoxicity (ADCC), and the degree of cytotoxicity has been correlated with autoantibody titers.

The role of antibody in Hashimoto's thyroiditis is clearly unresolved at present, and the same can be said for T-cell-mediated immunity.[53] The histologic appearance of affected glands is reminiscent of lesions of cell-mediated immunity, but may also be explained on the basis of ADCC. Many experiments *in vitro* have shown that T cells taken from patients with Hashimoto's disease are sensitized to thyroid antigens, but such studies are far from decisive in implicating T killer cells in the disease process.[54,55] *In vitro* cytotoxicity has also been demonstrated in situations where antibody does not seem to be involved.[56-58]

Graves' Disease

Graves' disease involves many organ systems. It is characterized by diffuse goiter, infiltrative ophthalmopathy and infiltrative dermopathy. Goiter is the most common finding, and Graves' disease is the leading cause of diffuse toxic goiter. It most commonly affects women in their third and fourth decades. Suggestions of an autoimmune etiology initially stemmed from the histologic observation of lymphocytic infiltrates in the thyroid and retro-orbital tissues, and the presence of antithyroid antibodies.

The characteristic functional abnormality of the thyroid in Graves' disease is hypersecretion that is not suppressible by exogenous hormone. The discovery of circulating IgG that is capable of stimulating the thyroid gland has therefore been of great interest in terms of a possible immunologic pathogenesis of the disease. Two stimulating IgG molecules have been described: long-acting thyroid stimulator (LATS) and LATS-protector (LATS-P).

LATS is a polyclonal IgG that can be found in the serum of approximately 50 per cent of patients with Graves' disease.[59] It is occasionally present in other thyroid disorders, but never in very high titers. Activity is most commonly assayed by measuring the release of labelled iodine from mouse thyroid glands *in vivo*. Compared to TSH, LATS activity is delayed in onset and then slowly builds over a long time course. Unlike TSH, it is an immunoglobulin produced by the patient's lymphocytes and is not subject to normal hormonal feedback.[60] These characteristics have earned it the designation of "long-acting thyroid-stimulating antibody."

LATS can mimic many of the biological activities of TSH on the thyroid gland, including iodine uptake and adenyl cyclase stimulation.[61] It appears to act by binding via its Fab portion to the thyroid receptor for TSH (Fig. 15-6).[62,63] Its antigenic target has not been precisely identified, although a 4S protein has recently been extracted from the thyroid which may be the target molecule. This protein can block LATS stimulation of mouse thyroid tissue, presumably by binding to the antigen-binding site of the immunoglobulin.[64]

These results initially suggested that

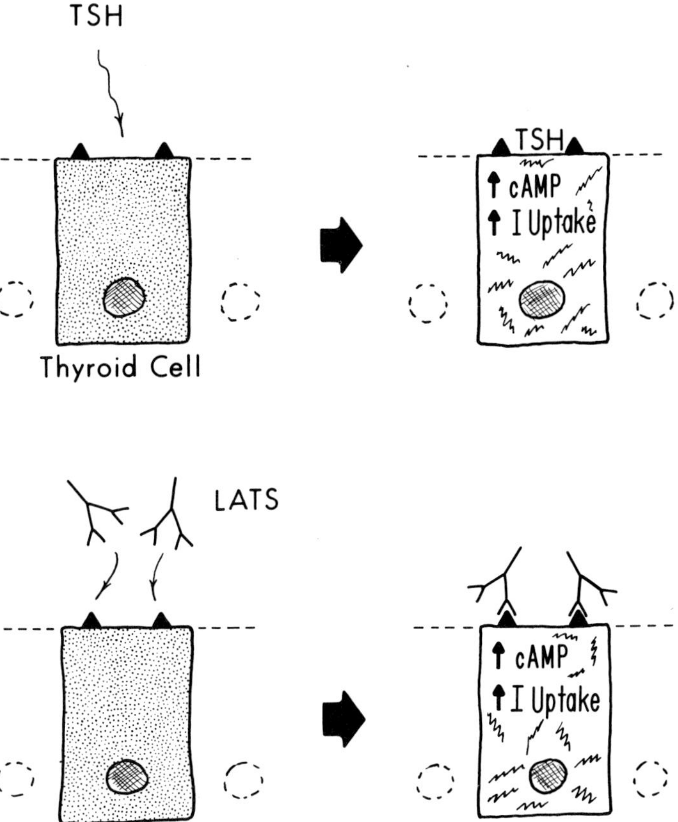

Fig. 15-6. The action of LATS on the thyroid mimics that of TSH.

LATS might be the agent primarily responsible for the nonsuppressibility and hypersecretion of the thyroid gland in Graves' disease. Thus, LATS can cross the placenta, causing a transient thyrotoxicosis in infants of mothers with Graves' disease.[65] However, there are reasons for believing that LATS alone cannot fully account for the thyroid dysfunction in affected patients. LATS titers do not always correlate with thyroid dysfunction and LATS may be present in the sera of patients with Graves' disease even when the gland is not hyperactive.[61] In addition, LATS is not found in all patients with active disease whereas it can be found in some people who have neither Graves' disease nor thyroid dysfunction.[66,67]

Another IgG with thyroid-stimulating function has been detected in the serum of patients with Graves' disease. In the mouse thyroid bioassay, this molecule can bind to the 4S "receptor" protein discussed above and prevent its inhibition of LATS stimulation (Fig. 15-7). This second IgG was therefore termed "LATS-protector" (LATS-P).[68]

LATS-P appears to have biological activities similar to LATS. It is distinguished from LATS by its specific activity for human thyroid (it therefore cannot be directly detected in the mouse thyroid assay). LATS-P is found in greater than 80 per cent of patients with Graves' disease, and thus has a higher disease association than LATS.[69] LATS-P has been associated with neonatal thyrotoxicosis and its titers are more closely correlated with thyroid hyperfunction than are LATS titers.[70,71]

The immunologic considerations of Graves' disease do not end with an examination of the thyroid. The possibility of an immunologic basis for the ophthalmopathy has been raised by a

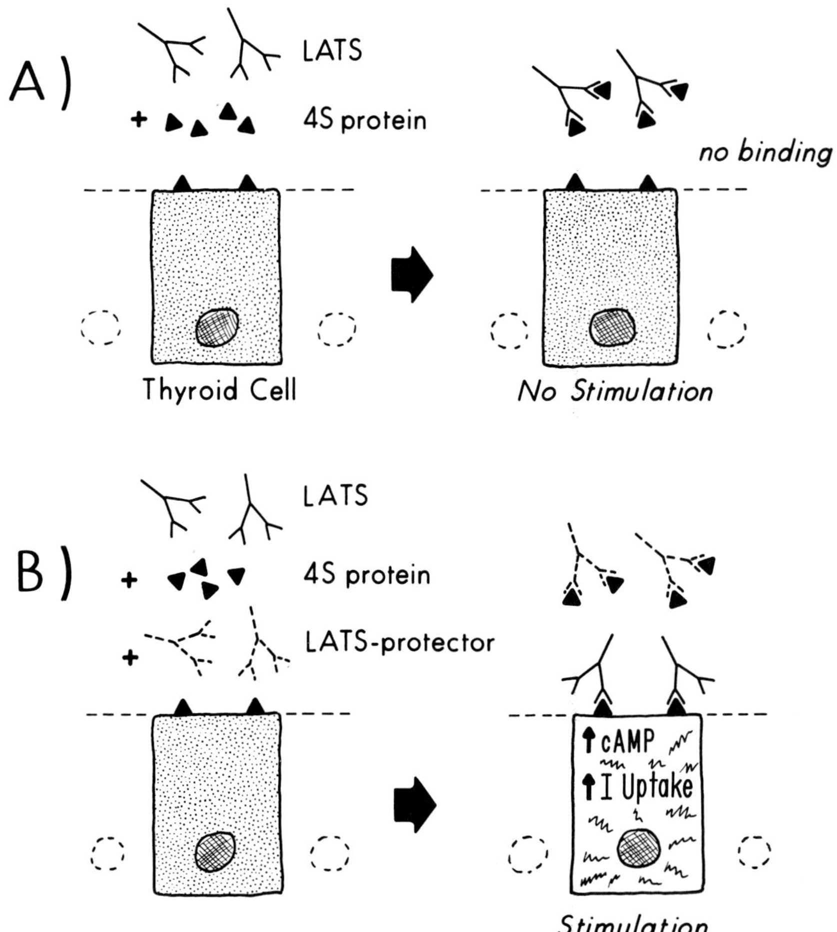

Fig. 15-7. LATS-protector. Both LATS and LATS-P bind to a 4S protein derived from human thyroid tissue. (A) The 4S protein binds to LATS, preventing it from stimulating the mouse thyroid cells. (B) LATS-P binds the free 4S protein, allowing the unbound $F(ab)_2$ portion of LATS to bind to and stimulate the mouse thyroid cells.

number of workers,[72] although little firm data is available at present. Complexes of thyroglobulin and antibody can bind to extraocular muscle membrane fractions, and it has been proposed that the extraocular myositis of Graves' disease may be triggered by the deposition of immune complexes within the muscle.[73] It has been further suggested that the complexes are composed of immunoglobulin and thyroglobulin, and that they make their way from the thyroid to the retro-orbital areas via lymphatic connections.[74]

An additional component of the ophthalmopathy is a proliferation of the adipose tissue of the retro-orbital region. This tissue appears to be responsive to stimulation by TSH and may therefore be responsive to thyroid-stimulating antibodies. Although exophthalmos-producing antibodies may be involved in the ocular abnormalities of Graves' disease, there is no firm evidence implicating either LATS or LATS-P in the ophthalmopathy.[75,76]

Genetics of the Autoimmune Thyroid Diseases

Many examples of multiple occurrences of Graves' disease and Hashimoto's disease within a single family have been reported. In addition, as many as 50 per cent of siblings of patients with thyroiditis possess antithyroid antibodies.[77] Relatives of patients with either Graves' disease or Hashimoto's disease have a significantly increased incidence of antithyroid antibodies.[78] No simple pattern of inheritance has yet been discerned and it is possible that a predisposition for antithyroid autoantibody production may be inherited in a polygenic fashion.[79]

ADRENAL DISEASE

Addison's disease is the name given to primary adrenal failure and the resulting deficiency in adrenocorticosteroid hormones. It is characterized by weakness, pigmentation of the skin and mucous membranes, weight loss, nausea, vomiting, hypotension and, less commonly, abdominal pain and salt craving. The majority of cases are currently classified as idiopathic. The histologic picture of idiopathic Addison's disease reveals a markedly atrophic gland with a loss of the normal glandular architecture. Mononuclear cell infiltrates dominated by the presence of small lymphocytes occur with varying degrees of intensity.

As many as 75 per cent of patients with Addison's disease have antiadrenal antibodies in their serum.[80] Antiadrenal antibodies are almost never found in the normal population, and only rarely in patients with other adrenal lesions such as tuberculous adrenal destruction. This observation suggests that the autoantibodies do not arise merely as reactants against antigens released during the process of glandular destruction. All the antigenic targets of the antiadrenal antibodies have not been identified but they appear to be present in the normal zona fasciculata and to include microsomal and mitochondrial constituents.[81]

DIABETES MELLITUS

Over the past several years, interest in a possible immunologic basis for diabetes mellitus has grown, sparked by observations of the immunopathology of other endocrinopathies as well as by the unexpectedly high frequency of autoimmune phenomena in diabetic patients.[82] However, the search for anti-islet-cell antibodies in these patients has been largely unrewarding.[83] On the other hand, some patients who have diabetes plus another disease of autoimmune origin do have antipancreatic autoantibodies.[84,85] These are complement-fixing IgG molecules which seem to affect all of the cells of the islets, not just the insulin-producing beta cells. *In vitro* assays of inhibition of leukocyte migration have revealed specific responsiveness to porcine pancreatic extract by cells taken from many diabetic patients.[86] This result presumably is due to the production of a lymphokine by the patient's lymphocytes which are sensitized to pancreatic antigens. The group with the highest frequency of positive responses are the young, insulin-dependent diabetics.

A small number of untreated patients have been detected who make anti-insulin antibodies.[87] These patients have postprandial hypoglycemia and an abnormal glucose tolerance test without abnormalities in fasting blood glucose levels. Recently, a small number of diabetics who have never taken exogenous insulin have been found to be immunologically sensitized against insulin.[88] In both groups of positive patients, the significance of these antibodies to the overall disease process has not been thoroughly evaluated.

The most common immunologic problem encountered in diabetes is not one of autoimmunity at all. Virtually every patient who takes exogenous insulin develops anti-insulin antibodies.[89] In the great majority of people these cause little trouble. Occasionally, however, a person may develop very high titers of insulin-binding antibodies and become insulin-resistant. This situation can be treated by giving less-antigenic forms of insulin (purified or porcine insulin) or with courses of corticosteroid therapy. Another complication of anti-insulin reactivity is the occurrence of IgE-mediated immediate-type hypersensitivity responses to administered insulin. This can be life-threatening and is fortunately very rare.

POLYGLANDULAR AUTOIMMUNE DISEASE

The co-existence of two or more glandular disorders in a single individual occurs with surprising frequency. For example, 40 per cent of patients with Addison's disease have a second endocrine abnormality, most commonly diabetes mellitus, Graves' disease, Hashimoto's thyroiditis or gonadal insufficiency.[81] The incidence of antithyroid antibodies in patients with idiopathic Addison's disease is even higher than the incidence of associated clinical thyroid disease. However, the incidence of antiadrenal antibodies in patients with thyroid disease and without adrenal insufficiency is very low. Thus, although antithyroid autoantibodies are often present without overt thyroid disease, the presence of antiadrenal antibodies usually means adrenal insufficiency.

Gonadal failure is common among females with idiopathic Addison's disease, and presents as ovarian failure. Testicular failure in males is such more unusual. Immunologic studies have shown that a majority of these patients have antigonadal antibodies.[90] These antibodies react with the steroid-producing gonadal cells and crossreact with antigens of the adrenal cortex. Such crossreactivity is in contrast to the organ-specific antithyroid antibodies that are often present in people with Addison's disease.

Patients with Addison's disease may also have autoantibodies directed against other tissues including the parathyroid glands and the gastric parietal cells.[91]

The reason for this impressive association of autoimmune phenomena is not known. A high correlation has been reported between HLA-B8 (as well as an HLA-D antigen) and Addison's disease,[92] and may reflect the linkage of an immune-response gene that controls reactivity to this group of endocrine-organ-related antigens.

PERNICIOUS ANEMIA AND ATROPHIC GASTRITIS

Pernicious anemia results from a failure to absorb vitamin B_{12} from the gastrointestinal tract. Typical findings include megaloblastic anemia, a progressive neurologic disorder termed "subacute combined degeneration" and atrophic gastritis. Biopsy of the gastric fundus reveals a lymphocytic infiltrate and an absence of parietal and chief cells. The volume of gastric secretions is reduced as is the amount of hydrochloric acid in the secretions. Atrophic gastritis is almost always seen in pernicious anemia, but it can occur without evidence of vitamin B_{12} deficiency. It is possible that pernicious anemia may represent a severe form of atrophic gastritis.

Gastric parietal cells ordinarily secrete a glycoprotein, called intrinsic factor, which has two active sites: one binds ingested vitamin B_{12} and the other binds to receptor sites in the distal ileum. The binding of intrinsic-factor–B_{12} complexes to the ileal receptors facilitates absorption of vitamin B_{12}. The secretion of intrinsic factor by the gastric parietal cells is controlled by humoral substances, notably gastrin. Pernicious anemia results from the lack of intrinsic-factor activity.

The importance of autoimmunity in pernicious anemia is suggested by the gastric histology as well as by several other findings.[93]

1. As many as 90 per cent of patients with pernicious anemia possess circulating antibodies against a cytoplasmic component of the gastric parietal cells. These auto-reactive antibodies can be IgG or IgA. A few per cent of normal young people have these antibodies; this rises to about 15 per cent of healthy people over 60 years of age.[94]

2. Between 40 and 60 per cent of patients with pernicious anemia have serum antibodies against intrinsic factor.[95] A slightly higher percentage of patients have antibodies against intrinsic-factor present in their gastric juice. Antibodies against intrinsic factor are found only rarely in the normal population. Two types of anti-intrinsic-factor antibodies have been defined.[96] "Blocking" antibodies, which prevent vitamin B_{12} from binding to intrinsic factor, are the most common. "Binding" antibodies attach to intrinsic factor and prevent the B_{12}–intrinsic-factor complex from binding to the ileal receptors (Fig. 15-8).

It is not known whether these antibodies are responsible for either the atrophic gastritis or the pernicious anemia. It has been observed that children of mothers with pernicious anemia who have passively acquired anti-intrinsic-factor antibodies transplacentally can present with vitamin B_{12} deficiency without gastric lesions.[97]

A large percentage of patients with pernicious anemia have other autoantibodies in addition to those we have already mentioned. Anti-thyroid antibodies are very common.[93] Relatives of patients with pernicious anemia have a higher-than-expected frequency of both thyroid and gastric parietal-cell autoantibodies, suggesting a genetic tendency toward autoimmune phenomena in these people.

GOODPASTURE'S SYNDROME

Goodpasture's syndrome is an uncommon disease which affects the lungs and kidneys primarily of young men.[98] The

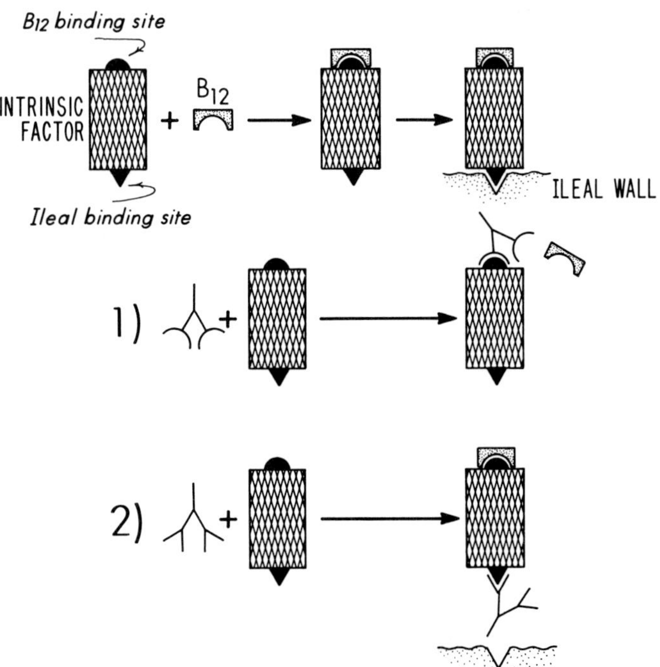

Fig. 15-8. Anti-intrinsic-factor antibody. Intrinsic factor is a bifunctional molecule, able to bind B_{12} and to attach to ileal receptor sites. (1) Blocking antibody binds to the B_{12} site on intrinsic factor. (2) Binding antibody binds to the part of intrinsic factor that attaches to the ileal receptor site.

patients most often present with hemoptysis secondary to pulmonary hemorrhage. This is quickly followed by the onset of rapidly progressive renal failure. Most patients die within a year of presentation. Pathologic findings include the following:

1. *The Lung.* The typical findings include intra-alveolar hemorrhage with hemosiderin-laden macrophages. The basement membrane of the alveolar septa appears abnormal although the alveolar cells seem to remain intact.

2. *The Kidneys.* The earliest findings are focal changes around the glomerular tufts, including the deposition of eosinophilic material and epithelial proliferation. These changes are followed by diffuse involvement of many glomeruli with marked epithelial proliferation leading to crescent formation. The glomerular capillaries can become occluded and there is often an interstitial inflammatory infiltrate. Electron microscopy reveals a glomerular basement membrane that is diffusely and irregularly thickened. However, discrete subendothelial and subepithelial deposits cannot be detected.[99,100]

Immunofluorescence studies reveal a *linear* deposition of IgG and C3 along the alveolar and glomerular basement membranes (Fig. 15-9).[101] The antibody is directed against an antigen of the basement membrane of both lung and kidney.[99] It is believed that the anti-basement-membrane antibodies mediate the tremendously destructive lesions in the lung and the kidney. This conclusion is supported by several animal studies. Administration of heterologous antibody against the glomerular basement membrane to an animal can reproduce the linear pattern of immunoglobulin staining and rapidly cause destructive changes in the kidney. Renal damage can be prevented by first

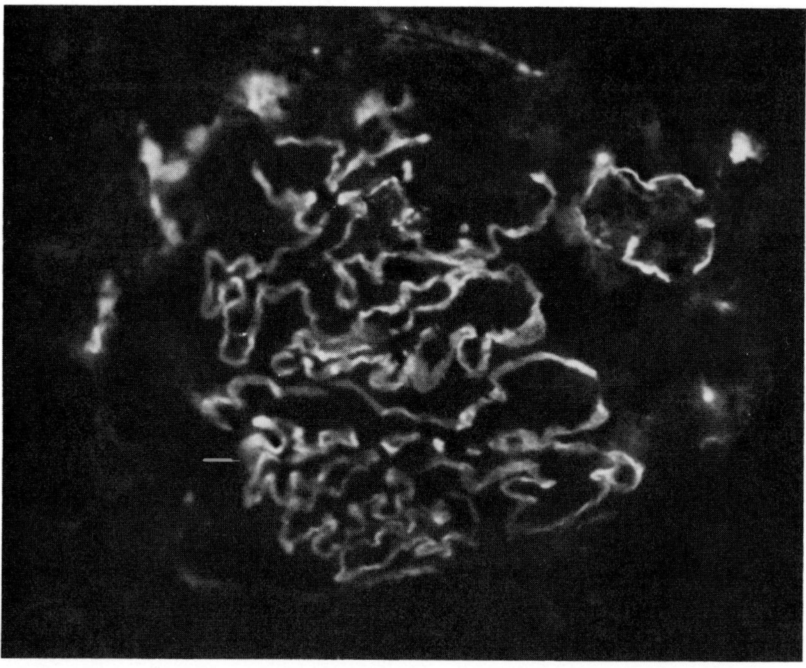

Fig. 15-9. Linear deposition of IgG along the glomerular basement membrane in the kidney of a patient with Goodpasture's syndrome. (Burkholder, P. M.: Atlas of Human Glomerular Pathology. New York, Harper and Row, 1974.)

decomplementing the animal, implicating complement in the destructive process.[101] The development of an autoimmune syndrome can be achieved by the injection of heterologous glomerular basement membranes in complete Freund's adjuvant into sheep.[102] The sheep produce antibodies against the glomerular basement membrane and develop a rapidly progressive glomerulonephritis with epithelial crescent formation. The injection of heterologous lung basement membrane in complete Freund's adjuvant into sheep will also produce a glomerulonephritis identical to that of Goodpasture's syndrome, complete with linear deposition of immunoglobulin along the basement membrane.[103] The glomerulonephritis of Goodpasture's syndrome thus appears to be truly autoimmune in nature and not the result of the deposition of circulating immune complexes.

REFERENCES

1. Schroeter, A. L., *et al.*: Immunofluorescence of cutaneous vasculitis associated with systemic disease. Arch. Dermatol., *104*:254, 1971.
2. Burnham, T. K., Neblett, T. R. and Fine, G.: The application of the fluorescent antibody technique to the investigation of lupus erythematosus and various dermatoses. J. Invest. Dermatol., *41*:451, 1963.
3. Provost, T. T., Pass, P., and Tomasi, T. B.: Evidence for the activation of complement via the C3 shunt in skin disease. Clin. Res., *20*:418, 1972.
4. Tuffanelli, D. L., Kay, D., and Fukayama, K.: Dermal-epidermal junction in lupus erythematosus. Arch. Dermatol., *99*:652, 1969.
5. Landry, M., and Sams, W. M.: Systemic lupus erythematosus: studies of the antibodies bound to skin. J. Clin. Invest., *52*:1871, 1973.
6. Koffler, D., Schur, P. H., and Kunkel, H. G.: Immunological studies concerning the nephritis of SLE. J. Exp. Med., *126*:607, 1967.
7. Gilliam, J. N.: The significance of cutaneous immunoglobulin deposits in lupus erythematosus and NZB/NZW F_1 hybrid mice. J. Invest. Dermatol., *65*:154, 1975.
8. McCreight, W. G., and Montgomery, H.: Cutaneous changes in lupus erythematosus. Arch. Dermatol., *61*:1, 1950.
9. Gilliam, J. N., Cheatum, D. E., Hurd, E. R., and Ziff, M.: The prognostic significance of the LE fluorescent band test. Arthritis Rheum., *16*:545, 1973.
10. Hashimoto, K., *et al.*: Identification of the substance binding pemphigus antibody and concanavalin A in the skin. J. Invest. Dermatol., *62*:423, 1974.
11. Jordan, R. F., Trifthausen, C. T., and Schroeter, A. L.: Direct immunofluorescent studies of pemphigus and bullous pemphigoid. Arch. Dermatol., *103*:486, 1971.
12. Tuffanelli, D. L.: Cutaneous immunopathology: recent observations. J. Invest. Dermatol., *65*:143, 1975.
13. Van Joost, T., Cormane, R. H., and Pondman, K. W.: Direct immunofluorescent study of the skin and occurrence of complement in pemphigus. Br. J. Dermatol., *87*:466, 1972.
14. Chorzelski, T. P., Von Weiss, J. F., and Lever, W. F.: Clinical significance of autoantibodies in pemphigus. Arch. Dermatol., *93*:570, 1966.
15. Lever, W. F., and Hashimoto, K.: the etiology and treatment of pemphigus and pemphigoid. J. Invest. Dermatol., *53*:373, 1969.
16. Bystryn, J. C., Abel, E., and Defeo, C.: Pemphigus foliaceus. Arch. Dermatol., *110*:857, 1974.
17. Jordan, R. E., *et al.*: Basement zone antibody in bullous pemphigoid. J.A.M.A., *200*:751, 1967.
18. Landry, M., Sams, W. M., and Jordon, R. E.: Bullous pemphigoid: elution of *in vivo*-fixed antibody J. Invest. Dermatol., *61*:348, 1973.
19. Chorzelski, T. P., *et al.*: Immunofluorescence studies in the diagnosis of dermatitis herpetiformis and its differentiation from bullous pemphigoid. J. Invest. Dermatol., *56*:373, 1971.
20. Mowbray, J. F., *et al.*: Circulating immune complexes in dermatitis herpetiformis. Lancet, *1*:400, 1973.
21. Van der Meer, J. B.: Granular deposits of immunoglobulin in the skin of patients with dermatitis herpetiformis. Br. J. Dermatol., *81*:493, 1969.
22. Provost, T. T., and Tomasi, T. B.: Evidence of the activation of complement via the alternate pathway in skin disease. Clin. Immunol. Immunopathol., *3*:178, 1974.
23. Seah, P. P., *et al.*: Alternate pathway complement fixation by IgA in the skin in dermatitis herpetiformis. Lancet, *2*:175, 1973.
24. Fraser, N. G., Dick, H. M., and Crichton, W. B.: Immunoglobulin in dermatitis herpetiformis and various other skin diseases. Br. J. Dermatol., *81*:89, 1969.
25. Gebhard, R. L., *et al.*: Dermatitis herpetiformis. J. Clin. Invest., *54*:98, 1974.
26. Brow, J. R., Parker, F., Weinstein, W. M., and Rubin, C. E.: The small intestinal mucosa in dermatitis herpetiformis. Gastroenterology, *60*:355, 1971.
27. Booth, C. C.: Enterocyte in celiac disease. Br. Med. J., *3*:725, 1970.
28. Benson, G. D., Kowlessar, O. D., and Sleisenger, M. H.: Adult celiac disease with

emphasis upon response to the gluten-free diet. Medicine, *43*:1, 1964.
29. Katz, J., Kantor, F. S., and Herskovic, T.: Intestinal antibodies to wheat fraction in celiac disease. Ann. Intern. Med., *69*:1149, 1968.
30. Kivel, R. M., Kearns, D. H., and Liebowitz, D.: Significance of antibodies to dietary proteins in serums of patients with nontropical sprue. N. Engl. J. Med., *271*:769, 1964.
31. Strober, W., Falchuk, Z. M., and Gebhard, R. L.: Gluten-sensitive enteropathy. Birth Defects, *11*:208, 1975.
32. Falchuk, Z. M., Gebhard, R. L., Sessoms, C., and Strober, W.: An *in vitro* model of gluten-sensitive enteropathy. J. Clin. Invest., *53*:487, 1974.
33. Loeb, P. M., Strober, W., Falchuk, Z. M., and Laster, L.: Incorporation of L-leucine-^{14}C into immunoglobulins by jejunal biopsies of patients with celiac sprue and other gastrointestinal diseases. J. Clin. Invest., *50*:559, 1971.
34. Falchuk, Z. M., and Strober, W.: Glutin-sensitive enteropathy: synthesis of antigliadin antibody *in vitro*. Gut, *15*:947, 1974.
35. Shiner, M., and Ballard, J.: Antigen-antibody reactions in jejunal mucosa in childhood celiac disease after gluten challenge. Lancet, *1*:1202, 1972.
36. Falchuk, Z. M., Rogentine, G. N., and Strober, W.: Predominance of histocompatibility antigen HLA-A5 in patients with gluten-sensitive enteropathy. J. Clin. Invest., *51*:1602, 1972.
37. Keuning, J. J., Pena, A. S., van Leewen, A., van Hooff, J. P. and van Rood, J. J.: HLA-DW3 associated with celiac disease. Lancet, *1*:506, 1976.
38. Rubin, W., Fauci, A. S., Sleisenger, M. H., and Jeffries, G. H.: Immunofluorescent studies in adult celiac disease. J. Clin. Invest., *44*:475, 1965.
39. Doniach, D.: Humoral and genetic aspects of thyroid autoimmunity. J. Clin. Endocrinol. Metab., *4*:267, 1975.
40. Torrigiani, G., Doniach, D., and Roitt, I. M.: Serum thyroglobulin levels in healthy subjects and in patients with thyroid disease. J. Clin. Endocrinol. Metab., *29*:305, 1969.
41. Bankhurst, A. D., and Torrigiani, G.: Lymphocytes binding human thyroglobulin in healthy people and its relevance to tolerance for autoantigens. Lancet, *1*:226, 1973.
42. Urbaniak, S. J., Penhale, W. J., and Irvine, W. J.: Circulating lymphocyte subpopulations in Hashimoto's thyroiditis. Clin. Exp. Immunol., *15*:345, 1973.
43. Roitt, I. M., Ling, N. R., Doniach, D., and Couchman, K. G.: The cytoplasmic auto-antigen of the human thyroid. Immunology, *7*:375, 1964.
44. Fagraeus, A., and Jonsson, J.: Distribution of organ antigens over the surface of thyroid cells as examined by the immunofluoresence test. Immunology, *18*:413, 1970.
45. Parker, R. H., and Beierwaltes, W. H.: Thyroid antibodies during pregnancy and in the newborn. J. Clin. Endocrinol. Metab., *21*:791, 1961.
46. Roitt, I. M., and Doniach, D.: Thyroid autoimmunity. Br. Med. Bull., *16*:152, 1960.
47. Rose, N. R.: Mechanisms of tissue damage in human and experimental autoimmune thyroiditis. *In* Grabar, P., and Miescher, P. (eds.): Mechanisms of Cell and Tissue Damage Produced by Immune Responses. P. 161. Schwabe and Co., Basel, 1961.
48. Nakamura, R. M., and Weigle, W.: Transfer of experimental autoimmune thyroiditis by serum from thyroidectomized donors. J. Exp. Med., *130*:263, 1969.
49. Clinton, B. A., and Weigle, W. O.: Cellular events during the induction of experimental thyroiditis in the rabbit. J. Exp. Med., *136*:1605, 1972.
50. Calder, E. A., Penhale, W. J., Barnes, E. W., and Irvine, W. J.: Evidence for circulating immune complexes in thyroid disease. Br. Med. J., *2*:30, 1974.
51. Kalderon, A. E., Bogaars, H. A., and Diamond, I.: Ultrastructural alterations of the follicular basement membrane in Hashimoto's thyroiditis. Am. J. Med., *55*:485, 1973.
52. Calder, E. A., *et al.*: Lymphocyte-dependent antibody-mediated cytotoxicity in Hasimoto's thyroiditis. Clin. Exp. Immunol., *14*:153, 1973.
53. Calder, E. A., and Irvine, W. J.: Cell-mediated immunity and immune complexes in thyroid disease. Clin. Endocrinol. Metab., *4*:287, 1975.
54. Lamki, L., Row, V. V., and Volpe, R.: Cell-mediated immunity in Graves' disease and in Hashimoto's thyroiditis as shown by the demonstration of MIF. J. Clin. Endocrinol. Metab., *36*:358, 1973.
55. Ehrenfeld, E., Klein, E., and Benezra, D.: Human thyroglobulin and thyroid extract as specific stimulators of sensitized lymphocytes. J. Clin. Endocrinol. Metab., *32*:115, 1971.
56. Laryea, E., Row, V. V., and Volpe, R.: The effect of blood leucocytes from patients with Hashimoto's disease on human thyroid cells in monolayer culture. Clin. Endocrinol., *2*:23, 1973.
57. Calder, E. A., Penhale, W. J., Barnes, E. W., and Irvine, W. J.: Cytotoxic lymphocytes in Hashimoto's thyroiditis. Clin. Exp. Immunol., *14*:19, 1973.
58. Podleski, W. K.: Cytotoxic lymphocytes in Hashimoto's thyroiditis. Clin. Exp. Immunol., *11*:543, 1972.
59. Lipman, L. M., *et al.*: Relationship of LATS to the clinical features in course of Graves' disease. Am. J. Med., *43*:486, 1967.
60. Wall, J. R., Good, B. F., Forbes, I. J., and Hetzel, B. S.: Demonstration of the production of the LATS by peripheral lymphocytes cultured *in vitro*. Clin. Exp. Immunol., *14*:555, 1973.
61. Kendall-Taylor, P.: LATS and human-specific thyroid stimulator; their relation to Graves' disease. Clin. Endocrinol. Metab., *4*:319, 1975.
62. Smith, B. R., and Hall, R.: Thyroid-stimulating

immunoglobulin in Graves' disease. Lancet, *2*:427, 1974.

63. Smith, B. R., Dorrington, K. J., and Munro, D. S.: The thyroid stimulating properties of LATS gamma G globulin subunits. Biochim. Biophys. Acta, *192*:277, 1969.
64. Smith, B. R.: The interaction of the LATS in thyroid tissue *in vitro*. J. Endocrinol., *46*:45, 1970.
65. McKenzie, J. M.: Neonatal Graves' disease. J. Clin. Endocrinol. Metab., *24*:660, 1964.
66. Bonnyns, M., *et al*.: LATS in thyroid function in relatives of patients with Graves' disease. Clin. Endocrinol., *3*:277, 1973.
67. Carneiro, L., Dorrington, K. J., and Munro, D. S.: Recovery of the LATS from serum from patients with thyrotoxicosis by concentration of IgG. Clin. Sci., *31*:215, 1966.
68. Adams, D. D., and Kennedy, T. H.: Evidence to suggest that LATS protector stimulates the human thyroid gland. J. Clin. Endocrinol. Metab., *33*:47, 1971.
69. Kendall-Taylor, P., Dirmikis, S., and Munro, D. S.: The detection and significance of LATS protector. Q. J. Med., *43*:619, 1974.
70. Dirmikis, S. M., *et al*.: Placental transmission of LATS-protector. Lancet, *2*:1579, 1974.
71. Adams, D. D., Kennedy, T. H., and Stewart, R. D. H.: Correlation between LATS-protector level and thyroid ^{131}I uptake in thyrotoxicosis. Br. Med. J., *2*:199 1974.
72. Doniach, D., and Florin-Christensen, A.: Autoimmunity in the pathogenesis of endocrine exophthalmos. Clin. Endocrinol. Metab., *4*:341, 1975.
73. Konishi, J., Herman, M. H., and Kriss, J. P.: Binding of thyroglobulin and thyroglobulin-anti-thyroglobulin immune complexes to extra-ocular muscle membrane. Endocrinology, *95*:434, 1974.
74. Kriss, J. P.: Radioisotopic thyroidolymphography in patients with Graves' disease. J. Clin. Endocrinol. Metab., *31*:315, 1970.
75. Der Kinderen, P. J.: EPS, LATS and exophthalmose. *In* Irvine, W. J. (eds.): Thyrotoxicosis. P. 221. Edinburgh, Livingstone, 1967.
76. Shillinglaw, J., and Utiger, R. D.: Failure of retro-orbital tissue to neutralize the biological activity of the LATS. J. Clin. Endocrinol. Metab., *28*:1069, 1968.
77. Hall, R., and Stanbury, J. B.: Familial studies of autoimmune thyroiditis. Clin. Exp. Immunol., *2*:719, 1967.
78. Roitt, I. M., and Doniach, D.: A reassessment of studies on the aggregation of thyroid autoimmunity in families of thyroiditis patients. Clin. Exp. Immunol., *2*:727, 1967.
79. Hall, R., Dingle, P. R., and Roberts, D. F.: Thyroid antibodies: a study of first degree relatives. Clin. Genet., *3*:319, 1972.
80. Nerup, J.: Addison's disease—serological studies. Acta Endocrinol., *76*:142, 1974.
81. Irvine, W. J., and Barnes, E. W.: Addison's disease, ovarian failure and hypoparathyroidism. Clin. Endocrinol. Metab., *4*:379, 1975.
82. MacCuish, A. C., and Irvine, W. J.: Autoimmunological aspects of diabetes mellitus. Clin. Endocrinol. Metab., *4*:435, 1975.
83. Doniach, D.: *In* Bastenic, V. A., and Gepts, W. (eds.): Immunology and Autoimmunity in Diabetes Mellitus. P. 170. Amsterdam, Excerpta Medica, 1974.
84. Bottazzo, G. F., Florin-Christensen, A., and Doniach, D.: Islet-cell antibodies in diabetes mellitus with autoimmune polyendocrine deficiencies. Lancet, *2*:1279, 1974.
85. MacCuish, A. C., Barnes, E. W., Irvine, W. J., and Duncan, L. J. P.: Antibodies to pancreatic islet cells in insulin-dependent diabetics with coexistent autoimmune disease. Lancet, *2*:1529, 1974.
86. Nerup, J., *et al*.: Antipancreatic cellular hypersensitivity in diabetes mellitus. Diabetes, *20*:424, 1971.
87. Hirata, Y., *et al*.: On insulin autoimmune syndrome. Tonyobyo (Suppl.), *15*:179, 1972.
88. MacCuish, A. C., *et al*.: Cell-mediated immunity in diabetes mellitus. Diabetes, *24*:36, 1975.
89. Berson, S. A., and Yalow, R. S.: Some current controversies in diabetes research. Diabetes, *14*:549, 1965.
90. Irvine, W. J., Chan, M. M., and Scarth, L.: Further characterization of auto-antibodies reactive with extra-adrenal steroid producing cells in patients with adrenal disorders. Clin. Exp. Immunol., *4*:489, 1969.
91. Blizzard, R. M., Chee, D., and Davis, W.: The incidence of adrenal and other antibodies in the sera of patients with idiopathic adrenal insufficiency. Clin. Exp. Immunol., *2*:19, 1967.
92. Thomsen, M., *et al*.: Mixed lymphocyte culture typing in juvenile diabetes mellitus and idiopathic Addison's disease. Transpl. Rev., *22*:125, 1975.
93. Irvine, W. J.: The association of atrophic gastritis with autoimmune thyroid disease. Clin. Endocrinol. Metab., *4*:351, 1975.
94. Roitt, I. M., Doniach, D., and Shapland, C.: Autoimmunity in pernicious anemia and atrophic gastritis. Ann. N.Y. Acad. Sci., *124*:644, 1965.
95. Strickland, R. G., Baur, S., Ashworth, L. A. E., and Taylor, K. B.: A correlative study of immunological phenomena in pernicious anemia. Clin. Exp. Immunol., *8*:25, 1971.
96. Roitt, I. M., Doniach, D., and Shapland, C.: Intrinsic-factor autoantibodies. Lancet, *2*:469, 1964.
97. Bar-Shany, S., and Herbert, V.: Transplacentally acquired antibodies to intrinsic factor with a vitamin B_{12} deficiency. Blood, *30*:777, 1967.
98. Proskey, A. J., *et al*.: Goodpasture's syndrome. Am. J. Med., *48*:162, 1970.
99. Poskitt, T. R.: Immunologic and electron microscopic studies in Goodpasture's syndrome. Am. J. Med., *49*:250, 1970.
100. Koffler, D., Sandson, J., Carr, R., and Kunkel, H. G.: Immunologic studies concerning the pulmonary lesions in Goodpasture's syndrome. Am. J. Pathol., *54*:293, 1969.

101. Hammer, D. K., and Dixon, F. J.: Experimental glomerulonephritis. J. Exp. Med., *117*:1019, 1963.
102. Steblay, R. W.: Glomerulonephritis induced in sheep by injections of heterologous glomerular basement membrane and Freund's complete adjuvant. J. Exp. Med., *116*:253, 1962.
103. Steblay, R. W., and Rudofsky, U.: Autoimmune glomerulonephritis induced in sheep by injection of human lung and Freund's adjuvant. Science, *160*:204, 1968.

16 Immunosuppressive Agents

Cecile R. Bassen, M.D.

In this chapter, we will look at several commonly employed immunosuppressive agents. We will examine these agents from two perspectives. (1) *What is known concerning their mechanisms of action.* Where do they intervene in the normal immune response? How is this intervention accomplished on a subcellular level? (2) *Aspects of their clinical use.* Does our knowledge of the mechanisms of action of these immunosuppressive agents explain their efficacy in various disease states?

Immunosuppressive agents are defined on an operational basis as drugs which are capable of inhibiting immune function. The term "immunosuppressive" implies inhibition of the specific mediators of the immune response as opposed to nonspecific "anti-inflammatory" action. As we shall see, however, the majority of immunosuppressants have anti-inflammatory effects in addition to immunosuppressive action, and the relative significance of these two components is often unclear.

The agents we will examine are corticosteroids, azathioprine, cyclophosphamide and antilymphocyte serum (see Fig. 16-1). Because the immunosuppressants differ considerably in their action in different species, we will confine our discussion to experiments done in man, unless it is otherwise noted.

CORTICOSTEROIDS

The glucocorticosteroids, or corticosteroids, are endogenous hormones produced by the adrenal cortex, the primary hormone in man being cortisol. These are potent hormones with multiple regulatory actions, including the control of carbohydrate metabolism. It is not clear what effect endogenous corticosteroids have on the immune response. Administered corticosteroids inhibit glucose uptake and other metabolic functions in lymphoid tissue and it is generally assumed that corticosteroids exert an inhibitory effect endogenously via this mechanism.[1] However, the magnitude and significance of this effect in the normally functioning individual is not known. At physiologic concentrations, *in vitro* corticosteroids clearly inhibit many metabolic functions in human lymphocytes,[2,3] but they may enhance others.[4]

Endogenous corticosteroids are known to affect circulating lymphocyte numbers. Man exhibits a normal diurnal variation in blood lymphocyte count which correlates inversely with the diurnal variation in plasma cortisol levels. Thus the

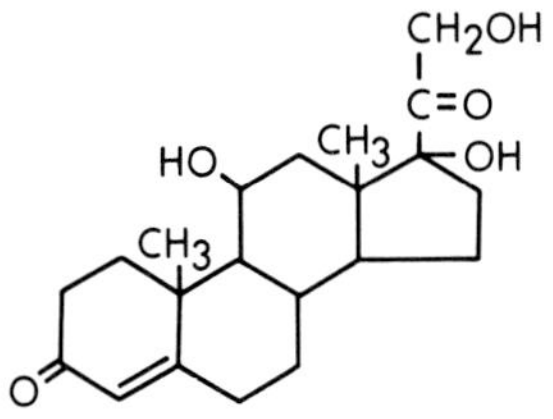

CORTISOL

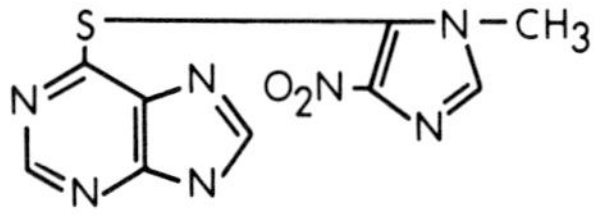

AZATHIOPRINE

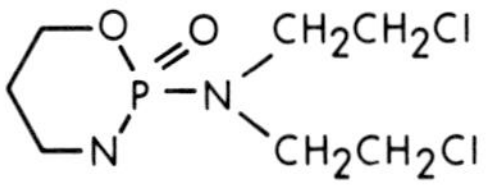

CYCLOPHOSPHAMIDE

Fig. 16-1. Chemical structures of the immunosuppressive agents.

absolute number of circulating lymphocytes is normally at a minimum in the early morning when cortisol levels are highest.[5] As first noted by Addison, lymphoid hyperplasia and lymphocytosis occur in the presence of adrenal insufficiency.[6,7]

Corticosteroids are cytotoxic for the lymphocytes of certain animal species, including the mouse, rat, rabbit and hamster.[8,9] In these species an increase in endogenous corticosteroids provoked by stress results in lymphopenia and involution of lymphoid tissue.[10] In the past it was assumed that this mechanism applied to man and was basic to the immunosuppressive action of exogenous corticosteroids. However, it is now known that corticosteroids are lymphocytotoxic only in certain species, referred to as corticosteroid-"sensitive" species. Corticosteroids are *not* lymphocytotoxic in man, guinea pigs or monkeys. These species are relatively corticosteroid-"resistant," since pharmacologic and even suprapharmacologic doses of corticosteroids produce only negligible lysis of their lymphocytes.[9,11]

What then is the mechanism of corticosteroid action in man? In the many years of research concerning the effects of corticosteroids as immunosuppressants, no simple and clear-cut answers have been found. However, much data has accumulated which shows that corticosteroids have multiple inhibitory effects on the human immune response. Some of these actions have been fairly well documented while others remain highly controversial.

IMMUNOSUPPRESSIVE ACTIONS

What happens when corticosteroids are administered to a normal individual? A single oral or intravenous pharmacologic dose of corticosteroids significantly changes the profile of the circulating white blood cells. There is a statistically significant decrease in the absolute number of circulating lymphocytes, monocytes and eosinophils, with an increase in the number of circulating neutrophils. The timing of this effect roughly corresponds to the change in plasma cortisol concentration.[12-14] Changes in the white blood cell differential are maximal approximately four to six hours after corticosteroid administration, with the blood count generally returning to normal at 24 hours. However, prolonged effects of up to 72 hours, outlasting any change in plasma cortisol concentration, have been found with high doses of certain corticosteroids.[14,15]

The degree of lymphocytopenia obtained is dose-dependent up to a point.[12,13] High doses of corticosteroids reduce lymphocyte numbers by a maximum of 50 to 75 per cent;[16] beyond this point, increasing the dose of corticosteroid has no further effect. A decrease in the absolute number of both B and T lymphocytes occurs, with T cells proportionately more affected.[13]

There is evidence from animal experiments that these changes are due to a redistribution of white blood cells, with sequestration of circulating T cells in the bone marrow.[17-19] In man, studies using labelled lymphocytes also suggest that corticosteroids act to selectively deplete recirculating lymphocytes from the intravascular space.[20] However, it is not known where in the extravascular space these cells are sequestered.

In addition to changes in white blood cell differential, pharmacologic doses of corticosteroids cause significant alterations in immune function. We will examine these effects in terms of corticosteroid action on the various white blood cells which participate in the immune response.

T Cells

T-cell function can be markedly impaired *in vivo* by a single dose of corticosteroids. Thus, skin test reactivity is diminished to a variety of antigens applied two hours after a high dose of corticosteroids.[21] Lymphocytes in culture from subjects before and after corticosteroid treatment show a significant decrease in responsiveness to mitogens, alloantigens and specific antigens.[12,14,22] These changes are transient and recovery of immune function is complete by 24 hours.[16,20,23]

The inhibition of T-cell function caused by *in vivo* corticosteroids appears to be related to corticosteroid-induced lymphocytopenia which follows a similar time course.[24] However, *in vitro* experiments suggest that more than sequestration is involved in corticosteroid suppression of T-cell function. Corticosteroids have been shown to inhibit T-cell response to mitogens, isoantigens and specific antigens when added directly to human lymphocytes in culture.[25,26]

In vitro studies show that the timing of corticosteroid administration relative to the addition of the stimulating mitogen or antigen is significant. In general, corticosteroids are most effective when added before or coincident with the stimulus; they may be totally ineffective when added afterwards.[25,27]

It is likely that corticosteroids differentially affect various subpopulations of T cells. There is strong evidence for this in corticosteroid-sensitive species.[9,28,29] In man, the fact that even very high doses of corticosteroids produce only partial sequestration of T cells and partial inhibition of T-cell function is consistent with the possibility that some T cells may be resistant to corticosteroids.[16,30] In addition, some T-cell functions appear to be relatively resistant to corticosteroids, in that they require higher doses for inhibition than do other functions.[27]

In addition to the inhibition of T-cell activation, corticosteroids appear to inhibit T-cell effector function indirectly. It has been shown *in vitro* that corticosteroids decrease human T-cell cytotoxicity by interfering with the effect of lymphotoxin on target cells.[31] When corticosteroids are added to guinea pig white blood cells, they interfere with normal MIF function without affecting MIF production.[32] Thus, some aspects of corticosteroid inhibition of T-cell function may not be due to corticosteroid effects on T cells at all, but rather to effects on other participants in the immune response. Of interest in this regard is evidence that corticosteroid-induced monocytopenia may play a role in *in vivo* suppression of T-cell function. It has been shown that the inhibition of the T-cell response to specific antigens produced by *in vivo* corticosteroid can be partially corrected by the addition of autologous monocytes to blood samples.[12]

B Cells

Demonstrable effects of corticosteroids on the humoral response are much less impressive than those on cell-mediated reactions. Corticosteroid treatment causes an increase in IgG catabolism[33] and seems to produce a delayed and prolonged depression of circulating IgG levels, over and above the effect due to the increased catabolic rate.[34,35] High-dose corticosteroid treatment of three or more weeks duration has been reported to inhibit significantly bone marrow production of IgG.[36] However, corticosteroids clearly fail to inhibit either primary or secondary antibody responses in man.[9,37]

Despite their lack of effect on the humoral response to a normal antigenic challenge, there is evidence that corticosteroids can specifically reduce the titers of circulating autoantibodies in patients with autoimmune diseases. We will return to this point later when we discuss corticosteroid treatment of antibody-mediated cytotoxic reactions. The effects of corticosteroids upon immunoglobulin production may be extremely complex, since *in vitro* studies have shown that whereas high pharmacologic doses of corticosteroids are inhibitory for immunoglobulin production, physiologic doses are stimulatory.[4,38]

Monocytes and Macrophages

Corticosteroids have multiple inhibitory effects on these cells. As already mentioned, *in vivo* corticosteroids cause a transient decrease in the number of circulating monocytes.[16,39] In addition, corticosteroids induce marked inhibition of monocyte bactericidal and fungicidal activity although phagocytosis and lysosomal degranulation remain normal.[40]

Other effects have been demonstrated with the use of corticosteroids *in vitro* but these remain controversial. They include (1) inhibition of monocyte random motility and chemotaxis,[40,41] and (2) inhibition of macrophage binding of red blood cells coated with IgG and C3.[41,42]

As we saw in the section on T cells, there is reason to believe that depletion and inhibition of monocytes may contribute significantly to corticosteroid inhibition of cell-mediated immunity. Further evidence in this regard comes from experiments in guinea pigs, a corticosteroid-resistant species like man. These studies show that inhibition of macrophage accumulation is significant in corticosteroid suppression of delayed hypersensitivity reactions.[43,44]

ANTI-INFLAMMATORY EFFECTS

A significant part of the "immunosuppressive" potency of corticosteroids may actually be due to nonspecific anti-inflammatory effects. Corticosteroids are potent inhibitors of the normal inflammatory response in man. Pretreatment with corticosteroids markedly diminishes the size of cellular inflammatory exudates in response to local trauma.[45,46] Chronic daily corticosteroid treatment results in significant inhibition of both neutrophilic and monocytic infiltrates.[39]

The anti-inflammatory action of corticosteroids appears to be multifaceted. Corticosteroids are known to be vasoconstrictive in man, and the vasoconstrictive capacity of any given topical corticosteroid appears to correlate well with its efficacy as an anti-inflammatory agent.[47-49] Corticosteroids have also been shown to inhibit granulocyte adherence;[50] this appears to prevent margination and thus prevents diapedesis of white blood cells.[51] There is also evidence that corticosteroids decrease vascular permeability in animals;[51] however, similar data is not available in man.

It has been suggested that corticosteroids may act to inhibit the synthesis and/or the action of a variety of soluble mediators of inflammation, including prostaglandins, histamine, kinins and complement.[52-57] Little is known about corticosteroid effects on these inflammatory substances. Corticosteroids do not appear to inhibit activation of either kinins or complement directly.[58-60] However, corticosteroid inhibition of exudate formation is likely to result in diminished histamine release with decreased complement and kinin activation and thus in a markedly lower level of inflammation. In addition, animal studies suggest that corticosteroids may alter plasma and tissue levels of these inflammatory substrates.[57,58]

Neutrophils

The neutrophil is the major type of cell present in acute inflammatory reactions. Several studies have provided evidence that corticosteroids have multiple inhibitory effects on neutrophil functions, including chemotaxis, phagocytosis, metabolic activation and bacterial killing.[41,61-68] However, many of these studies are mutually contradictory, and corticosteroids do not appear consistently to inhibit any of these functions.[14,41,64,69-72] The most significant effect of corticosteroids on neutrophils appears to be inhibition of neutrophil egress from the circulation into areas of inflammation.[39,45] As already mentioned, this may be due to inhibition of granulocyte adherence.[50]

In summary, corticosteroids cause transient lymphocytopenia, monocytopenia and eosinopenia, most probably by inducing sequestration of these cells. Corticosteroids appear to suppress normal T-cell function both directly by inhibiting T-cell activation and indirectly by interfering with the effect of lymphokines on target cells. Although corticosteroids do not suppress the normal humoral response, they do reduce autoantibody titers and may nonspecifically inhibit IgG production. Corticosteroids also inhibit some aspects of monocyte and macrophage function. They are potent anti-inflammatory agents and prevent accumulation of neutrophils and monocytes in inflammatory exudates.

SUBCELLULAR MECHANISMS OF CORTICOSTEROID ACTION

We have seen that corticosteroids exert potent specific effects on various mediators of the immune response. What are the mechanisms by which corticosteroids accomplish these actions?

The immunosuppressive properties of corticosteroids are merely part of a spectrum of activities that these hormones carry out. All of these activities appear to be mediated by the same subcellular mechanisms. To understand the manner in which corticosteroids function as immunosuppressive agents we must first examine the way that they and other steroid hormones function in general.

Cytoplasmic Receptors for Corticosteroids

It is believed that all steroid hormones act to regulate cell function throughout the body via one basic mechanism. Target cells for these hormones contain cytoplasmic receptors specific for the hormone in question (Fig. 16-2). Steroids combine with and modify these cytoplasmic proteins. Noncovalent reversible binding of the steroid hormone allosterically modifies and activates the receptor so that the steroid-receptor complex is capable of entering the nucleus. Once inside the nucleus, the steroid-receptor complex is believed to combine with the chromatin. The exact nature of this bind-

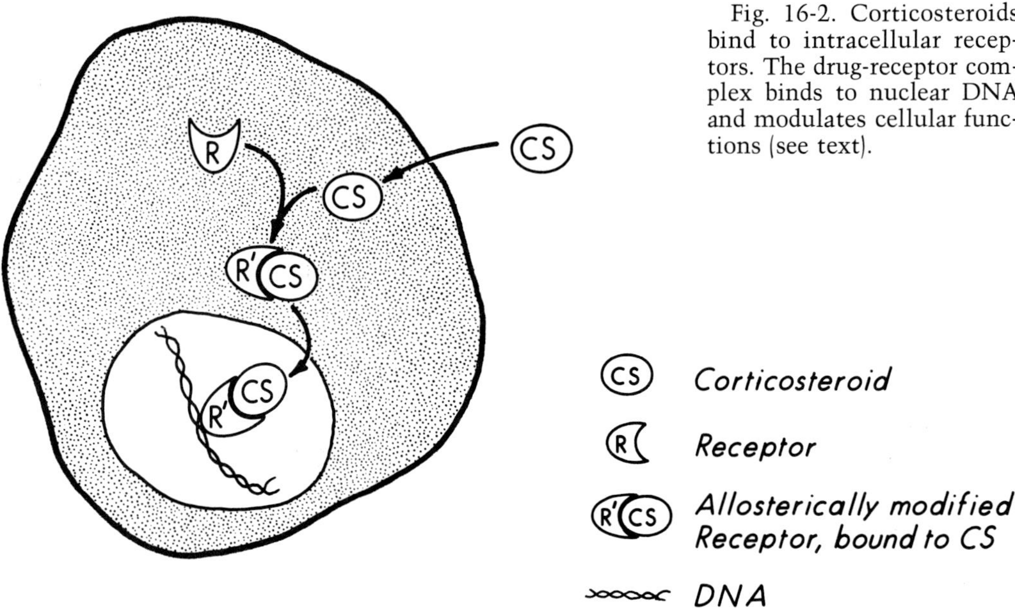

Fig. 16-2. Corticosteroids bind to intracellular receptors. The drug-receptor complex binds to nuclear DNA and modulates cellular functions (see text).

ing is not understood, and it may vary with the specific hormone-receptor complex. By binding to the chromatin, the complex exerts a regulatory influence on DNA transcription, leading to specific alterations in enzyme synthesis and cell metabolism.[73]

It appears that most, if not all, corticosteroid effects are mediated through cytoplasmic receptors. There is a strong correlation between the ability of corticosteroids to affect a given cell type or tissue and the presence of cytoplasmic receptors in that tissue. The biological potency of the various corticosteroids has also been shown to reflect their relative affinities of binding with cytoplasmic receptors.[74]

Cytoplasmic receptors for corticosteroids have been demonstrated in normal lymphocytes of many species. Human lymphocytes normally contain a low concentration of cytoplasmic receptors for corticosteroids; this has been suggested as an explanation for the relative resistance of human lymphocytes to corticosteroid lysis.[27] Thus, human ALL cells which are sensitive to corticosteroid lysis exhibit approximately ten times as much corticosteroid-binding activity as either normal human lymphocytes or corticosteroid-resistant ALL cells.[75] As ALL patients become refractory to corticosteroid therapy they show a loss of corticosteroid-binding activity over time.[75]

It has been proposed that the resistance of a given lymphocyte to corticosteroid inhibition may be related to the maturity of that cell.[37] In corticosteroid-sensitive species, immature T cells are sensitive to corticosteroid lysis whereas mature functional T cells are not.[9] Human T cells are less sensitive to corticosteroid inhibition after mitogenic stimulation.[27] Thus, maturation or commitment of a T cell may involve a loss of corticosteroid receptors. The increased number of corticosteroid receptors seen in ALL cells may therefore reflect the immaturity of these cells.

What effect do corticosteroids have on lymphocyte metabolism? Studies of normal human lymphocytes have shown that pharmacologic levels of corticosteroids *in vitro* significantly inhibit many aspects of both stimulated and resting cell metabolism including DNA, RNA and protein synthesis and glucose utilization.[76-79] Some of these effects may be mediated via the induction of inhibitory molecules.[80-82] It is far from clear how these effects translate into specific immunosuppressive activity. Even less is known concerning the subcellular effects of corticosteroids on macrophages and neutrophils.

It is well established and widely accepted that corticosteroid – target-cell interaction occurs via cytoplasmic receptors. Two additional mechanisms of corticosteroid immunosuppression have been proposed which may or may not involve cytoplasmic receptors: increase in intracellular cyclic AMP, and membrane stabilization.

Corticosteroids and Cyclic AMP

Corticosteroids are known to be permissive for other endogenous hormones, especially those that utilize cAMP as a second messenger.[1] There is evidence that the immunosuppressive action of corticosteroids may be accomplished in part via a permissive effect involving cAMP. This nucleotide has been found to have significant inhibitory effects on the immune response (see Chap. 4).[83]

It has been shown that corticosteroids augment the stimulatory effect of beta-adrenergics and prostaglandin E_1 on intracellular cyclic AMP levels in human lymphocytes.[78,84] There is also evidence that *in vitro* corticosteroids can directly increase cyclic AMP.[84-86] However, this latter effect remains controversial.[78,87] Whether direct or indirect, increases in intracellular cyclic AMP in lymphocytes and other white blood cells could explain many of the known immunosuppressive and anti-inflammatory effects of corticosteroids (fur further discussion see type I reactions, below).

Membrane Stabilization

It has been suggested that many of the anti-inflammatory actions of corticosteroids could be accomplished by direct corticosteroid stabilization of lysosomes and other cell membranes.[88-91] Lysosomal stabilization could also result in an inhibitory effect on lymphocyte activation.[92-94] There is evidence that corticosteroids *in vitro* can inhibit lysosomal discharge in human neutrophils under certain circumstances.[89,91] However, the clinical applicability of these findings is quite controversial.[39,64] In general, corticosteroids do not appear to significantly stabilize lysosomes in human white blood cells.[95] From studies on patients with rheumatoid arthritis,[96,97] there is some evidence that corticosteroids do stabilize synovial membranes. However, the weight of the evidence argues against membrane stabilization as a significant mechanism of corticosteroid action in man.

CLINICAL APPLICATIONS

Since 1949, when the first reports on the clinical use of corticosteroids in inflammatory disease were published,[98,99] it has been appreciated that corticosteroids are effective in diminishing the signs and symptoms of inflammation, such as fever, malaise, joint swelling and tenderness. In the ensuing years, corticosteroids were enthusiastically endorsed by physicians and employed therapeutically in a wide variety of disease states. It has since become clear, however, that corticosteroids afford symptomatic relief in many disease processes without otherwise altering their natural course. Thus, in a great many clinical situations, corticosteroids provide palliation rather than cure.[100]

In diseases, such as infections, where a normal immune response is beneficial and necessary to the well-being of the host, corticosteroids may actually increase the severity of the disease while minimizing its symptoms. In addition, by suppressing the normal immune response, corticosteroids may increase susceptibility to infections. It has been reported that patients treated with corticosteroids are predisposed to infections of almost all etiologies.[101] It is unclear how much of this susceptibility is due to the underlying diseases for which these patients are being treated. However, chronic treatment with daily corticosteroids appears to increase the incidence of infection, in at least certain disease states, in a dose-dependent fashion.[101] Thus infection is a potential, but by no means invariable, complication of corticosteroid immunosuppression.

The immunosuppressive actions of corticosteroids are beneficial in those disease states where the immune response is pathologic. As we shall see, corticosteroids can induce remissions in some of these diseases, while in others they are merely palliative. The variable course of some diseases makes therapeutic intervention difficult to assess; in these instances the true efficacy of corticosteroids remains unclear.

A comprehensive review of corticosteroid therapy of diseases involving immune mechanisms is beyond the scope of this book. We will limit ourselves to a brief review of the efficacy of corticosteroids in various types of immune reactions, concentrating on diseases where the effect of corticosteroids on specific immune mechanisms has been extensively investigated. As we shall see, it is often impossible to trace the therapeutic effect of corticosteroids to a specific immune intervention; frequently multiple mechanisms appear to be involved.

Type I Reactions: IgE-Mediated Immediate Hypersensitivity

Corticosteroids have been shown to be useful in the treatment of various IgE-mediated hypersensitivity disorders such as allergic rhinitis,[102] atopic dermatitis,[103] chronic extrinsic asthma,[104,105] status asthmaticus[106] and drug reactions.[107] Corticosteroid therapy of these diseases, although effective, is purely palliative. It must therefore be continuous for as long as the disease persists.[108] Topical corticosteroids are effective although they do not seem to be systemically absorbed, suggesting that the action of corticosteroids in these disorders is local.

Corticosteroids most probably relieve the symptoms of atopic dermatitis and allergic rhinitis by nonspecific anti-inflammatory effects including vasoconstriction and decreased vascular permeability. This may be mediated, in part, by decreased histamine production and facilitation of beta-adrenergic stimulation.[57]

The situation is more complex in the treatment of asthma. The major effect of corticosteroids appears to be anti-inflammatory. Probable actions include: (1) a decrease in bronchial edema and bronchorrhea, possibly associated with a decreased release of histamine and/or SRS-A,[110,111] (2) relaxation of bronchial smooth muscle either by permissive action to increase the response of smooth muscle to beta-adrenergics or possibly by a direct effect,[111,112] and (3) inhibition of histamine and/or alpha-adrenergic-mediated bronchoconstriction.[113] These anti-inflammatory effects may be largely accomplished by corticosteroid-mediated increases in intracellular cyclic AMP.[57,114] There is evidence that corticosteroids significantly diminish beta-adrenergic blockade in asthmatics and thus potentiate the effects of exogenous catecholamines.[84,86,112]

Corticosteroids may also act to inhibit specific immune phenomena which occur in asthma, including lymphocytic infiltration of bronchial walls and deposition of immunoglobulin complexes in the bronchial basement membrane.[115] In addition, there is indirect evidence that corticosteroids may decrease serum IgE concentrations. It appears significant that few asthmatic children on long-term corticosteroid therapy have elevated IgE levels, and that the serum levels of IgE in these children tend to rise when corticosteroids are discontinued.[116]

It is important to stress that corticosteroids are generally effective in the extrinsic or atopic form of asthma but not in the purely intrinsic form.[110] The presence of high levels of eosinophils in the blood and sputum appears to be associated with an increased probability of response to corticosteroids.[104] It has been suggested that the total eosinophil count can be used as a guide to corticosteroid dosage.[117] Asthmatic patients who are relatively resistant to corticosteroids, requiring high doses for symptomatic relief, show a decreased eosinopenic response to corticosteroids as well as a decreased half-life of plasma cortisol.[118] Those patients who spontaneously become more responsive to corticosteroid therapy exhibit an increased eosinopenic response.[119]

Of interest is the observation that adrenal insufficiency may be associated with an unmasking of the symptoms of allergic rhinitis, eczema or asthma.[109,120] Both adrenalectomy and treatment with adrenal cortical inhibitors have been found to increase the severity of immediate hypersensitivity reactions in animals.[107,121] It appears, therefore, that endogenous as well as exogenous corticosteroids may have some palliative effect in the various manifestations of IgE-mediated hypersensitivity.

Type II Reactions: Antibody-Mediated Cytotoxicity

Although there is evidence that corticosteroids do not inhibit the normal humoral immune response,[9,37] corticosteroids are often effective in the treatment of type II autoimmune diseases. Corticosteroid therapy is associated with a high rate of long-term remission in these disorders, making it the treatment of choice for autoimmune hemolytic anemia[122] and severe or progressive pemphigus vulgaris.[123]

Corticosteroid therapy induces remission in approximately 80 per cent of patients with autoimmune hemolytic anemia (AIHA) mediated by warm-reacting antibodies; some 30 to 70 per cent of these patients will remain in either long-term or permanent remission.[122] Clinical improvement with decreased hemolysis is usually seen two to three weeks after the initiation of therapy. Patients with positive indirect Coombs' tests (indicating free serum anti-red-blood-cell antibody) are generally less responsive to corticosteroids.[122]

Several mechanisms of action are thought to be involved in corticosteroid-induced remissions of AIHA. (1) Inhibition of autoantibody production clearly occurs in some but not all patients who enter remission, with reversion of the positive direct Coombs' test to negative.[122] (2) Corticosteroids appear to inhibit erythrophagocytosis in the absence of any change in the amount of cell-bound antibody.[42,124,125] (3) Corticosteroids may also decrease the degree of antibody binding to red blood cells.[125] However, this phenomenon, seen *in vivo*, has not been confirmed by studies *in vitro*.[126]

Corticosteroids are equally effective in the treatment of diffuse pemphigus vulgaris, which is otherwise associated with a very poor prognosis.[123] During corticosteroid therapy, a decrease in the amount of skin deposition of intercellular antibody is seen, which roughly parallels in time course the improvement seen clinically. These antibodies may become undetectable in patients with corticosteroid-induced remission.[127] Of interest is the fact that in this disease, as in many others, large doses of corticosteroids are required initially to induce remission.[123] In most patients, remission can then be maintained on very small doses of corticosteroids, which do not affect delayed hypersensitivity responses.[123,127] Discontinuance or further tapering of these maintenance doses may lead to renewed disease which once again requires large doses of corticosteroids for control. The mechanism for this commonly observed phenomenon is unclear.

In idiopathic thrombocytopenic purpura (ITP) there is a strong inverse correlation between platelet-bound IgG and platelet count. It has been shown that patients with ITP who respond to corticosteroid treatment with an increase in platelet count have a concomitant reduction in platelet-surface IgG to within the normal range.[128] However, abnormal serum platelet antibodies are not necessarily affected. Thus, the therapeutic effect of corticosteroids in this disease may be related to factors other than antibody production per se.

In summary, corticosteroids are effective in inducing remissions in type II autoimmune disease. In some of these diseases, such as pemphigus vulgaris, there appears to be a good correlation between corticosteroid efficacy and a decrease in autoantibody titers. In other diseases, including autoimmune hemolytic anemia and ITP, a decrease in autoantibody titers may occur but additional mechanisms, such as inhibition of reticuloendothelial system clearance, are probably involved. It is intriguing that corticosteroids appear to be capable of inhibiting autoantibody production despite their lack of inhibition of the normal humoral response. There is no explanation for this dichotomy at present.

Type III Reactions: Immune Complex Disorders

Corticosteroids are widely used in the treatment of immune complex disorders. It is generally agreed that their major effect on immune complex disease is anti-inflammatory.[129] Corticosteroids appear to provide marked symptomatic relief in these disorders without altering the fundamental disease processes.[130]

It is clear that corticosteroids fail to alter the natural course of rheumatoid arthritis.[130] This appears to be true for the most part in systemic lupus erythematosus as well, despite the fact that corticosteroid therapy is often associated with decreases in antinuclear antibody titers and in the frequency of positive LE cell preparations.[131,132] However, it remains highly controversial as to whether or not corticosteroids alter the course of lupus glomerulonephritis.[133-136] There are reports which indicate that high-dose corticosteroid therapy can significantly improve renal function and prolong survival in patients with this disease.[134-136]

Type IV Reactions: Cell-Mediated Reactions

Corticosteroids are potent inhibitors of cell-mediated immune reactions. They are used clinically in the treatment of allergic contact dermatitis[137] and for both prophylaxis against and treatment of graft rejection. Renal-transplant recipients are universally treated with combination immunosuppressive therapy which includes corticosteroids.[138,139] We will defer further discussion of the role of corticosteroids in the treatment of graft recipients until the section on combination immunosuppression.

AZATHIOPRINE

Azathioprine (AZA) is a synthetic purine analogue which functions as an antimetabolite and an immunosuppressive agent. It is a derivative of 6-mercaptopurine (6-MP) and, like 6-MP, has little or no intrinsic activity. All the thiopurines must be metabolically activated; they are thought to become functional upon transformation to the ribonucleotide form.[140]

The thiopurines interfere with all stages of purine metabolism, inhibiting DNA, RNA and protein synthesis in both quiescent and activated cells. Due to these actions they are cytotoxic agents. However, their immunosuppressive effects are felt to be independent of cytotoxic activity since they can be elicited at lower dosages.[140] Thus AZA is effective in the treatment of autoimmune disease at doses which do not cause lymphocytopenia, leukopenia or bone marrow depression.[140,141]

It has not been established to what extent the various thiopurines differ in their immunosuppressive actions. AZA is believed to be metabolized to 6-MP *in vivo* but its metabolic effects, although similar, are not identical to those of 6-MP.[140] AZA is generally preferred to 6-MP as an immunosuppressant because its toxicity is lower.[140]

Data on the mechanisms of AZA immunosuppression is inconclusive, providing no solid evidence for any primary site of action. There is evidence that AZA can inhibit T-cell function both *in vitro*[142,143] and *in vivo*.[144] However, AZA therapy results at best in only partial inhibition of T-cell function; in patients treated with AZA their response to specific antigens may be suppressed, but mitogen and alloantigen responsiveness does not appear to be affected.[144,145] In addition, patients treated with standard immunosuppressive doses of AZA may fail to exhibit significant suppression of cell-mediated immunity despite a clinical response to therapy.[146,147]

There is little evidence for any consistent effect of AZA on the normal humoral response. Although there have been several reports that AZA inhibits the humoral immune response and/or decreases serum immunoglobulin levels,[140,141,146,148] other studies have reported negative findings.[145-147,149] The fact that treatment with AZA is associated with an increased incidence of viral infections but not with an increase in bacterial infections has been taken as evidence against any major inhibition of humoral immunity.[139] Of interest, however, is a report that lymphocytes from patients treated with AZA fail to proliferate normally when challenged with pokeweed mitogen or anti-immunoglobulin serum.[145] It has also been reported that patients with inflammatory bowel disease treated with AZA show a significant decrease in plasma-cell infiltration on rectal lamina propria biopsy and a decrease in antibody-dependent cytotoxic activity.[150]

Part of the "immunosuppressive" effect of AZA may be due to a nonspecific anti-inflammatory action.[140,146,151] In animals, thiopurines appear to inhibit both monocyte production and function.[152,153] Similar data is not available in man.

It has been theorized that AZA immunosuppression is due to inhibition of rapidly dividing cells.[150] AZA may sterilize proliferating cell populations, causing "reproductive death."[154] It is also possible that chronic AZA administration prevents normal replacement of cells lost by attrition. This would be consistent with its delayed clinical efficacy and the fact that relapses which occur when AZA is discontinued are also delayed.[155,156]

Clinical Use

Although the data concerning its immunosuppressive actions is unimpressive, AZA has proved to be effective in the treatment of autoimmune disease. Due to its potential toxicity it is generally reserved for situations where corticosteroids alone are inadequate or ineffective. AZA is widely used at present in the combination immunosuppressive therapy of lupus glomerulonephritis and in renal-transplant recipients. It is also used to treat patients with rheumatoid arthritis who are refractory to other modes of therapy.[151,157,158]

Although AZA often fails to inhibit the normal humoral response, AZA treatment of patients with autoimmune disease is frequently associated with a decrease in autoantibody titers.[141,146,147,159] However, changes in autoantibody titers and other laboratory parameters of disease activity during AZA therapy do not always correlate with the degree of clinical improvement.[151,152,158,159]

Various reports attest to a lack of correlation between a clinical response to AZA and demonstrable inhibition of either cellular or humoral immunity in individual patients with autoimmune disease.[141,151,160] Thus the mechanisms by which AZA achieves its clinical efficacy remain unclear.

Lupus Nephritis. There is evidence that AZA is beneficial in the treatment of lupus nephritis. Significant improvement in renal function and histology has been documented in patients with lupus glomerulonephritis treated with a combination of AZA and corticosteroids.[133,161] Complete resolution of subendothelial deposits may be seen, associated with transformation from a predominantly proliferative to a membranous form of glomerulonephritis.[133] Controlled clinical studies have found that combined AZA and prednisone therapy is more effective than prednisone alone in terms of decreasing morbidity and mortality and improving renal function in patients with lupus nephritis.[160,162] However, other studies which have obtained good results with corticosteroid treatment have failed to find that AZA therapy confers significant additional benefit.[136,163-165]

Transplantation. The use of AZA in renal transplantation is discussed in the section of this chapter on combined immunosuppression.

CYCLOPHOSPHAMIDE

Cyclophosphamide (CPA), a phosphoric acid ester diamide, is the most potent immunosuppressant among the synthetic alkylating agents.[166] By alkylating and cross-linking DNA nucleotides, CPA causes latent damage which becomes lethal when cells enter DNA synthesis. It is especially toxic for cells with a high rate of mitosis, including lymphocytes and bone marrow cells among others.

When CPA is administered to man in standard immunosuppressive doses it causes a decrease in the absolute number of circulating B and T cells.[167,168] Long-term CPA therapy generally results in moderate to marked lymphopenia; total depletion of small lymphocytes from the circulation may be obtained.[169] CPA also decreases the number of circulating monocytes and polymorphonuclear leukocytes, although to a lesser degree.[170,171]

CPA must be metabolically activated *in vivo* and appears to have little, if any, activity *in vitro*.[166] Many of its effects are delayed in onset. There is generally a lag of several weeks before significant lymphopenia is seen, and months may be required.[167,168] Inhibition of lymphocyte function is similarly delayed.[172] This differs considerably from the immediate noncumulative effect of corticosteroids on lymphocytes.

CPA appears capable of inhibiting both B- and T-cell function in man. Investigators have reported inhibition of T-cell transformation by mitogens and specific antigens in CPA-treated individuals.[166,172] Lethal injury or inability of residual T cells to complete mitosis may be involved.[173]

Unlike corticosteroids and AZA, CPA is clearly able to inhibit the normal humoral response in man,[174] although it is ineffective if administered before a given antigen.[175] In certain circumstances, CPA also appears to be capable of inducing specific unresponsiveness to individual antigens.[175,176] Serum immunoglobulin levels often decrease during CPA therapy[169,170,172,177] and significant decreases in autoantibody titers are generally seen.[170,172]

Several investigators have reported that there is no change in the relative percentage of circulating B and T cells during CPA-induced lymphopenia.[168,178] However, in at least some patients with autoimmune disease on low-dose CPA maintenance therapy, B cells are depleted to a greater extent than T cells and B-cell function is preferentially inhibited.[179-181] Since CPA is most likely to affect cells which are actively dividing, it is possible that in low doses it could differentially inhibit those immune cells involved in disease activity, whether these be B or T cells.

CPA appears to have little direct effect on inflammation.[171,179] The dose of CPA can generally be adjusted so that lymphopenia is obtained without a significant leukopenia, and leukopenia does not appear to be necessary in order to obtain a good clinical response.[169,180]

Clinical Use

Clinical response to CPA frequently requires several months of therapy.[172] This lag period is compatible with the delayed effects of CPA on lymphocyte number and function.[169] However, on an individual basis there appears to be no direct correlation between clinical response to CPA and either the severity of lymphopenia or the degree of immunosuppression attained.[169,172,177]

CPA has been reported to be clinically effective in rheumatoid arthritis.[182-186] It is the drug of choice in the treatment of Wegener's granulomatosis.[171,187] CPA treatment of Wegener's granulomatosis has been associated with the disappearance of circulating immune complexes and the healing of renal lesions; long-term and possibly permanent remissions may be achieved.[171,187,188]

When used in conjunction with corticosteroids, CPA appears to be beneficial in the treatment of lupus nephritis.[170,189-191] There is evidence that CPA may be more effective than AZA in this disease.[190] However, the effectiveness of either cytotoxic agent relative to corticosteroid therapy alone remains controversial.[164]

CPA is also commonly used as an immunosuppressive agent for patients receiving bone marrow and renal transplants.[139,192] It has been of some value in controlling graft-versus-host disease in bone marrow recipients.[192] Despite the differences between AZA and CPA which we have outlined, it appears that CPA and AZA may be used interchangeably in renal transplantation[138] and in several of the autoimmune diseases.

ANTILYMPHOCYTE SERUM

Antilymphocyte serum is produced by injecting human lymphocytes into an animal and subsequently collecting its serum. If the immunoglobulin fraction is extracted from the collected serum and used alone, the product is referred to as antilymphocyte globulin (ALG). Unlike the other immunosuppressive agents we have discussed, antilymphocyte serum (ALS) is not a pure chemical compound. It is a complex biological product with inherent variability. Every batch of ALS differs somewhat from the next one. This variability is increased by the use of different animal species and different antigen sources.

ALG comprises the active fraction of ALS. It is assumed to act by binding to specific antigens on the lymphocyte surface. There is evidence that different antigens may be preferentially recognized on B and T lymphocytes.[193] Absorption of ALS with B cells leaves a serum which is fairly specific for T lymphocytes.[194]

ALS has multiple effects upon human lymphocytes *in vitro*. These include: inhibition of lymphocyte stimulation by specific antigens, alloantigens and mitogens; inhibition of lymphocyte cytotoxicity, both direct and antibody-mediated; inhibition of lymphocyte mobility and migration; inhibition of rosette formation; inhibition of plaque-forming cells; agglutination; lymphocyte opsonization; and complement-dependent cytotoxicity.[195] In high concentrations, ALS also has a direct mitogen-like effect causing blast transformation and proliferation.[195] The relative significance of these effects in terms of the *in vivo* immunosuppressive potency of ALS remains unclear. Some *in vitro* parameters (in particular rosette inhibition and opsonization) appear to correlate with the *in vivo* potency of a given batch of ALS whereas others do not.[195]

ALS is thought to be cytotoxic for lymphocytes *in vivo* as well as *in vitro*. Administration of ALS to human subjects causes a transient lymphocytopenia with selective depletion of small lymphocytes from the circulation.[196] There is evidence that both opsonization and direct lysis may be involved.[195,197] The relative contribution of lymphocytotoxicity to ALS immunosuppression is not known. In man, ALS-induced immunosuppression clearly outlasts lymphopenia,[196] suggesting that functional inhibition of lymphocytes is also involved.

The major effect of ALS is felt to be on cell-mediated immunity. Treatment of human subjects with ALS results in suppression of positive delayed hypersensitivity skin test reactions.[196] Blast transformation to PPD, PHA and in the MLR is also suppressed by ALS *in vivo*.[196,198] Suppression of cell-mediated immunity after ALS therapy can be prolonged for several weeks or more.[198,199]

ALS inhibition of T-cell function *in vitro* is reversible and demonstrably independent of lymphocyte destruction.[195,200,201] "Blindfolding" (blocking of antigen recognition sites) has been proposed as a possible mechanism of action. However, ALS remains inhibitory when it is added some time after a stimulatory antigen or mitogen;[200,202,203] thus other mechanisms must be involved.

The effect of ALS on the human humoral immune response has not been well characterized. Evidence from animal experiments suggests that ALS has virtually no direct inhibitory effect on B cells.[195,204] However, in man treatment with ALS has resulted in therapeutic response and remission with disappearance of autoantibodies in both type II and type III autoimmune disease.[205,206]

Animal data suggest that, in addition to its immunosuppressive action, ALS has a nonspecific anti-inflammatory effect.[195] A decrease in complement titers has been seen in human patients treated with ALS.[199,207] ALG may compete with inflammatory reactions for available complement and thus serve to diminish their intensity.

Clinical Use

Due to its method of production, several problems are encountered in the administration of ALS. At least one half of the patients treated with horse anti-human-lymphocyte globulin develop antibodies to equine IgG.[195,208] These antibodies interfere with intramuscular absorption of ALS and induce rapid clearance of ALS from the plasma, thus significantly diminishing its activity.[208] The appearance of antibodies in some patients has been correlated with a loss of suppression of preexisting delayed hypersensitivity reactions.[208] An immune response to ALS may also result in toxic side effects including anaphylactoid symptoms, serum sickness and, rarely, immune complex glomerulonephritis.[195,199] Another problem is specificity. ALS frequently contains antibodies against nonlymphoid antigens including red cells, platelets and kidney antigens; these are a potential source of significant toxicity.[195] Finally, the inherent variability of ALS makes assessment of its clinical efficacy difficult.

The primary use of ALS has been in the immunosuppression of renal-transplant recipients. ALS has also been used in bone marrow recipients both to prevent the development of graft-versus-host reactions and to reverse established graft-versus-host disease.[198,209,210] In addition, ALS has been used on a sporadic basis to treat patients with autoimmune diseases resistant to more conventional therapy. There have been no controlled clinical trials concerning the efficacy of ALS in autoimmune disease. There is a case report of ALG therapy resulting in significant clinical improvement in dermatomyositis, with resolution of lymphoid infiltrates on muscle biopsy.[211] ALG therapy (alone or with CPA) has also been reported to induce remission in pure red-cell aplasia, with disappearance of circulating autoantibodies.[206]

COMBINED IMMUNOSUPPRESSIVE THERAPY

Combination immunosuppression is employed clinically in situations where no one immunosuppressant has proved adequate. The use of various combinations is empirical; it is based on clinical efficacy and patient tolerance rather than on theoretical considerations. The management of the immunosuppressed patient involves a continuous battle to suppress undesired immune processes without destroying vital immune defenses against infectious agents. This involves considerable adjustment of dosages for each individual patient with frequent modifications over time. Wide individual variations in disease course and response to therapy make it difficult to assess immunosuppressive regimens. In this setting it is extremely difficult to determine whether one protocol is superior to another.

The current major use of long-term combination immunosuppressive therapy is in renal transplantation. Renal transplantation first became practical with the introduction of combination immunosuppression in the early 1960's, when azathioprine and prednisone were found to be reasonably effective when used together.[138] This has remained the basic regimen. Common variations include the substitution of CPA for azathioprine and the addition of ALG for the first few months postoperatively.

Immunosuppression of transplant recipients must be continued indefinitely, although the initial doses required for effective immunosuppression can be tapered over time. In general, an attempt is made to taper corticosteroids to a minimum while the cytotoxic drug used is continued at a standard dose, adjusted to avoid significant leukopenia and other toxic side effects. Occasionally corticosteroids may be discontinued altogether; however, attempts to taper or discontinue corticosteroids can precipitate rejection.[138,212]

Three basic types of rejection occur in transplant recipients despite immunosuppression (see Chap. 9). Intense short-term treatment with high-dose corticosteroids is effective in reversing approximately 80 per cent of acute cell-mediated rejection crises.[213] However, hyperacute rejection and chronic rejection are essentially irreversible.[138]

The frequency of renal rejection and of various complications of therapy has led to clinical trials with triple drug therapy. It was hoped that the addition of a third agent might allow decreased doses of corticosteroids and azathioprine, with a potential reduction in toxic side effects. Combined corticosteroid, azathioprine and ALG therapy is in fairly widespread use at present. A controlled trial of azathioprine and corticosteroids with and without ALG in cadaveric transplantation showed that the addition of ALG was associated with a decreased frequency of graft failure due to rejection, increased graft survival and improved renal function in surviving grafts. There was, however, no decrease in fatalities due to infections or other drug complications.[214,215]

The most striking benefit of ALG appears to be a decrease in the incidence of acute rejection episodes.[215] It has been suggested that this may be due to the marked inhibitory effect of ALG on T cells.[216] Addition of ALG to azathioprine and prednisone results in a significant decrease in the number of circulating T cells and the degree of mitogen responsiveness *in vitro*.[216] In addition to prophylaxis against rejection, ALG is also effective in reversing acute rejection crises.[217]

The value of ALG in renal transplantation is still controversial.[205] It remains to be demonstrated whether or not triple drug therapy will be associated with an ultimate increase in patient survival.[138]

Except for questions of individual toxicity there is no demonstrated or apparent advantage to the substitution of CPA for azathioprine in either double or triple drug therapy.[138] Despite the differences between these drugs that we have already enumerated, they seem to serve equivalent functions in the immunosuppression of allograft rejection.

REFERENCES

1. Baxter, J. D., and Forsham, P. H.: Tissue effects of glucocorticoids. Am. J. Med., *53*:573, 1972.
2. Rauch, H. C., Loomis, M. E., Johnson, M. E., and Favour, C. B.: *In vitro* suppression of polymorphonuclear leukocyte and lymphocyte glycolysis by cortisol. Endocrinology, *68*:375, 1961.
3. Tormey, D. C., Fudenberg, H. H., and Kamin, R. M.: Effect of prednisolone on the synthesis of DNA and RNA by human lymphocytes *in vitro*. Nature, *213*:281, 1967.
4. Smith, R. S., Sherman, N. A., and Middleton, E., Jr.: Effect of hydrocortisone on immunoglobulin synthesis and secretion by human peripheral lymphocytes *in vitro*. Int. Arch. Allergy Appl. Immunol., *43*:859, 1972.
5. Elmadjian, F., and Pincus, G.: A study of the diurnal variations in circulating lymphocytes in normal and psychotic subjects. J. Clin. Endocrinol., *6*:287, 1946.
6. Addison, T.: On the Constitutional and Local Effects of Disease of the Suprarenal Capsules. London, S. Highly, 1855.
7. Gordon, A. S.: Some aspects of hormonal influences upon the leukocytes. Ann. N.Y. Acad. Sci., *59*:907, 1955.
8. Dougherty, T. F.: Effect of hormones on lymphatic tissue. Physiol Rev., *32*:379, 1952.
9. Claman, H. N.: Corticosteroids and lymphoid cells. N. Engl. J. Med., *287*:388, 1972.
10. Seyle, H.: Thymus and adrenals in the response of the organism to injuries and intoxications. Br. J. Exp. Pathol., *17*:234, 1936.
11. Claman, H. N., Moorhead, J. W., and Benner, W. H.: Corticosteroids and lymphoid cells *in vitro*. I. Hydrocortisone lysis of human, guinea pig and mouse thymus cells. J. Lab. Clin. Med., *78*:499, 1971.
12. Fauci, A. S., and Dale, D. C.: The effect of *in vivo* hydrocortisone on subpopulations of human lymphocytes. J. Clin. Invest., *53*:240, 1974.
13. Yu, D. T. Y., *et al.*: Human lymphocyte subpopulations: Effect of corticosteroids. J. Clin. Invest., *53*:565, 1974.
14. Webel, M. L., Ritts, R. E., Jr., Taswell, H. F., Donadio, J. V., and Woods, J. E.: Cellular immunity after intravenous administration of methylprednisolone. J. Lab. Clin. Med., *83*:383, 1974.
15. Novak, E., Stubbs, S. S., Seckman, C. E., and Hearron, M. S.: Effects of a single large intravenous dose of methylprednisolone sodium succinate. Clin. Pharmacol. Ther., *11*:711, 1970.
16. Fauci, A. S.: Corticosteroids and circulating lymphocytes. Transplant. Proc., *7*:37, 1975.
17. ———: Mechanisms of corticosteroid action on lymphocyte subpopulations I. Redistribution of circulating T and B lymphocytes to bone marrow. Immunology, *28*:669, 1975.
18. Cohen, J. J.: Thymus-derived lymphocytes sequestered in the bone marrow of hydrocortisone treated mice. J. Immunol., *108*:841, 1972.
19. Moorhead, J. W., and Claman, H. N.: Thymus-derived lymphocytes and hydrocortisone. Identifications of subsets of theta-bearing cells and redistribution to bone marrow. Cell. Immunol., *5*:74, 1972.
20. Fauci, A. S., and Dale, D. C.: Alternate day prednisone therapy and human lymphocyte subpopulations. J. Clin. Invest., *55*:22, 1975.
21. Coburg, A. F., *et al.*: Disappearance rates and immunosuppression of intermittent intravenously administered prednisolone in rabbits and human beings. Surg. Gynecol. Obstet., *131*:933, 1970.
22. Cheigh, J. S., Stenzel, K. H., Riggio, R. R., Katz, E. B., and Rubin, A. L.: Effects of intravenous methylprednisolone on mixed lymphocyte cultures in normal humans. Transplant. Proc., *7*:31, 1975.
23. Chai, H., and Gilbert, A.: The effect of alternate-day prednisone on the white blood count in children with chronic asthma. J. Allergy Clin. Immunol., *51*:65, 1973.
24. Fauci, A. S., Dale, D. C., and Balow, J. E.: Glucocorticosteroid therapy: Mechanisms of action and clinical considerations. Ann. Intern. Med., *84*:304, 1976.
25. Caron, G. A.: Prednisolone inhibition of DNA synthesis by human lymphocytes induced *in vitro* by PHA. Int. Arch. All. Appl. Immunol., *32*:191, 1967.
26. Heilman, D. H., and Leichner, J. P.: Effect of cortisol on the transformation of human blood lymphocytes by antigens and allogeneic

leucocytes. *In* Schwarz, M. R. (ed.): Proc. 6th Leucocyte Culture Conf. P. 581. New York, Academic Press, 1972.

27. Bach, J. F.: Corticosteroids. *In* The Mode of Action of Immunosuppressive Agents. P. 21. Amsterdam, North Holland, Publ., 1975.
28. Cohen, J. J., and Claman, H. N.: Thymus-marrow immunocompetence V. Hydrocortisone-resistant cells and processes in the hemolytic antibody response of mice. J. Exp. Med., *133*:1026, 1971.
29. Cohen, I. R., Stavy, L., and Feldman, M.: Glucocorticoids and cellular immunity *in vitro*. Facilitation of the sensitization phase and inhibition of the effector phase of a lymphocyte antifibroblast reaction. J. Exp. Med., *132*:1055, 1970.
30. Heilman, D. H.: Failure of hydrocortisone to inhibit blastogenesis by pokeweed mitogen in human leucocyte cultures. Clin. Exp. Immunol., *11*:393, 1972.
31. Peter, J. B.: Cytotoxins produced by human lymphocytes: inhibition by anti-inflammatory steroids and anti-malarial drugs. Cell. Immunol., *2*:199, 1971.
32. Balow, J. E., and Rosenthal, A. S.: Glucocorticoid suppression of macrophage migration inhibitory factor. J. Exp. Med., *137*:1031, 1973.
33. Griggs, R. C., Condemi, J. J., and Vaughan, J. H.: Effect of therapeutic dosages of prednisone on human immunoglobulin G metabolism. J. Allergy Clin. Immunol., *49*:267, 1972.
34. Butler, W. T.: Corticosteroids and immunoglobulin synthesis. Transplant. Proc., *7*:49, 1975.
35. Butler, W. T., and Rossen, R. D.: Effect of methylprednisolone on immunoglobulin metabolism in man. Fed. Proc., *32*:1028A, 1973.
36. McMillan, R., Longire, R., and Yelenosky, R.: The effect of corticosteroids on human IgG synthesis. J. Immunol., *116*:1592, 1976.
37. Bach, J. F.: Recent advances in steroid therapy. *In* Hamburger, J., Crosnier, J., and Maxwell, M. H.: Advances in Nephrology. Vol. 5, p. 173. 1975.
38. Ambrose, C.: The essential role of CS in the induction of the immune response *in vitro*. *In* Wolstenholme, G. E. W., and Knight, J.: Hormones and the Immune Response. (Ciba Foundation Study Group 36) P. 100. London, J. A. Churchill, 1970.
39. Dale, D. C., Fauci, A. S., and Wolff, S. M.: Alternate day prednisone-leukocyte kinetics and susceptibility to infections. N. Engl. J. Med., *291*:1154, 1974.
40. Rinehart, J. J., Sagone, A. L., Balcerzak, S. P., Ackerman, G. A., and LoBuglio, A. F.: Effects of CS therapy on human monocyte function. N. Engl. J. Med., *292*:236, 1975.
41. Rinehart, J. J., Balcerzak, S. P., Sagone, A. L., and LoBuglio, A. F.: Effect of CS on human monocyte function. J. Clin. Invest., *54*:1337, 1974.
42. Schreiber, A. D., Parsons, J., McDermott, P., and Cooper, R. A.: Effect of CS on the human monocyte IgG and complement receptors. J. Clin. Invest., *56*:1189, 1975.
43. Weston, W. L., Mandel, M. J., Krueger, G. C., and Claman, H. N.: Differential suppressive effect of hydrocortisone on lymphocytes and mononuclear macrophages in delayed hypersensitivity of guinea pigs. J. Invest. Dermatol., *59*:345, 1972.
44. Weston, W. L., Mandel, M. J., Yedley, J. A., Krueger, G. C., and Claman, H. N.: Mechanisms of cortisol inhibition of adoptive transfer of tuberculin sensitivity. J. Lab. Clin. Med., *82*:366, 1973.
45. Bishop, C. R., *et al.*: Leukokinetic studies XIII. A non-steady state kinetic evaluation of the mechanism of cortisone-induced granulocytosis. J. Clin. Invest., *47*:249, 1968.
46. Boggs, D. R., Athens, J. W., Carthwright, G. E., and Wintrobe, M. M.: The effect of adrenal glucocorticosteroids upon the cellular composition of inflammatory exudates. Am. J. Pathol., *44*:763, 1964.
47. McKenzie, A. W., and Stoughton, R. B.: Method for comparing percutaneous absorption of steroids. Arch. Dermatol., *86*:608, 1962.
48. Greeson, T. P., Levan, N. E., Freedman, R. I., and Wong, W. H.: CS-induced vasoconstriction studied by xenon 133 clearance. J. Invest. Dermatol., *61*:242, 1973.
49. Maiback, H., and Stoughton, R. B.: Topical CS. *In* Azarnoff, D. L.: Steroid Therapy. P. 174. Philadelphia, W. B. Saunders, 1975.
50. MacGregor, R. R., Spagnuolo, P. J., and Lentnek, A. L.: Inhibition of granulocyte adherence by ethanol, prednisone, and aspirin measured with an assay system. N. Engl. J. Med., *291*:642, 1974.
51. Ebert, R. H., and Barclay, W. R.: Changes in connective tissue reaction induced by cortisone. Ann. Intern. Med., *37*:506, 1952.
52. Juhlin, L., and Michaelsson, G.: Cutaneous vascular reactions to prostaglandins in healthy subjects and in patients with urticaria and atopic dermatitis. Acta Derm. Venereol., *49*:251, 1969.
53. Greaves, M. W., and McDonald-Gibson, W.: Prostaglandin biosynthesis by human skin and its inhibition by CS. Br. J. Pharmacol., *46*:172, 1972.
54. Schayer, R. W.: A unified theory of glucocorticoid action II. On a circulatory basis for the metabolic effects of glucocorticoids. Perspect. Biol. Med., *10*:409, 1967.
55. Cline, M. J., and Melmon, K. L.: Plasma kinins and cortisol: a possible explanation of the anti-inflammatory action of cortisol. Science, *153*:1135, 1966.
56. Atkinson, J. P., and Frank, M. M.: Effect of cortisone therapy on serum complement components. J. Immunol., *111*:1061, 1973.
57. Kirkpatrick, C., and Rosenthal, A. S.: Glucocorticoids and allergic reactions. *In* Azarnoff, D. L.: Steroid Therapy. P. 238. Philadelphia, W. B. Saunders, 1975.
58. Gewurz, H., Wernick, P. R., Quie, P. G., and

Good, R. A.: Effects of hydrocortisone succinate on the complement system. Nature, *208*:755, 1965.

59. Eisen, V., Greenbaum, L., and Lewis, G. P.: Kinins and anti-inflammatory steroids. Br. J. Pharmacol., *34*:169, 1968.
60. Lefer, A. M., and Inge, T. F., Jr.: Lack of interactions between glucocorticoids and the kallikrein-kinin system. Proc. Soc. Exp. Biol. Med., *145*:658, 1974.
61. Ketchel, M. M., Favour, C. B., and Sturgis, S. H.: The *in vitro* action of hydrocortisone on leukocyte migration. J. Exp. Med., *107*:211, 1958.
62. Rebuck, J. W., and Mellinger, R. C.: Interruption by topical cortisone of leukocytic cycles in acute inflammation in man. Ann. N.Y. Acad. Sci., *56*:715, 1953.
63. Crepea, S. B., Magnin, G. E., and Seastone, C. V.: Effect of ACTH and cortisone on phagocytosis. Proc. Soc. Exp. Biol. Med., *77*:704, 1961.
64. Mandell, G. L., Rubin, W., and Hook, E. W.: The effect of an NADH oxidase inhibitor (hydrocortisone) on polymorphonuclear leukocyte bactericidal activity. J. Clin. Invest., *49*:1381, 1970.
65. Chretien, J. H., and Garaguai, V. F.: CS effect on phagocytosis and NBT reduction by human polymorphonuclear neutrophils. J. Reticuloendothel. Soc., *11*:358, 1972.
66. Ruutu, T., and Kosunen, T. U.: *In vitro* effect of anti-inflammatory agents on phagocytosis and bacterial killing by human neutrophilic leukocytes. Acta Pharmacol. Toxicol., *31*:226, 1972.
67. Cooper, M. R., DeChatelet, R., and McCall, C. E.: The *in vitro* effect of steroids on polymorphonuclear leukocyte metabolism. Proc. Soc. Exp. Biol. Med., *141*:986, 1972.
68. Miller, D. R., and Kaplan, H. G.: Decreased nitroblue tetrazolium dye reduction in the phagocytes of patients receiving prednisone. Pediatrics, *45*:861, 1970.
69. Lotz, M.: The effect of adrenal steroids and sterile filtrates of bacteria on chemotaxis of polymorphonuclear leukocytes *in vitro*. Lab. Invest., *12*:593, 1963.
70. Allison, F., Jr., and Adcock, M. H.: Failure of pretreatment with glucocorticoids to modify the phagocytic and bactericidal capacity of human leukocytes for encapsulated type I pneumococcus. J. Bacteriol., *89*:1256, 1965.
71. Renner, E. D., Webel, N. L., and Ritts, R. E., Jr.: The effect of methylprednisolone on leukocyte function. J. Reticuloendothel. Soc., *14*:530, 1973.
72. Matula, G., and Paterson, P. Y.: Spontaneous *in vitro* reduction of nitroblue tetrazolium by neutrophils of adult patients with bacterial infection. N. Engl. J. Med., *285*:311, 1971.
73. Feldman, D., Funder, J. W., and Edelman, I. S.: Subcellular mechanisms in the actions of adrenal steroids. Am. J. Med., *53*:545, 1972.
74. Cake, M. H., and Litwack, G.: The glucocorticoid receptor. *In* Litwack, G.: Biochemical Actions of Hormones. Vol. 3, p. 317. New York, Academic Press, 1975.
75. Lippman, M. E., Halterman, R. H., Levanthal, B. G., Perry, S., and Thompson, E. B.: Glucocorticoid-binding proteins in human acute lymphoblastic leukemic blast cells. J. Clin. Invest., *52*:1715, 1973.
76. Rosenfeld, M., G., *et al.*: Control of transcription of RNA rich in polyadenylic acid in human lymphocytes. Proc. Natl. Acad. Sci. U.S.A., *69*:2306, 1972.
77. Werthamer, S., Pachter, B., and Amaral, L.: Protein synthesis in human leukocytes and lymphocytes 4. The effect of cortisol on RNA and protein synthesis in lymphocytes. Life Sci. [II], *10*:1039, 1971.
78. Mendelsohn, J., Multer, M. M., and Boone, R. F.: Enhanced effects of prostaglandin E1 and dibutycyl cyclic AMP upon human lymphocytes in the presence of cortisol. J. Clin. Invest., *52*:2129, 1973.
79. Hedeskow, C. J., and Esmann, V.: Major metabolic pathways of glucose in normal human lymphocytes and the effect of cortisol. B and B Acta, *148*:372, 1967.
80. Hallahan, C., Young, D. A., and Munck, A.: Time course of early events in the action of glucocorticoids on rat thymus cells *in vitro*. J. Biol. Chem., *248*:2922, 1973.
81. Frengley, P. A., Lichtman, M. A., and Peck, W. A.: Specificity and sensitivity of cortisol-induced changes in alpha aminoisobutyric acid transport in human leukemic small lymphocytes and leukemic myeloblasts. J. Clin. Invest., *52*:1518, 1973.
82. Baran, D. T., Lichtman, M. A., and Peck, W. A.: Alpha aminoisobutyric acid transport in human leukemic lymphocytes: *in vitro* characteristics and inhibition by cortisol and cycloheximide. J. Clin. Invest., *51*:2181, 1972.
83. Bourne, H. R., *et al.*: Modulation of inflammation and immunity by cyclic AMP. Science, *184*:19, 1974.
84. Parker, C. W., Huber, M. G., and Baumann, M. L.: Alterations in cyclic AMP metabolism in human bronchial asthma III. Leukocyte and lymphocyte responses to steroids. J. Clin. Invest., *52*:1342, 1973.
85. Coffey, R. G., Logsdon, P. J., and Middleton, E., Jr.: Effect of glucocorticosteroids on leukocyte adenyl cyclase and ATPase of asthmatic and normal children. J. Allergy Clin. Immunol., *49*:87A, 1972.
86. Logsdon, P., Middleton, E., Jr., and Coffey, R. G.: Stimulation of leukocyte adenyl cyclase by hydrocortisone and isoproterenol in asthmatic and non-asthmatic subjects. J. Allergy Clin. Immunol., *50*:45, 1972.
87. Thompson, E. B., and Lippman, M. E.: Mechanism of action of glucocorticoids. Metabolism, *23*:159, 1974.
88. de Duve, C., Wattiaux, R., and Wibo, M.: Effects of fat-soluble components on lysosomes *in vitro*. Biochem. Pharmacol., *9*:97, 1962.

89. Goldstein, I. M.: Effect of steroids on lysosomes. Transplant. Proc., *7*:21, 1975.
90. Weissmann, G., Sessa, G., and Weissmann, S.: The action of steroids and triton X-100 upon phospholipid/cholesterol structures. Biochem. Pharmacol., *15*:1537, 1966.
91. Weissmann, G.: Effects of CS on the stability and fusion of biomembranes. *In* Austen, K. F., and Lichtenstein, L. M.: Asthma. P. 221. 1973.
92. ———: Lysosomal mechanisms of tissue injury in arthritis. N. Engl. J. Med., *286*:141, 1972.
93. Hirschhorn, R., Grossman, J., Troll, W., and Weissmann, G.: The effect of epsilon amino caproic acid and other inhibitors of proteolysis upon the response of human peripheral blood lymphocytes to PHA. J. Clin. Invest., *50*:1206, 1971.
94. Hirschhorn, R., Brittinger, G., Hirshhorn, K., and Weissmann, G.: Studies on lysosomes XII. Redistribution of acid hydrolases in human lymphocytes stimulated by PHA. J. Cell Biol., *37*:412, 1968.
95. Persellin, R. H., and Ku, L. C.: Effect of steroid hormones on human PMN leukocyte lysosomes. J. Clin. invest., *54*:919, 1974.
96. Lewis, D. A., and Day, E. H.: Biochemical factors in the actions of steroids on diseased joints in rheumatoid arthritis. Ann. Rheum. Dis., *31*:374, 1972.
97. Bitensky, L., Butcher, R. G., Johnstone, J. J., and Chayen, J.: Effect of glucocorticoids on lysosomes in synovial lining cells in human rheumatoid arthritis. Ann. Rheum. Dis., *33*:57, 1974.
98. Hench, P. S., Kendall, E. C., Slocumb, C. H., and Polley, H. F.: The effect of a hormone of the adrenal cortex and of pituitary ACTH on rheumatoid arthritis. Preliminary report. Proc. Staff Meetings Mayo Clin., *24*:181, 1949.
99. Hench, P. S., *et al.*: The effects of the adrenal cortical hormone 17-hydroxy-11-dehydrocorticosterone on the acute phase of rheumatic fever. Preliminary report. Proc. Staff Meetings May Clin., *24*:277, 1949.
100. Cope, C. L.: C.S. therapy in specific diseases. *In* Adrenal Steroids and Disease. P. 569. Philadelphia, J. B. Lippincott, 1972.
101. Dale, D. C., and Petersdorf, R. G.: CS and infectious diseases. *In* Azarnoff, D. L.: Steroid Therapy. P. 209. Philadelphia, W. B. Saunders, 1975.
102. Patterson, R.: Rhinitis. Med. Clin. North Am., *58*:43, 1974.
103. Sulzberger, M. B.: Atopic dermatitis—Part III. *In* Fitzpatrick, T. B., *et al.*: Dermatology in General Medicine. P. 687. New York, McGraw-Hill, 1971.
104. Livingstone, J. L., and Davies, J. P.: Steroids in the long term treatment of asthma. Lancet, *1*:1310, 1961.
105. Ellu-Micallef, R., Barthwick, R. C., and McHardy, G. J. R.: The time course of response to prednisolone in chronic bronchial asthma. Clin. Sci. Mol. Med., *47*:105, 1974.
106. Medical Research Council: Controlled trial of effects of cortisone acetate in status asthmaticus. Lancet, *2*:798, 1956.
107. Criep, L. H.: Clinical Immunology and Allergy. Ps. 231–254; 282–307. New York, Grune & Stratton, 1969.
108. Richerson, H. B.: Symptomatic treatment of adults with bronchial asthma. Med. Clin. North Am., *58*:135, 1974.
109. Brown, H. M., Storey, G., and George, W. H. S.: Beclomethasone dipropionate: a new steroid aerosol for the treatment of allergic asthma. Br. Med. J., *1*:585, 1972.
110. Kettel, L. J., and Morse, J. O.: Corticosteroids in the treatment of pulmonary disease. *In* Azarnoff, D. L.: Steroid Therapy. P. 287. Philadelphia, W. B. Saunders, 1975.
111. Aviado, D. M., and Carrilo, L. R.: Antiasthmatic action of corticosteroids: a review of the literature on their mechanism of action. J. Clin. Pharmacol., *10*:3, 1970.
112. Townley, R. G., Reeb, R., Fitzgibbons, T., and Adolphson, R.: The effect of corticosteroids on the β adrenergic receptors in bronchial smooth muscle. J. Allergy, *45*:118, 1970.
113. Townley, R. G., Honrath, T., and Guirgis, H. M.: The inhibitory effect of hydrocortisone on the alpha adrenergic responses of human and guinea pig isolated respiratory smooth muscle. J. Allergy Clin. Immunol., *49*:88, 1972.
114. Kaliner, M., and Austen, K. F.: A sequence of bronchial events in the antigen induced release of chemical mediators from sensitized human lung tissue. J. Exp. Med., *138*:1077, 1973.
115. Callerane, M. L., *et al.*: Immunoglobulins in bronchial tissues in asthma with special reference to IgE. J. Allergy, *47*,187, 1971.
116. Kuman, L., Newcomb, R. W., Ishizaka, K., Middleton, E., Jr., and Hornbrook, M. M.: IgE levels in sera of children with asthma. Pediatrics, *47*:848, 1971.
117. McCombs, R. P.: Disease due to immunologic reactions in the lungs. N. Engl. J. Med., *286*:1186, 1972.
118. Schwartz, H. J., Lowell, F. C., and Melby, J. C.: Steroid resistance in bronchial asthma. Ann. Intern. Med., *69*:493, 1968.
119. Lowell, F. C.: Changing steroid resistance in asthma. J. Allergy, *45*:131, 1970.
120. Green, M., and Lim, K. H.: Bronchial asthma with Addison's disease. Lancet, *1*:1159, 1971.
121. Hicks, R.: The effects of drug induced adrenocortical deficiency and of mineralocorticoid drugs on anaphylaxis in the guinea pig. J. Pharm. Pharmacol., *20*:497, 1968.
122. Atkinson, J. P., and Frank, M. M.: Glucocorticoids in the treatment of hemolytic disorders. *In* Azarnoff, D. L.: Steroid Therapy. P. 49. Philadelphia, W. B. Saunders, 1975.
123. Lever, W. F.: Pemphigus. *In* Fitzpatrick, T., *et al.*: Dermatology in General Medicine. P. 644. New York, McGraw-Hill, 1971.
124. Atkinson, J. P., Schreiber, A. D., and Frank, M. M.: Effect of CS and splenectomy on the im-

mune clearance and destruction of erythrocytes. J. Clin. Invest., *52*:1509, 1973.

125. Rosse, W. F.: Quantitative immunology of immune hemolytic anemia II. The relationship of cell-bound antibody to hemolysis and the effect of treatment. J. Clin. Invest., *50*:734, 1971.
126. Evans, R. S., Bingham, M., and Boehni, P.: Autoimmune hemolytic disease. Arch. Intern. Med., *108*:338, 1961.
127. Rabhan, N. B., and Kopf, A. W.: Alternate day prednisone therapy for pemphigus vulgaris—preliminary report. Arch. Dermatol., *103*:615, 1971.
128. Dixon, R., Rosse, W., and Ebert, L.: Quantitative determination of antibody in idiopathic thrombocytopenic purpura. N. Engl. J. Med., *292*:230, 1975.
129. Claman, H. N.: How CS work. J. Allergy Clin. Immunol., *55*:145, 1975.
130. Gifford, R. H.: CS therapy for rheumatoid arthritis. *In* Azarnoff, D. L.: Steroid Therapy. P. 78. Philadelphia, W. B. Saunders, 1975.
131. Yount, W. J., Utsinger, P. D., Hadler, N. M., and Gammon, W. R.: CS therapy of the collagen vascular disorders. *In* Azarnoff, D. L.: Steroid Therapy. P. 269. Philadelphia, W. B. Saunders, 1975.
132. Shulman, L. E., and Harvey, A. M.: Systemic lupus erythematosus. *In* Hollander, J. L., and McCarty, D. J., Jr.: Arthritis and Allied Conditions. P. 893. Philadelphia, Lea & Febiger, 1972.
133. Hecht, B., Siegel, N. J., Kashgarian, M., and Hayslett, J. P.: Lupus nephritis: natural history and treatment. *In* Suki, W. N., and Eknoyan, G.: The Kidney in Systemic Disease. P. 21. New York, Wiley, 1976.
134. Pollak, V. E., Pirani, C. L., and Schwartz, F. D.: The natural history of the renal manifestations of SLE. J. Lab. Clin. Med., *63*:537, 1964.
135. Ackerman, G. L.: Alternate day steroid therapy in lupus nephritis. Ann. Intern. Med., *72*:511, 1970.
136. Donadio, J. V., Jr., Holley, K. E., Wagon, R. P., Ferguson, R. H., and McDuffie, F. C.: Treatment of lupus nephritis with prednisone and combined azathioprine and prednisone. Ann. Intern. Med., *77*:829, 1972.
137. Feuerman, E., and Levy, A.: A study of the effect of prednisone and an anti-histamine on patch test reactions. Br. J. Dermatol., *86*:68, 1972.
138. Starzl, T. E., Porter, K. A., Husberg, B. S., Ishikawa, M., and Putnam, C. W.: Renal homotransplantation—Part I. Curr. Probl. Surg., April, 1974.
139. Hamburger, J., Crosnier, J., Dormont, J., and Bach, J. F.: Renal Transplantation—Theory and Practice. P. 77. Boston, Williams & Wilkins, 1972.
140. Bach, J. F.: Thiopurines, the Mode of Action of Immunosuppressive Agents. P. 93. Amsterdam, North-Holland Publ., 1975.
141. Swanson, M. A., and Schwartz, R. S.: Immunosuppressive therapy: the relationship between clinical response and immunologic competence. N. Engl. J. Med., *277*:163, 1967.
142. Bach, M. A., and Bach, J. F.: Activities of immunosuppressive agents *in vitro*—different timing of azathioprine and methotrexate in inhibition and stimulation of mixed lymphocyte reaction. Clin. Exp. Immunol., *11*:89, 1972.
143. Smith, J. L., and Forbes, I. J.: Inhibition of protein synthesis in human lymphocytes by thiopurines. Aust. J. Exp. Biol. Med. Sci., *48*:267, 1970.
144. Zweiman, B., Abdou, N. I., Casella, S. R., Lisak, R. P., and Silverberg, D. H.: Azathioprine-induced selective immunosuppression in man. Clin. Res., *20*:523, 1972.
145. Abdou, N. I., Zweiman, B., and Casella, S. R.: Effects of azathioprine therapy on bone marrow-dependent and thymus-dependent cells in man. Clin. Exp. Immunol., *13*:55, 1973.
146. Deman, E. J., Denman, A. M., Greenwood, B. M., Gall, D., and Heath, R. B.: Failure of cytotoxic drugs to suppress immune responses of patients with rheumatoid arthritis. Ann. Rheum. Dis., *29*:220, 1970.
147. Levy, J., Barnett, E. V., MacDonald, N. S., Klinenberg, J. R., and Pearson, C. M.: The effect of azathioprine on gammaglobulin synthesis in man. J. Clin. Invest., *51*:2233, 1972.
148. Maibach, H. I., and Epstein, W. L.: Immunologic responses of healthy volunteers receiving azathioprine. Int. Arch. Allergy, *27*:102, 1965.
149. Lee, A. K. Y., MacKay, I. R., Rowley, M. J., and Yap, C. Y.: Measurement of antibody-producing capacity to flagellin in man. Clin. Exp. Immunol., *9*:507, 1971.
150. Campbell, A. C., *et al.*: Immunosuppression in the treatment of inflammatory bowel disease. Clin. Exp. Immunol., *16*:521, 1974.
151. Dodson, W. H., and Bennett, J. C.: Possible usefulness of azathioprine in severe rheumatoid arthritis. J. Clin. Pharmacol., *9*:251, 1969.
152. Van Furth, R., Thompson, J., and Gassmann, A. E.: The kinetics of mononuclear phagocytes during normal steady-state conditions, acute infection, and the effects of glucocorticosteroids and azathioprine. *In* Braun, W., and Ungar, J.: Non-specific Factors Influencing Host Resistance—A Re-examination. P. 79. Basel, Karger, 1973.
153. Phillips, S. M., and Zweiman, B.: Mechanisms in the suppression of delayed hypersensitivity in the guinea pig by 6-MP. J. Exp. Med., *137*:1494, 1973.
154. Berenbaum, M. C.: Immunosuppressive agents and allogeneic transplantation. J. Clin. Pathol., *20*:471, 1967.
155. Yu, D. T. Y., *et al.*: Lymphocyte characteristics in rheumatic patients and the effect of azathioprine therapy. Arthritis Rheum., *17*:37, 1974.
156. Sharon, E., Kaplan, D., and Diamond, H. S.:

Exacerbation of SLE after withdrawal of azathioprine therapy. N. Engl. J. Med., *288*:122, 1973.
157. Hunter, T., Urowitz, M. B., Gordon, D. A., Smythe, H. A., and Osryzlo, M. A.: Azathioprine in rheumatoid arthritis. A long term follow-up study. Arthritis Rheum., *18*:15, 1975.
158. Urowitz, M. B., Gordon, D. A., Smythe, H. A., Pruzanski, W., and Ogryzlo, M. A.: Azathioprine treatment of rheumatoid arthritis. Double-blind crossover study. Arthritis Rheum., *14*:419, 1971.
159. Drinkard, J. P., *et al.*: Azathioprine and prednisone in the treatment of adults with lupus nephritis. Medicine, *49*:411, 1970.
160. Sztejnbok, M., Stewart, A., Diamond, H., and Kaplan, D.: Azathioprine in the treatment of systemic lupus erythematosus—a controlled study. Arthritis Rheum., *14*:639, 1971.
161. Hayslett, J. P., Kashgarian, M., Cook, C. D., and Spargo, B. H.: The effect of azathioprine on lupus glomerulonephritis. Medicine, *51*:393, 1972.
162. Cade, R., *et al.*: Comparison of azathioprine, prednisone and heparin alone or combined in treating lupus nephritis. Nephron, *10*:37, 1973.
163. Donadio, J. V., Jr., Holley, K. E., Wagoner, R. D., Ferguson, R. H., and McFuffie, F. C.: Further observations on the treatment of lupus nephritis with prednisone and combined prednisone and azathioprine. Arthritis Rheum., *17*:573, 1974.
164. Decker, J. L., Kippel, J. H., Plotz, P. H., and Steinberg, A. D.: Cyclophosphamide or azathioprine in lupus glomerulonephritis—a controlled trial: Results at 28 months. Ann. Intern. Med., *83*:606, 1975.
165. Hahn, B. H., Kantor, O. S., and Oaterland, C. K.: Azathioprine plus prednisone compared with prednisone alone in the treatment of SLE—report of a prospective controlled trial in 24 patients. Ann. Intern. Med., *83*:597, 1975.
166. Bach, J. F.: Alkylating agents. *In* The mode of Action of Immunosuppressive Agents. P. 173. Amsterdam, North-Holland Publ., 1975.
167. Hurd, E. R., and Giuliano, V. J.: The effect of cyclophosphamide on B and T lymphocytes in patients with connective tissue disease. Arthritis Rheum., *18*:67, 1975.
168. Clements, P. J., Yu, D. T. Y., Levy, J., Paulus, H. E., and Barnett, E. V.: Effects of cyclophosphamide on B and T lymphocytes in rheumatoid arthritis. Arthritis Rheum., *17*:347, 1974.
169. Hurd, E. R., and Ziff, M.: Parameters of improvement in patients with rheumatoid arthritis treated with CPA. Arthritis Rheum., *17*:72, 1974.
170. Steinberg, A. D., *et al.*: CPA in lupus nephritis: a controlled trial. Ann. Intern. Med., *75*:165, 1971.
171. Wolff, S. M., Fauci, A. S., Horne, R. G., and Cale, D. C.: Wegener's granulomatosis. Ann. Intern. Med., *81*:513, 1974.
172. Alepa, F. P., Zvaifler, N. J., and Sliwinski, A. J.: Immunologic effects of CPA treatment in rheumatoid arthritis. Arthritis Rheum., *13*:754, 1970.
173. Winkelstein, A., Mikulla, J. M., Nankin, H. R., Pollock, B. H., and Stolzer, B. L.: Mechanism of immunosuppression: effects of CPA on lymphocytes. J. Lab. Clin. Med., *80*:506, 1972.
174. Santos, G. W., Owens, A. H., Jr., and Sensenbrenner, L. L.: Effect of selected cytotoxic agents on antibody production in man: a preliminary report. Ann. N.Y. Acad. Sci., *114*:404, 1964.
175. Santos, G. W., Burke, P. J., Sensenbrenner, L. L., and Owens, A. H., Jr.: Rationale for the use of CPA as an immunosuppressant for marrow transplants in man. *In* Bertelli, A., and Mooaco, A. P.: Pharmacological Treatment in Organ and Tissue Transplantation. Int. Congress Series No. 197. P. 24. Amsterdam, Excerpta Medica Foundation, 1970.
176. Stein, R. S., and Colman, R. W.: Hemophilia with factor VIII inhibitor–elimination of anamnestic response. Ann. Intern. Med., *79*:84, 1973.
177. Strong, J. S., Bartholomew, B. A., and Smyth, C. J.: Immunoresponsiveness of patients with rheumatoid arthritis receiving CPA or gold salts. Ann. Rheum. Dis., *32*:233, 1973.
178. Keith, H. I., and Currey, H. L. F.: Rosette formation by peripheral blood lymphocytes in rheumatoid arthritis. Ann. Rheum. Dis., *32*:202, 1973.
179. Fauci, A. S., Dale, D. C., and Wolff, S. M.: CPA and lymphocyte subpopulation in Wegener's granulomatosis. Arthritis Rheum., *17*:355, 1974.
180. Horwitz, D. A.: Selective depletion of immunoglobulin bearing lymphocytes by CPA in rheumatoid arthritis and systemic lupus erythematosus. Arthritis Rheum., *17*:363, 1974.
181. ——: Selective depletion of human circulating B lymphocytes by CPA. Fed. Proc., *32*:980, 1973.
182. Fosdick, W. M., Parsons, J. L., and Hill, D. F.: Preliminary report: long term CPA therapy in rheumatoid arthritis. Arthritis Rheum., *11*:151, 1968.
183. Levy, J., Paulus, H. E., and Bangert, R.: Comparison of azathioprine and CPA in the treatment of rheumatoid arthritis. Arthritis Rheum., *18*:412, 1975.
184. Townes, A. S., Sowa, J. M., and Shulman, L. E.: Controlled trial of CPA in rheumatoid arthritis: an 18 month double-blind crossover study. Arthritis Rheum., *15*:129A, 1972.
185. Ainland, D. M., and Decker, J. L.: A controlled trial of CPA in rheumatoid arthritis: a preliminary report. Arthritis Rheum., *12*:680, 1969.
186. Cooperating Clinics Committee of the American Rheumatism Association: A controlled trial of CPA in rheumatoid arthritis. N. Engl. J. Med., *283*:843, 1970.
187. Reza, M. J., Dornfeld, L., Goldberg, L. S., Blue-

stone, R., and Pearson, C. M.: Wegener's granulomatosis—long term follow-up of patients treated with CPA. Arthritis Rheum., *18*:501, 1975.

188. Howell, S. B., and Epstein, W. V.: Circulating immunoglobulin complexes in Wegener's Granulomatosis. Am. J. Med., *60*:259, 1976.
189. Cameron, J. S., Boulton-Jones, M., Robinson, R., and Ogg, C.: Treatment of lupus nephritis with CPA. Lancet, *2*:846, 1970.
190. Steinberg, A. D., and Decker, J. L.: A double blind controlled trial comparing CPA, azathioprine and placebo in the treatment of lupus glomerulonephritis. Arthritis Rheum., *17*:923, 1974.
191. Hadidi, T.: CPA in systemic lupus erythematosus. Ann. Rheum. Dis., *29*:673, 1970.
192. Santos, G. W., *et al.*: Marrow transplantation in man following CPA. Transplant. Proc., *3*:400, 1971.
193. Zimmerman, B.: Lymphocyte plasma membranes V. Specificity and mitogenicity of absorbed antilymphocyte sera. J. Immunol., *115*:701, 1975.
194. Woody, J. N., Ahmed, A., Knudsen, R. C., Strong, D. M., and Sell, K. W.: Human T-cell heterogeneity as delineated with a specific human thymus lymphocyte antiserum. J. Clin. Invest., *55*:956, 1975.
195. Bach, J. F.: Antilymphocyte sera. *In* The Mode of Action of Immunosuppressive Agents. P. 227. Amsterdam, North-Holland Publ., 1975.
196. Reveillard, J. P., and Brochier, J.: Selective deficiency of cell-mediated immunity in humans treated with antilymphocyte globulins. Transplant. Proc., *3*:725, 1971.
197. Chanard, J., Bach, J. F., Assailly, J., and Funck-Brentano, J. L.: Hepatic homing of labelled lymphocytes in man. Br. Med., *2*:502, 1972.
198. Storb, R., *et al.*: Treatment of established human graft vs. host disease by antithymocyte globulin. Blood, *44*:57, 1974.
199. Traeger, J., *et al.*: Studies of anti-lymphocyte globulins made from thoracic duct lymphocytes—two and a half years' experience in kidney transplantation. *In* Bertelli, A., and Monaco, A. P.: Pharmacologic Treatment in Organ and Tissue Transplantation. Int. Congress Series No. 197. P. 315. Amsterdam, Excerpta Medica Foundation, 1970.
200. Owen, F. L., and Fanger, M. W.: Studies on the human T-lymphocyte population I. The development and characterization of a specific anti-human T-cell antibody. J. Immunol., *113*:1128, 1974.
201. Gallagher, M. T., Richie, E. R., and Trentin, J. J.: Inhibition of allograft reactivity *in vitro* and *in vivo* by Fab fragments obtained from ALG. Transplant. Proc., *5*:869, 1973.
202. Eijswoogel, V. P., Dubois, M. J. G. J., Schellekens, P. Th. A., and Van Loghem, J. J.: The stimulating and suppressive properties of anti-lymphocyte serum on lymphocyte transformation *in vitro*. Transplant. Proc., *1*:408, 1969.
203. Lundgren, G.: Induction and suppression of the cytotoxic activity of human lymphocytes *in vitro* by heterologous antilymphocyte serum. Clin. Exp. Immunol., *5*:381, 1969.
204. Editorial. Current status of antilymphocyte globulin. Br. Med. J., *1*:644, 1975.
205. Pirofsky, B., Reid, R. H., Bardana, E. J., Jr., and Bayracki, C.: Antithymocyte antisera therapy in non-surgical immunologic disease. Transplant. Proc., *3*:769, 1971.
206. Marmont, A., Peschle, C., Sanguinetti, M., and Condorelli, M.: Pure red cell aplasia: reponse of three patients to cyclophosphamide and/or antilymphocyte globulin and demonstration of two types of serum IgG inhibitors to erythropoiesis. Blood, *45*:247, 1975.
207. Botha, M. C.: Serologic observations relating to the clinical use of horse anti-human lymphocyte globulin. *In* Bertelli, A., and Monaco, A. P.: Pharmacologic Treatment in Organ and Tissue Transplantation. Int. Congress Series No. 197. P. 265. Amsterdam, Excerpta Medica Foundation, 1970.
208. Butler, W. T., and Rossen, R. D.: Increasing effectiveness of antilymphocytic globulin by prevention of antibody formation to horse IgG. Transplant. Proc., *3*:733, 1971.
209. Gengozian, N., Edwards, C. L., Vodopick, H. A., and Hubner, K. F.: Bone marrow transplantation in a leukemic patient following immunosuppression with antithymocyte globulin and total body irradiation. Transplantation, *15*:446, 1973.
210. Mathe, G., *et al.*: Bone marrow graft in man after conditioning by antilymphocyte serum. Transplant. Proc., *3*:325, 1971.
211. Brendel, W., Land, W., and Pichlmayr, R.: Intravenous treatment with horse anti-human lymphocyte globulin in organ transplantation and autoimmune diseases. *In* Bertelli, A., and Monaco, A. P.: Pharmacologic Treatment in Organ and Tissue Transplantation. Int. Congress Series No. 197. P. 208. Amsterdam, Excerpta Medica Foundation, 1970.
212. Turcotte, J. G., Dickerman, R. M., and Harper, M. L.: Minimum steroid requirements in the late post-transplant period. Transplant. Proc., *7*:83, 1975.
213. Kountz, S. L.: Clinical transplantation—an overview. Transplant. Proc., *5*:59,1973.
214. Sheil, A. G. R., *et al.*: A controlled trial of antilymphocyte globulin therapy in man. Transplant. Proc., *4*:501, 1972.
215. ——: Causes of allograft failure in recipients treated with and without antilymphocyte globulin. Transplant. Proc., *5*:561, 1973.
216. Thomas, F., *et al.*: Studies of thymus-derived and bone marrow-derived lymphocytes in renal transplant patients. Am. Surg., *41*:738, 1975.
217. Traeger, J., Touraine, J. L., Fries, D., and Berthous, F.: Evaluation of intravascular route for administration of antilymphocyte globulin in humans. Transplant. Proc., *3*:749, 1971.

Appendix A: Complement

THE CLASSICAL PATHWAY

The classical complement pathway involves eleven components, all of which are glycoproteins. They are all fairly large molecules and their molecular weights as well as their serum concentrations are shown in *Table A-1*.[1] C3 is the most abundant of the complement components. Several of the complement components are heat-labile, including C1q, C1r, C2, C6 and C8.[2] This property is often applied experimentally to heat inactive complement in a serum sample.

Initiation

The classical pathway is initiated by the binding of C1q to either IgM or IgG. The Fc segments of immunoglobulin molecules express the C1q binding site, which for IgG is part of the C_{H2} domain.[3] IgG_3 and IgG_1 bind C1q well, IgG_2 binds C1q poorly, and IgG_4 does not bind C1q at all.[4] However, the Fc fragment of IgG_4 is capable of binding C1q even though the intact molecule is not,[5] indicating that the $F(ab)_2$ portion of the intact molecule may prevent complement fixation by the Fc segment.

One molecule of pentameric IgM can activate the complement pathway whereas at least two adjacent molecules of IgG appear to be required.[6] The requirement for proximity between IgG molecules for complement activation may be important in certain clinical situations. Thus, anti-RhD IgG generally does not activate complement, probably because the D antigen is sparsely distributed on the red-cell surface. On the other hand, IgG directed against the more densely distributed ABO antigens will often activate complement.[7]

Recent elucidation of the structure of C1q offers a graphic illustration of why activation may involve multiple binding to more than one Fc segment.[8] Figure 2-15 shows that C1q resembles a six-flower bouquet. It has been proposed that the six globular carboxy-terminal heads are the Fc combining sites.[9]

The C1 component is actually a com-

Table A-1. Properties of the Classical Complement Components

Component	*Serum Conc. (μg./ml.)*	*Sedimentation Coeff.(S)*	*Mol. Wt.*
C1q	150–200	11	400,000
C1r	——	7.5	180,000
C1s	~ 100	4.5	86,000
C2	~ 25	4.5	117,000
C3	1600	9.5	180,000
C4	640	10	206,000
C5	~ 80	8.7	180,000
C6	~ 75	5.5	95,000
C7	~ 55	6.0	110,000
C8	~ 80	8.0	163,000
C9	~ 250	4.5	79,000

plex of C1q, C1r and C1s which are bound together in the presence of calcium (Fig. A-1).[10] It is felt that the binding of C1q to complement-fixing immunoglobulin molecules produces a conformational change in the C1q component (Fig. A-2). The altered C1q then activates the C1r proenzyme to an active enzyme, $C\overline{1}r$.[11] The substrate of $C\overline{1}r$ is C1s which is cleaved to give the activated $C\overline{1}s$.[12] $C\overline{1}s$ is an active serine esterase[13] analogous to trypsin, and is comprised of two subunits.

C4, C2 and the Formation of the C3 Esterase

$C\overline{1}s$ can cleave (1) C4 into a large fragment, C4b, and a small fragment, C4a, and (2) C2 into large (C2a) and small (C2b) fragments.[14,15] These cleavages result in the production of the molecular complex, $C\overline{4b2a}$, which is an active esterase.[16] This occurs in the following way (Fig. A-3). The cleavage of C4 exposes a membrane-binding site on C4b. C4b will attach to the antigen against which the initiating antibody has been directed,[17] but at a different site than that occupied by the antibody-C1 complex.[18] C2a will bind to C4b and this complex is capable of cleaving C3.[16,19] C3 is the only natural substrate of $C\overline{42}$. The enzymatic site of the esterase is believed to reside in the C2a component.[20] Nevertheless, it is only the bimolecular complex $C\overline{42}$ that is capable of cleaving C3.

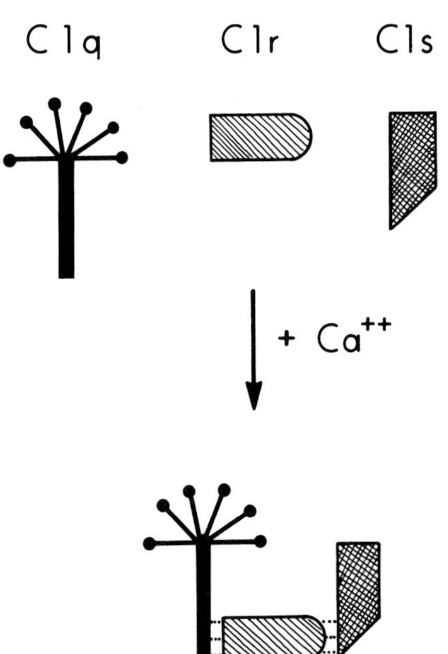

Fig. A-1. The C1 molecule is composed of three parts, C1q, C1r and C1s, which associate in the presence of calcium.

C3 Activation

The C3 esterase, $C\overline{42}$, can split C3 into C3a and C3b (Fig. A-4). C3a is a small fragment of C3 with a molecular weight of about 9,000. Some molecules of C3b associate with the membrane-bound $C\overline{42}$ complex but, like C4b, C3b is also capable of nonspecifically binding to the surface of the antigen.[19] The association of C3b with $C\overline{42}$ modulates the activity of the C3 convertase, shifting its substrate spectrum to C5. The $C\overline{423b}$ complex is referred to as C5 convertase.[21]

C5 through C9

C5 convertase ($C\overline{423b}$) cleaves C5 in a manner that is analogous to the cleavage of C3 by $C\overline{42}$ (Fig. A-5). A small fragment, C5a, is split off, leaving behind the major C5b fragment. The C5b fragment then can bind one molecule each of C6 and C7. This trimolecular complex can bind nonspecifically to membranes via the C5b component.[22] As with the other complement components that bind nonspecifically to membranes (C4b and C3b), C5b can bind to sites distant from the C5 convertase. This is illustrated by the finding that the terminal complement components can attach to, and initiate the lysis of, cells that do not bind C1-4.[23] The phenomenon of complement-mediated lysis of unsensitized cells via the nonspecific adsorption of $C\overline{5b67}$ has been termed reactive lysis.[24] One can imagine the dangers of such a phenomenon in the destruction of "innocent" host cells during an immune response. How-

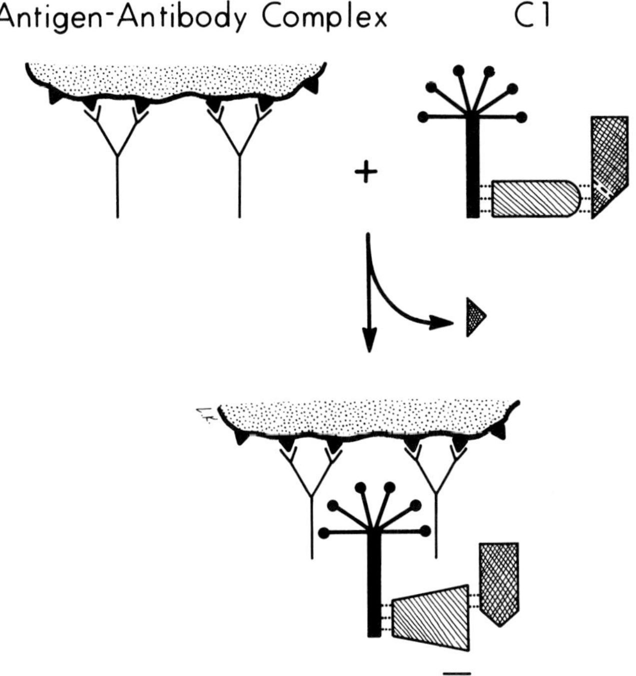

Fig. A-2. C1 is activated by antigen-antibody complexes when it reacts with the Fc portion of the antibody.

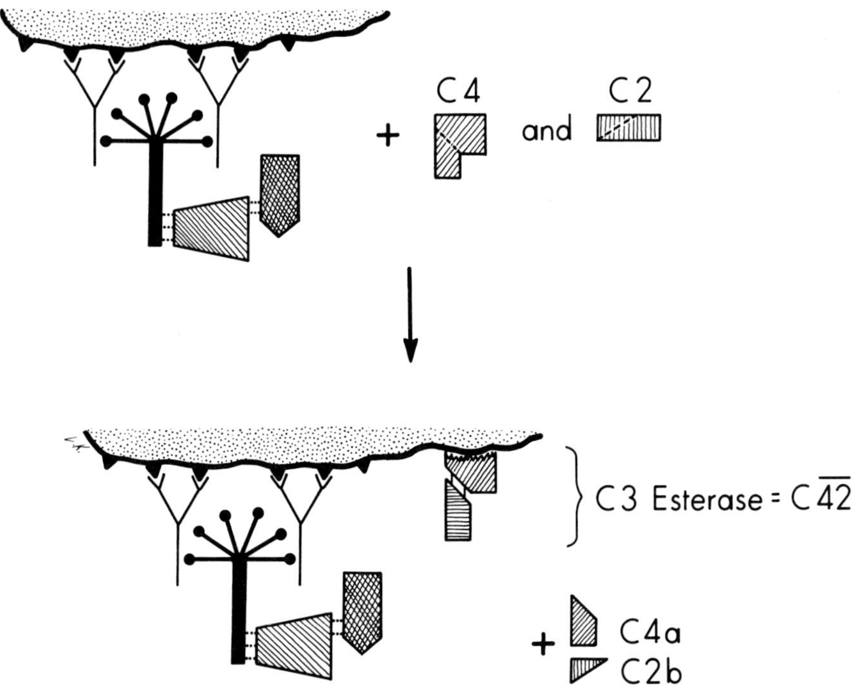

Fig. A-3. Formation of the C3 esterase.

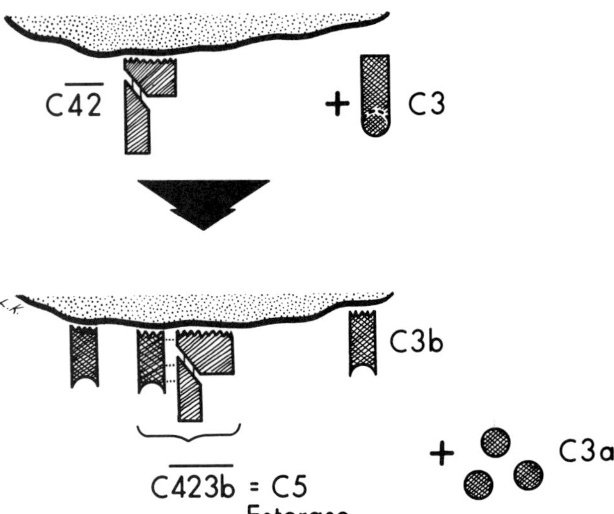

Fig. A-4. The activation of C3 by C$\overline{42}$ and the formation of the C5 esterase.

ever, the free complex is unstable and its ability to adsorb to cells decays rapidly.[25]

The C$\overline{5b67}$ complex provides the binding site for one molecule of C8 (Fig. A-6).[26]

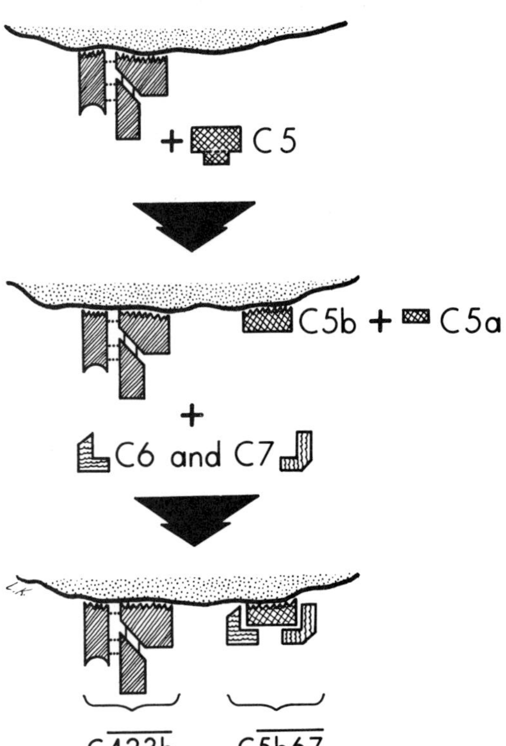

Fig. A-5. The activation of C5 and formation of the C$\overline{5b67}$ complex.

With the addition of C8, the 4-component complex induces a low-grade lesion in the membrane to which it is attached.[27] The C$\overline{5b678}$ complex can also bind C9.[26] Six molecules of C9 can be bound, forming a 10-component complex with a molecular weight of greater than 1,000,000.[26] The lysis of the cell by C$\overline{5b678}$ is greatly enhanced by the additional binding of the C9 molecules. Whether or not C9 is actually required to complete cell lysis is not known.

Mechanisms of Lysis

The precise mechanism by which the C$\overline{5b6789}$ complex induces cell lysis is unknown. C8 is required but may not itself make contact with the membrane. It has often been suggested that the lytic event is caused by an enzymatic attack on the membrane, although the evidence for this is slight.[28] An alternate hypothesis is that some part of the C$\overline{5b678}$ complex can insert itself into the membrane and thereby disrupt its structural integrity.[1] Some part of the C5b molecule is a likely candidate for this insertion.

The lesions produced by complement have been visualized by electron microscopy (Figure 1-15).[29] These lesions may represent hydrophilic "holes" that de-

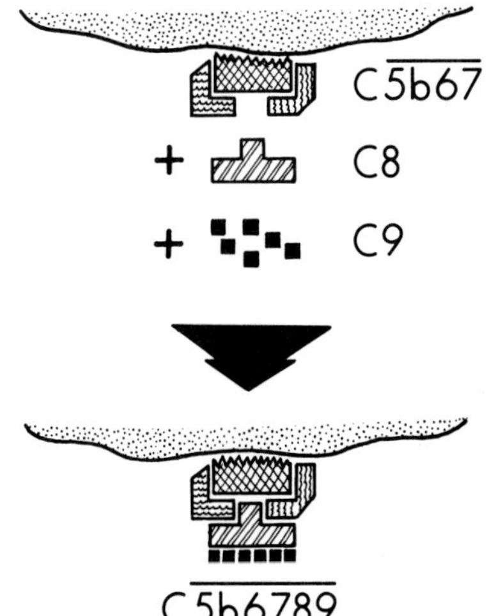

Fig. A-6. Formation of the lytic complex C$\overline{5b6789}$.

stroy the osmotic barrier of the membrane and allow it to become leaky to intra- and extracellular ions.[30] The destruction of this barrier results in cell death.

Amplification in the Complement Pathway

Complement has been described as a cascade, much like the blood coagulation system. There are several points along the pathway at which one molecule or molecular complex leads to the activation of many subsequent molecules. The C$\overline{1}$ complex is capable of generating many C$\overline{42}$ complexes. C$\overline{42}$ can generate many molecules of C3b. However, only one molecular complex of C$\overline{423b}$ can be generated for each C$\overline{42}$. Each C$\overline{423b}$ complex can activate a considerable number of molecules of C5, thereby producing many molecules of C$\overline{5b\text{-}9}$.[1]

Many, and perhaps most, of the molecules of C3b formed do not associate with C$\overline{42}$ in such a way as to produce an active C5 convertase. Therefore, although the amplification cascade proceeds up through the cleavage of C5, there may be more molecules of C3 split and activated than there are activated molecules of C5.

Immune Adherence

C4b and C3b can mediate immune adherence. An antigen coated with either of these molecules can attach to cells bearing surface receptors for these components. This observation indicates that C3b and C4b are bifunctional molecules. We have already seen that the activation of C4 and C3 produces fragments (C4b and C3b respectively) that readily bind to the surface of antigens. Presumably, activation results in the formation of a binding site that allows these molecules to "stick" to the surface of antigens. Activation also results in the exposure of the adherence sites by which the fragments specifically bind to their respective receptors on phagocytes and lymphocytes (see Fig. A-7).

THE PROPERDIN PATHWAY

The details of the properdin pathway are still incompletely understood and information concerning the early events of properdin pathway activation is rapidly changing. As mentioned in Chapter 1, the properdin pathway provides a means of generating a C3 esterase, analogous to C$\overline{42}$. The following is the list of the important components of the properdin pathway (see Table A-2):

1. *Properdin* is a glycoprotein consisting of four similar subunits and having a molecular weight of about 185,000. Properdin appears to exist in both inactive and biologically active ($\overline{P}$) forms.[31]

2. *C3 proactivator Convertase (C3PAse)* appears to be a single-chain molecule with a molecular weight of about 24,000.[1] C3 proactivator convertase is also referred to as factor D.[32] This molecule may also exist in an active and inactive form. The nature of the activation process is not known but the activated form possesses enzymatic activity.[33]

3. *C3 Proactivator (C3PA)*[33] is also called factor B and "glycine-rich beta-

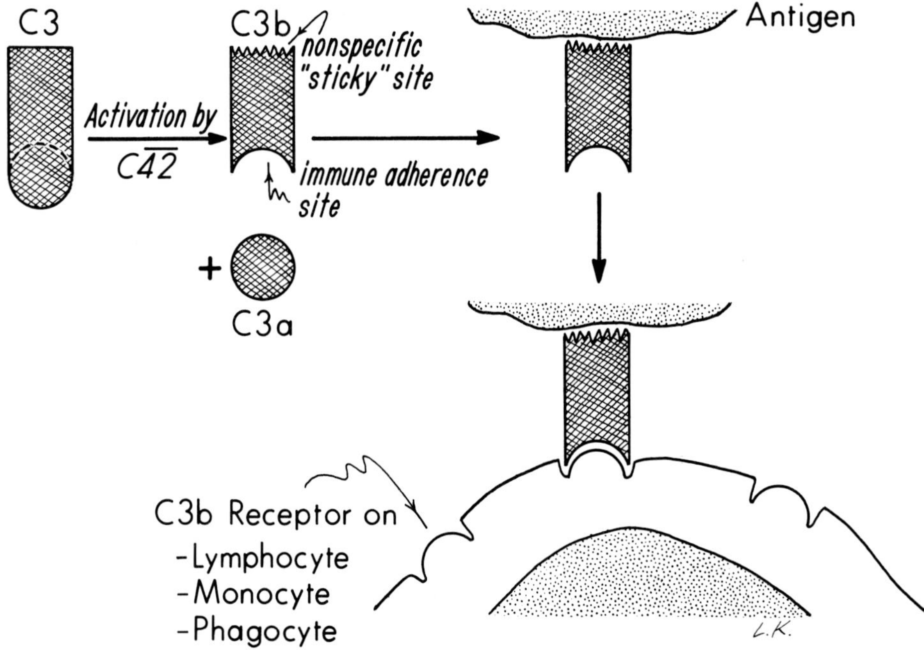

Fig. A-7. Activation of C3 by C$\overline{42}$ produces C3b, a bifunctional molecule. One end binds nonspecifically to antigens, the other binds to C3b receptors on lymphocytes or other receptor-bearing cells.

globulin."[34,35] The molecule has a molecular weight of about 93,000. It is activated to produce C3 activator (C3A) by cleavage which removes an inert 30,000 molecular weight fragment.[36]

4. *C3b.* This molecule, which is the major fragment of activated C3, is a crucial component of the properdin pathway.[37]

The Activation Sequence (Fig. A-8)

The presence of C3b may be an essential step in the activation of the alternate C3 esterase. C3b binds to C3PA which allows C3PA to be acted upon by the activated C3PAse ($\overline{D}$). This results in the cleavage of C3PA (B) leaving the fragment that is referred to as Bb in association with C3b as the bimolecular complex $\overline{\text{C3bBb}}$.[1] This complex possesses the enzymatic C3 splitting activity. The actual esteratic site is on the Bb molecule.[38]

$\overline{\text{C3bBb}}$ is a labile complex and dissociates readily. The function of P seems to be to bind to and stabilize this complex.[39] The $\overline{\text{C3bBb}}$ complex can be assembled on cell surfaces. For example, erythrocytes can be coated with C3b and, in the presence of B and $\overline{D}$, can activate more C3 as well as the rest of the com-

Table A-2. Properties of the Components of the Properdin Pathway

Component	*Symbol*	*Sedimentation Coeff.(S)*	*Mol. Wt.*
Properdin	P	5.4	184,000
C3	C3	9.5	180,000
C3b	C3b	9.0	172,000
C3 proactivator	C3PA, B	5–6	93,000
C3 activator	C3A, $\overline{B}$	4	63,000
C3 proactivator convertase	C3PAse, $\overline{D}$	3	24,000

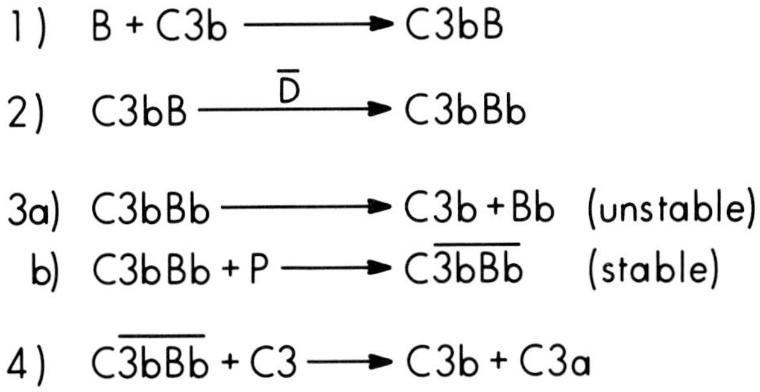

Fig. A-8. The properdin pathway: activation of the alternate C3 esterase.

1) $B + C3b \longrightarrow C3bB$

2) $C3bB \xrightarrow{\overline{D}} C3bBb$

3a) $C3bBb \longrightarrow C3b + Bb$ (unstable)

b) $C3bBb + P \longrightarrow \overline{C3bBb}$ (stable)

4) $\overline{C3bBb} + C3 \longrightarrow C3b + C3a$

plement sequence (C5–9) leading to the lysis of the red cell.[40]

The role of C3b in the properdin pathway illustrates an important positive feedback cycle in the generation of the alternate C3 convertase.[37] As $\overline{C3bBb}$ is generated, C3 is split, leading to the production of more C3b which, in the presence of B and $\overline{D}$, would generate more $\overline{C3bBb}$ and therefore more C3b and so on (Fig. A-9).

We have avoided the question of how factor D and properdin become activated since no definite answer to this has yet emerged. It is well documented that a variety of substances such as immunoglobulin, endotoxin, inulin and others can activate the properdin pathway, but the manner in which they accomplish this is not yet understood.

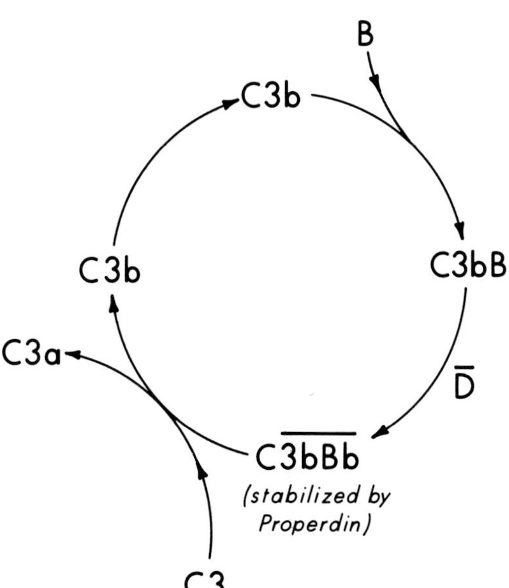

Fig. A-9. The C3b feedback cycle in the properdin pathway.

There is another factor which may play a role in the activation of the properdin pathway. This is the C3 nephritic factor which has been reported to be present in the sera of several patients with membranoproliferative glomerulonephritis.[41] It is a nonimmunoglobulin gammaglobulin with a molecular weight of about 150,000 and is capable of activating the properdin complement pathway. C3NeF may be a normal serum component that is found in high amounts in these patients. One of its functions may be similar to that of properdin in stabilizing $\overline{C3bBb}$.

CONTROLS OVER COMPLEMENT ACTIVATION

In Chapter 1 we mentioned the existence of several inhibitors of complement activity that are present in normal serum.

1. *C1 Esterase Inhibitor* forms a stable one-to-one complex with C1s and inhibits the enzymatic activity of that component.[42] The consequences of the absence of this inhibitor in hereditary angioneurotic edema are discussed in Chapter 10, The Immunodeficiency Diseases.

2. *C3b Inactivator or KAF.* This molecule splits C3b into two factors, C3c and C3d[43] resulting in the loss of enzymatic activity of both $\overline{C423b}$ and $\overline{C3bBb}$.[37,44] This cleavage also results in

the loss of the C3b immune adherence function.[45] KAF may also split and inactivate C4b.

3. *A Serum Carboxypeptidase* can inactivate both C5a and C3a.[46] Finally, C42 and C5b67 decay rapidly in the serum, limiting the range and time span of action of these molecules.[25,47]

MOLECULAR STRUCTURE OF COMPLEMENT COMPONENTS

Very recent work has begun to elucidate the molecular structure of various complement components. The electron micrographs of C1q (discussed earlier) have followed a greater conceptualization of the structure-function relationship of that molecule. Structural analysis of C3 has resulted in the following model (Fig. A-10):[1,48] C3 convertase splits the small C3a fragment from the alpha chain producing C3b. KAF can then further degrade the alpha chain by producing two sequential cleavages:

1. The first cleavage occurs very rapidly with the removal of a 25,000 molecular weight fragment and the loss in the ability of C3b to participate in the properdin pathway.

2. The second cleavage occurs more slowly as KAF cleaves off an additional 14,000 molecular weight piece. At this time it is not exactly clear which KAF cleavage products are C3d and C3c although the C3c is the larger molecule and contains both the beta and some part of the alpha chain.

There is little firm data on the structure of the other complement components. It has been suggested, however, that C4 and C5 have structures analogous to the C3 molecule.

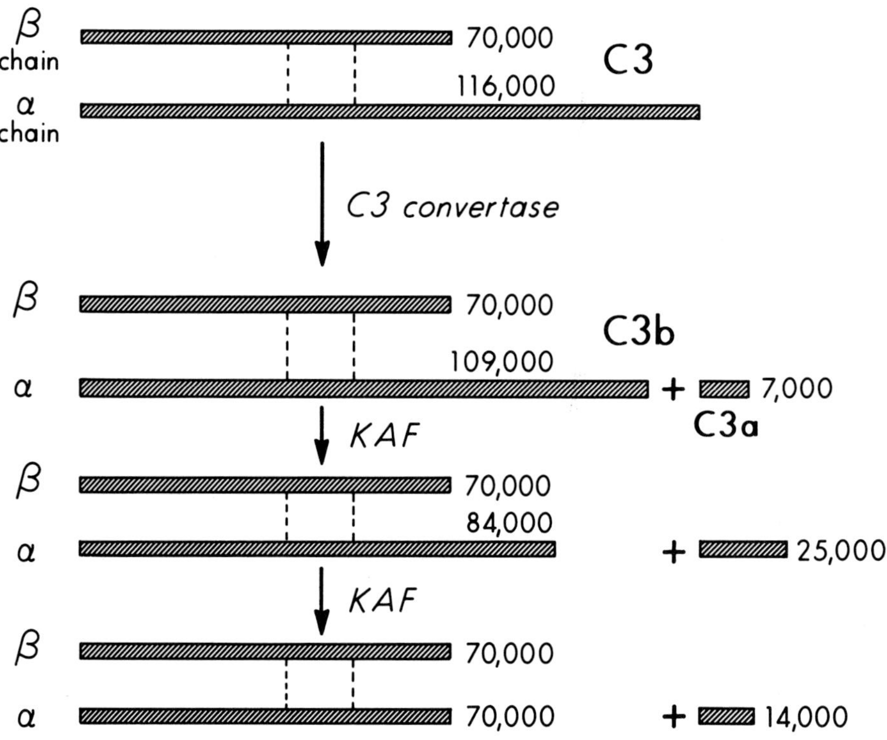

Fig. A-10. Structure and sequential enzymatic degradation of C3.

REFERENCES

1. Müller-Eberhard, H. J.: Complement. Ann. Rev. Biochem., *44*:697, 1975.
2. Lachmann, P. J.: *In* Hobart, M. J., and McDowell, I. (eds.): The Immune System: A Course. P. 54. Oxford, Blackwell Scientific Publications, 1975.
3. Kehoe, J. M., and Fougereau, M.: Immunoglobulin peptide with complement fixing activity. Nature, *224*:1212, 1969.
4. Augener, W., Grey, H. M., Cooper, N. R., and Müller-Eberhard, H. J.: The reaction of monomeric and aggregated immunoglobulins with C1. Immunochemistry, *8*:1011, 1971.
5. Isenman, D. E., Dorrington, K., and Painter, R. H.: The structure and function of immunoglobulin domains. J. Immunol., *114*:1726, 1975.
6. Borsos, T., and Rapp, H. J.: Complement fixation on cell surfaces by 19S and 7S antibodies. Science, *150*:505, 1965.
7. Rosse, W. F.: The detection of small amounts of antibody on the red cell in autoimmune hemolytic anemia. Ser. Haematol., *7*:358, 1974.
8. Knobel, H. R., Villiger, W., and Isliker, H.: Chemical analysis and electron microscopy studies of human C1q prepared by different methods. Eur. J. Immunol., *5*:78, 1975.
9. Isliker, H., *et al.*: Interaction of C1q with IgG and fragments thereof. Adv. Biosci., *12*:270, 1974.
10. Lepow, I. H., *et al.*: Chromatographic resolution of the first component of human complement into 3 activities. J. Exp. Med., *117*:983, 1963.
11. Valet, G., and Cooper, N. R.: Isolation and characterization of the proenzyme form of the C1r subunit of the first complement component. J. Immunol., *112*:1667, 1974.
12. Sakai, K., and Stroud, R. M.: Purification, molecular properties, and activation of C1 proesterase, C1s. J. Immunol., *110*:1010, 1973.
13. ———: The activation of C1s with purified C1r. Immunochemistry, *11*:191, 1974.
14. Patrick, R. A., Taubman, S. B., and Lepow, I. H.: Cleavage of the fourth component of human complement (C4) by activated C1s. Immunochemistry, *7*:217, 1970.
15. Polley, M. J., and Müller-Eberhard, H. J.: The second component of human complement: its isolation, fragmentation by C′1 esterase, and incorporation into C′3 convertase. J. Exp. Med., *128*:533, 1968.
16. Müller-Eberhard, H. J., Polley, M. J., and Calcott, M. A.: Formation and functional significance of a molecular complex derived from the second and the fourth component of human complement. J. Exp. Med., *125*:359, 1967.
17. Müller-Eberhard, H. J., and Lepow, I. H.: C′1 esterase effect on activity and physicochemical properties of the fourth component of complement. J. Exp. Med., *121*:819, 1965.
18. Schreiber, R. D., and Müller-Eberhard, H. J.: Fourth component of human complement: description of a 3 polypeptide chain structure. J. Exp. Med., *140*:1324, 1974.
19. Müller-Eberhard, H. J., Dalmasso, A. P., and Calcott, M. A.: The reaction mechanism of β_{1c}-globulin (C′3) in immune hemolysis. J. Exp. Med., 123:33, 1966.
20. Cooper, N. R.: Enzymes of the complement system. Prog. Immunol., *1*:567, 1971.
21. Goldlust, M. B., Shin, H. S., Hammer, C. H., and Mayer, M. M.: Studies of complement complex C5b,6 eluted from EAC-6: reaction of C5b,6 with EAC4b,3b and evidence on the role of C2a and C3b in the activation of C5. J. Immunol., *113*:998, 1974.
22. Arroyave, C. M., and Müller-Eberhard, H. J.: Interactions between human C5, C6, and C7 and their functional significance in complement-dependent cytolysis. J. Immunol., *111*:536, 1973.
23. Gotze, O., and Müller-Eberhard, H. J.: Lysis of erythrocytes by complement in the absence of antibody. J. Exp. Med., *132*:898, 1970.
24. Thompson, R. A., and Lachmann, P. J.: Reactive lysis: the complement-mediated lysis of unsensitized cells. J. Exp. Med., *131*:629, 1970.
25. Kolb, W. P., and Müller-Eberhard, H. J.: The membrane attack mechanism of complement. J. Exp. Med., *138*:438, 1973.
26. Kolb, W. P., Haxby, J. A., Arroyave, C. M., and Müller-Eberhard, H. J.: Molecular analysis of the membrane attack mechanism of complement. J. Exp. Med., *135*:549, 1972.
27. Stolfi, R. L.: Immune lytic transformation: a state of irreversible damage generated as a result of the reaction of the eighth component in the guinea pig complement system. J. Immunol., *100*:46, 1968.
28. Delage, J. M., Lehner-Netsch, G., and Simard, J.: The tributyrinase activity of C7. Immunology, *24*:671, 1973.
29. Humphrey, J. H., and Dourmashkin, R. R.: The lesions in cell membranes caused by complement. Adv. Immunol., *11*:75, 1969.
30. Mayer, M. M.: Mechanism of cytolysis by complement. Proc. Natl. Acad. Sci. U.S.A., *69*:2954, 1972.
31. Fearon, D. T., Austen, K. F., and Ruddy, S.: Properdin factor D II. Activation to D by properdin. J. Exp. Med., *140*: 426, 1974.
32. Hunsicker, L. G., Ruddy, S., and Austen, K. F.: Alternate complement pathway: factors involved in cobra venom factor (CoVF) activation of the third component of complement (C3). J. Immunol., *110*:128, 1973.
33. Fearon, D. T., Austen, K. F., and Ruddy, S.: Properdin factor D: characterization of its active site and isolation of the precursor form. J. Exp. Med., *139*:355, 1974.
34. Goodkofsky, I., and Lepow, I. H.: Functional relationship of factor B in the properdin system to C3 proactivator of human serum. J. Immunol., *107*:1200, 1971.
35. Boenisch, T., and Alper, C. A.: Isolation and properties of a glycine-rich γ-glycoprotein of human serum. Biochim. Biophys. Acta, *214*:135, 1970.
36. Vogt, W.: Activation, activities and phar-

macologically active products of complement. Pharmacol. Rev., *26*:125, 1974.
37. Müller-Eberhard, H. J., and Götze, O.: C3 proactivator convertase and its mode of action. J. Exp. Med., *135*:1003, 1971.
38. Götze, O., and Müller-Eberhard, H. J.: The C3-activator system: an alternate pathway of complement activation. J. Exp. Med., *134*:90s, 1971.
39. Fearon, D. T., and Austen, K. F.: Properdin: binding to C3b and stabilization of the C3b-dependent C3 convertase. J. Exp. Med., *142*:856, 1975.
40. Fearon, D. T., Austen, K. F., and Ruddy, S.: Formation of a hemolytically active cellular intermediate by the interaction between properdin factors B and D and the activated third component of complement. J. Exp. Med., *138*:1305, 1973.
41. Vallota, E. H., *et al.*: Characteristics of a non-complement-dependent C3-reactive complex formed from factors in nephritic and normal serum. J. Exp. Med., *131*:1306, 1970.
42. Pensky, J., Levy, L. R., and Lepow, I. H.: Partial purification of a serum inhibitor of C'1-esterase. J. Biol. Chem., *236*:1674, 1961.
43. Ruddy, S., and Austen, K. F.: C3b inactivator of man. J. Immunol., *107*:742, 1971.
44. Alper, C. A., Rosen, F. S., and Lachmann, P. J.: Inactivator of the third component of complement as an inhibitor in the properdin pathway. Proc. Natl. Acad. Sci. U.S.A., *69*:2910, 1972.
45. Tamura, N., and Nelson, R. T., Jr.: Three naturally-occurring inhibitors of components of complement in guinea pig and rabbit serum. J. Immunol., *99*:582, 1967.
46. Bokisch, V. A., and Müller-Eberhard, H. J.: Anaphylatoxin inactivator of human plasma: its isolation and characterization as a carboxypeptidase. J. Clin. Invest., *49*:2427, 1970.
47. Mayer, M. M.: Highlights of complement research during the past twenty-five years. Immunochemistry, *7*:485, 1970.
48. Gitling, J., Rosen, F. S., and Lachmann, P. J.: The mechanism of action of the C3b inactivator on its natural substrate the major fragment of the third component of complement. J. Exp. Med., *141*:221, 1975.

Appendix B: Isotypes and Allotypes of the Light Chains

Isotypes are antigenic specificities present on the immunoglobulins of all individuals. Several isotypic variants have been identified on the λ chain. Some have been defined serologically; some only by amino acid sequencing.

An allotype is an antigenic specificity present on a relatively high percentage of immunoglobulin molecules that represents the expressed gene product or products of a given allele. Thus far the only system of allelic markers defined for light chains is the Inv allotypic markers expressed on κ chains. Three Inv antigens have been detected. Inv(1) is associated with a leucine at position 191 and Inv(3) with a valine at the same position. The Inv(2) antigen is more complexly defined. The antiserum directed against this antigen detects both leucine at position 191 and alanine at position 153 (positions 191 and 153 are located on adjacent polypeptide loops and are within 10 Å of each other). Most immunoglobulins which express leucine at position 191 also express alanine at position 153, and therefore both antigens Inv(1) and Inv(2) are detected on these molecules. This serologically defined phenotype is appropriately termed Inv(1,2). Occasionally position 153 is occupied by valine, a larger amino acid than alanine. In these situations the Inv(2) antiserum is sterically prevented from recognizing the leucine at position 191 and is therefore unreactive. Antisera to the Inv(1) antigen do not appear to include position 153 in their site of reactivity and can therefore still bind to the leucine at position 191. Such molecules which react only with Inv(1) antisera are of the phenotype Inv(1). This phenotype is extremely rare, being found in fewer than 2 per cent of Caucasians. Molecules bearing the Inv(3) antigen (valine at position 191) react only with Inv(3) antiserum and are thus of the phenotype Inv(3). There are thus three phenotypes possible for κ chains:

1. Inv(1) representing leucine at 191 and valine at 153
2. Inv(1,2) representing leucine at 191 and alanine at 153, and
3. Inv(3) representing valine at 191 and alanine at 153.

A person inherits only one of these phenotypes from each parent, and therefore these are true alleles.

Table B-1. Isotypic Variants of the λ Chain*

Isotype	*Position*	*Amino Acid Residue*
Oz +	193	Lys
–		Arg
Kern +	156	Gly
–		Ser
Mz +	147/174	Val/Asn
–		Ala/Lys
Mcg +	116/118/167	Asn/Thr/Lys
–		Ala/Ser/Thr

*Solomon, A: N. Engl. J. Med., *294*(1):17, 1976.

Appendix C: Tests and Assays

Essential to the rapid increase in knowledge in immunology over the past several years has been the development of a variety of laboratory techniques that have enabled researchers to measure and monitor the many elements and functions of the immune system.

TESTS EMPLOYING THE INTERACTION OF ANTIGEN WITH ANTIBODY

PRECIPITATION REACTIONS

The classical precipitation curve discussed in Chapter 7 was introduced as an aid to understanding the molecular composition of immune complexes. Forty years ago the use of such tube precipitin curves was the only way to obtain quantitative information about specific antibodies. Polysaccharide antigens could be added to a solution containing an unknown quantity of antibodies until equivalence was reached. All the antibody would then be in the precipitate, and all the protein in the precipitate would be antibody. The quantity of precipitated protein could then be calculated by classical chemical methods to give an estimate of the amount of specific antibody present in the original solution. Of course, this method only worked for quantitating antibodies to nonprotein antigens.

The phenomenon of immune complex precipitation has since been applied to a wide range of techniques for detecting specific antigen-antibody interactions.

Double Diffusion Gel Precipitation

Perhaps the single most useful modification of the precipitation reaction has been the precipitation of antigen-antibody complexes in gels. This technique was described by Ouchterlony and has been termed double diffusion gel precipitation or Ouchterlony analysis. The experimental design is simple: an agar dish is set up and two circular wells are made. A specific antiserum is placed in one cell, a test antigen in the other. Both the antibody molecules and the antigen will diffuse randomly in all directions from their respective wells into the gel (Fig. C-1). This diffusion will result in constantly widening circles of the contents of each well. At some place in between the two wells the two diffusing species will meet. If the test antigen is the specific target of the antiserum, *immune complexes* will form and will *precipitate*. This precipitate is visible as an opaque line in the agar gel (see Fig. C-2). If the antigen is not an appropriate target of the

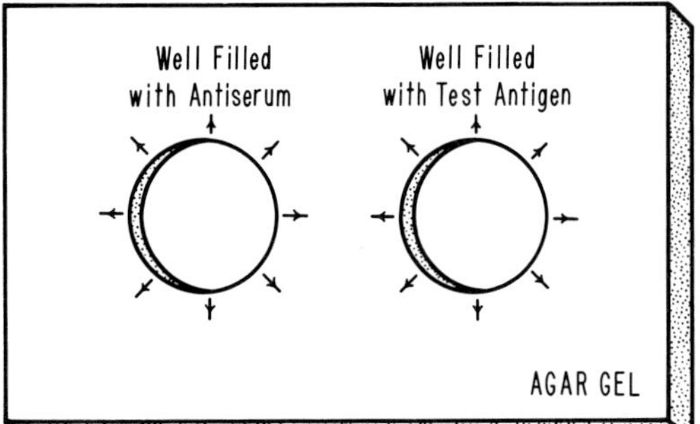

Fig. C-1. Ouchterlony gel and wells for antigen and antiserum. Both reagents diffuse into the gel.

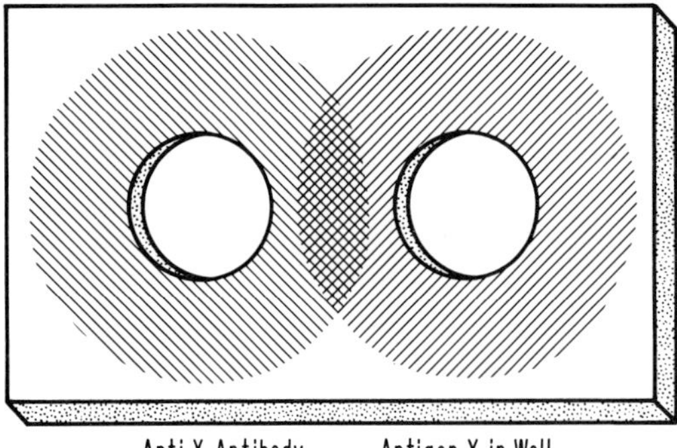

Fig. C-3. If antiserum and antigen do not combine, they will continue to diffuse past each other and no precipitin band will form.

antiserum, no immune complexes will form and no band will be seen (Fig. C-3). This technique therefore offers a way to either test the specificity of an antiserum against a known antigen or to test the identity of an antigen with a known antiserum.

The precipitin band is a semipermeable barrier. The specific antibody *and* the specific antigen that comprise the immune complex of the band are not able to diffuse past the line. This is because there is always free antibody just to the antibody side of the line and free antigen just to the other side. Any antigen attempting to cross the line will be immediately bound by antibody and the resulting complex will precipitate onto the band. On the other hand, this opaque line is perfectly permeable to any other antigen or antibody molecule, and any such molecule will freely diffuse across the precipitate as if the visible line were not even there. This selective permeability allows us to test the identity of two or more antigens as follows:

In the agar plate shown in Figure C-4 there are three wells, two containing antigen X and one containing antibody against X as shown. A line is formed in the shape of a smooth curve because the precipitate forms uniformly at the inter-

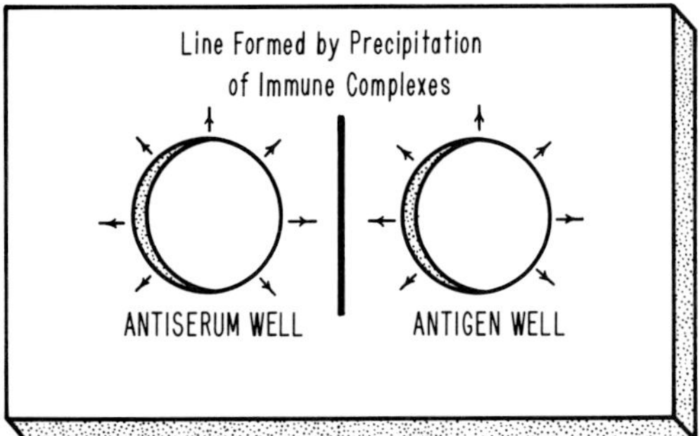

Fig. C-2. Formation of a precipitin band composed of insoluble antigen-antibody complexes.

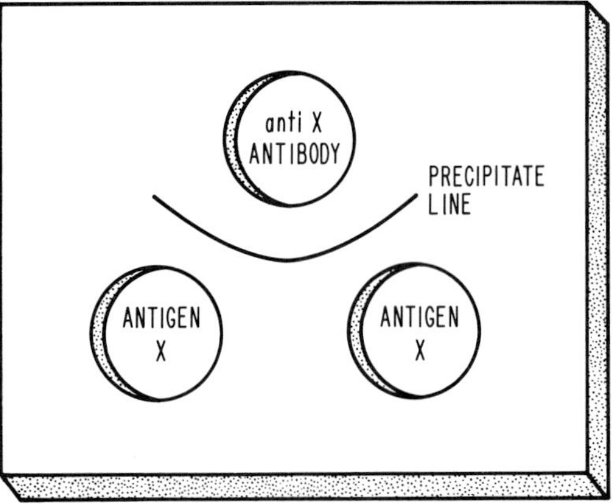

Fig. C-4. Smooth curve of precipitation between antiserum and two antigen wells filled with the same antigen.

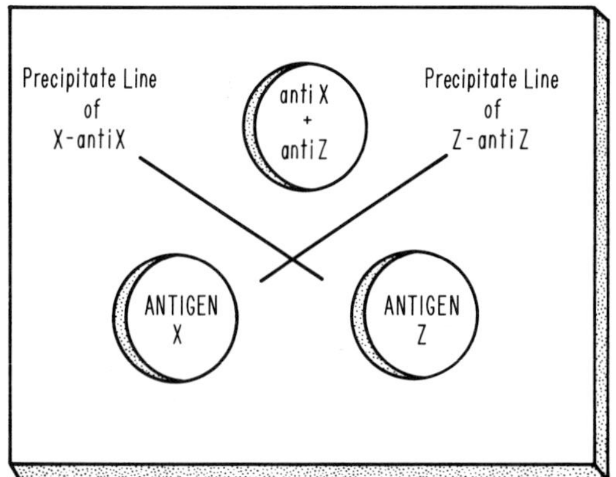

Fig. C-5. Distinct precipitin bands formed by two unrelated antigen-antibody complexes.

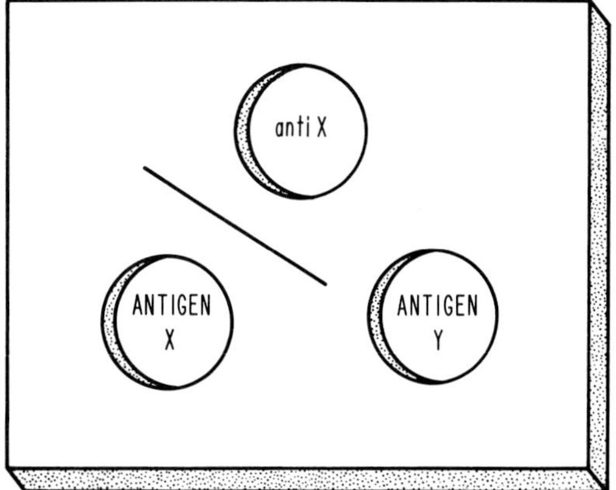

Fig. C-7. Single precipitin band.

section of the three widening diffusion circles.

In another experiment, shown in Figure C-5, the antigen wells are filled separately with two unrelated antigens, X and Z, and the antibody well is filled with a mixed antiserum against both X and Z. In this case no single precipitate is formed by the interception of the three diffusion circles. Instead, there are two separate precipitates: Z-anti-Z and X-anti-X (see Fig. C-5). Note that the two lines *cross*. This is because X and anti-X effectively "ignore" the line formed by Z and anti-Z and vice versa. The principle of selective permeability allows us to view the crossing of two precipitating lines as evidence that there is no identity between the components of one precipitate with the components of the other.

A third example also employing three wells illustrates a situation that combines aspects of the previous two. In one antigen well is placed a molecule with determinants X and Y and in the other a molecule with determinants Y and Z. The antiserum well contains antibody against X and antibodies against Y. As above, each precipitin system must be viewed separately. The Y-anti-Y line will give the same type of curve as in the first example (see Fig. C-6). We can add to this the X-anti-X line (see Fig. C-7). Putting together these two independent patterns we get the curve shown in Figure C-8. The

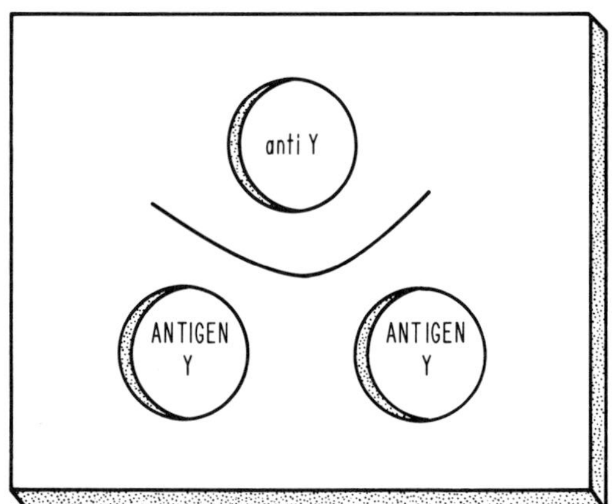

Fig. C-6. Smooth precipitin band.

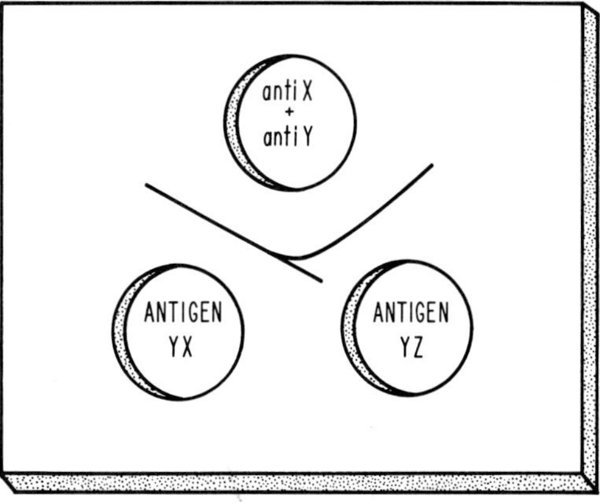

Fig. C-8. Combination of Figures C-6 and C-7 showing partial identity of antigen YX and antigen YZ.

spur indicates the nonidentity of the antigens in the two wells. The smooth curved line, however, indicates that the molecules in the two wells do share certain determinants. This pattern therefore is indicative of the *partial identity* of XY and YZ. If anti-Z were added to the antiserum well the pattern of precipitation shown in Figure C-9 would emerge.

There are other characteristics of the precipitin line formed by this double diffusion method that can tell us about the nature of the interacting constituents. These include the shape, width and position of the line with respect to the two diffusing substances. The shape and position of the lines are largely a function of the diffusion characteristics of the molecules in the gel. If both the antigen and the antibody diffuse with equal speed, the precipitate will be a straight line halfway between the two wells (Fig. C-10). If, as is more likely, the antibody and the antigen have different rates of diffusion, the precipitate will form a curved line that is concave toward, and closer to, the more slowly diffusing molecule (Fig. C-11). The more the disparity between diffusion rates, the more accentuated these changes will be. In general, the larger a molecule is, the slower it will diffuse.

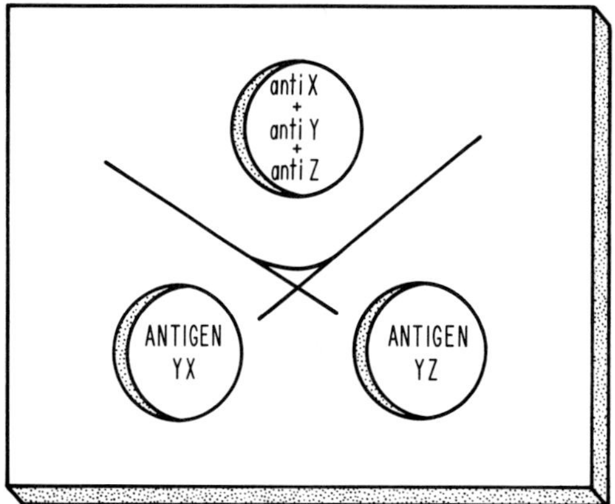

Fig. C-9. Complex pattern formed by the addition of anti-Z to the antiserum well in Figure C-8.

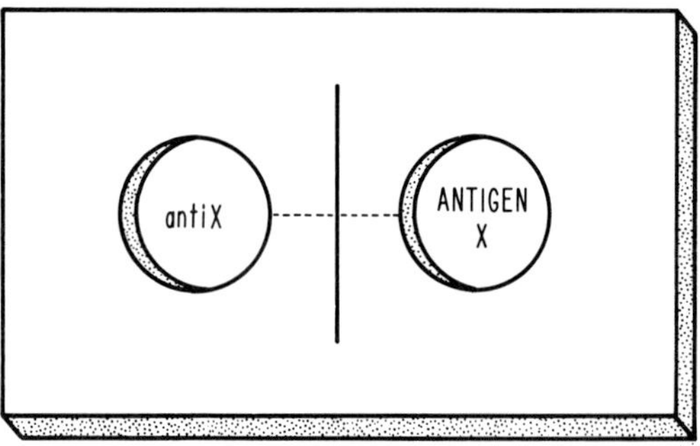

Fig. C-10. Precipitin band shown as a straight line equidistant from both antibody and antigen wells when both species share the same diffusion characteristics.

These principles can be illustrated by using the example of the three-well agar plate. Antigen X and antigen Y are placed in one well. Antigen Y is placed in another. The antiserum well contains anti-X and anti-Y antibodies. One of two precipitate patterns can result, depending upon the diffusion rates of each molecule (see Figs. C-12 and C-13).

The concentration of each reagent affects the width of the precipitate line that is produced. If one component is in large excess of the other, the line will be "fuzzy" and will spread from the first line of contact toward the well with the more dilute component (see Fig. C-14). Fuzzy precipitant bands are therefore indicative of gross imbalances in the concentration of the antigen and the antibody.

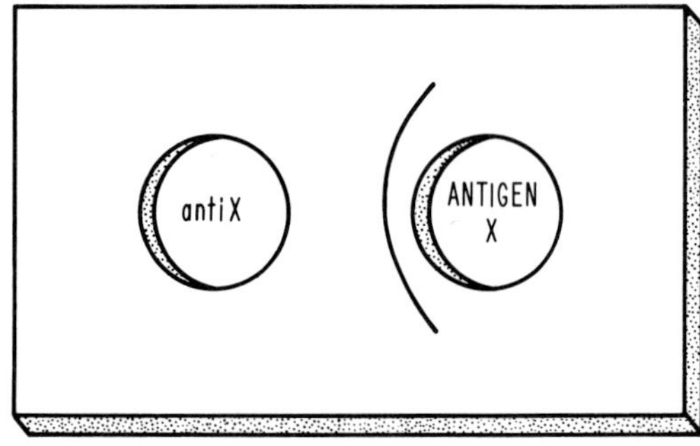

Fig. C-11. Curved precipitin band formed as a result of the slower diffusion of antigen X with respect to anti-X.

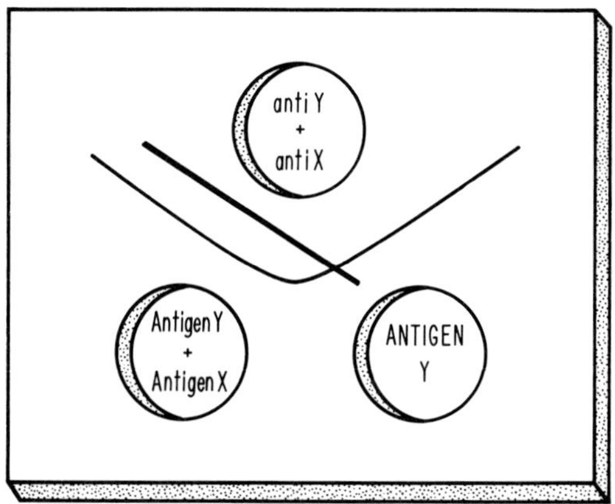

Fig. C-12. Complex precipitin bands formed when antigen X diffuses more rapidly than antigen Y.

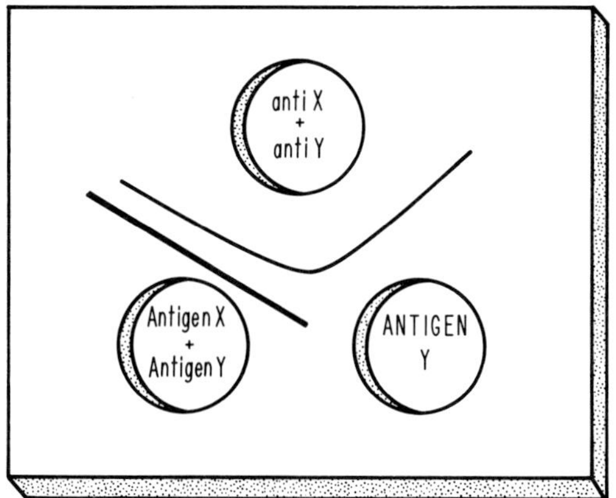

Fig. C-13. Complex precipitin bands where antigen X diffuses more slowly than antigen Y.

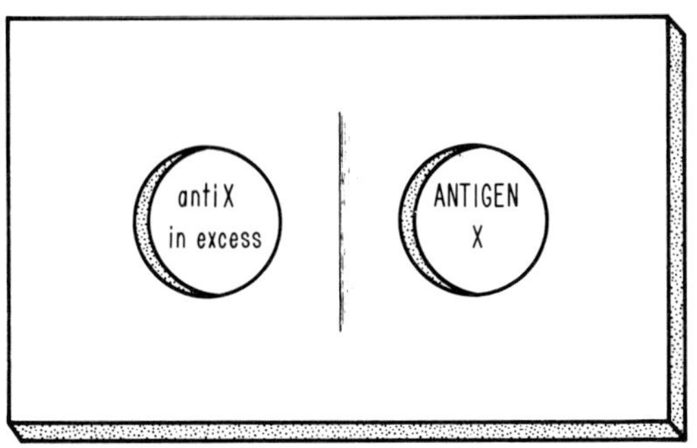

Fig. C-14. Inequality in concentration of antibody and antigen leads to slurred precipitin bands.

Immunoelectrophoresis

A mixture of charged molecules can be separated by their mobility in an electric field. Human serum can be separated into many of its components by placing a sample of serum onto an agar gel and allowing the various molecules to migrate into the gel under the influence of an electric field. The separated molecules can be stained and identified according to their individual mobilities as seen in Figure C-15.

The principle of the specificity of antigen-antibody precipitation reactions was applied by Grabar in 1953 to the identification of molecules that have been separated by electrophoresis. The agar strip containing the separated molecules (e.g., human serum) is placed next to a trough which contains polyspecific antisera against human serum components. The electrophoresed molecules and the antibodies diffuse toward each other in the gel and form specific precipitin bands whenever a specific antigen-antibody reaction occurs (see Fig. C-16). Many distinct lines are formed. This technique has allowed the identification of many more specific serum components than are recognizable by simple serum electrophoresis.

The immunoelectrophoretic pattern of normal human serum is now well recognized, and specific bands have been associated with specific serum molecules. The absence of a particular band, for example transferrin, indicates the absence of that molecule from the serum (i.e., atransferrinemia). Immunoelectrophoresis can be used to obtain a qualitative impression as to the presence or absence of the major immunoglobulin classes. A simple serum electrophoresis, for example, may reveal a sharp peak and immunoelectrophoresis may identify this as a monoclonal immunoglobulin "spike" indicative of any of a variety of immunoproliferative states, including multiple myeloma, Waldenström's mac-

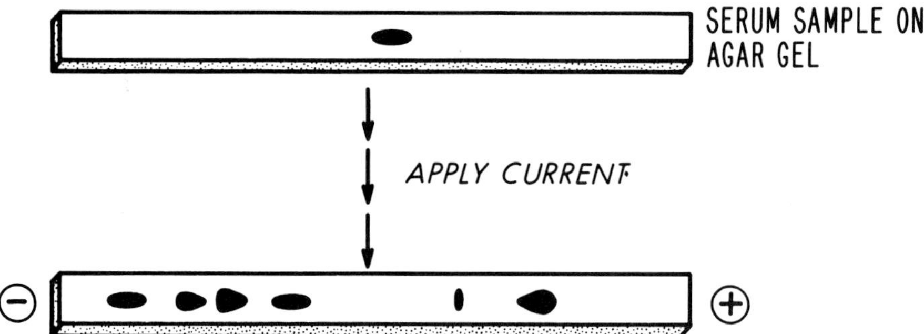

Fig. C-15. Schematic of the principle of serum electrophoresis. Serum sample is separated into its component parts according to their different mobilities in an electric field.

roglobulinemia, benign monoclonal gammopathy and others (see Fig. 12-10).

If radioactive antigen or antibody is used in this technique, the appropriate precipitant bands will be radiolabelled. Autoradiography can then be done to visualize bands containing amounts of antigen or antibody that are too small to visualize directly. This modification is termed *radioimmunoelectrophoresis*.

Counter Electrophoresis

The Ouchterlony double diffusion technique, although useful, is nevertheless inefficient in that most of the antigen and antibody diffuse in directions away from each other and thus are never detected. For this reason the Ouchterlony technique is not a sensitive way to detect small quantities of either reagent. The technique of counter electrophoresis provides a way of specifically directing the movement of antigen and antibody toward each other in an electric field (see Fig. C-17). This technique only works if the antibody and antigen molecules under study have different isoelectric pH's so that a pH intermediate between the two will result in each molecule having an opposite net charge. The charged molecules are each placed on the side distal to the electrode toward which they will

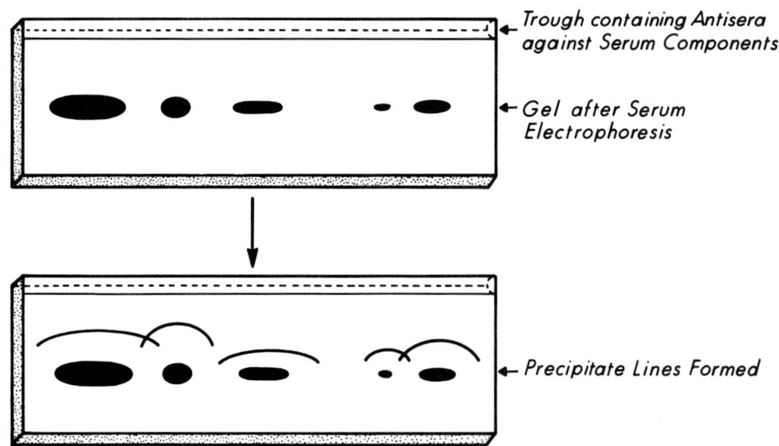

Fig. C-16. Immunoelectrophoresis. Polyspecific antisera in the trough and the separated serum components in the gel diffuse toward each other to form precipitin bands when appropriate antibody-antigen complexes are formed.

Fig. C-17. Counter electrophoresis. In this example the pH of the gel is chosen so that the antigen has a net negative charge and the antibody has a net positive charge. Accordingly, the antibody will migrate to the right and the antigen to the left. A precipitin band will form where they cross.

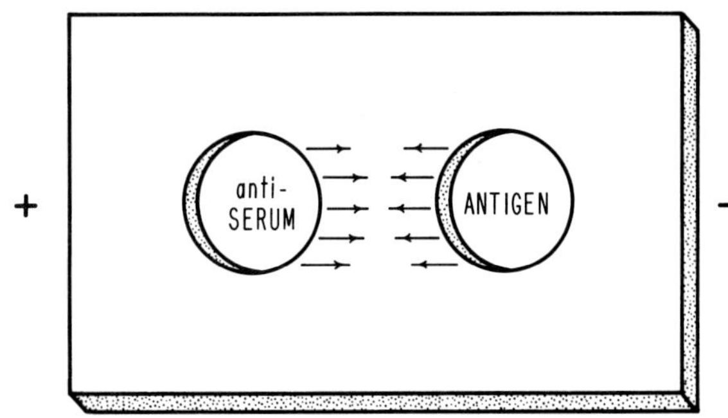

migrate so that their paths will cross and precipitation will occur. This method is not only more sensitive than the Ouchterlony plates, but it is also faster. It has found its greatest clinical application in the detection of the Australia antigen of the hepatitis B virus.

Methods Employing Single Diffusion Gel Precipitation

These methods employ gels into which either the antibody or, less commonly, the antigen is uniformly incorporated into the agar. Only one of the reagents either diffuses or is electrophoresed through the gel.

Single Radial Immunodiffusion

In this commonly employed technique antiserum is diffusely incorporated at a relatively low concentration into a gel. A single well is made in the gel into which target antigen is placed. As antigen diffuses into the gel, it forms a progressively widening circle of precipitate. The diameter of the precipitant ring is directly proportional to the concentration of antigen in the well (see Fig. C-18). This important direct relationship between antigen concentration and ring diameter allows onc to calculate the concentration of a known antigen. This can be done by standardizing ring size produced in the same gel with antigens of known concentration and plotting a straight line (see Fig. C-19). This technique can be very accurate and is often the method of choice for quantitating a variety of substances such as immunoglobulin classes and subclasses and serum complement components.

Rocket Electrophoresis

Antigen is electrophoresed across a gel that is impregnated with a specific antiserum as in the single radial immunodiffusion technique. Usually a series of wells is placed at one end of the gel, into which a range of dilutions of antigen is placed. The precipitate patterns shown in Figure C-20 are formed after electrophoresis. The distance from the starting point to the tip of the arc is directly proportional to the antigen concentration. This method is faster than single radial immunodiffusion. Since one does not want the antiserum and the antigen to migrate in the same direction under

Fig. C-18. Single radial immunodiffusion. Antibody is incorporated throughout the gel and the diameter of the precipitin ring is proportional to the concentration of the Ig in the well.

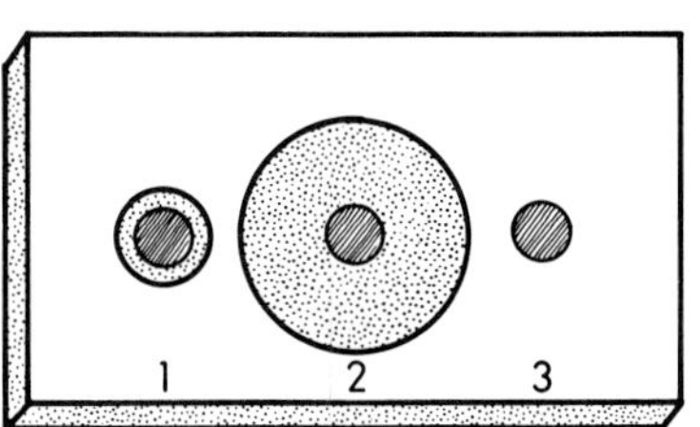

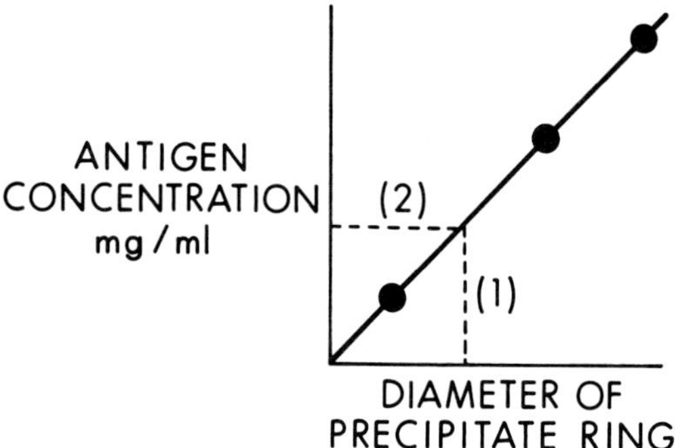

Fig. C-19. Calculation of antigen concentration by measurement of the diameter of the ring in single radial immunodiffusion. The points shown represent standardization points obtained by measuring the ring diameter using known antigen concentrations. A straight line is drawn and the concentration of any test antigen can be determined by measuring the ring diameter (1) and extrapolating to the appropriate antigen concentration (2).

the influence of the electric field, this technique is usually not used for quantitating immunoglobulin concentrations.

Two-Dimensional Immunoelectrophoresis

In this technique a normal electrophoresis is first accomplished as is shown in Figure C-15. The separated components are then placed next to a gel which is impregnated with polyspecific antisera (as in immunoelectrophoresis). The separated components are then electrophoresed a second time into the gel so that specific precipitant arcs are formed (see Fig. C-21). In effect, this method allows quantitation of immunoelectrophoresis.

AGGLUTINATION REACTIONS

Agglutination involves the specific clumping of antigenic particles by antisera. Among the differences between agglutination and precipitation are:

1. Target antigens in agglutination reactions are part of *insoluble* molecules which are in *suspension*. With precipitation the antigens are *soluble* and are in *solution*.
2. Agglutination particles are *larger*.
3. Agglutination may be a more sensitive way to detect small amounts of antibody.
4. Agglutination occurs within a few hours whereas precipitation may take as long as several days.

In general, the particles to be agglutinated are many times larger than the agglutinating antibodies. The larger the antibody molecule, the better it can agglutinate. Thus, IgM is a good agglutinin whereas IgG will rarely agglutinate particles by itself.

The titer of agglutinating antibodies is measured by taking a given concentration of target particles and mixing with progressively more dilute solutions of antibody. The final dilution at which visible clumping occurs is referred to as the specific antibody titer. Thus if agglutina-

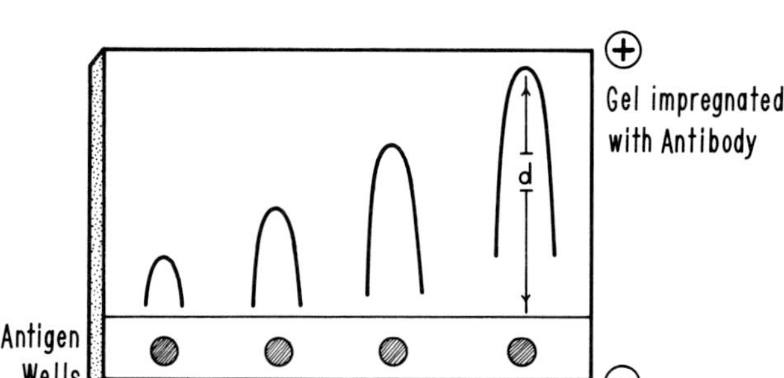

Fig. C-20. Rocket electrophoresis. The distance (d) from the antigen wells to the apex of the precipitin arcs is proportional to the antigen concentration.

Fig. C-21. Two-dimensional electrophoresis. Serum electrophoresis gel (A) is placed next to the gel (B) impregnated with polyspecific antisera. The separated serum components are then electrophoresed into the gel to produce the pattern shown.

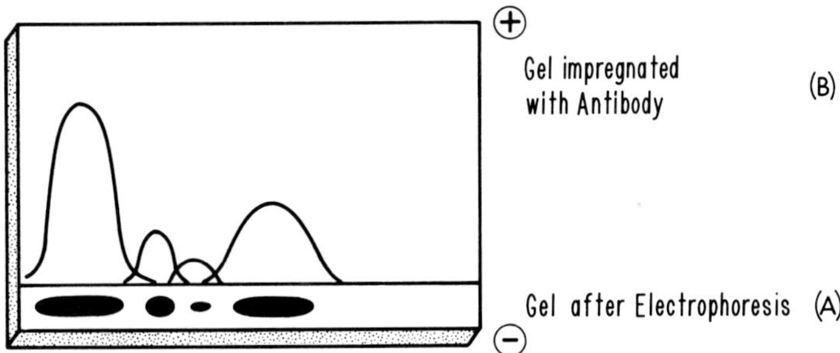

tion occurs down to a dilution of 1 to 256, the titer will be 256. Occasionally, there is a phenomenon of *prozone* in which very concentrated solutions of antisera fail to agglutinate the particles despite agglutination at somewhat lower concentrations.

Most agglutination assays are done in tubes in which varying solutions of antisera are added to given volumes of a standard particle suspension. The tubes are inspected for visible *clumping*. Brief periods of centrifugation may be used to detect smaller aggregates. Sedimentation of nonagglutinated particles results in a packed "button" at the bottom of the tube. Sedimentation of aggregates can be seen as diffuse loose precipitates (Fig. C-22).

Agglutination can be visualized on slides where one drop of each of a variety of antisera dilutions is added to one drop of particles in suspension. Small, coarse aggregates rapidly appear. The advantages of this technique are its speed and the small amount of material that is needed (Fig. C-23).

Agglutination tests can be used to detect the presence of antibodies directed against infectious agents in the sera of patients.

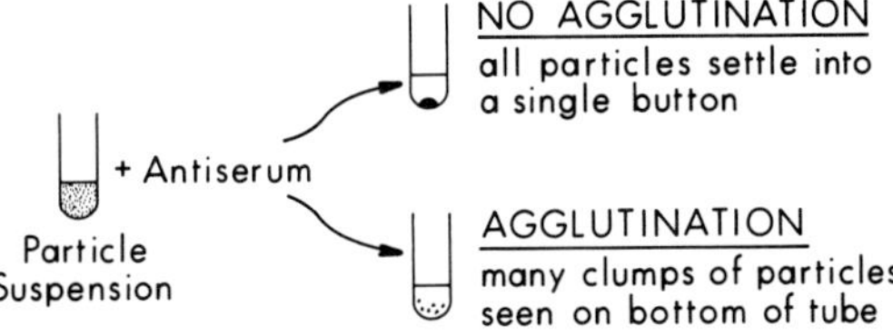

Fig. C-22. Agglutination reaction.

One of the most commonly employed agglutination tests is the *latex fixation test*, most often used to detect IgM rheumatoid factor. Polystyrene latex particles are coated with human IgG. In suspension these coated particles appear as a milk-white liquid. Serum is added and, if IgM anti-IgG is present, the particles will be agglutinated. This will result in the production of a coarse agglomerate. The dilutions of serum can be tested in order to arrive at a rheumatoid factor titer.

Hemagglutination

The clumping of red blood cells is one of the most commonly employed applications of the agglutination technique. Some of the characteristics of red-cell agglutination were discussed in Chapter 14. Blood-grouping and -typing can rapidly be accomplished by testing for agglutination with known antisera. Similarly, blood can be crossmatched by screening the recipient's serum for antidonor agglutinins.

The direct Coombs' test employs agglutination to determine the presence of IgG on the red-cell surface (see Fig. 14-17). The red cells to be tested are mixed with a solution of anti-human IgG antiserum. If the target cells have IgG on their surface, they will be agglutinated. By using serial dilutions of the Coombs' test reagent, an anti-red-cell antibody titer can be obtained. The indirect

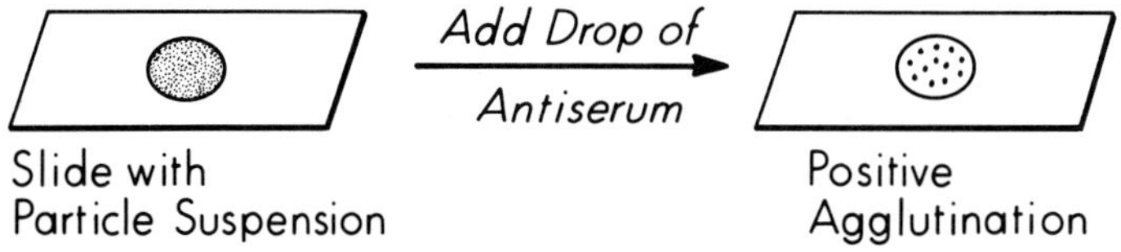

Slide with Particle Suspension — Add Drop of Antiserum → Positive Agglutination

Fig. C-23. Slide agglutination reaction.

Coombs' test employs the same principle to test the patient's serum for the presence of circulating anti-red-cell antibodies (see Fig. 14-18). The serum must first be reacted with test erythrocytes and then the Coombs' reagent can be added.

Because the agglutination of red cells is so readily visible, these cells have been used in much the same way as latex particles to test for rheumatoid factor. Tests that employ the red cell as the indicator of (rather than the direct target of) agglutination are called *passive hemagglutination* techniques (Fig. C-24). In these tests, the target antigens are adsorbed onto the red-cell surface. Polysaccharide antigens readily adhere to erythrocytes; protein antigens are more difficult to attach. However, if the red cells are first treated with dilute tannic acid (producing "tanned" red cells), protein antigens will readily stick to their surface. Treatment of the red cell with chromium chloride can also be used for this purpose.

A variety of antigens can be adsorbed to these indicator cells. For example, this technique has been used for the detection of antithyroglobulin antibodies. Thyroglobulin is attached to modified erythrocyte surfaces. The serum of a patient suspected of having such autoantibodies is then added to the antigen-coated red-cell suspension. Agglutination indicates the presence of the antibody. This method is called *direct passive hemagglutination* (Fig. C-24A). Certain IgG antisera may attach to antigen-coated red cells but will not lead to agglutination. In these situations a Coombs' reagent (anti-IgG antibody) can be added which will then secondarily cause a positive test. This is referred to as *indirect passive hemagglutination* (Fig. C-24B).

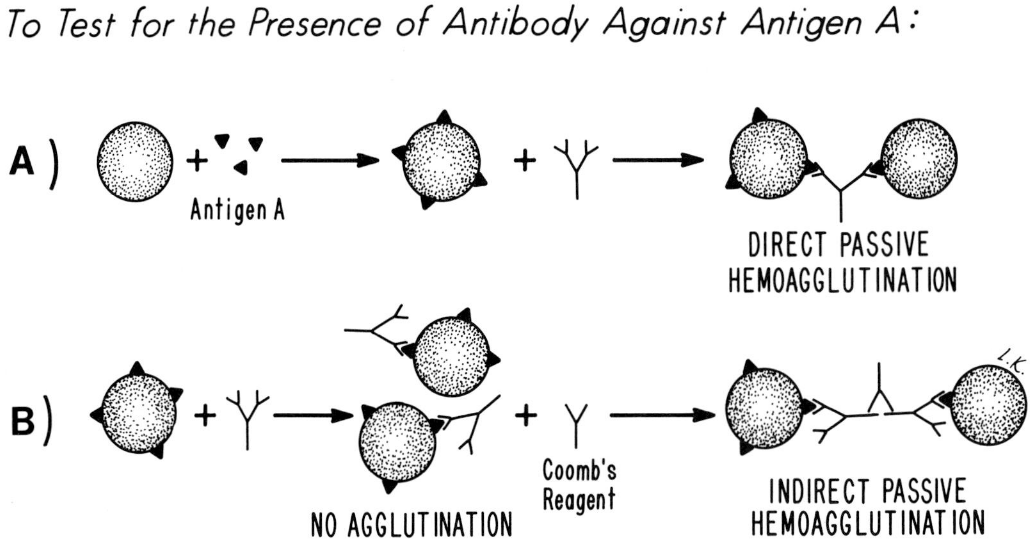

To Test for the Presence of Antibody Against Antigen A:

A) Antigen A → DIRECT PASSIVE HEMOAGGLUTINATION

B) NO AGGLUTINATION — Coomb's Reagent → INDIRECT PASSIVE HEMOAGGLUTINATION

Fig. C-24. Passive hemagglutination. (A) direct, (B) indirect.

The agglutination techniques detect the presence of specific antibody. The tests can be reversed in order to detect levels of specific antigen. The antigen to be tested for is first adsorbed onto red cells. A known quantity of specific hemagglutinating antibody is then mixed with the serum being tested for the presence of the known antigen. If the antigen is in the serum it will combine with the antibody and only the remaining free antibody will be left to agglutinate the coated red cells. The more antigen present in the test serum, the lower the titer of remaining agglutinating antibody. In this way the titer of serum antigen can be measured. This test is called the *inhibition of passive hemagglutination*.

OTHER TECHNIQUES FOR EXAMINING ANTIGEN-ANTIBODY INTERACTIONS

Two different techniques have been employed in order to assess the antigen-binding capacity of a given sample of antisera. These are the Farr and the immunocoprecipitation techniques. Both of these begin with a test antisera to which is added an excess of radioactively labelled antigen. The excess of antigen allows each antibody combining site to be saturated with a separate antigen molecule. The antigen-antibody complexes are then separated from the remaining soluble antigen and the complexed antigen can be quantitated, revealing the antigen-binding capacity of the antisera (Fig. C-25).

In the *Farr* technique, the precipitation of antigen-antibody complexes is brought about by adding ammonium sulfate. This technique is a useful separation procedure providing the free antigen does not precipitate as well.

The *immunocoprecipitation* technique uses a more specific means of separating the complexes from the free antigen. Here anti-immunoglobulin antiserum is added to the reaction mixture. Large complexes will form that contain the original antigen-antibody complexes, thus sep-

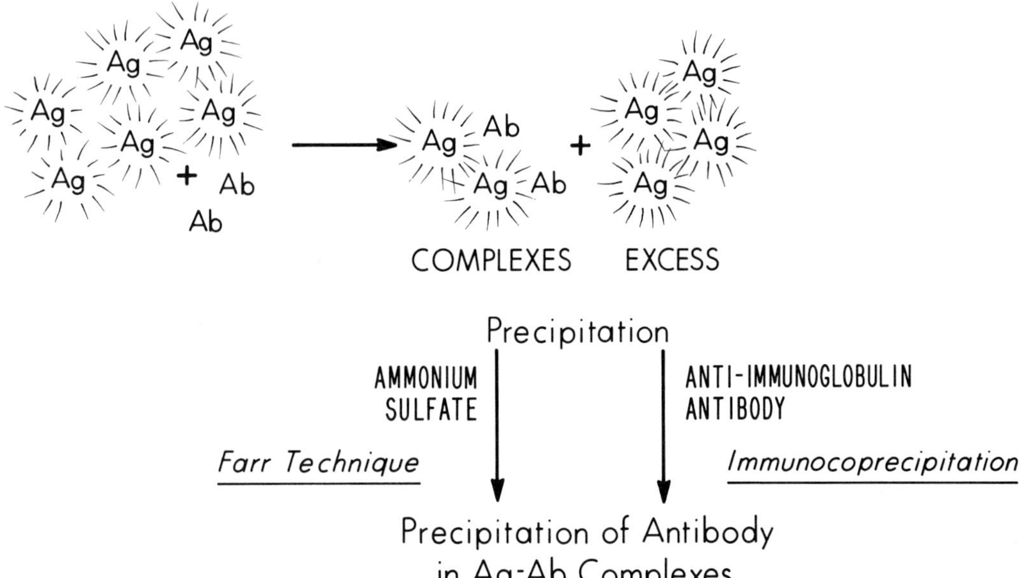

Fig. C-25. Precipitation techniques employing radioactively-labelled antigen. (1) The Farr technique. Antigen-antibody complexes are precipitated in ammonium sulfate solutions. (2) Immunocoprecipitation technique. Antigen-antibody complexes are precipitated by anti-Ig antibody.

arating the complexed antigen from the free antigen. This technique can be modified by employing antisera against specific immunoglobulin classes or subclasses and thereby allowing one to determine the distribution of antibody activity within the antiserum.

Radioimmunoassays are being used more and more both in clinical medicine and in experimental science to detect very small quantities of antigen (Fig. C-26). This technique is similar to the ones described above. A known amount of excess radioactively labelled antigen is added to a given amount of a specific antibody and the complexes are precipitated. The ratio of radioactive label in the supernatant to the precipitate is measured. The actual test is then run by mixing the known amount of radioactive antigen with an unknown amount of the same antigen that is not radioactive. This mixture is then added to the known antibody solution and complexes are precipitated. Again, the ratio of radioactive label in the precipitate to the supernatant is determined. The ratio will have changed because the unknown quantity of unlabelled antigen has distributed itself between the bound and free compartments. The new ratio, when compared to the old, can give a measure of the amount of unlabelled antigen that has been added.

TESTS INVOLVING COMPLEMENT

Complement Component Titers

The amount of individual components in body fluids can be measured by the specific immunoassays mentioned above, such as the two-dimensional single gel diffusion method. This type of physical measurement is most commonly employed to detect C3 and C4. By immunoelectrophoresis these two components can be readily detected in human serum. They have been named according to their electrophoretic mobility as β_1C (C3) and β_1E (C4).

More commonly, a *functional* assay is used to quantitate the level of complement activity in a given fluid sample. The most widely available functional assay measures the activity of the whole complement sequence. The titer obtained is called the CH_{50}. This name reflects the nature of the test in which the titer refers to the dilution of serum that will lyse 50 per cent of a standardized population of antibody-coated sheep red blood cells. The more dilutions one is able to make before less than 50 per cent of the cells are lysed, the higher the serum titer of complement (CH_{50}).

This technique measures the classical pathway. A total absence of activity of one of the components as occurs in a vari-

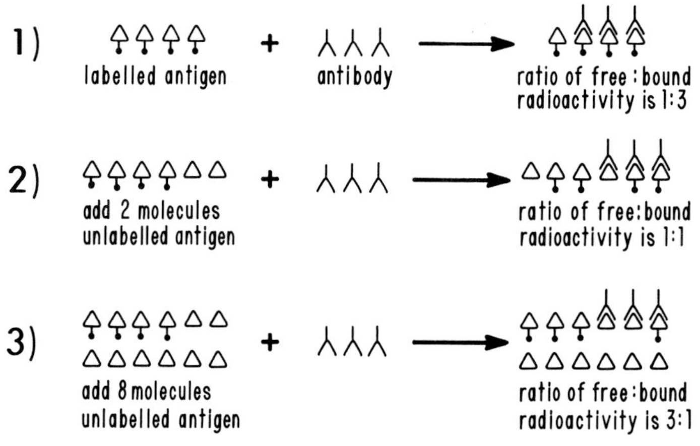

Fig. C-26. Radioimmunoassay. As the amount of unlabelled antigen is increased, the ratio of labelled antigen free in the supernatant to that bound in the precipitate also increases due to competition for antibody binding by the unlabelled antigen. One can then calculate the amount of unlabelled antigen from the observed ratios.

ety of the complement deficiency diseases will result in a CH_{50} of zero. This procedure does not give any information as to which specific component is depressed. In certain centers, a modification of the CH_{50} technique can be employed which will reveal which component (or components) is depressed.

Complement Fixation

This test is a valuable and sensitive tool for antigen detection and enjoys wide clinical application. The principle of the test is simple (Fig. C-27). Antibodies react to the target antigen in the presence of complement. The antigen-antibody complexes will fix the complement components and effectively "use them up." Antibody-coated red cells are then added to the solution. These will be lysed by the remaining complement. The amount of remaining complement is inversely proportional to the amount of antigen-antibody complexes in the solution. Therefore, the amount of red-cell lysis, which can be easily quantitated, is also inversely proportional to the concentration of antigen-antibody complexes. This technique allows one to identify an antigen given an antiserum of known specificity since complement will only be fixed and consumed if the unknown antigen can combine with the antiserum.

IMMUNOFLUORESCENCE

Immunofluorescence, originally developed by Coons, has become a versatile tool for the localization of specific antigen, either in tissue section or on individual cells. The reagents used are specific antisera which are reacted with

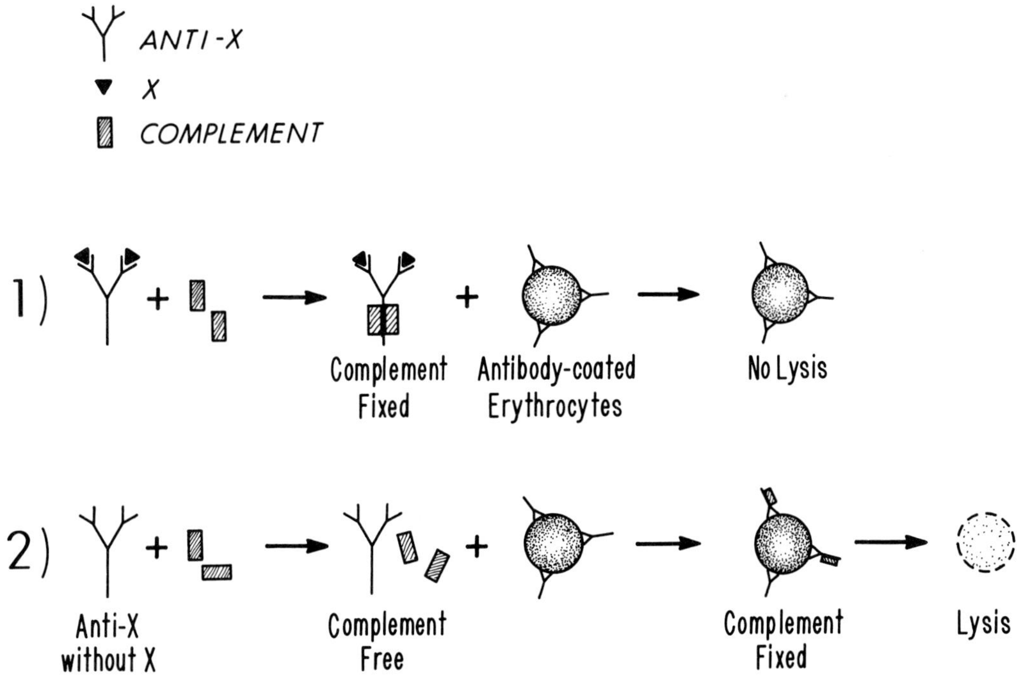

Fig. C-27. Complement fixation test for detecting the presence of antigen.(1) In the presence of antigen, antigen-antibody complexes will form and "use up" the complement that is present. Antibody-coated red cells which are subsequently added will not be lysed because the serum is now complement-depleted. (2) Without antigen, no antigen-antibody complexes are formed and complement remains in the serum. The addition of antibody-coated red cells leads to complement fixation on the red cells and lysis.

agents called fluorochromes. These fluorochromes can be attached to the immunoglobulin molecules without changing the antigen-binding capacity of the antibodies. Fluorochromes can be excited by ultraviolet light of a specific wave length to emit visible light. Each individual fluorochrome will emit light of a different wave length given identical incident stimulation. There are two commonly used fluorochromes: fluorescein, which emits a yellow-green light, and rhodamine, which emits an orange-red light. One can visualize the localized fluorescence after a specific labelled antiserum is reacted with a tissue section or cell. The presence and localization of the fluorescence indicates the distribution of the target antigen.

Direct Method

This employs a fluorochrome conjugated to a specific antibody that is specific for the antigen that one is trying to localize. This technique is useful to detect and localize unknown antigens by the use of known antibodies. One interesting application of fluorochrome-labelled antigen-specific antisera is the ability to detect specific antigen-binding lymphocytes. This can be employed if one wishes to determine the number of lymphocytes in a given preparation that will bind a specific antigen, X. The lymphocytes are fixed to a slide and the antigen is allowed to bind to those cells with receptors for X. The slide is then overlaid with fluorescent anti-X antiserum which will react with exposed determinants on X only on those lymphocytes that have already bound X (see Fig. C-28). This technique is called the *sandwich method* because the antigen is sandwiched between the lymphocyte receptor and the fluorescent antiserum.

Indirect Method

This variation tests for the presence of an antibody against a known antigen. The reagent used is less specific than in the first method. In this case, a fluorochrome is conjugated to anti-immunoglobulin antibody. A patient's serum can be tested for the presence of particular antibodies by first reacting the serum with tissue or cells that have the target antigen and then overlaying with the solution of fluorochrome-conjugated anti-immunoglobulin. Only if the patient's serum contains the specific antibody will the fluorescent reagent attach to the test material.

One common example of this test is the fluorescent anti-nuclear antibody test

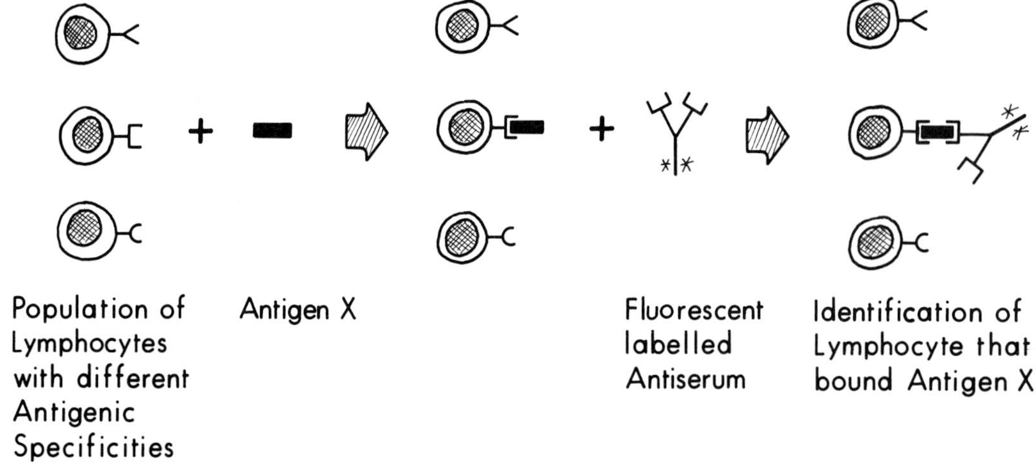

Fig. C-28. Sandwich technique of direct immunofluorescence.

employed in systemic lupus erythematosus (see Fig. 8-13). One technique uses sections of mouse liver as the source of nuclei. The patient's serum is reacted with the tissue and then fluorochrome-labelled anti-immunoglobulin is added. If the patient's serum contains antinuclear antibodies, the fluorescent reagent will bind to them on the tissue section. As discussed in Chapter 8, this test may show several patterns of antinuclear antibody localization. This indirect technique has several advantages over the direct technique:

1. One reagent (anti-immunoglobulin antibody) can be used to test for many antigen-antibody interactions.
2. It is more sensitive since a single antigen site which is bound by one specific antibody can then be the target for several labelled anti-immunoglobulin antibody molecules.
3. If the conjugated antiserum is made specific for particular classes or subclasses of immunoglobulin, one can ascertain not only the presence of particular antibodies but their class and subclass as well.

Two very important specific uses of fluorochrome-labelled anti-immunoglobulin antisera are: (1) the detection of lymphocytes that bear surface immunoglobulin (see Chap. 3), and (2) the presence of immunoglobulin deposition in tissues in a variety of disease states. The immunoglobulin deposited in a particular tissue may be the result of immune complex deposition as in lupus nephritis or poststreptococcal glomerulonephritis (see Chap. 7).

Alternatively, the antibody may be directed against a self-component in the tissue section such as in Goodpasture's syndrome (see Chap. 15).

The indirect method is commonly adjusted so that the conjugated antiserum is directed against complement components. Thus one can detect the deposition or fixation of complement, either in tissues or on the surface of cells.

TESTS AND ASSAYS OF CELLS AND THEIR FUNCTIONS

PHYSICAL TESTS

There are a variety of ways to identify specific cell types of interest to the immunologist. The microscopic distinction among cells was discussed in Chapter 1. Thus we saw how the microscopist can distinguish the resting lymphocyte, transformed "immunoblast," plasma cells, monocytes, macrophages and the other blood elements. Many other techniques, more specific to immunology, are employed to distinguish among populations and subpopulations of cells. Identification of specific surface markers is one example. The most carefully studied markers were discussed in Chapter 3.

Surface Markers

Surface Immunoglobulin. Surface Ig is most commonly detected by a direct immunofluorescence technique. The reagent is a fluorochrome-labelled anti-immunoglobulin which can be directed against specific heavy-chain isotypes and allotypes, light chains or idiotypes.

Fc Receptors. These receptors are usually detected by the use of heat-aggregated human IgG which has been conjugated to a fluorochrome. The Fc portions of the aggregated IgG molecules will bind to cell-surface Fc receptors and the cells will fluoresce.

Complement Receptors. A rosetting technique is used for the detection of complement receptors. The reagent is prepared by mixing red cells with anti-red-cell antibody in the presence of complement. The anti-red-cell antibody will fix complement components on the red-cell surface. These complement-coated cells can then be mixed with the cell population in which one wants to identify complement receptors. Those cells with the appropriate receptors will bind several coated red cells around them, thus forming a rosette. The surface immunoglobulin can be removed from the red-cell surface in several ways in order to avoid detecting cells with Fc receptors only. One of these techniques uses cold-reacting antibody which can be removed from the red cell merely by warming the culture (see Fig. 3-6).

Spontaneous Sheep Erythrocyte Rosettes. There are several ways to perform this assay. The essential scheme involves the mixture of lymphocytes with sheep erythrocytes. Variations involve the time course and temperature of incubation employed in the formation of the rosettes.

Cell Separation Procedures

Density Gradients. Lymphocytes have different buoyant densities. When a particle is sedimented (either under the influence of gravity or centrifugal force) the sedimenting force is opposed by a buoyant force. If the particle is sedimenting through a medium of progressively increasing density, it will sink until it reaches a level that matches the buoyant density of the particle.

The most commonly employed technique for lymphocyte separation by density uses discontinuous gradients of solutions of either albumin or Ficoll-Isopaque. The gradients are prepared by layering progressively less concentrated solutions upon each other within a tube. The cells to be separated are then layered on top of the gradient and sedimented in a centrifuge. Using a discontinuous 17 to 35 per cent albumin gradient, peripheral blood lymphocytes can be divided into T cells (in the middle 23 to 27% fractions) and B cells (in the bottom 27 to 35% fractions).

Ficoll-Isopaque gradients are often used in the separation of mononuclear cells (lymphocytes and monocytes) from the other blood elements.

Electrophoresis. Free-flow electrophoresis has been used in animals to separate B and T lymphocytes. In mice, clear separations have been accomplished between low-mobility B cells and high-mobility T cells. Although some investigators have reported similar separations with human lymphocytes, others have found the overlap between B- and T-cell mobility to be too great to permit ready separation.

Affinity Columns. Columns are constructed so that a solution of cells can be filtered through the column material, most often glass or synthetic beads. The beads can be coated with either specific antigens or antisera. Those cells that will bind to the coated beads will be retained by the column. The eluate will contain only those subpopulations of cells that are unable to specifically interact with the beads. Table C-1 shows the subpopulations of cells removed by passage through columns with beads coated with different substances. With some affinity columns, the retained cells can later be eluted from the column. Such a procedure will result in a reasonably pure subpopulation of cells, all of which have surface affinity to the specific column.

A mixed peripheral blood sample can be passed through a glass-bead column in which the beads have not been modified. A subpopulation of adherent cells will stick to the column. Many of these cells are mononuclear phagocytic cells (i.e., monocytes).

Columns have also been used that are packed with glass wool or nylon fibers. These columns selectively retain surface Ig-bearing lymphocytes and monocytes although the percentage of these cells removed on one pass is considerably less than 100 per cent.

Table C-1. Affinity Columns

Beads Are Coated With	*Adherent Cell Population*
Anti-Ig whole Ig	Cells with surface Ig or Fc receptors
Anti-Ig $F(ab)_2$	Cells with surface Ig
Aggregated IgG	Cells with Fc receptors
Activated C3	Cells with C3 receptors
Specific haptens	Cells with hapten-specific receptors

Separation of Monocyte-Macrophages. A variety of techniques have been used to separate monocytes from lymphocytes. Unfortunately, it is very difficult to obtain pure preparations of lymphocytes free from mononuclear phagocytes. Many of these techniques involve the preferential ability of monocyte-macrophages to adhere to several surfaces and to phagocytose particles. Although monocytes will adhere to glass, not all monocytes can be removed in this way and a percentage of lymphocytes, primarily B cells, seems to adhere as well. Another way to separate mononuclear phagocytes is with the use of iron filings. These can be added to a mixed cell population and are primarily taken up by phagocytes. The iron-laden cells are then removed magnetically or by sedimentation, and the remaining cell population is largely free of mononuclear phagocytes.

Rosette Sedimentation. Specific subpopulations of cells can be separated by forming specific erythrocyte rosettes and sedimenting the large rosettes away from the unrosetted cells. This technique can separate T-cell SRBC rosettes or complement erythrocyte rosettes.

FUNCTIONAL TESTS

Mitogenesis. See Chapter 4.

Mixed Lymphocyte Reaction. See Chapters 4 and 8.

Cell-Mediated Lymphocytolysis. See Chapter 8.

Lymphokine Production. See Chapters 1, 4 and 6.

Index